BASIC SCIENCE of CANCER

Editors

Gary D. Kruh, MD, PhD
Member
Medical Science Division
Fox Chase Cancer Center
Philadelphia, PA

Kenneth D. Tew, PhD, DSc
Chairman, Department of Pharmacology
G. Willing Pepper Chair in Cancer Research
Fox Chase Cancer Center
Philadelphia, PA

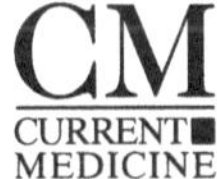
Current Medicine, Inc.

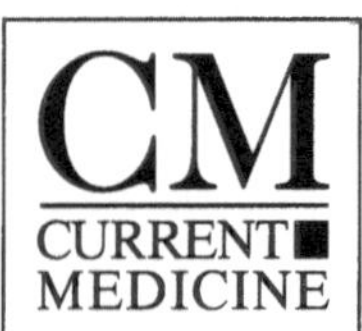

Current Medicine, Inc.
400 Market Street
Suite 700
Philadelphia, PA 19106

Managing Editor: Charles C. Field
Editorial Supervisor: Fran Klass
Developmental Editor: Kathleen Gilbert
Editorial Assistant: Annmarie D'Ortona
Art Director: Jerilyn Kauffman
Cover Design: Christine Keller-Quirk
Design and Layout: Christine Keller-Quirk
Illustration Director: Ann Saydlowski
Illustrator: Nicole Mock
Production Manager: Lori Holland
Assistant Production Manager: Simon Dickey
Indexer: Dorothy Hoffman

Basic science of cancer / editors, Gary Kruh, Kenneth Tew.
p.cm.
Includes bibliographical references and index.
ISBN 978-1-4684-8439-7 ISBN 978-1-4684-8437-3 (eBook)
DOI 10.1007/978-1-4684-8437-3
1. Oncology. 2. Cancer. 3. Carcinogenesis. 4. Cancer--Genetic aspects. 5. Cancer cells. I. Kruh, Gary. II. Tew, Kenneth D.
RC254.B37 2000
616.99'4--dc21
99-42518
CIP

For more information please call 1-800-427-1796
or email us inquiry@phl.cursci.com.

www.current-science-group.com

ISBN 978-1-4684-8439-7

Although every effort has been made to ensure that drug dosages and other information are presented accurately in this publication, the ultimate responsibility rests with the prescribing physician. Neither the publishers nor the author can be held responsible for errors or for any consequence arising from the use of the information contained therein. Any product mentioned in this publication should be used in accordance with the prescribing information prepared by the manufacturers. No claims or endorsements are made for any drug or compound at present under clinical investigation.

5 4 3 2 1

PREFACE

This volume covers a range of highly interrelated topics dealing with the development of human cancer and its treatment. The material is handled in a fashion such that it is accessible to oncologists and other health care professionals who are not scientists, with emphasis on explaining modern cancer research techniques in nontechnical language. Chapters deal with the known dominant- (oncogenes) and negative-acting (tumor suppressor) genes involved in cancer etiology, the identification of novel cancer genes, the interplay of the environment and somatic mutations in these genes (carcinogenesis), and the mechanisms associated with the action of oncogenes and tumor suppressor genes (signal transduction, cell cycle control, transcriptional control, DNA repair, and apoptosis). Additional chapters involve the mechanisms of action of drugs used to treat cancer (pharmacology of antineoplastic agents), the obstacles to successful use of chemotherapeutic agents (drug resistance), modern techniques used in the identification of new agents (approaches to new drug discovery), and the genetic basis of individual variations in response to anticancer agents (pharmacogenetics). Together these topics focus the attention of the reader on areas that are at the forefront of cancer research.

Gary D. Kruh, MD, PhD
Department of Medical Oncology
Fox Chase Cancer Center

Kenneth D. Tew, PhD, DSc
Chairman, Department of Pharmacology
G. Willing Pepper Chair in Cancer Research
Fox Chase Cancer Center

CONTRIBUTORS

Jonathan Chernoff, MD, PhD
Member
Fox Chase Cancer Center
Philadelphia, Pennsylvania

Louis P. Deiss, MD
Assistant Professor
Molecular Genetics
University of Illinois at Chicago
College of Medicine
Chicago, Illinois

Dwayne Dexter, PhD
Penn State College of Medicine
Hershey, Pennsylvania

Leonard C. Erickson, MD
Professor
Pharmacology
Associate Director, Cancer Center
Indiana University School of Medicine
Indianapolis, Indiana

Elizabeth Petri Henske, MD
Associate Member
Medical Oncology
Fox Chase Cancer Center
Philadelphia, Pennsylvania

Tan A. Ince, MD, PhD
Department of Pathology
Harvard University
Massachusetts General Hospital
Boston, Massachusetts

Lawrence M. Kauvar, PhD
President
Trellis Bioinformatics, Inc.
San Francisco, California

Mark R. Kelley, PhD
Professor
Pediatrics, Section of Hematology/Oncology and Department of Biochemistry & Molecular Biology
Associate Director, Wells Center for Pediatric Research
Herman B. Wells Center for Pediatric Research
Indiana University Medical School
Indianapolis, Indiana

Deanne King, BS
MD and PhD Graduate Student
Medical University of South Carolina
Charleston, South Carolina

Matthias H. Kraus
Department of Experimental Oncology
European Institute of Oncology
Milan, Italy

Warren D. Kruger, PhD
Associate Member
Population Science
Fox Chase Cancer Center
Philadelphia, Pennsylvania

Wen-Ching Lee, PhD
Brooklyn, New York

James Norris, PhD
Professor and Vice Chairman
Microbiology and Immunology
Medical University of South Carolina
Charleston, South Carolina

Tracey L. Plank, PhD
Postdoctoral Fellow
Medical Oncology
Fox Chase Cancer Center
Philadelphia, Pennsylvania

Kathleen W. Scotto, MD
Department of Pharmacology
Memorial Sloan-Kettering Cancer Center
New York, New York

Randy Strich, PhD
Member
Institute of Cancer Research
Fox Chase Cancer Center
Philadelphia, Pennsylvania

Joseph R. Testa, PhD
Director
Human Genetics Program
Fox Chase Cancer Center
Philadelphia, Pennsylvania

Kenneth D. Tew, PhD
Chairman
Department of Pharmacology
Fox Chase Cancer Center
Philadelphia, Pennsylvania

Fruma Yehiely, PhD
Resident Assistant Professor
Molecular Genetics
University of Illinois at Chicago
Chicago, Illinois

CONTENTS

CHAPTER

1

Techniques for Identifying Cancer Genes

Wen-Ching Lee
Joseph R. Testa

Tumorigenesis is a multistep process involving a series of acquired genetic changes, including the activation of proto-oncogenes and the inactivation of tumor suppressor genes (TSGs). Cancer genes usually are identified based on their mechanisms of action. Proto-oncogenes encode various components of the signaling pathways that promote cell growth. A proto-oncogene can become oncogenic if it is expressed in excessive amounts or in inappropriate tissues; such forms of expression may be associated with a chromosomal translocation or gene amplification. Mutations in the coding region of a proto-oncogene, or translocation-mediated fusion of a proto-oncogene with another gene, also can result in protein products that have altered functions and thus become oncogenic. In contrast to dominantly acting oncogenes, TSGs are involved in tumorigenesis in a recessive manner. Their gene products provide signals that constrain cell proliferation, and one functional copy of the gene in each cell is sufficient to provide normal growth control. Only when both alleles of the TSG are inactivated by mutations or deletions does the neoplastic phenotype manifest itself in a cell.

In this chapter, various cytogenetic and molecular biology techniques frequently employed to identify cancer genes are introduced. For simplicity of illustration, most techniques are presented as strategies for identifying either proto-oncogenes or TSGs. However, many techniques mentioned in the proto-oncogene section are equally applicable for isolating TSGs and vice versa. Also discussed in this chapter are several differential cloning techniques that take advantage of differences between normal and tumor cells, either at the genomic DNA level or at the expression level, that can be used to identify potential cancer genes.

IDENTIFICATION OF ONCOGENES

Chromosomal Translocation

Many nonrandom chromosomal translocations have been identified in leukemias, lymphomas, and sarcomas by using chromosome banding analysis. Incorporation of certain DNA-specific dyes into metaphase chromosomes, typically following a proteolytic digestion step, creates a staining pattern of transverse, alternating light and dark bands. The unique banding pattern of each human chromosome permits accurate differentiation of chromosomes and thus the detection of chromosomal abnormalities in cancer cells.

Giemsa (G)-banding, the most commonly used banding technique, is illustrated in Figure 1-1*A*. A mitotic inhibitor, such as Colcemid (Gibco BRL, Gaithersburg, MD), is added to the cell culture to arrest the cells during mitosis. The cells then are harvested, swollen in a hypotonic solution, and collected by centrifugation. The collected cells are dispersed in fixative and dropped onto microscope slides in such a way that the cells remain separated and evenly dispersed on the slide. The slides are air-dried, treated with trypsin, and stained with Giemsa. The slides then are examined under a microscope (Fig. 1-1*B*) and individual metaphase spreads are photographed. Chromosomes can be cut from the photograph and arranged into a karyotype based on the size and banding pattern of each chromosome (Fig. 1-1C). A diagrammatic representation of the G-banding pattern of normal human chromosomes is shown in Figure 1-1*D*.

Aberrant karyotypes are observed frequently in tumor cells. The association of consistent chromosomal abnormalities with certain types of cancer has proved to be valuable for the identification of cancer genes and the elucidation of their mechanisms of action. A well-known example is the Philadelphia chromosome, the first consistent chromosomal aberration observed in a human neoplasm (Figs. 1-2 and 1-3*A*). The Ph chromosome results from a reciprocal translocation between chromosomes 9 (band q34) and 22 (band q11) and is abbreviated t(9;22)(q34;q11). This cytogenetic abnormality is detected in 95% of patients with chronic myelogenous leukemia and in some patients with acute lymphocytic leukemia or acute myelogenous leukemia. Cloning of the Philadelphia chromosome translocation breakpoint revealed that the *ABL* proto-oncogene at chromosome band 9q34 is fused with the *BCR* gene located at 22q11 (Fig. 1-3*B*). This fusion gene produces a chimeric BCR-ABL protein that retains the tyrosine kinase domain of ABL and that has altered functional activity because the N-terminal regulatory sequences of ABL are replaced by sequences from the BCR protein.

Fluorescence in situ hybridization (FISH; Fig. 1-4) is another cytogenetic technique that can be used to identify chromosomal translocations. Hybridization involves binding of a labeled nucleic acid probe to unlabeled target DNA by complementary base pairing. In this procedure, the target is chromosomal DNA from tumor cells that has been fixed on microscope slides using the procedure illustrated in Figure 1-1*A*. However, because FISH can be performed on both metaphase spreads and interphase nuclei, it may not be necessary to add mitotic inhibitors to increase the number of cells arrested in metaphase. In addition, after the slides are air-dried, they are treated with formamide to denature the chromosomal DNA and incubated with specific denatured probes prepared by nick translating or random priming a cloned piece of DNA in the presence of a nucleotide derivative. The commonly used nucleotide derivatives in this procedure are deoxynucleotides covalently linked to reporter molecules such as biotin or digoxigenin. The probes hybridized to the chromosomal DNA on the slides can be detected by using fluorochrome-conjugated molecules such as avidin and antibodies that can bind the reporter specifically. Multiple layers of the reporter and its binding molecule may be used to increase the local concentration of the fluorochrome at the target site so that the signal is enhanced. Chromosomes then can be counterstained with a fluorescent DNA dye to reveal individual nuclei or metaphase chromosomes. Multiple probes, labeled with different reporter molecules, can be hybridized to the same slide and distinguished by their specific reporter binding molecules conjugated to different fluorochromes. A fluorescence microscope is used to visualize fluorescent signals on metaphase and interphase nuclei. A cooled charge-coupled device (CCD) camera may be used to acquire images of individual stains or fluorochromes, and the electronic images are merged with a specialized computer imaging software package.

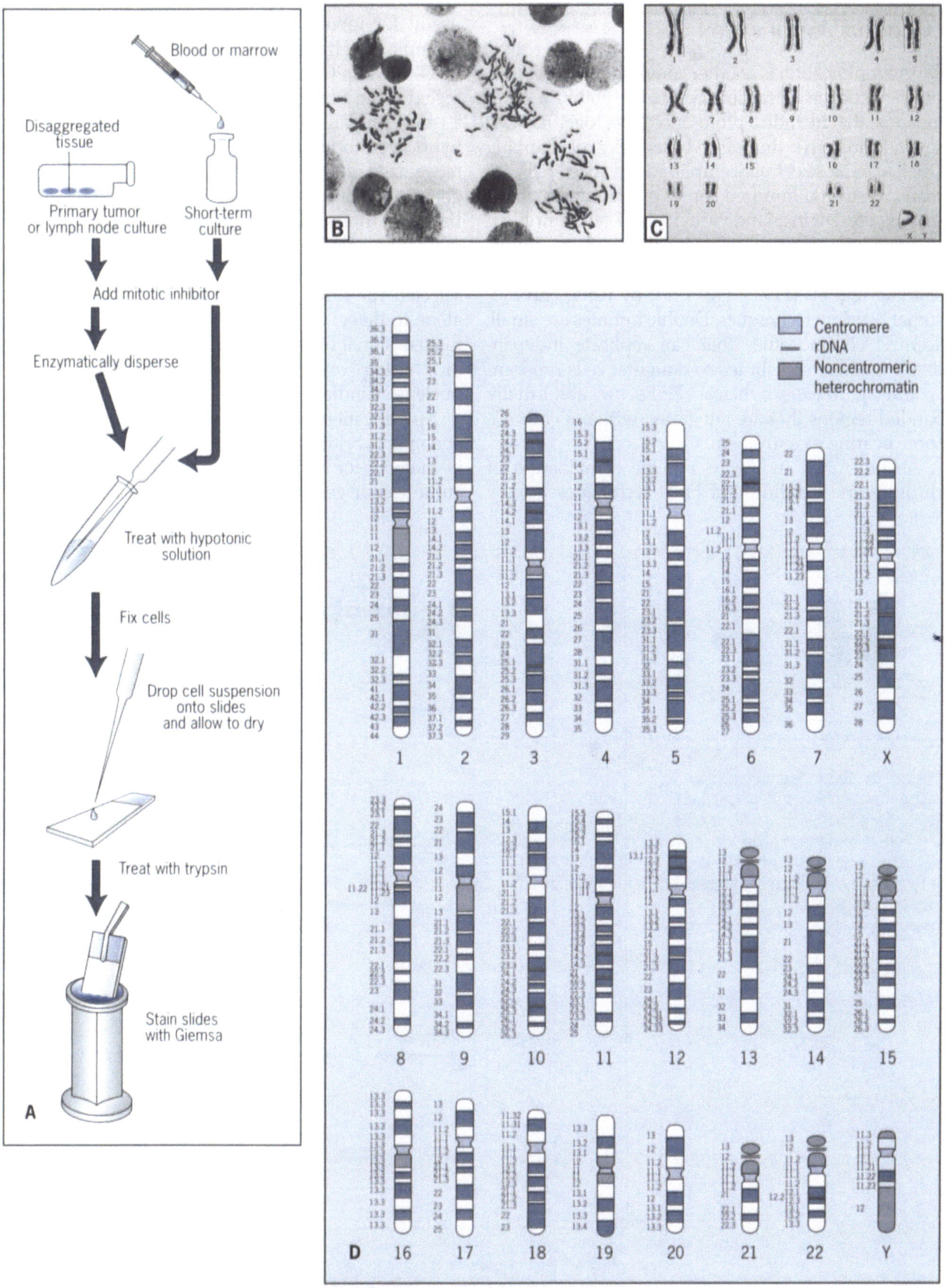

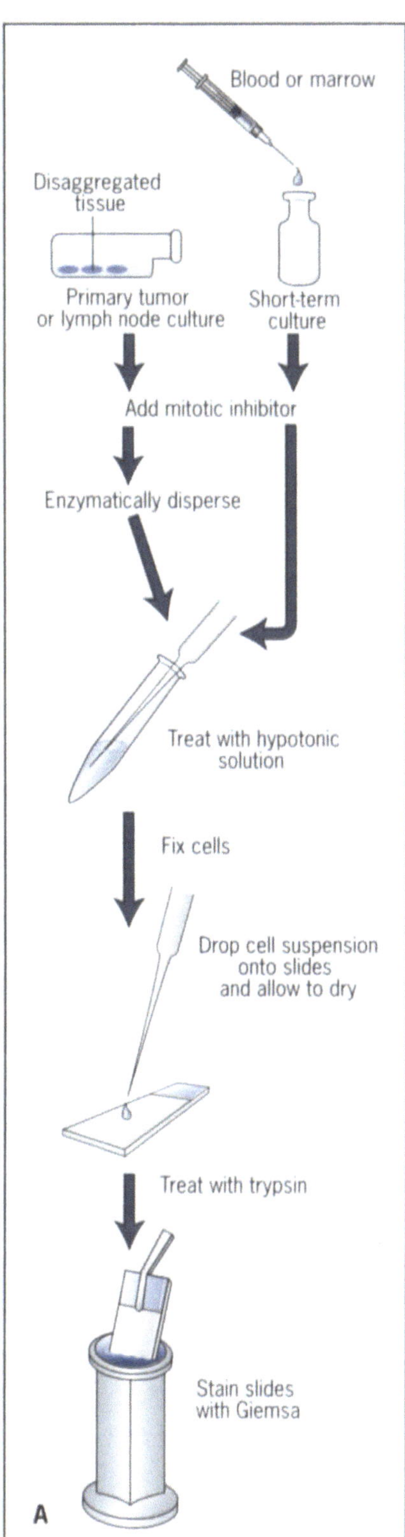

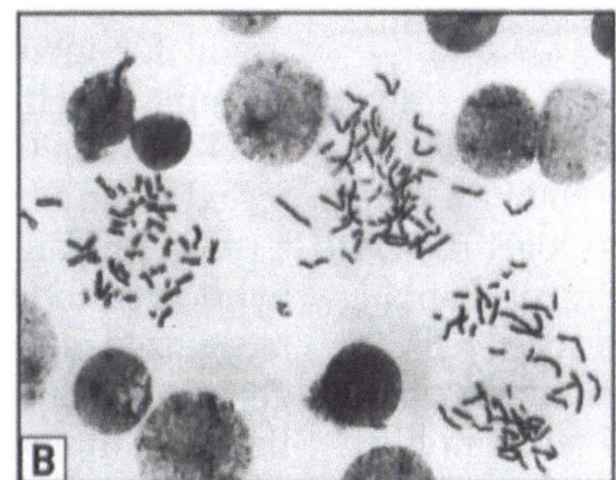

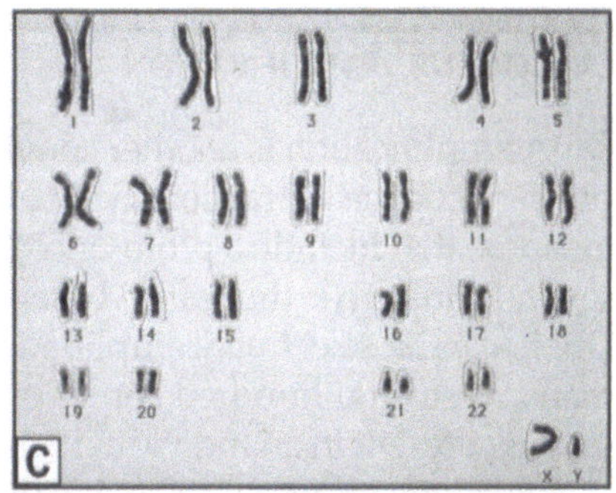

Centromere
rDNA
Noncentromeric heterochromatin

1 2 3 4 5 6 7 X

8 9 10 11 12 13 14 15

D 16 17 18 19 20 21 22 Y

Figure 1-1. Chromosomal banding. **A,** Giemsa (G)-banding technique. **B,** G-banded metaphase spreads obtained using the protocol in *panel A* (original magnification ×120). In addition to metaphases, other nondividing nuclei are also present. **C,** Normal G-banded karyotype of a human man (46, XY). **D,** Diagram showing G-banding pattern for normal human chromosomes.

Oncogene Amplification

DNA amplification is another common mechanism of proto-oncogene activation. Segments within a chromosome that include a proto-oncogene, together with several hundred thousand base pairs of flanking DNA, can be selectively amplified in cancer cells. As many as several hundred copies of a proto-oncogene may be present in an individual tumor cell. Amplified chromosome segments can be detected as double minute chromosomes (Fig. 1-5) or homogeneously staining regions (HSRs; Fig. 1-6*A*) by using chromosomal banding techniques. Double minutes are small, acentric chromosomes that can replicate independently and are distributed to daughter cells randomly during mitosis, whereas HSRs are abnormally banded regions that are integrated within a chromosome bearing a centromere.

As illustrated in Figure 1-6, the combination of chromosome banding and FISH techniques is very useful for identifying amplified oncogenes. In this example, an HSR identified in a lung cancer cell line by G-banding (Fig. 1-6*A*, upper panel) was microdissected using a micromanipulator (Fig. 1-6*A*, *B*). When a probe prepared from the microdissected DNA was hybridized to metaphases from the same cell line, it recognized not only the HSR, but also the proto-oncogene at its native chromosomal location (Fig. 1-6C). Because thousands of human genes have been mapped to specific chromosome locations, candidate genes previously mapped to this location can be selected for further testing. FISH also can be used alone to detect or screen for DNA amplification. An intense signal on a metaphase marker chromosome, or a "string" of signals located in a single interphase nucleus, is indicative of amplification.

Amplifications also can be detected by comparative genomic hybridization (CGH), a molecular cytogenetic method for identifying DNA imbalances in the entire tumor genome in a single experiment (Fig. 1-

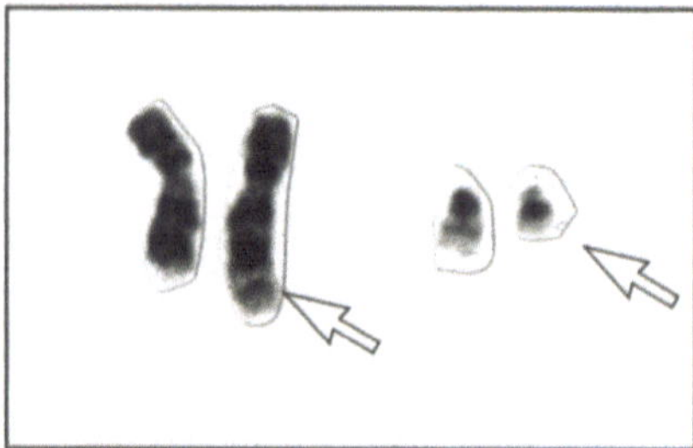

Figure 1-2. G-banded partial karyotype from a chronic myelogenous leukemia patient with a Philadelphia chromosome translocation: t(9;22)(q34;q11). *Arrows* indicate the breakpoints of the rearranged chromosomes.

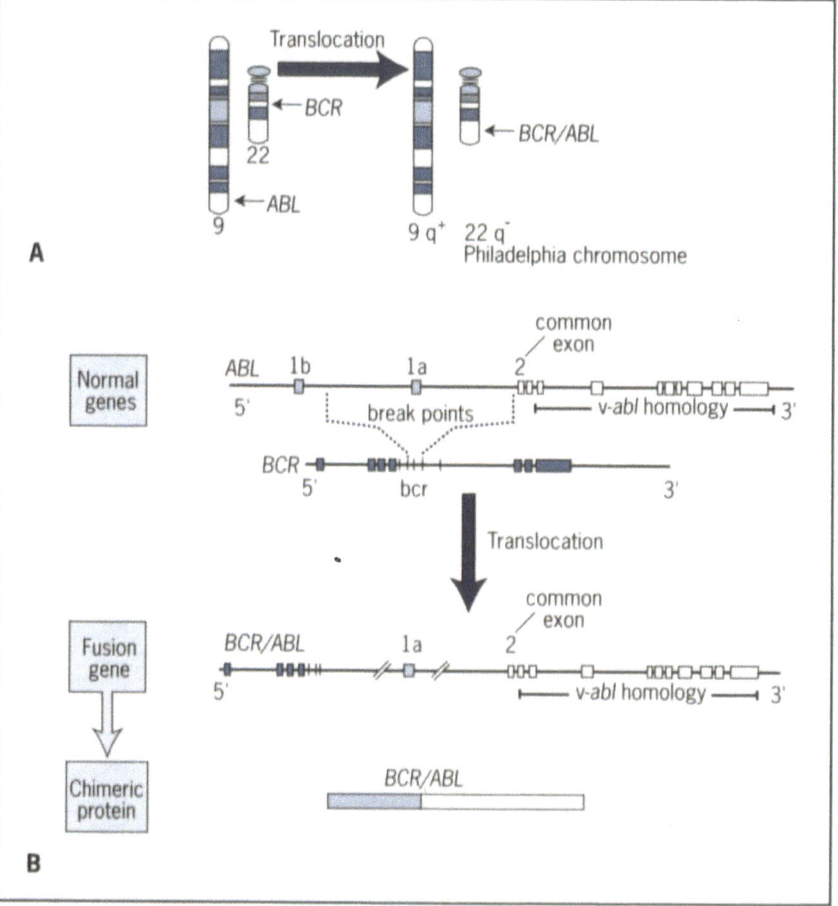

Figure 1-3. Philadelphia chromosome translocation. **A,** A reciprocal translocation results in the Philadelphia chromosome (22q-) and 9q+. **B,** The translocation fuses *ABL* and *BCR* gene sequences and results in the synthesis of a chimeric protein. The molecular breakpoint within *ABL* in different Philadelphia chromosomes is variable but is restricted to the region encompassed by the two *vertical dashed lines.* The major breakpoint cluster region (bcr) of the *BCR* gene is also indicated.

7A). Equal amounts of normal and tumor DNA are labeled individually with different reporter molecules and then are hybridized as a mixture to normal metaphase spreads. FISH signals from individual reporter molecules are measured, and a ratio profile then can be calculated using image-processing software. Because identical amounts of tumor and normal reference DNA are used in the hybridization, a ratio of 1 is expected if there are no genomic imbalances in the tumor. Chromosome regions in which the ratio profile

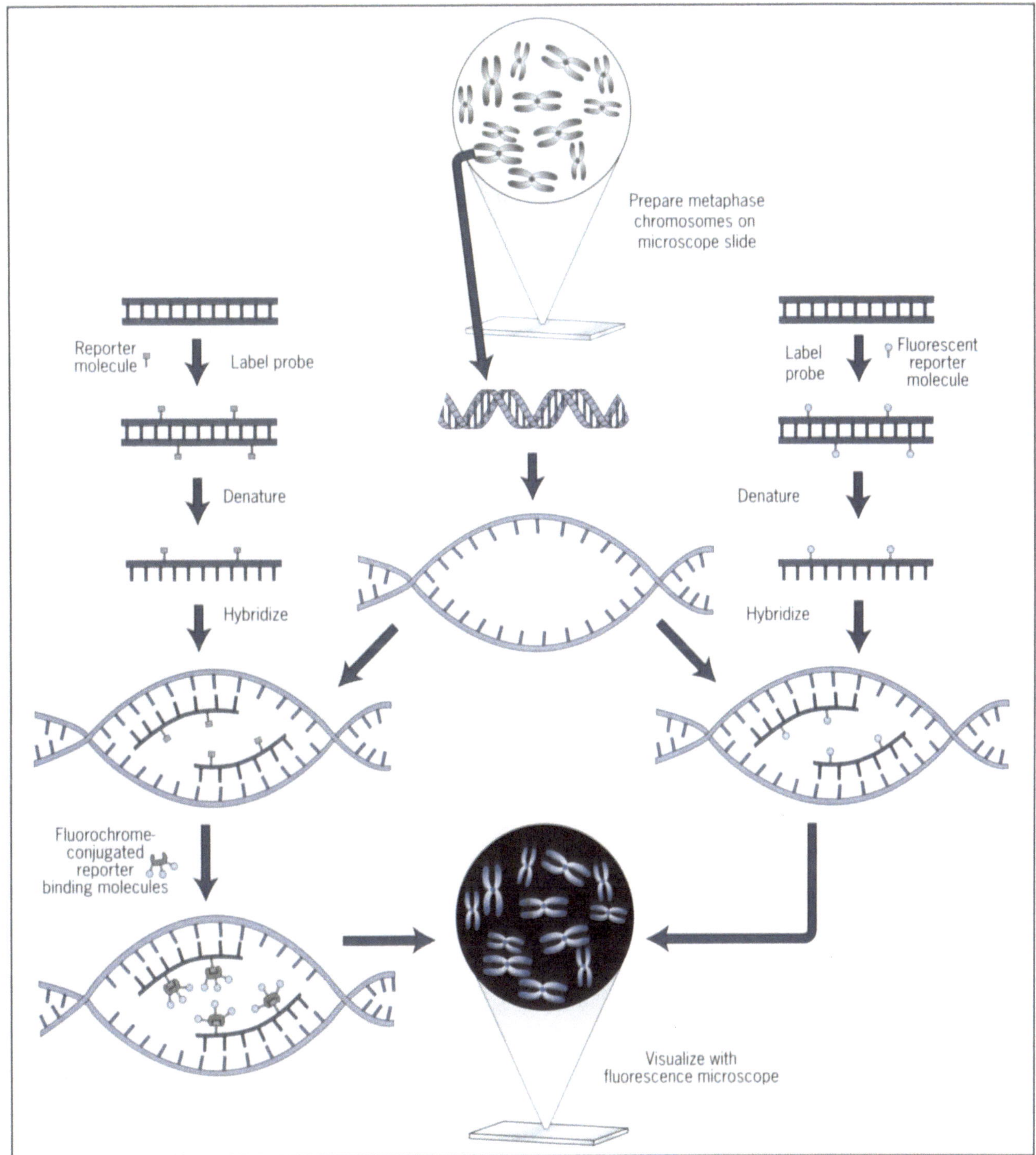

Figure 1-4. Technique of fluorescence in situ hybridization on metaphase chromosomes. Metaphase spreads are prepared on a microscope slide. Chromosomal DNA is denatured into single strands and hybridized with a denatured probe labeled with reporter molecules. Fluorochromes can be incorporated into the probe directly (using labeled deoxynucleotides [dNTPs]) or conjugated onto molecules that bind the reporter molecules specifically. The chromosomal location of the hybridized probe then can be visualized with a fluorescence microscope.

deviates from this expected value represent net DNA gain or loss in the tumor cells. A DNA amplification event will give rise to a very strong tumor signal (*ie*, a very high tumor–normal ratio) at the region where the chromosomal segment is amplified. Conversely, an underrepresentation of the tumor signal (*ie*, a low tumor–normal ratio) would pinpoint a chromosome region where DNA is deleted from the tumor genome. A CGH fluorescence ratio profile of the entire genome of a lung cancer cell line is shown in Figure 1-7*B*.

Among the numerous molecular biology techniques used for identifying cancer genes, Southern blot analysis is perhaps the most widely used. Southern blot analysis (Fig. 1-8) can directly assay the copy number of a cloned DNA segment in the genome of tumor cells; thus, it frequently is used for screening and detecting proto-oncogene amplification. In this procedure, genomic DNA is first digested with one or more restriction enzymes. The resulting DNA fragments are size fractionated by agarose gel electrophoresis. The porous gel acts as a molecular sieve; when the negatively charged DNA fragments migrate toward the positive electrode, the movement of large fragments is retarded much more than that of smaller ones. After electrophoresis, a complex mixture of DNA fragments is arranged in the gel according to size. The gel then is soaked in strong alkali to denature the DNA fragments into single strands. Because agarose gels are fragile and the DNA can diffuse within the gel, it is common practice to transfer the denatured DNA fragments to a nitrocellulose or charged nylon filter, to which single-stranded DNA can bind tightly. The filter then is incubated in a solution containing the denatured, labeled probe so that the probe can bind to its complementary sequences in the immobilized target DNA. After excess probe is washed away, the bound probe can be detected. Traditionally, probes have been labeled radioactively with nucleotides containing ^{32}P, and detected by exposure to radiographic film. Recent improvements in various

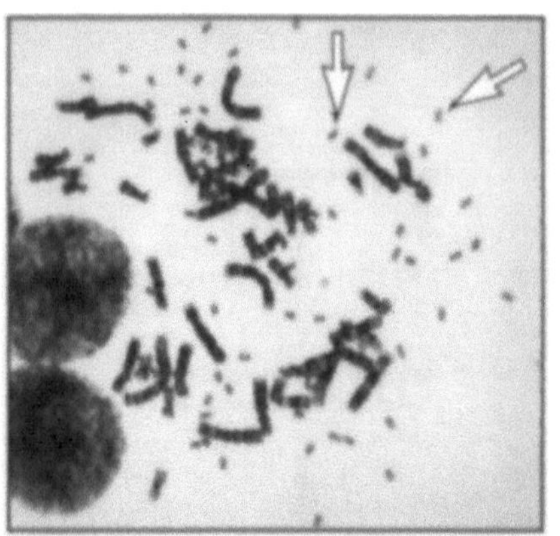

Figure 1-5. G-banded metaphase spread from a lung cancer cell displays numerous double minute chromosomes (*arrows*).

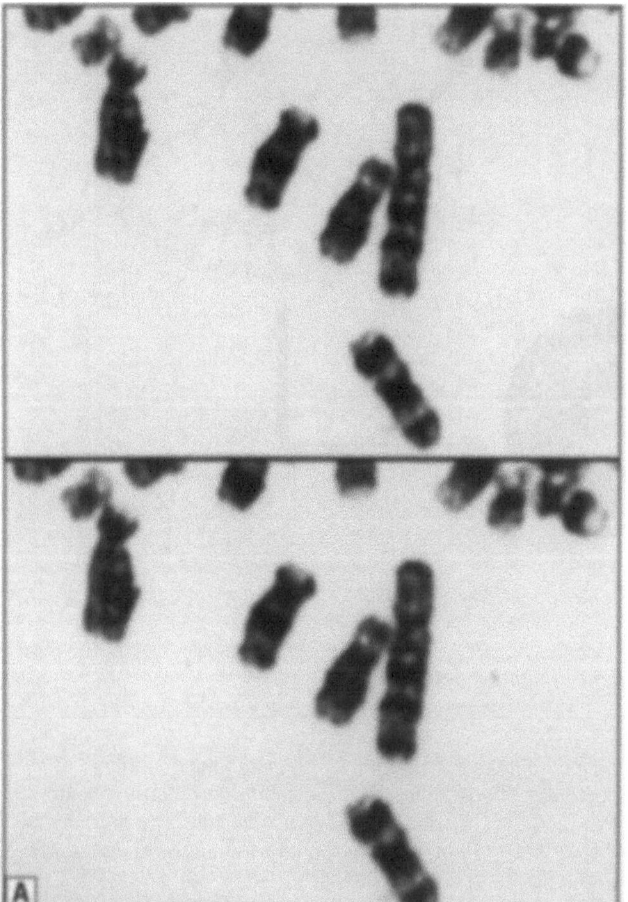

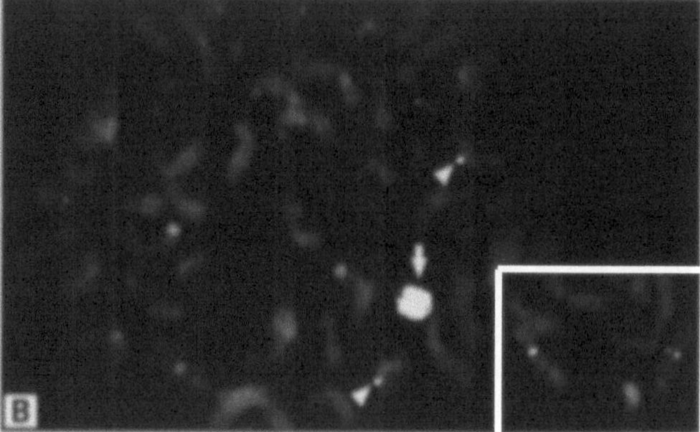

Figure 1-6. Microdissection of a homogenously staining region (HSR) from a lung cancer cell line and chromosomal localization of amplified DNA. **A,** Portion of a G-banded metaphase spread before (*top*) and after (*bottom*) microdissection of the HSR (*bracket*). **B,** The fluorescence in situ hybridization (FISH) probe derived from microdissected DNA hybridizes to the HSR (*arrow*) and normal 7p (*arrowheads*) of another metaphase from the same lung tumor cell line. **Inset,** FISH mapping of the same HSR microdissection probe to normal metaphase chromosomes, localizing the native position at 7p12-13. (*From* Taguchi *et al.* [1]; with permission.)

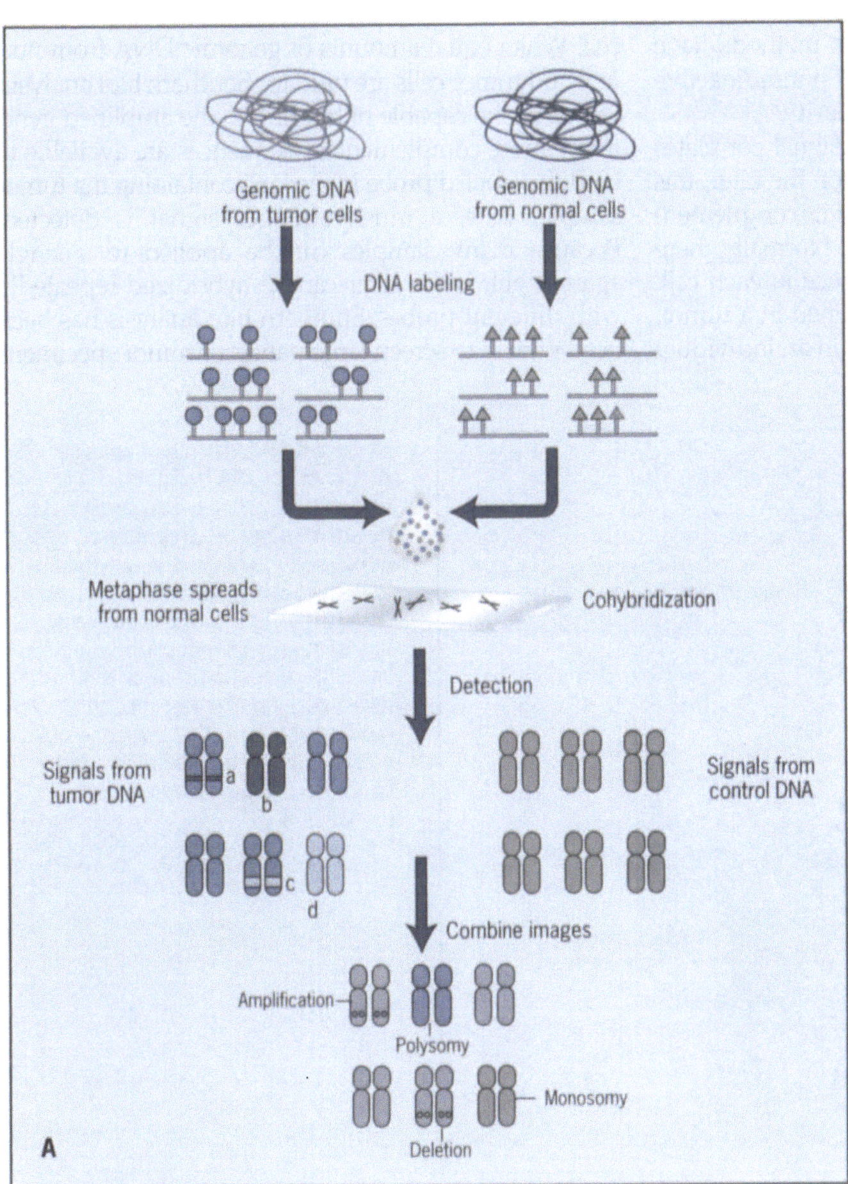

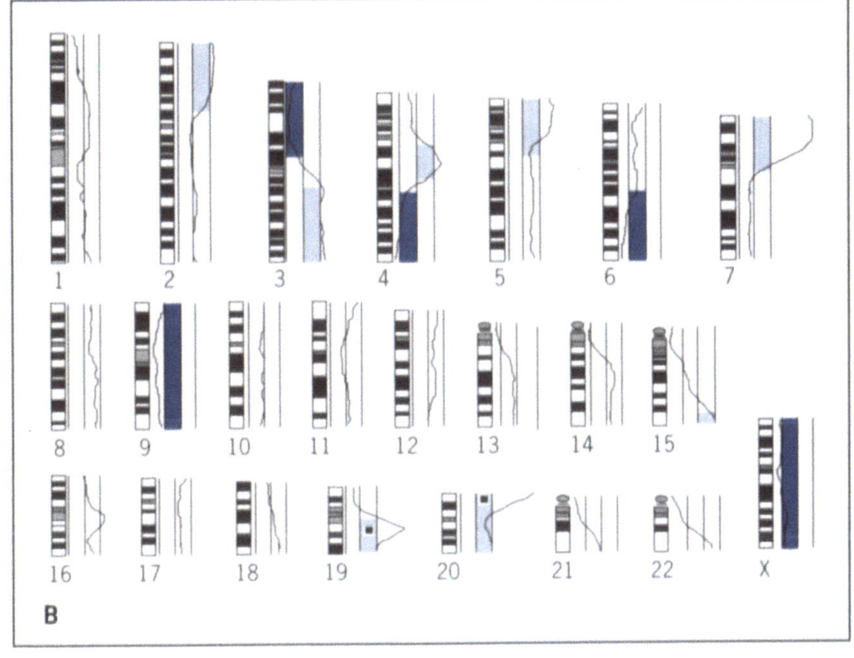

Figure 1-7. A, The comparative genomic hybridization (CGH) technique. Equal amounts of normal and tumor DNA are labeled with different reporter molecules and hybridized together to normal metaphase spreads. Fluorescence in situ hybridization signals are measured individually and combined into a fluorescence ratio image. Regions deviating from the expected ratio can be easily identified. **B,** CGH fluorescence ratio profile of a lung cancer cell line displaying overrepresentation (*light blue rectangles*) of part or all of chromosome arms 2p, 3q, 4q, 5p, 7p, and 15q; amplification (*solid square*) of portions of 19q and 20p; and underrepresentation (*dark blue rectangles*) of part or all of 3p, 4q, 6q, 9, and X. The profile represents the average fluorescence ratios calculated for each chromosome from a total of 18 metaphase spreads. (*From* Testa *et al.* [2]; with permission.)

nonradioactive labeling and detection methods have greatly enhanced the sensitivity of nonradioactive probes and thus increased their popularity.

Generally, the strength of a probe signal correlates with the amount of the labeled probe on the filter; this in turn depends on the copy number of its complementary sequence immobilized on the filter. Normally, there are only two copies of a given sequence in each cell. However, if a proto-oncogene is amplified in a tumor, more than two copies may be present in an individual cell. When equal amounts of genomic DNA from normal and tumor cells are used for Southern blot analysis, with a probe capable of binding to the amplified gene, many more complementary sequences are available to bind the labeled probe in the lane containing the tumor sample; thus, a much stronger signal is detected. Because many samples can be applied to a single agarose gel, and a filter can be hybridized repeatedly with different probes, Southern blot analysis has been used widely to screen large panels of tumor specimens

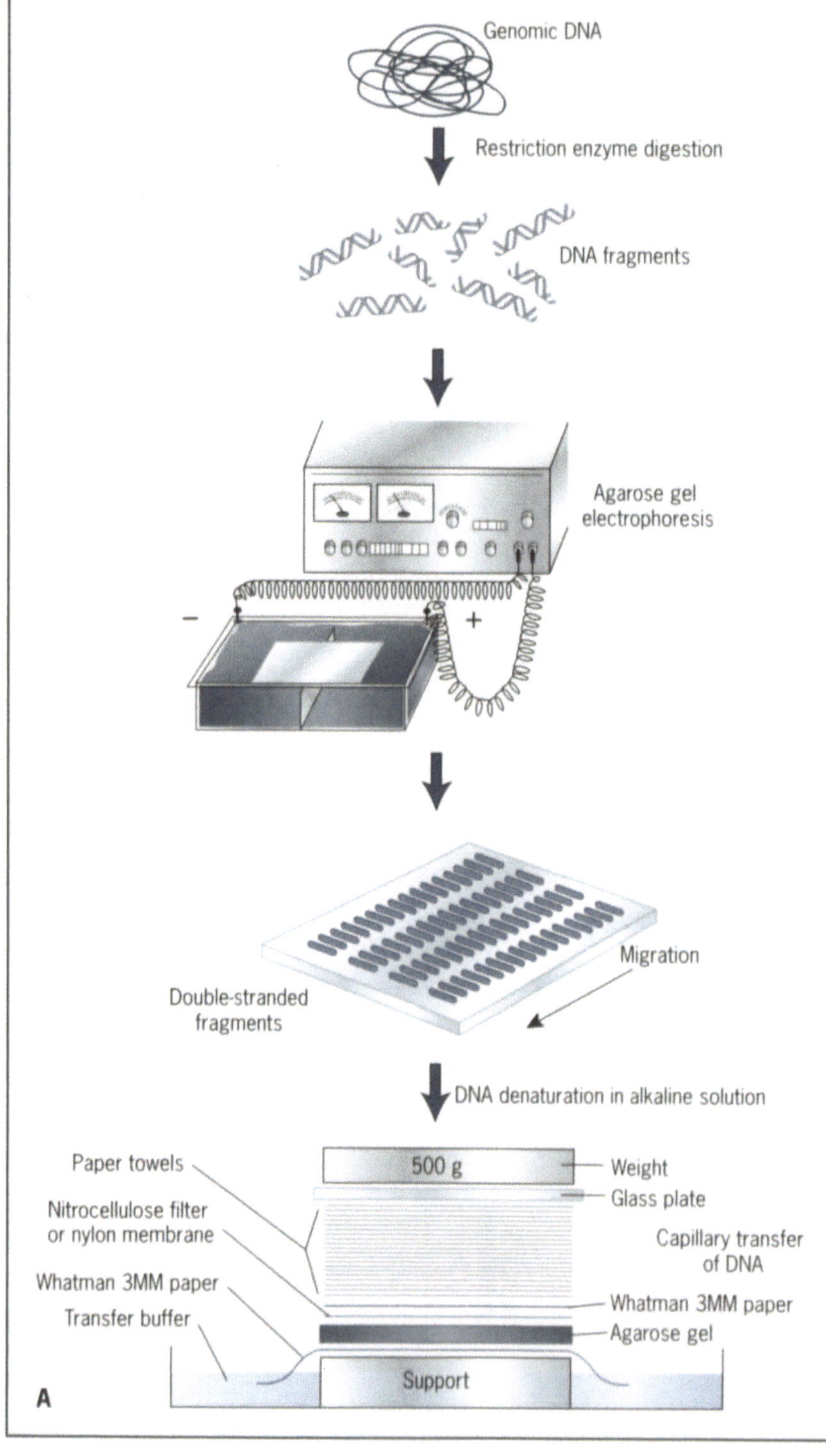

Figure 1-8. Southern blot analysis. **A**, Genomic DNA is digested with restriction enzymes, size fractionated by agarose gel electrophoresis, denatured, and transferred to a nylon filter for hybridization (**B**). After the radiolabeled probe binds to its complementary sequences immobilized on the filter, the unbound probe is washed away, and the filter is exposed to radiographic film. The positions of the bound probe are detected as dark bands on the developed film. (*continued*)

for gene amplification. An example of this type of experiment is shown in Figure 1-9. A probe prepared from the genomic region containing the *AKT2* proto-oncogene, which encodes a serine/threonine kinase, detected amplification in several ovarian cancer cell lines and primary tumors, whereas the *ERCC1* DNA repair gene, located near *AKT2* on chromosome 19, was not amplified in any of the samples.

OVEREXPRESSION

Oncogenes are often overexpressed in tumor cells. Overexpression results from genetic changes such as gene amplification, chromosomal translocation, and viral insertion. Amplification of a proto-oncogene provides excessive amounts of template for transcription and thereby increases the amount of mRNA in the cell. Transcription from a single copy of a proto-oncogene can be increased greatly by other mechanisms, *eg*, by relocating the proto-oncogene to the vicinity of a strong transcriptional control element through a chromosomal translocation event or by rendering its transcription under the control of a strong viral promoter through a retroviral insertion event.

Northern blot analysis is commonly used to measure the steady-state level of mRNA. The Northern blot is a variant of the Southern blot in which RNA is analyzed instead of DNA. Because the secondary structure of nucleic acids can affect their mobility in agarose gels, it is common practice to size fractionate RNA under denaturing conditions. Total RNA or poly(A)$^+$ mRNA samples are usually denatured by heating in a solution containing a chemical denatu-

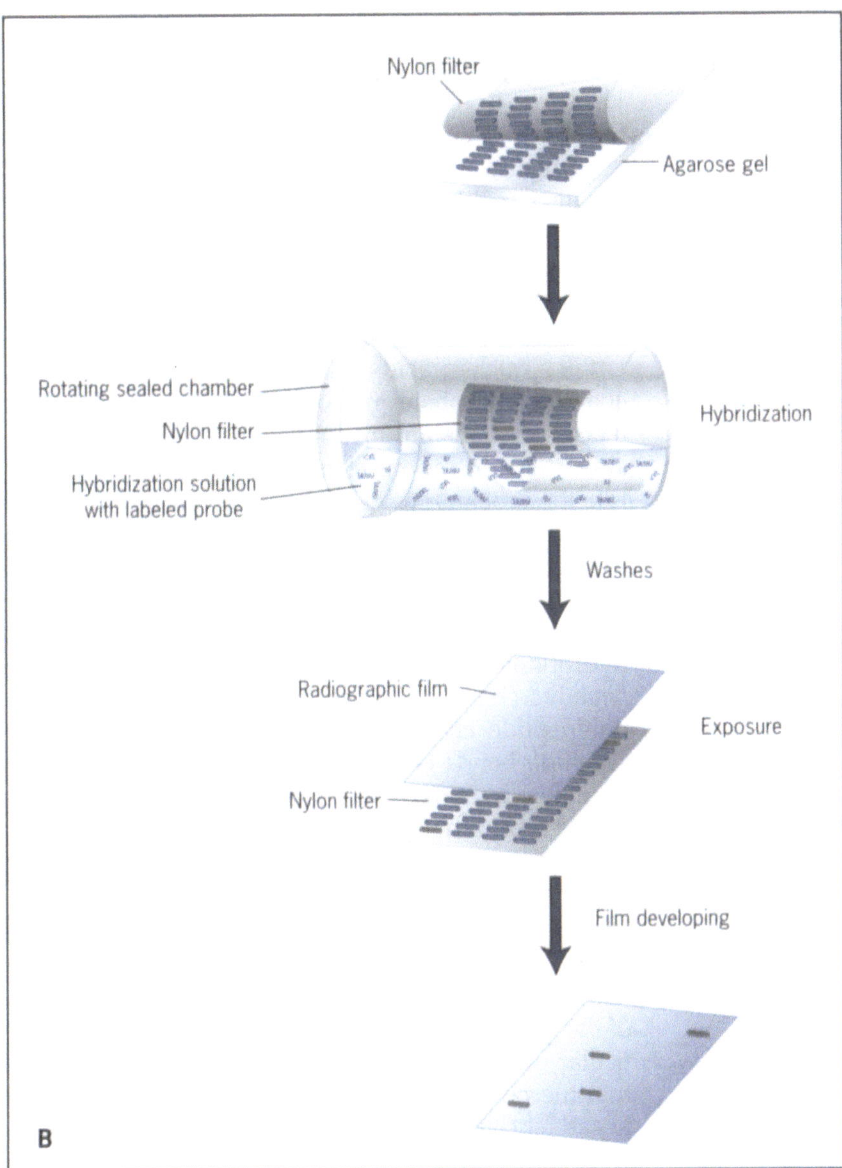

Figure 1-8. *(continued)*

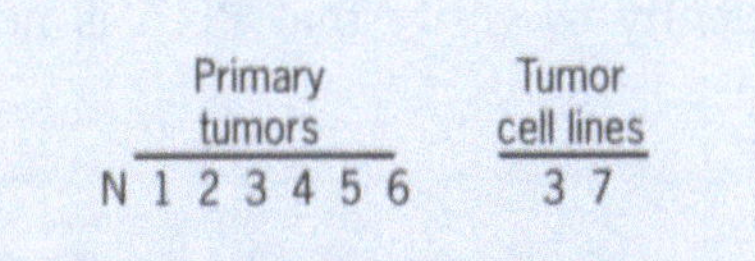

Figure 1-9. Southern blot analysis of ovarian carcinomas. Genomic DNA from normal placenta (N), six primary ovarian carcinomas, and two cell lines were digested with *Eco*RI. Hybridization with a genomic *AKT2* probe is shown in the upper portion of the figure. The lower portion shows rehybridization with a control probe for *ERCC1*, located on the same chromosome arm (*ie*, 19q) as *AKT2*. Amplification of *AKT2* is clearly seen in primary tumors 2 and 5 and both cell lines; no *ERCC1* amplification is detected. (*From* Cheng *et al.* [3]; with permission.)

rant, such as formamide, before being loaded onto an agarose gel. The gel also contains a high concentration of the chemical denaturant to ensure that RNA molecules remain free of secondary structure during electrophoresis and are separated based solely on size. After electrophoresis, RNA molecules are transferred to a filter and can be analyzed using hybridization and detection procedures similar to those described for Southern blot analysis.

Figure 1-10 shows a typical Northern blot analysis. Total RNA was isolated from a series of ovarian carcinoma cell lines and cultured, normal human ovarian surface-epithelial cells. Equal amounts of RNA from these two sources were electrophoresed in a denaturing gel. Because the majority of RNA molecules in living cells are ribosomal RNAs (rRNAs), the 28S and 18S rRNAs are readily visible when the gel is stained with the fluorescent nucleic acid dye ethidium bromide (Fig. 1-10C). These rRNAs are checked frequently to verify that RNA is not degraded and to ensure that each lane contains comparable amounts of RNA. The RNA in the gel was transferred to a nylon filter and hybridized with ^{32}P-labeled nucleic acid probes. When hybridized with a probe prepared from a complementary DNA (cDNA) clone of the *AKT2* oncogene, more intense (*ie*, darker) bands are seen in two cancer cell lines compared with those seen in the normal cells (Fig. 1-10*A*), indicating that *AKT2* is overexpressed in the two cancer cell lines. However, when the same filter is rehybridized with a probe for the housekeeping gene glyceraldehyde-3-phosphate dehydrogenase, comparable levels of expression are observed in the normal cell lines and in both cancer cell lines (Fig. 1-10*B*). Because housekeeping genes are responsible for maintaining basic cellular functions, their expression usually remains quite constant even when cells become malignant. In fact, the expression of glyceraldehyde-3-phosphate dehydrogenase and other housekeeping genes often is used as a control for equivalent loading of samples.

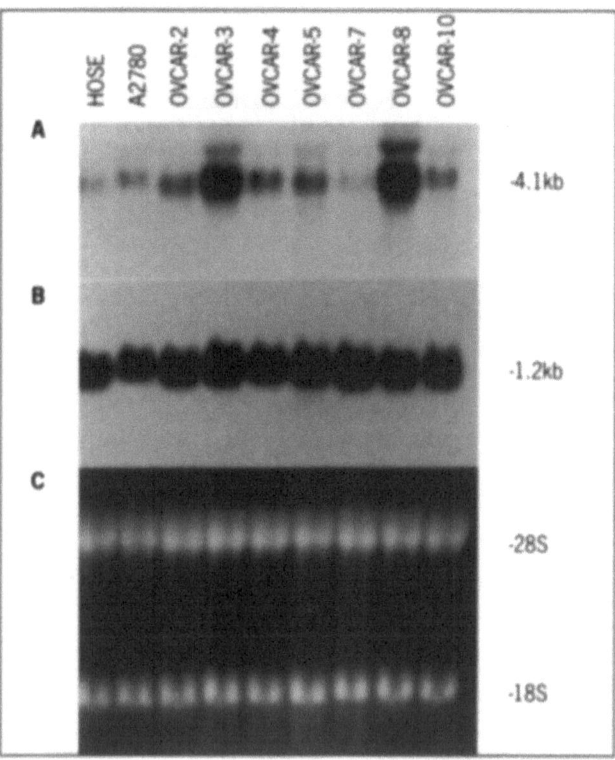

Figure 1-10. Northern blot analysis of ovarian carcinoma cell lines. Total RNA extracted from normal human ovarian surface epithelial cells in early passage (HOSE) and eight ovarian carcinomas cell lines are analyzed. **A,** Hybridization of the filter with the *AKT2* complementary DNA probe. **B,** Rehybridizat-ion with a glyceraldehyde-phosphate dehydrogenase control probe. **C,** Ethidium bromide–stained gel; the positions of 28S and 18S ribosomal RNA are marked. *Panel B* and *panel C* indicate equivalent loading of RNA among lanes. Overexpression of *AKT2* is evident in tumor cell lines 3 and 7 (OVCAR-3, OVCAR-8). (*From* Cheng *et al.* [3]; with permission.)

Overexpression also can be accessed at the protein level. The technique most frequently used to measure the steady-state levels of proteins is Western blot analysis, which is also known as immunoblotting (Fig. 1-11) because antibodies are used to detect the protein of interest in this process. Similar to the nucleic acid blotting techniques, the proteins are size fractionated by gel electrophoresis and transferred to a nitrocellulose filter before the detection of specific protein molecules. Unlike nucleic acids, which contain a negatively charged phosphate group in each of their building blocks, proteins are made of amino acids containing side chains of various charges and polarities. To separate the proteins based solely on size, they are usually first denatured by heating in a solution containing sodium dodecyl sulfate (SDS) and a reducing agent such as beta-mercaptoethanol or dithiothreitol. SDS, a powerful, negatively charged detergent, binds to hydrophobic regions of proteins, coating them with negative charges and unfolding them into extended polypeptide chains. The reducing agent breaks the disulfide bonds between constituent polypeptides in multi-subunit proteins so that each of the polypeptides can be analyzed separately. It also breaks intramolecular disulfide linkages such that all polypeptides become linear molecules. Proteins are commonly size fractionated by SDS–polyacrylamide gel electrophoresis (SDS-PAGE). The gel is prepared by polymerizing and cross-linking acrylamide monomers; the pore size of the gel can be adjusted to separate proteins of a particular size range. The gel also contains SDS to ensure that the polypeptide chains remain embedded in the negatively charged SDS and move toward the positive electrode. Because small polypeptides can migrate through the pores of the gel much faster then large ones, a complex mixture of proteins is fractionated into a series of discrete bands that are arranged in order of molecular weight. The gel can be stained with a dye such as Coomassie blue to reveal all the major protein bands. To detect a particular protein with its specific antibody, the fractionated proteins have to be electrotransferred from the gel to a sheet of nitrocellulose or a nylon filter. Electrotransfer can be performed using a tank or by using a semi-dry transferring apparatus. After proteins are immobilized on the filter, identification of a specific protein usually is achieved by an indirect immunochemical method (Fig. 1-11*B*). First, the filter is incubated with a primary antibody that is capable of binding to the protein of interest. Following washes to remove excess primary antibody, the filter is incubated with a secondary antibody that recognizes the primary antibody specifically. Secondary antibodies are conjugated to a reporter molecule, such as a radioactive isotope, enzyme, or fluorescent dye, for final detection. Most Western blot analyses are performed with secondary antibodies conjugated to peroxidase or alkaline phosphatase. These enzymes usually are detected by their ability to catalyze soluble substrates to form insoluble color or phosphorescent products that precipitate where the enzymes are located. Western blot analysis is quantitative because the strength of the amplified signal is proportional to the number of antigen molecules immobilized on the filter.

Figure 1-12 demonstrates how Western blot analysis was used to detect overexpression of the *AKT2*

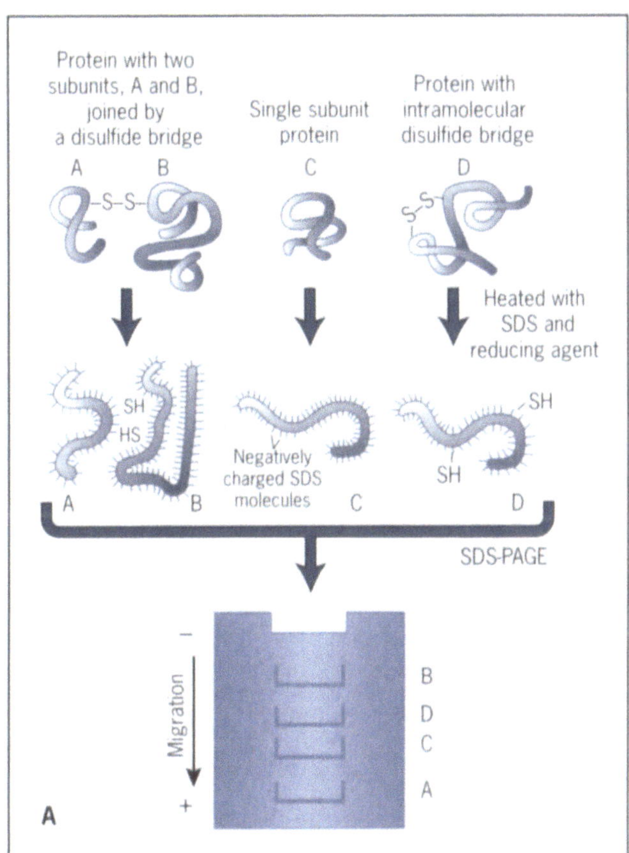

Figure 1-11. Western blot analysis. **A,** A mixture of proteins is denatured in the presence of sodium dodecyl sulfate (SDS) and β-mercaptoethanol and then size fractionated by SDS–polyacrylamide gel electrophoresis (SDS-PAGE). **B,** Indirect immunochemistry can be used to detect the protein of interest on the filter.

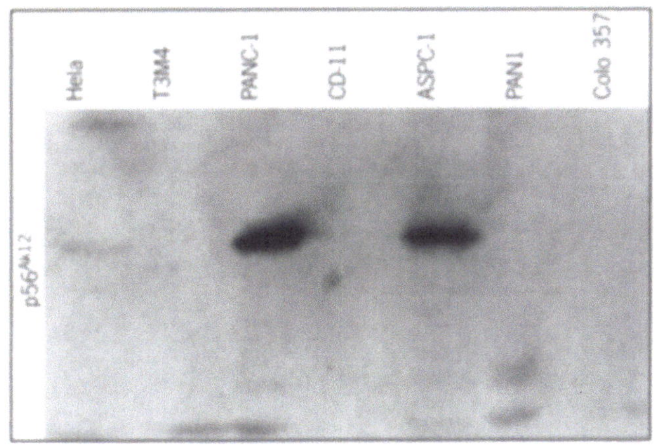

Figure 1-12. Western blot analysis of cancer cell lines. Polyclonal anti-AKT2 antibody was used to analyze cell lysates prepared from HeLa cells and six pancreatic carcinoma cell lines. Note high levels of *AKT2* in PANC-1 and ASPC-1 compared with other cell lines, indicating that *AKT2* is overexpressed in these two cell lines. (*From* Cheng *et al.* [4]; with permission.)

oncogene in two pancreatic cancer cell lines. Equivalent amounts of protein extracted from various pancreatic carcinoma cell lines and HeLa cells were separated by SDS-PAGE and transferred to a nylon filter. The AKT2 protein levels were assessed using a polyclonal antibody raised in rabbits against purified AKT2 protein. The level of *AKT2* expression varies among cell lines; the AKT2 protein is not detectable in several cell lines and is barely visible in HeLa cells, whereas expression of AKT2 is highly elevated in the PANC-1 and ASPC-1 cell lines. The indirect immunochemical method employed in Western blot analysis is also frequently used to detect a protein of interest in situ. For example, an antibody can be used to measure the level and subcellular localization of the protein under investigation in cultured cells or paraffin sections of histologic samples.

Gene Transfer

Gene transfer is an approach used to transform normal cells in culture by transfection of tumor cell DNA containing a transforming gene. In this procedure (Fig. 1-13), genomic DNA extracted from human tumor cell lines or primary tumor specimens is used to transfect NIH 3T3 cells. Each NIH 3T3 cell in the culture receives a small portion of the tumor DNA. If a cell obtains the tumor DNA containing the transforming gene, it will outgrow the other cells and form a focus on the culture dish. The identification of sequences from tumor DNA that are retained in transformed cells has led to the discovery of numerous tumor-associated oncogenes.

IDENTIFICATION OF TUMOR SUPPRESSOR GENES

The Two-Hit Theory

Cell fusion experiments provided the earliest evidence for the involvement of TSGs in tumorigenesis. When human tumor cells were fused with normal cells, the resulting somatic cell hybrids usually lost many of their malignant properties, indicating that the neoplastic phenotype in these tumor cells was recessive. In other words, the neoplastic transformation of the tumor cells used in the fusion resulted from the loss of a critical, growth-regulating TSG. A normal copy of this gene contributed by the normal cells during the fusion process was sufficient to restore cell growth control and thus revert the neoplastic phenotype. This "two-hit" hypothesis was first proposed as a genetic explanation for familial and sporadic retinoblastomas, which are rare, aggressive childhood tumors of the retina. As illustrated in Figure 1-14, the first mutation in the familial form is inherited from one of the parents and is present at conception; therefore, all cells in an affected individual, including those of the retina, carry this mutation. A second mutation occurring in the retinal cells gives rise to retinoblastoma. Because the number of cells in the retina is so large that the second mutation is virtually certain to occur in at least one cell, tumors develop early in life and at multiple sites. The two-hit hypothesis also explains why a genetically recessive event can lead to a dominant inheritance. In contrast, two somatic mutations in the retinal cells are required for the sporadic retinoblastoma to form. The chance that a single retinal cell undergoes the two necessary mutations is very small, thus accounting for the solitary nature and the later age of onset of sporadic cases.

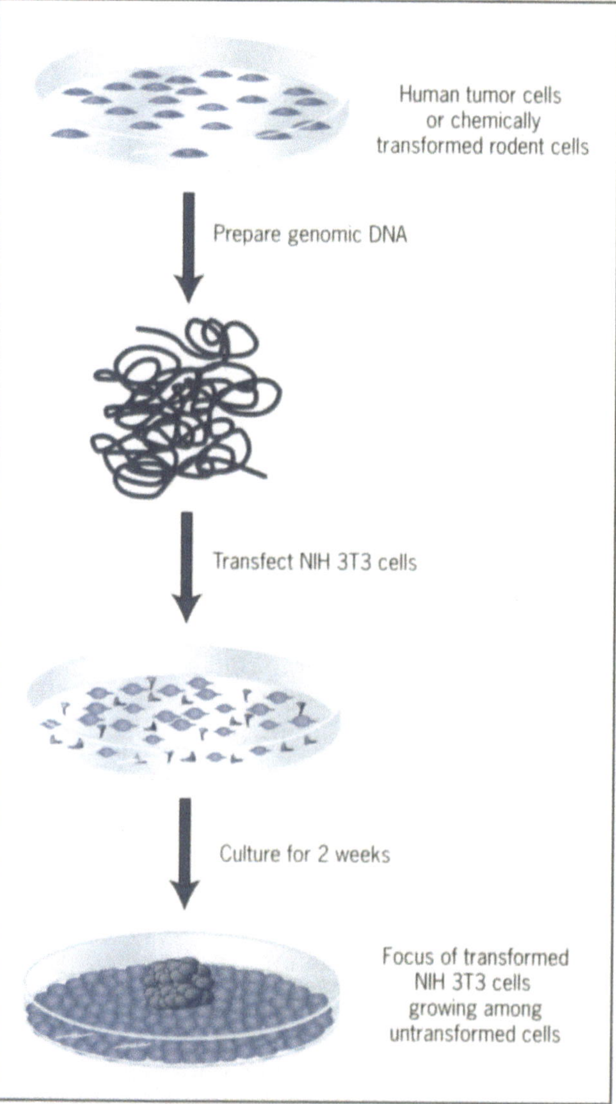

Figure 1-13. Gene transfer technique. The oncogene in tumor DNA can transform NIH 3T3 cells in culture. (*Adapted from* Bishop and Hanafusa [7]; with permission.)

DELETION MAPPING

Because each cell generally needs only one functional copy of a TSG to maintain its normal growth, it takes two mutation events (knocking out both alleles of the same gene) to transform a cell. In familial tumors, a point mutation or other intragenic change confined to the TSG is usually inherited. Elimination of the remaining wild-type allele of the TSG may occur by several mechanisms. One mechanism involves a somatic mutation event, but the frequency of these events is only 10^{-6} to 10^{-7} per cell generation, so inactivation of the second copy of the TSG by this mechanism is relatively rare. Several chromosomal mechanisms, such as chromosomal nondisjunction (leading to loss of a whole chromosome), mitotic recombination, and interstitial deletion, occur at much higher frequencies and thus represent more likely ways that the second copy of a TSG can be eliminated. In fact, loss of all or part of a chromosome containing a relevant TSG locus is frequently observed in both familial and sporadic tumors. Homozygous deletions of TSGs are also occasionally found in sporadic tumors. Therefore, mapping the sites deleted in tumor cells can provide important clues to the likely locations of TSGs.

Deletion mapping can be performed at the cytogenetic or molecular level. Two cytogenetic techniques mentioned previously—karyotypic analysis (*see* Fig. 1-1) and CGH (*see* Fig.1-7)—can be used to detect deletions. Figure 1-15*A* shows the karyotype of a cell line derived from a pleural malignant mesothelioma, a neoplasm associated with asbestos exposure. Numerous deletions involving different chromosomes can be identified in this case. Because tumorigenesis is a multistep process involving a series of genetic changes, karyotypes of solid tumors are usually quite complex and contain many chromosomal abnormalities. However, after many specimens of the same type of tumor are examined, recurrent sites of chromosomal loss can be identified as shown in Figure 1-15*B*. Presumably, each deletion encompasses a putative TSG locus; thus, the TSG must be located in the minimal region common to all the deletions, *ie*, within the shortest region of overlapping deletions.

At the DNA level, deletions are identified by loss of heterozygosity (LOH) analysis using polymorphic genetic markers. Heterozygosity exists when the two alleles at a polymorphic site are different. If one allele is deleted from the cell, heterozygosity at this locus is lost. Early LOH studies were carried out using restriction fragment length polymorphism (RFLP) markers. RFLPs are produced by the presence or absence of a restriction site due to polymorphic variations in DNA sequences (Fig. 1-16). RFLPs are usually analyzed for LOH by hybridizing Southern blots of restriction digests of normal and tumor DNAs with radiolabeled probes. As shown in Figure 1-17, Southern blot analysis was performed using paired normal and mesothelioma DNAs digested with the restriction enzyme *Eco*RI. The RFLP marker MYCL, located at chromosome 1p32, was analyzed. Both patients are heterozygous at this locus because the probe detects two different alleles in the normal DNA samples.

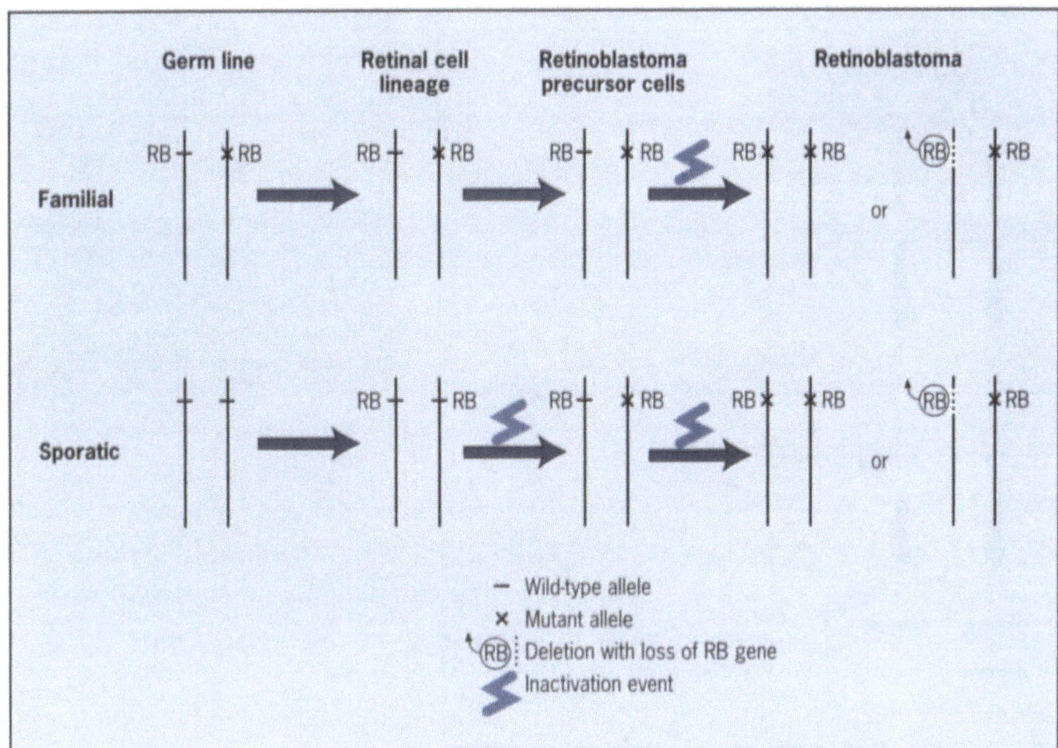

Figure 1-14. The genetic mechanism of familial and sporadic retinoblastoma. Patients with the familial form of the disease inherit the first *RB1* mutation (indicated by an X), and a second hit in the remaining allele in retinal cells gives rise to tumors. In sporadic cases, both inactivation events are somatic.

Heterozygosity is maintained in the tumor from patient 1, whereas only one allele is present in the tumor from patient 2, indicating that the other allele was deleted during tumorigenesis.

The usefulness of RFLP analysis is limited because only two alleles exist; the restriction site is present or it is absent. The development of the DNA amplification method polymerase chain reaction (PCR) has led to the use of polymorphic microsatellite DNA sequences to create a new set of highly informative multi-allelic markers. PCR is a rapid and versatile in vitro method for selectively amplifying a specific target DNA sequence or sequences within a source of DNA. PCR consists of many cycles of a primer extension reaction,

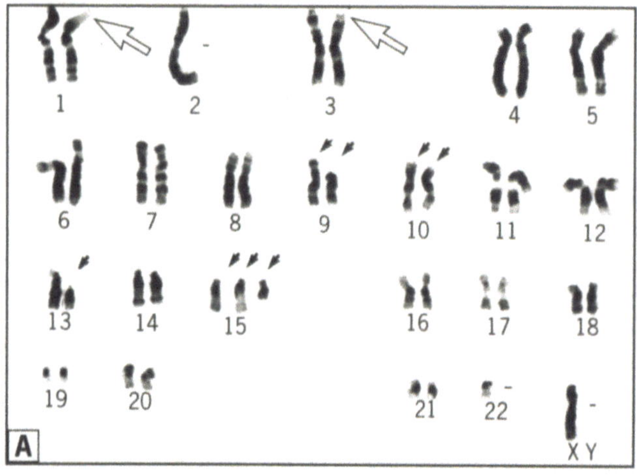

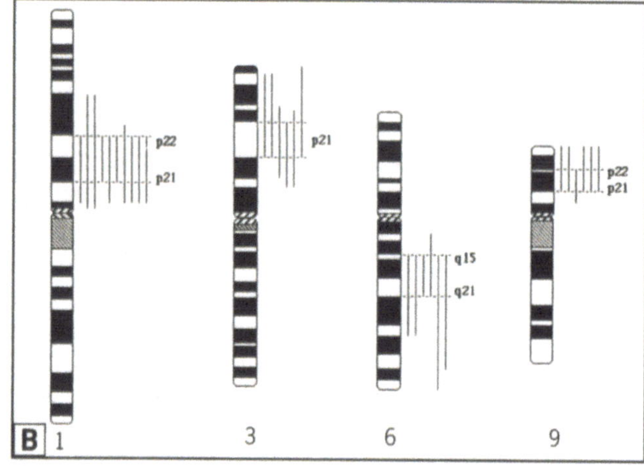

Figure 1-15. Cytogenetic deletion mapping. **A,** Karyotype of a G-banded metaphase spread from a malignant mesothelioma cell line. Arrows indicate the rearranged chromosomes, including interstitial deletions of 1p and 3p, two different unbalanced rearrangements of 9p, and several other numerical and structural alterations. **B,** Schematic representation of regional losses of 1p, 3p, 6q, and 9p resulting from the karyotypic study of 20 mesotheliomas. *Vertical lines* indicate deleted segments in individual tumor specimens or cell lines. The smallest region of overlapping deletions is located between the two horizontal lines. (*From* Taguchi *et al.* [8]; with permission.)

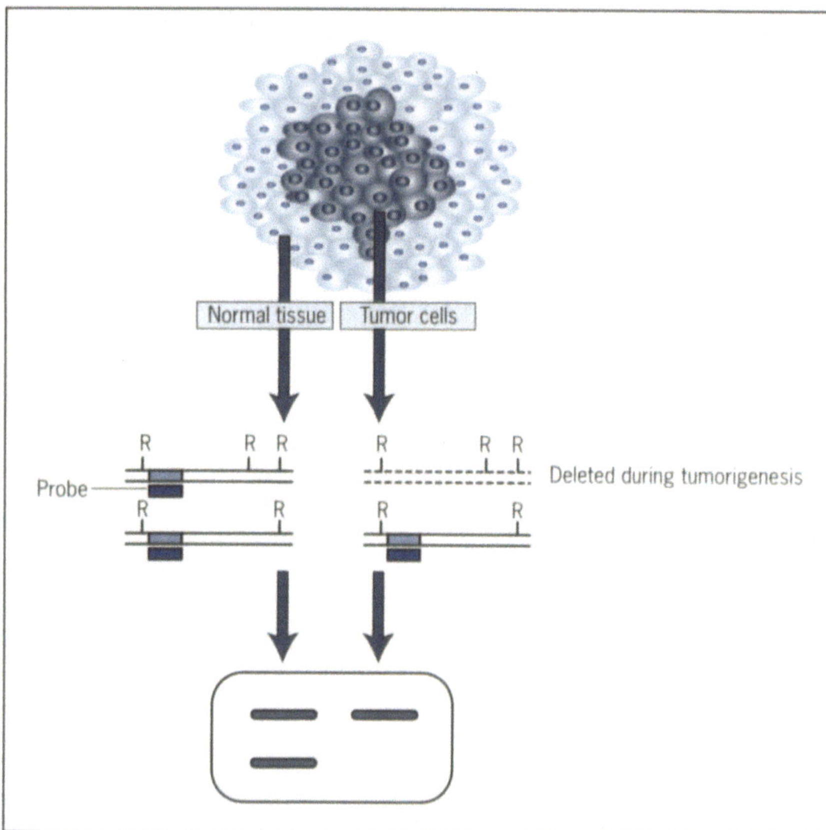

Figure 1-16. Loss of heterozygosity analysis using restriction fragment length polymorphism (RFLP) markers. RFLP results from the presence or absence of a restriction site (R) due to polymorphic differences in DNA sequences. Different alleles of a polymorphic locus can be distinguished by a probe on a Southern blot. The example shown indicates individual heterozygosity at this locus, because two different alleles are identified in normal cells. If one copy of this chromosomal region is deleted during tumorigenesis, the heterozygosity at this locus is lost in the tumor cells.

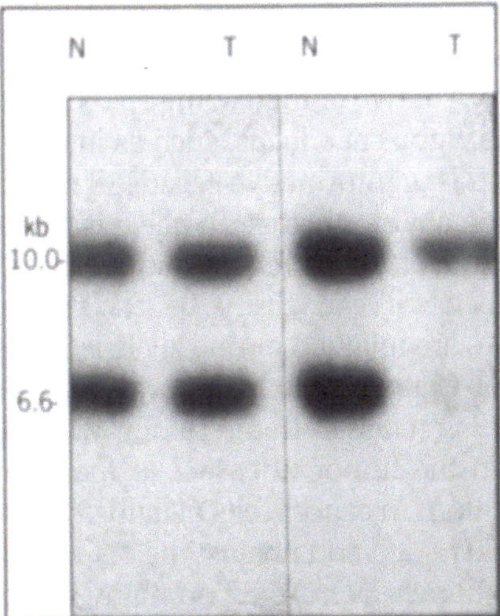

Figure 1-17. Restriction fragment length polymorphism (RFLP) analysis of malignant mesothelioma. Southern blotting was performed using paired normal and tumor DNA digested with *Eco*RI, and the filter was hybridized with an RFLP marker probe. Heterozygosity was retained in the tumor from case 1 (*left*) but lost in the tumor from case 2 (*right*). N—normal DNA; T—tumor DNA.

as illustrated in Figure 1-18. The primers are short, synthetic oligonucleotides, often 15 to 30 nucleotides long, that correspond to sequences immediately flanking the target region. In addition to DNA and an excess amount of primers, the PCR reaction mixture contains a heat-stable DNA polymerase and DNA building blocks (*ie,* dATP, dTTP, dCTP, and dGTP). Each reaction cycle starts by heat denaturing the double-stranded DNA template into single strands. The temperature is then reduced to allow the primers to anneal to their complementary sequences in the target DNA. Finally, the DNA polymerase extends from the 3′ end of the annealed primers to form a new DNA strand complementary to the original template. These newly formed double helices are used as templates in the next cycle. The number of target DNA molecules is doubled in each cycle, and each cycle takes only a few minutes; therefore, it is possible to generate millions of copies of the desired target sequences from a single DNA molecule in a matter of hours.

Microsatellite DNA comprises a collection of small arrays of short tandemly repeated DNA sequences (often 1 to 4 bp) that are interspersed throughout the

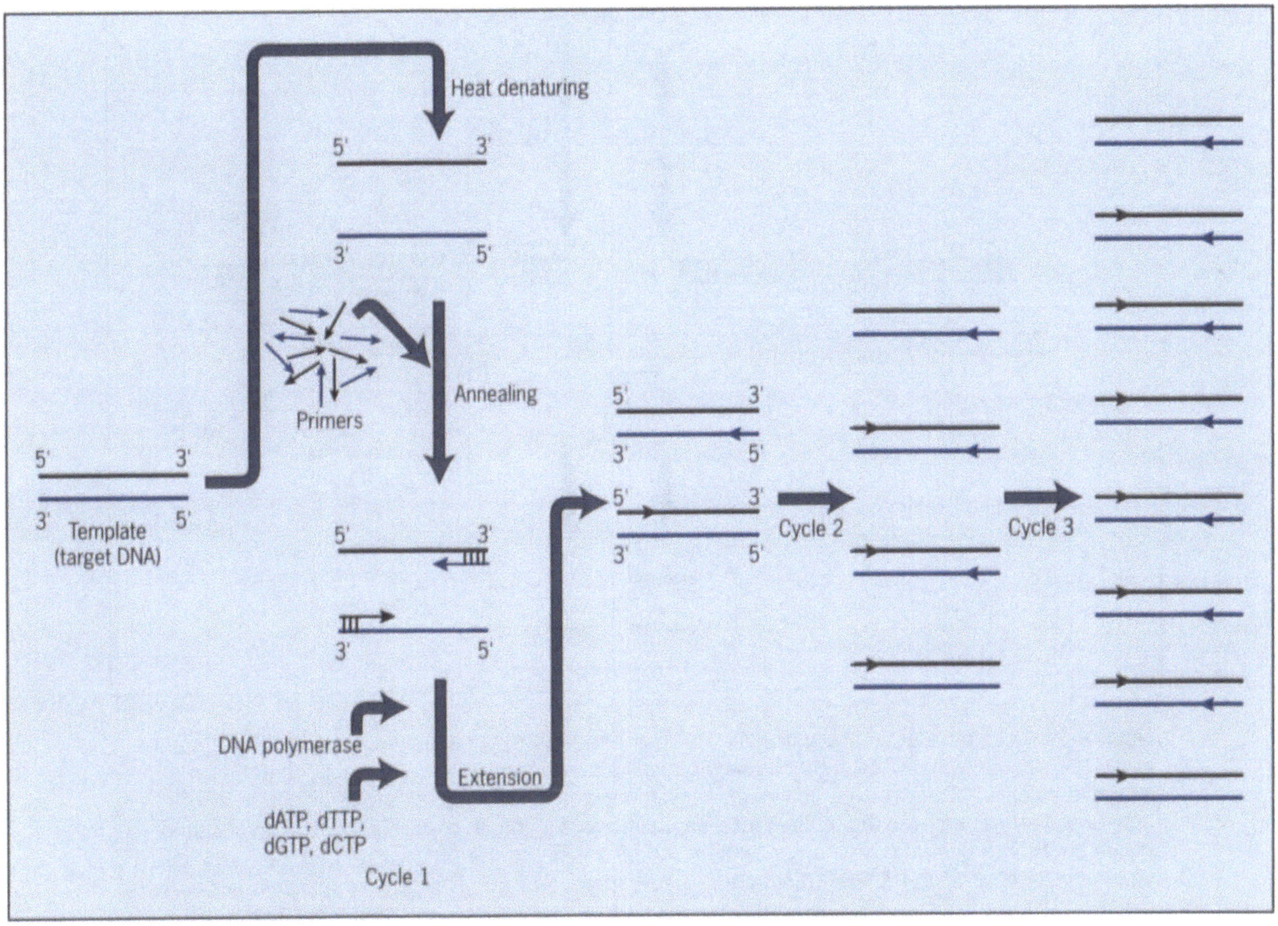

Figure 1-18. Polymerase chain reaction. Each cycle is composed of three steps: heat denaturation of the template, annealing, and extension of the primers to produce new double-stranded DNA. The number of the target DNA molecules is doubled after each cycle.

genome. The number of repeats at each locus is highly variable, probably due to slippage during DNA replication. PCR makes it possible to use this short tandem repeat polymorphism (STRP) in microsatellite DNA to generate highly polymorphic genetic markers. The primer pairs for STRP markers are designed to hybridize to the unique sequences flanking the tandem repeats (Fig. 1-19). The PCR products from different alleles vary in length based on the number of repeats and can be resolved by denaturing PAGE. Frequently, one of the PCR primers included in the PCR mixture is labeled with ^{32}P, or radiolabeled deoxynucleotides such as alpha^{32}P-dATP or ^{35}S-dATP are included in the PCR mixture so that the PCR products can be seen using autoradiography. STRPs are the predominant tool for LOH analysis in cancer because of their multi-allelic and highly polymorphic nature and because of the speed and simplicity of the PCR technique.

Figure 1-20 shows an autoradiograph of an STRP analysis of six paired samples of normal and tumor (mesothelioma) DNA at two chromosome 1p loci. If an individual is homozygous at a locus, such as in case 2 at *D1S519*, this locus is uninformative because it cannot provide information about whether an allele is lost in the tumor cells. Conversely, if an individual is heterozygous at a locus, it can easily be ascertained whether both alleles are retained or one allele is lost in the tumor cells. For example, the heterozygosity seen in case 1 at *D1S519* is retained in the tumor, whereas LOH is detected in the tumor of case 3 at the same locus. Because deletions in cancer cells usually involve a long chromosomal region and not just the TSG locus, LOH analysis is routinely performed on many tumor specimens to delineate the common region of deletion. For example, as shown in Figure 1-21, primary tumor specimens or cell lines from 50 malignant mesothe-

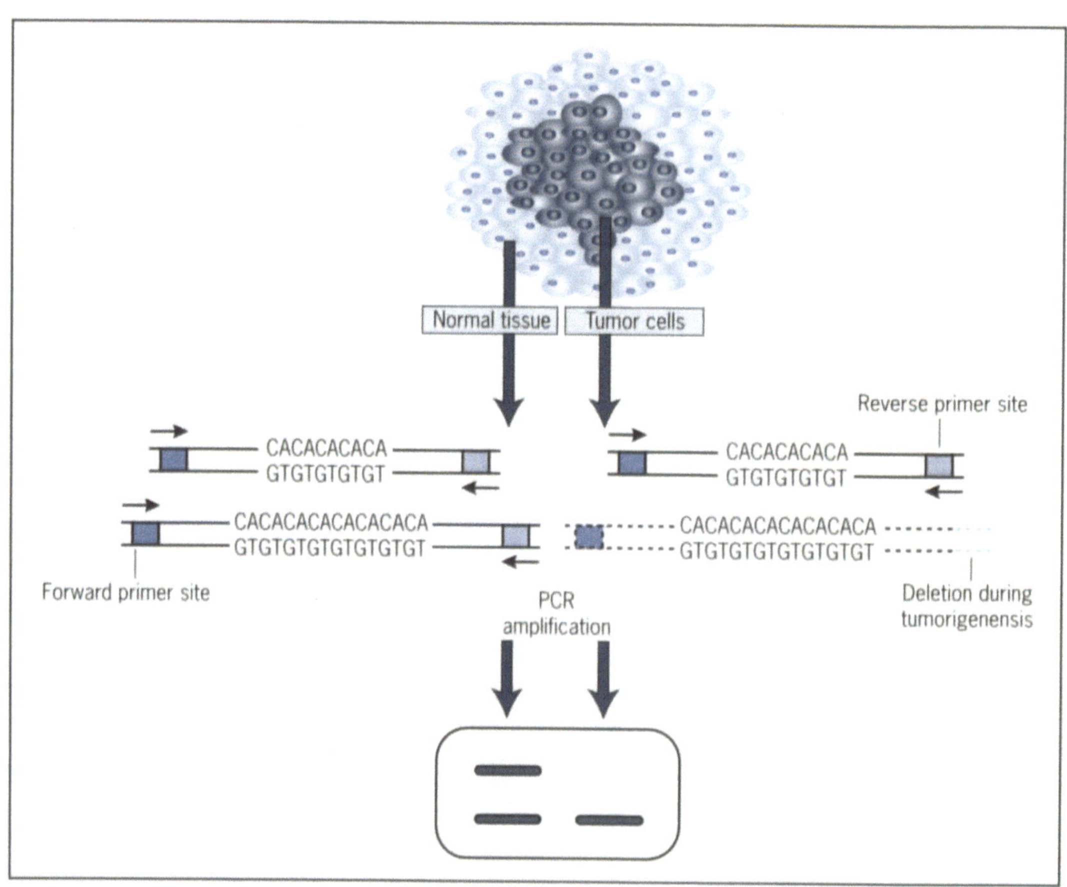

Figure 1-19. Loss of heterozygosity analysis using short tandem repeat polymorphism (STRP) markers. STRP results from the different numbers of copies of the tandem-repeat sequence (CA in this example) in different alleles. The polymerase chain reaction (PCR) primers are designed to bind the unique sequences flanking the tandem repeats; therefore, the length of the PCR products are determined by the numbers of copies of the tandem-repeat sequence. Heterozygosity at a locus can be visualized by separating the PCR products on a polyacrylamide gel. This heterozygosity is not retained in tumor cells if one copy of this chromosomal region has been deleted during tumorigenesis.

1
2
3
4
5
6
N T N T N T N T N T N T
D1S519
D1S550

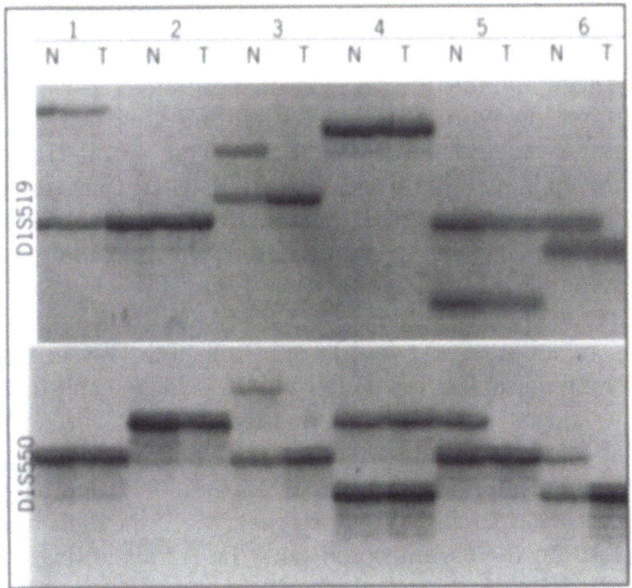

Figure 1-20. Short tandem repeat polymorphism analysis of malignant mesothelioma. Six pairs of normal (N) and tumor (T) DNA samples were examined at two chromosome 1p loci: *D1S519* and *D1S550*. The PCR products were visualized by autoradiography because α-^{35}S-dATP was included in the PCR mixtures. Loss of heterozygosity can be identified clearly in several cases (*eg*, cases 3 and 6 at both loci).

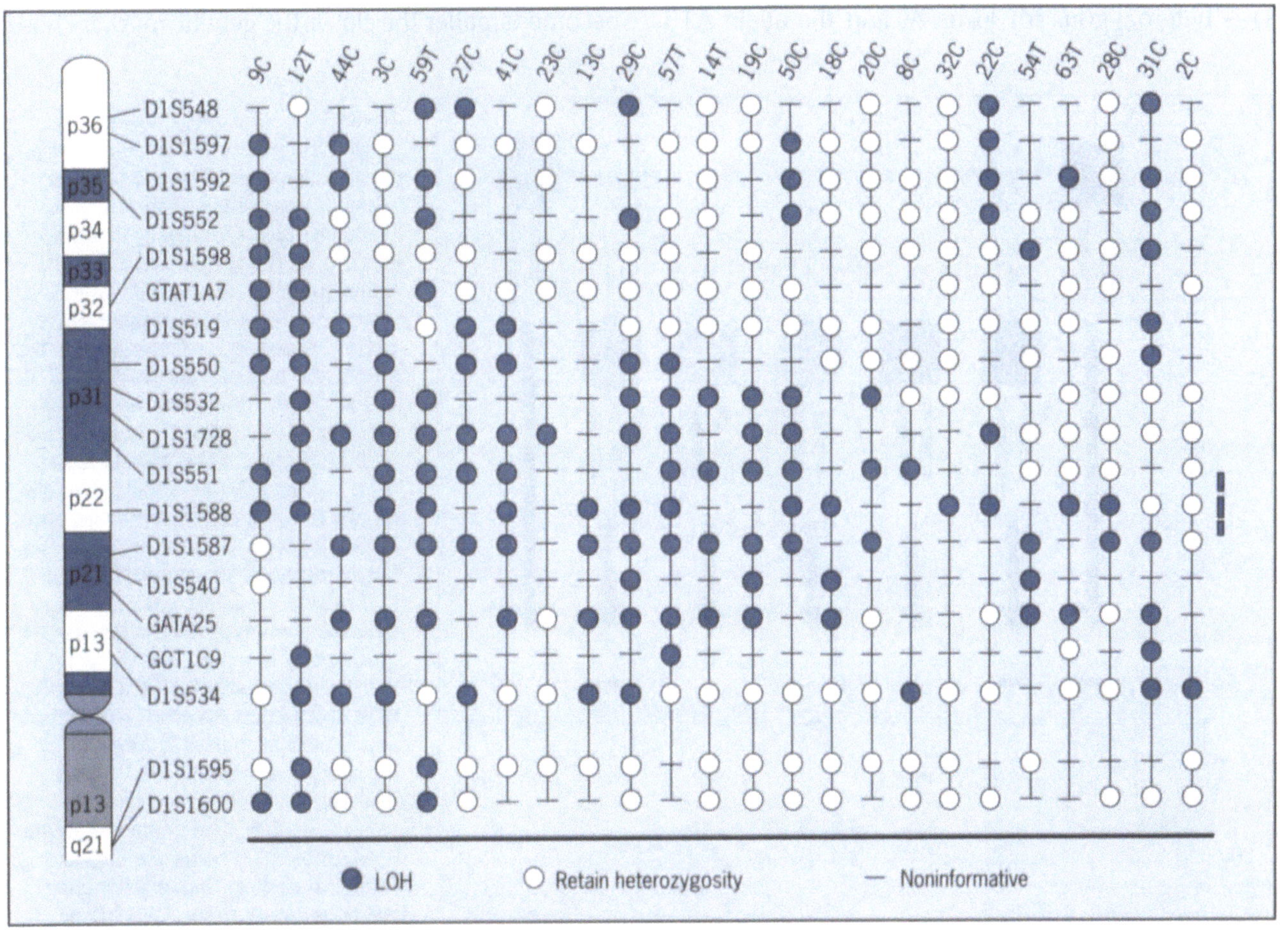

9C 12T 44C 3C 59T 27C 41C 23C 13C 29C 57T 14T 19C 50C 18C 20C 8C 32C 22C 54T 63T 28C 31C 2C
p36
p35
p34
p33
p32
p31
p22
p21
p13
p13
q21
D1S548
D1S1597
D1S1592
D1S552
D1S1598
GTAT1A7
D1S519
D1S550
D1S532
D1S1728
D1S551
D1S1588
D1S1587
D1S540
GATA25
GCT1C9
D1S534
D1S1595
D1S1600
LOH
Retain heterozygosity
Noninformative

Figure 1-21. Loss of heterozygosity (LOH) analysis of chromosome 1 at 19 short tandem repeat polymorphism loci in malignant mesothelioma. Primary tumor specimens (T) or cell lines (C) from 50 malignant mesotheliomas were examined. Thirty-seven cases showed allelic losses at one or more loci in 1p, and the 24 cases exhibiting interstitial and/or terminal deletion of 1p are shown. Case numbers are indicated at the *top*. The shortest region of overlapping deletions is indicated at the *right* by *vertical dashes*. (*Adapted from* Lee *et al.* [9]; with permission.)

liomas were examined for LOH at 19 STRP loci on chromosome 1. Thirty-seven cases (74%) showed allelic losses at one or more loci in 1p. By analyzing the LOH patterns of the cases exhibiting interstitial or terminal deletions, the shortest region of overlapping deletions among all of the cases can be determined.

Linkage Analysis

Familial cancers provide another approach for locating TSGs—linkage analysis (Fig. 1-22). In familial cancers, the defective TSG is transmitted from generation to generation in a Mendelian fashion, as are genetic markers. If a genetic marker is located on the same chromosome as the TSG under investigation, and if these two loci are linked, a specific allele of this genetic marker and the defective TSG are usually inherited together in the family. For example, as shown in Figure 1-22*A*, the affected father (subject I-1) is heterozygous for locus A, and the allele A1 is located on the same chromosome as the defective TSG (T-). The homologous chromosomes segregate during the meiotic division of spermatogenesis. The offspring who inherited the chromosome carrying the A1 allele, such as the eldest son (subject II-1) and the younger daughter (subject II-5), usually also have inherited the mutated TSG and thus would be affected. The offspring who inherited the chromosome carrying the A2 allele and the wild-type TSG (T+), such as the elder daughter (subject II-3) and the youngest son (subject II-4), would not be affected. The second son (subject II-2) also inherited the A2 allele and thus would be expected to be unaffected. However, he is affected because he inherited a recombined chromosome resulting from a crossover event between the A and TSG loci during meiosis that placed the defective TSG on the chromosome with the A2 allele (Fig. 1-22*B*). Because the frequency of genetic recombination between two loci is roughly proportional to their physical distance, the chance of recombination becomes smaller the closer the genetic marker chosen

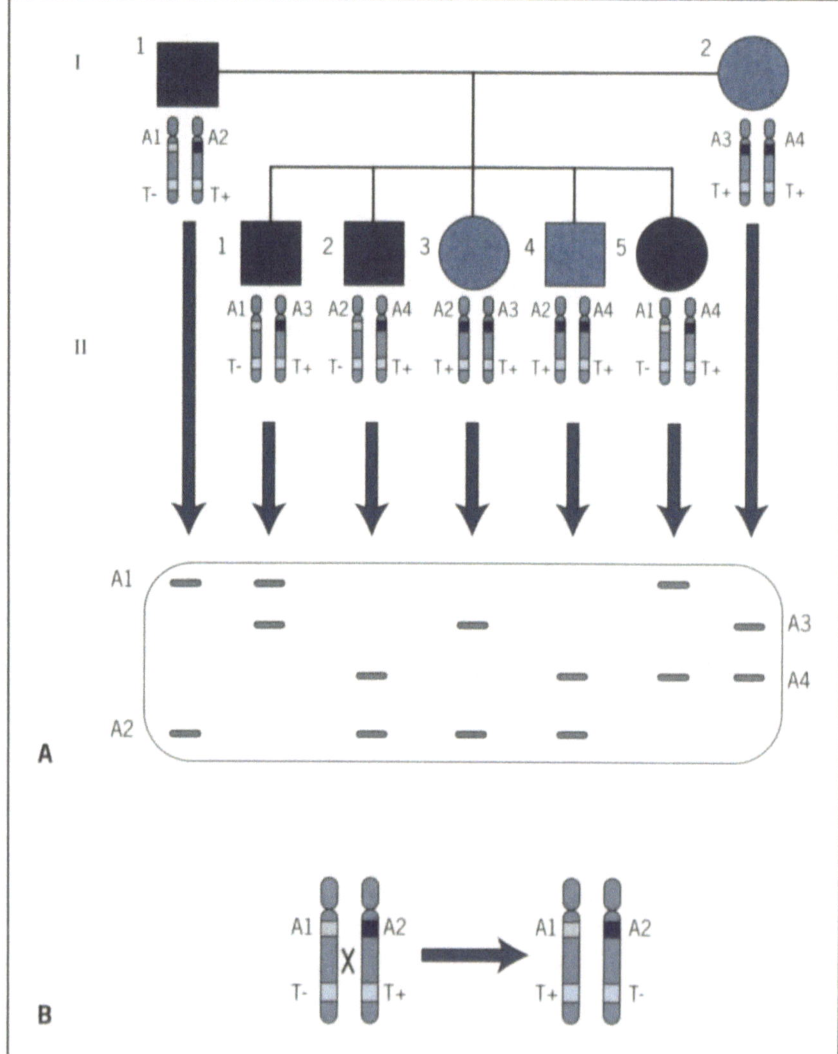

Figure 1-22. Linkage analysis. If a genetic marker is linked to a tumor suppressor gene (TSG), a specific allele of this genetic marker and the defective TSG are usually inherited together in the family. The affected father (*panel A*, subject I-1) is heterozygous for a short tandem repeat polymorphism locus (locus A) with two alleles, A1 and A2. The defective TSG (T-) is located on the same chromosome as the A1 allele. The unaffected mother (subject I-2) is also heterozygous for locus A with another two alleles, A3 and A4, and has the wild-type TSG (T+) on both chromosomes. All family members are typed for locus A to correlate the allelic type with the disease phenotype. The offspring (generation II) inherited a chromosome carrying either A1 and T- (and thus affected) or A2 and T+ (and thus unaffected) from their father, except the second son (subject II-2), who inherited the recombined chromosome (*panel B*). The chance of genetic recombination becomes smaller when the genetic marker chosen for testing is closer to the TSG locus; thus, the position of the TSG can be located by typing the family to find the most tightly associated loci.

for testing is to the TSG locus. Therefore, it is now common practice to locate the TSG in cancer-susceptible families by scanning the whole genome with STRP markers to determine which genetic marker locus is tightly associated with the cancer susceptibility phenotype.

Positional Cloning

Positional cloning refers to the cloning of a gene based solely on its subchromosomal location, as shown schematically in Figure 1-23. As mentioned previously, potential locations of TSGs can be identified by mapping the regions deleted in tumors using karyotypic analysis or LOH analysis, and linkage analysis in cancer-susceptible families. Often the initial localization defines a relatively large region of 10 cM or more. Additional genetic markers within this region then are tested to narrow down the candidate region, preferably to 1 to 2 cM, which is roughly equivalent to 1 to 2 million bp. The next step in positional cloning is to establish a contiguous array of overlapping genomic DNA fragments covering the entire candidate region (physical mapping), followed by construction of a transcript map of all expressed sequences within the region (transcript mapping). Candidate genes then can be selected from the transcripts located within the map. Selection is usually based on various types of information, such as sequence homology to known genes or expression patterns. Finally, evidence such as the presence of function-inactivating mutations within the gene in tumor cells and affected members of cancer families, or the capability of the gene to restore the normal phenotype when transfected into cancer cells is used to verify that a candidate gene is a TSG

Physical Mapping

The physical mapping step in positional cloning is often carried out by chromosome walking (Fig. 1-24). A probe is prepared from a genetic marker that is

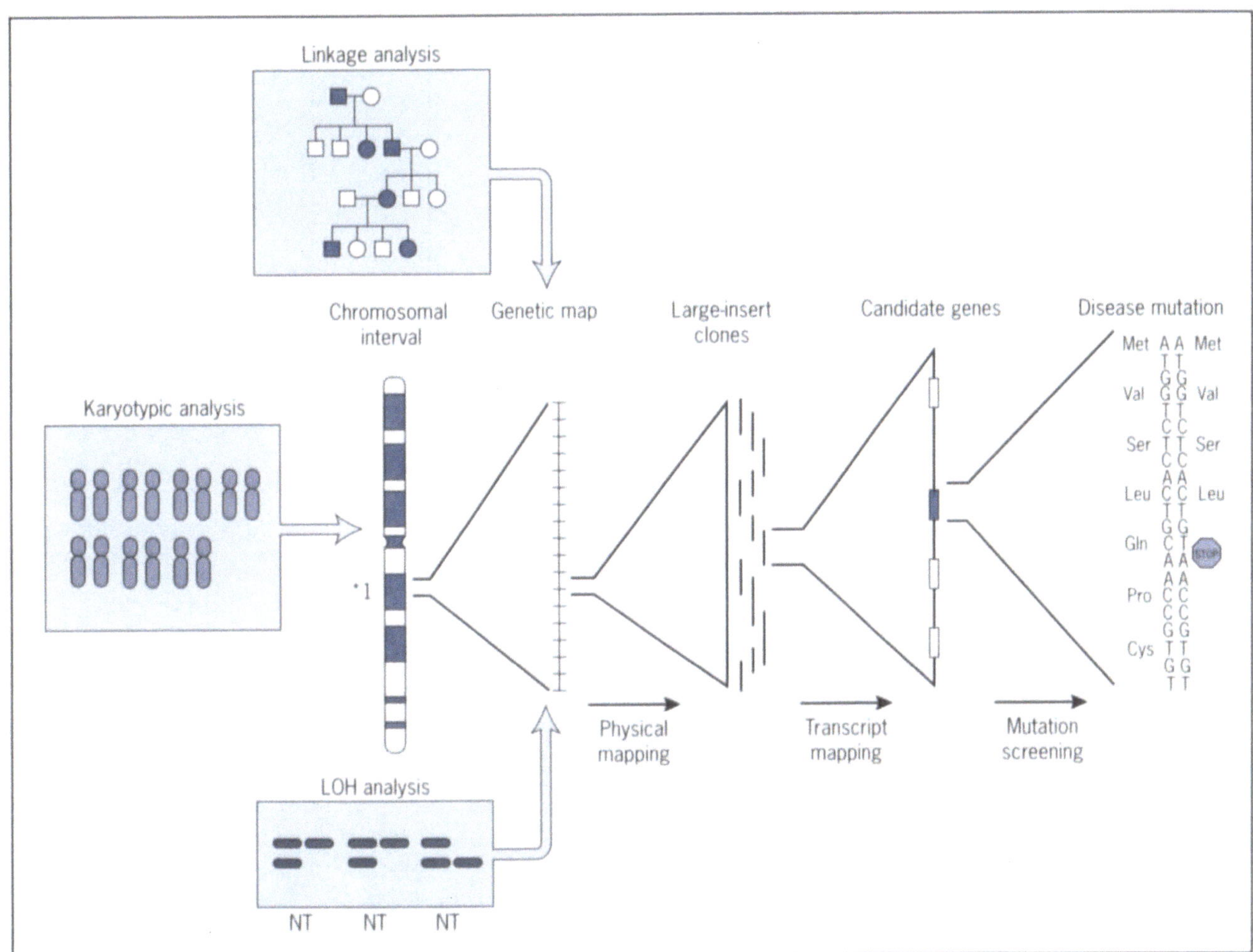

Figure 1-23. The major steps of positional cloning. LOH—loss of heterozygosity.

most closely linked to the candidate TSG locus as shown by linkage analysis or that defines the shortest region of overlapping deletions as shown by deletion mapping. The probe is hybridized to a genomic library to identify a clone that contains sequences that overlap with the genetic marker. A new probe, prepared from the end of the genomic DNA fragment in the first clone, is then used to identify another overlapping clone from the genomic library. This process is repeated until a clone that overlaps with a genetic marker on the other side of the candidate TSG locus is obtained. For simplicity, the diagram presented in Figure 1-24 depicts monodirectional walking. However, chromosome walking is commonly carried out bidirectionally, starting from both flanking genetic markers and walking toward each other until the region between the markers is covered by overlapping clones.

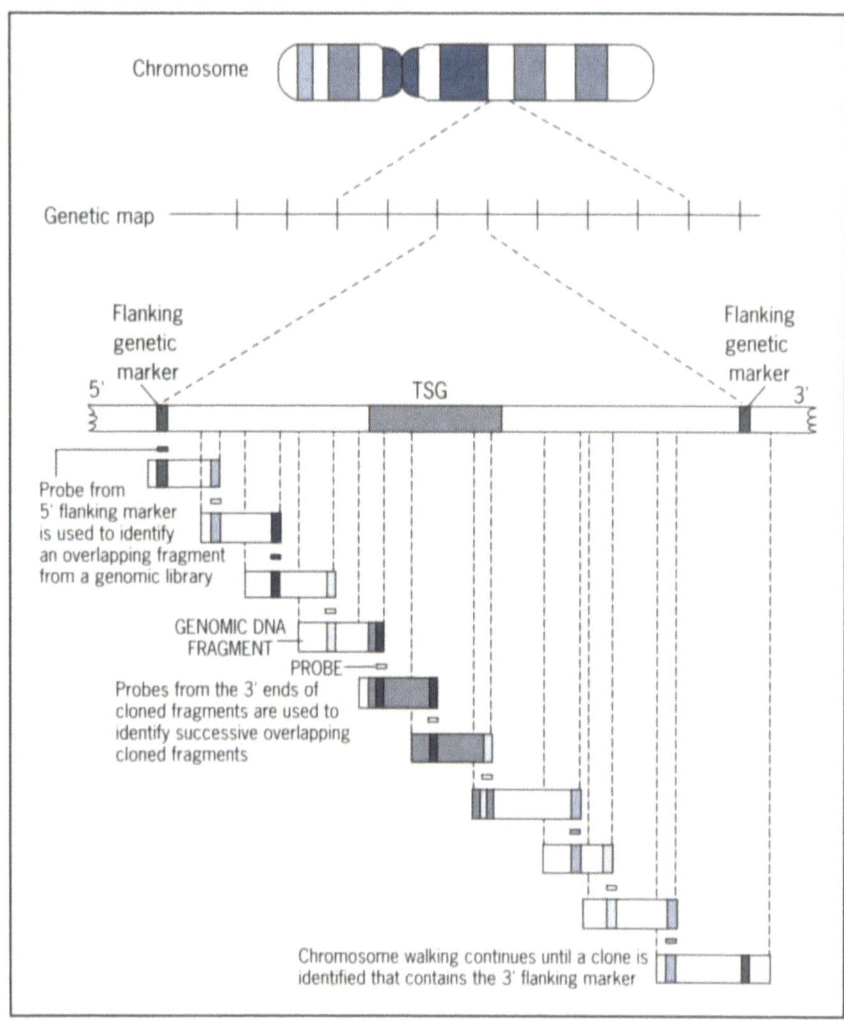

Figure 1-24. Chromosome walking. A clone contig spanning the entire region of interest can be constructed by screening a genomic DNA library for overlapping fragments. (*Adapted from* Micklos and Freyer [10]; with permission). TSG—tumor suppressor gene.

Table 1-1. Cloning vectors commonly used in positional cloning

Cloning vector	Insert size (kb)
Cosmid	30–45
Bacteriophage P1	70–100
P1 artificial chromosome (PAC)	130–150
Bacterial artificial chromosome (BAC)	70–300
Yeast artificial chromosome (YAC)	200–2000

Because the regions to be mapped by chromosome walking frequently span millions of base pairs, cloning systems for manipulating large fragments of human genomic DNA are essential. Table 1-1 lists the types and capacities of cloning vectors commonly used in positional cloning. Among these vectors, cosmids and yeast artificial chromosomes (YACs) are the primary tools for physical mapping.

Cosmids, which are derived from bacteriophage lambda, were the first vectors specifically designed for cloning large fragments of mammalian DNA. The essential components of a cosmid vector include a drug resistance marker, an origin of replication, unique restriction cloning sites, and the ligated cohesive end (*cos*) site of bacteriophage lambda (Fig. 1-25*A*). After restriction enzyme–digested source DNA fragments are linked to cosmid molecules in a ligation reaction, the *cos* sites are cleaved and the intervening DNA is packaged into mature bacteriophage particles in an in vitro lambda packaging reaction. When infecting *Escherichia coli,* the recombinant DNA in the bacteriophage particle is injected into the cell, circularized via the phage cohesive ends, and replicated as a plasmid. Because this in vitro packaging process is very efficient, cosmid vectors can be used to construct high-complexity libraries from small amounts of source DNA, such as that from flow-sorted chromosomes. In addition, purification of cosmid DNA and maintenance of cosmid libraries are quite simple. The main disadvantages of cosmids that limit their use in long-range mapping of complex genomes are their relatively small capacity for foreign DNA inserts (30 to 45 kb) and frequent instability of clones.

The YAC system is at the other end of the vector spectrum for insert size (Table 1-1). The YAC vector contains all of the basic functional units of yeast chromosomes: a centromere, two telomeres, and an autonomous replication sequence that functions as an origin of replication (Fig. 1-25*B*). DNA fragments over 1 million bp long can be cloned between the two arms of the vector and propagated in yeast as linear chromosomes. This huge insert capacity has made a tremendous contribution to the rapid progress in long-range contig mapping of the human genome. The major obstacles in using this system include the presence of abundant chimeric clones in YAC libraries, low transformation efficiency, and occasional insert instability. DNA manipulation in yeast systems is also more complicated than that in bacterial systems.

Several alternative systems have been developed in an effort to overcome the shortcomings of the cosmid and YAC cloning systems. Generally, there is a trade-off between insert size and the efficiency of cloning. The bacteriophage P1 system uses the same cloning strategy as that of the cosmid vectors but is capable of accepting inserts as large as 100 kb. However, its in vitro packaging process is much more elaborate and its cloning efficiency is intermediate between that of cosmids and YACs. The bacterial artificial chromosome (BAC) system is based on the well-studied *E. coli* fertility plasmid (F-factor). Human genomic DNA fragments greater than 300 kb have been ligated to the pBAC vector and introduced into bacterial cells by electroporation. Although there is no selectable marker in the pBAC vector and DNA recovery from the clones is relatively low, the BAC system is gaining popularity because of its ability to maintain individual large insert clones with a high degree of structural stability. The PAC system is a combination of the P1 and BAC systems; the PAC vector is derived from bacteriophage P1, but the recombinant DNA is introduced into *E. coli* by electroporation. Although the PAC system offers much easier manipulation of cloned DNA than the BAC system, its insert capacity is much smaller.

Transcript Mapping

The identification of transcribed sequences within clone contigs covering specific chromosomal regions of interest has been a major rate-limiting step in positional cloning. In principle, methods commonly used for locating genes within cloned DNA are based on their capability of expression or their evolutionary conservation of coding regions and important regulatory sequences (Table 1-2).

One approach that uses the expression characteristics of coding sequences to identify genes is to search for cDNA clones from one or more cDNA libraries that are capable of hybridizing to cloned genomic fragments. Cosmid clone inserts are frequently directly labeled and used as hybridization probes for screening cDNA libraries. Larger clones, such as YACs can be used as hybridization probes but are associated with more technical difficulty and less efficiency. Therefore, methods have been developed to selectively amplify cDNA sequences capable of hybridizing to large genomic inserts. Figure 1-26 illustrates two variations of the direct cDNA selection technique. One approach starts with the immobilization of target genomic DNA (purified YAC or cosmid) on nylon-filter discs. Repeat sequences within the target DNA can be quenched by prehybridization with sheared total human DNA. All of the cDNA inserts in a cDNA library are then amplified by PCR and hybridized to the target DNA on the discs. The second approach differs only in that the hybridization is carried out in solution. The target genomic DNA is biotinylated so that any cDNA specifically bound to the target DNA can be captured by streptavidin-coated magnetic beads. After washing to remove non-specifically bound sequences, the specific cDNAs remaining on the nylon-filter discs or the magnetic beads can be eluted and amplified by PCR. The

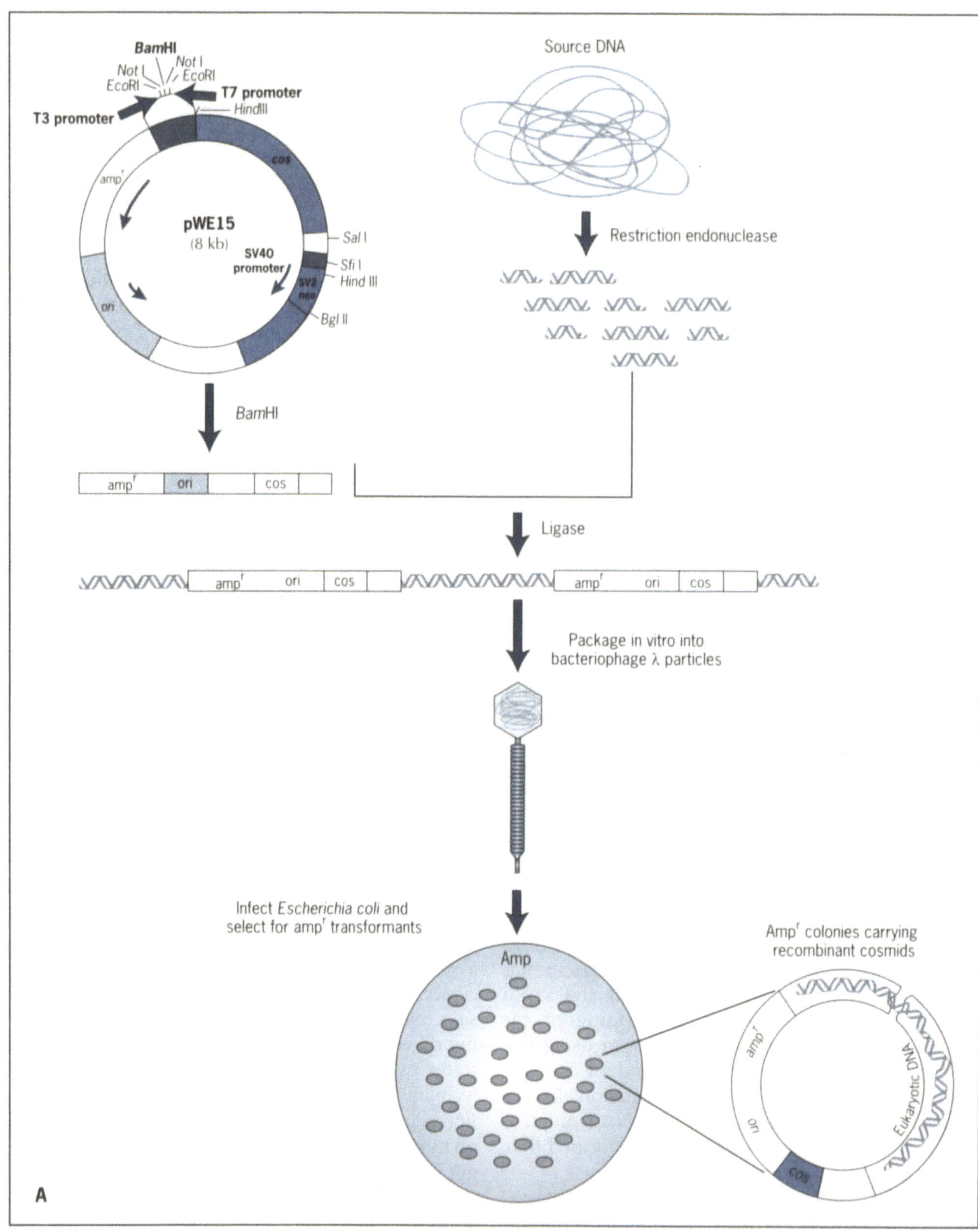

Figure 1-25. Cloning systems for physical mapping. **A,** The cosmid system. *(continued)*

amplified products can be cloned and analyzed or used for another round of hybridization for further enrichment of the specific cDNA sequences.

The main concern in using cDNA libraries for transcript mapping is that to be detected, all of the genes located within the region of interest must be expressed in the tissues from which the libraries were made. To overcome this problem, a method called "exon trapping" was devised that identifies exons directly from genomic clones by their ability to engage in an artificial RNA splicing assay (Fig. 1-27). In this procedure, the target genomic sequences are subcloned into a specially designed vector, between splice donor and splice acceptor sites. The recombinant DNA is then transfected into a strain of monkey cells known as COS cells. If an exon is present in the genomic sequence cloned into the vector, it will be transcribed and spliced into mature mRNA. A cDNA copy of this mRNA can then be synthesized with reverse transcriptase and PCR amplified with primers specific for the vector exon sequences. The extra exon provided by the genomic insert leads to PCR products of a larger size than that of the vector alone, that can be identified easily by agarose gel electrophoresis.

The sequence characteristics of coding regions and important control elements provide another direction for the initial localization of genes within cloned genomic segments. Coding DNAs are under selection pressure to preserve sequences of important biologic functions and thus are much more strongly conserved among species than are noncoding DNAs. This sequence conservation feature can be detected using a zoo blot, which is a Southern blot of genomic DNA samples from a wide variety of species (Fig. 1-28). Human genomic DNA fragments can be used to probe a zoo blot at a reduced hybridization stringency; those fragments that cross-hybridize to other species are generally found to contain coding sequences. However, this method requires subcloning of large DNA fragments and hybridization of individual subclones to the zoo blots, making it impractical for mapping very large regions.

Conversely, CpG island identification provides a rapid means for locating potential sites of genes within long DNA fragments. CpG islands are short stretches of hypomethylated GC-rich DNA frequently found at the 5′ end of vertebrate genes. It is estimated that more than half of human genes are associated with such sequences. The CpG island structure of the *RB1* gene is shown in Figure 1-29*A*. CpG islands usually have recognition sites for a variety of rare cutter restriction endonucleases that cleave at GC-rich sequences containing one or two CpG dinucleotides. Therefore, a cluster of such rare cutter sites is indicative of a CpG island and can be detected by restriction mapping of cloned DNA. In addition, a

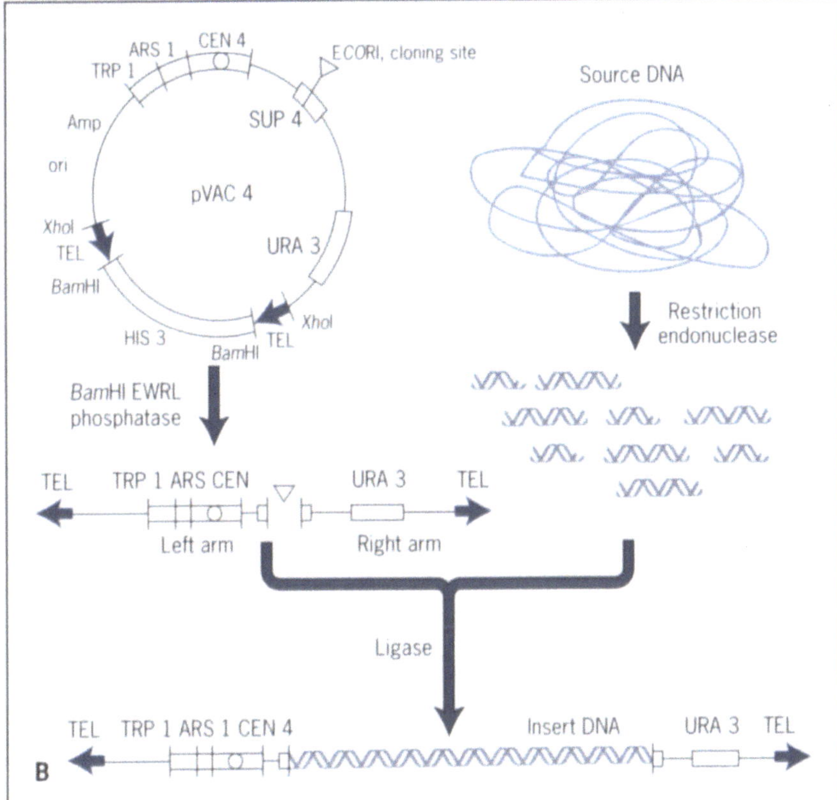

Figure 1-25. (*continued*) **B,** The yeast artificial chromosome system.

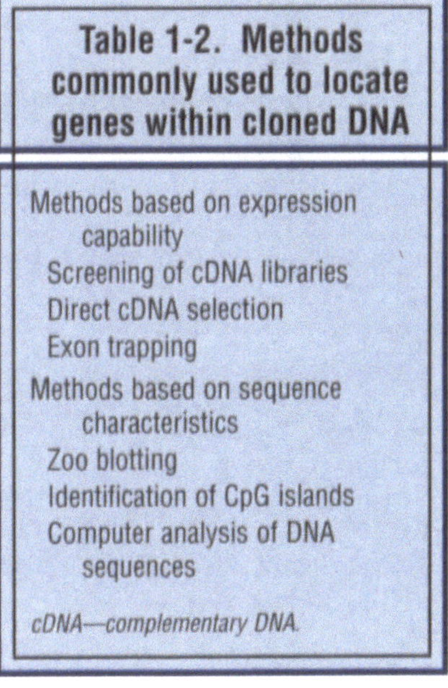

Table 1-2. Methods commonly used to locate genes within cloned DNA

Methods based on expression capability
- Screening of cDNA libraries
- Direct cDNA selection
- Exon trapping

Methods based on sequence characteristics
- Zoo blotting
- Identification of CpG islands
- Computer analysis of DNA sequences

cDNA—complementary DNA.

technique known as island rescue PCR has been devised to selectively amplify CpG islands and their adjacent sequences from human YACs (Fig. 1-29*B*). This method involves digestion of YAC DNA with a rare cutter restriction endonuclease, ligation of an adaptor, and PCR amplification of sequences between the adaptor and an *Alu* repeat that is in the vicinity of the cloned CpG island. The *Alu* repeat refers to a family of highly repetitive sequences with a copy number of about 750,000. Because these repeats are dispersed mainly throughout the euchromatic regions of the human genome, there is a high likelihood that an *Alu* repeat will be located in the vicinity of a CpG island. The products from island rescue PCR can be cloned and analyzed.

If the sequence of the cloned DNA has been determined, computer analysis also can be used to predict the likely locations of transcripts. There are two types

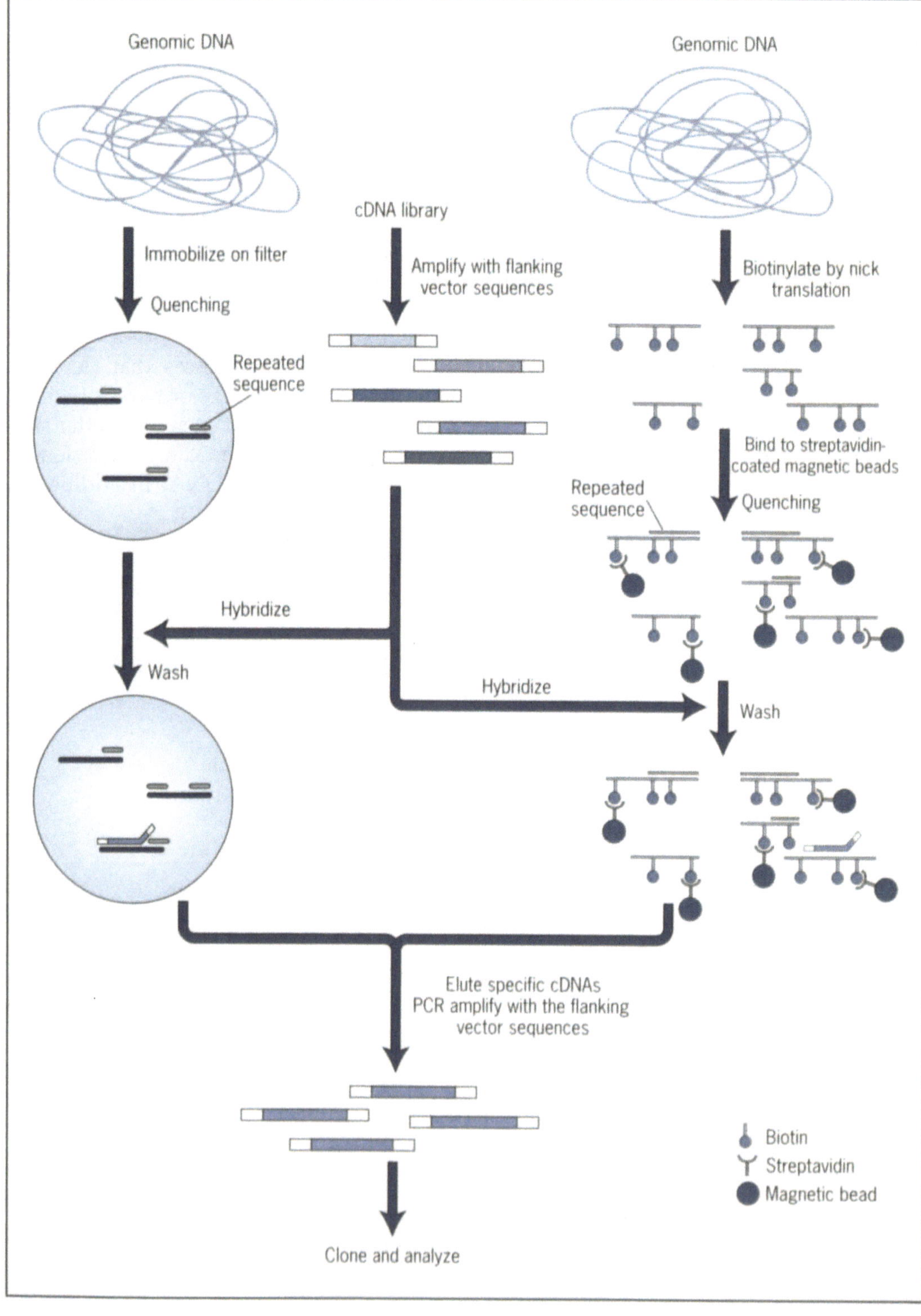

Figure 1-26. Direct complementary DNA (cDNA) selection techniques. The target genomic DNA can be immobilized on nylon-filter discs (*left*) or biotinylated and then immobilized by binding to streptavidin-coated magnetic beads (*right*). All the cDNA inserts in a cDNA library are amplified by polymerase chain reaction (PCR), and the sequences capable of hybridizing to the target DNA are selected.

of software used to examine whether a sequence is likely to represent part of a gene. The first type compares the nucleotide sequence of the cloned DNA and its deduced amino acid sequence in all three reading frames to all available DNA and protein sequences. Any significant sequence homology detected, between or within species, may indicate the presence of an exon or other gene-associated sequences. The second type of software is designed to recognize sequence patterns that are characteristic of genes or biologically important elements. For example, likely locations of exons can be predicted

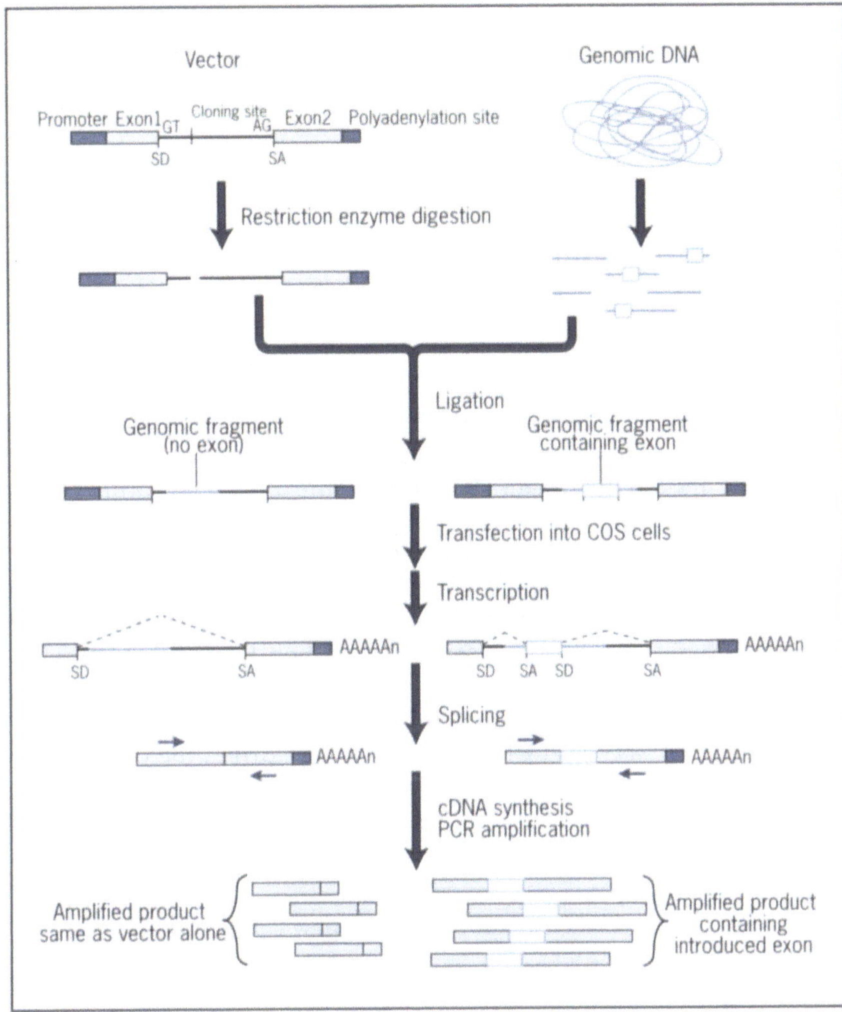

Figure 1-27. Exon trapping technique. Genomic DNA is subcloned into the cloning site located between two exons and then transfected into COS cells. If the genomic insert contains an exon with functional splice donor (SD) and splice acceptor (SA) sequences, the exon will be spliced into mature mRNA and, following complementary DNA (cDNA) synthesis, can be amplified by polymerase chain reaction (PCR) using primers specific for vector exon sequences.

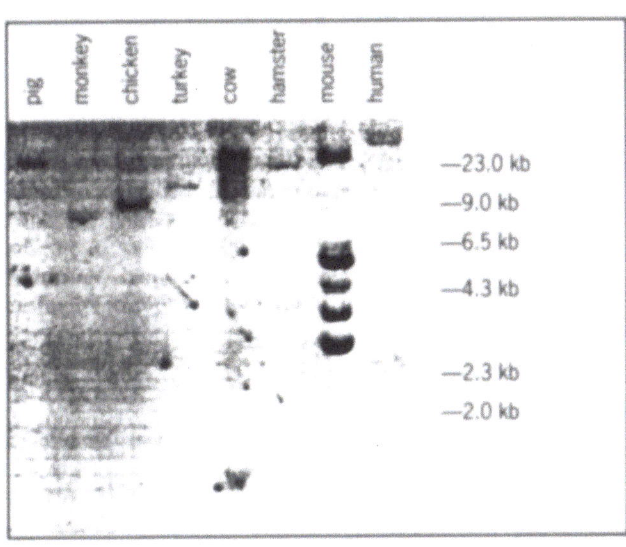

Figure 1-28. Zoo blot analysis. A complementary DNA clone from the neurofibromatosis type 2 gene (*NF2*) was used as the hybridization probe against a Southern blot of genomic DNA samples from the indicated species. (*Adapted from* Claudio *et al.* [11]; with permission.)

by scanning for conserved sequences of exon/intron boundaries, splice branch sites, and relatively long open reading frames. It should be noted that the exon-trapping technique and all methods based on sequence characteristics provide information only about possible locations of genes. Further experiments are necessary to verify that the predicted gene sequences are actually expressed.

Positional Candidate Gene Approach

Positional cloning has been applied successfully to isolate many disease genes, including TSGs involved in familial and sporadic tumors. However, both physical mapping and transcript mapping are very time-consuming and labor-intensive processes. Thus, the positional candidate gene approach is also commonly employed for gene identification. After the likely location of a TSG has been determined by linkage or deletion analysis, potential candidates are selected directly from the transcripts already mapped to the region under investigation. Obviously, the success of this approach depends heavily on the density of known transcripts located within the chromosomal region of interest, and thus it is gaining popularity with the progression of the Human Genome Project. As of 1998, more than 30,000 human genes have been mapped. With the completion of the Human Genome Project, projected to occur ahead of schedule in the year 2000, the candidate gene approach probably will become the method of choice for disease gene identification.

Mutation and Methylation

After a gene is selected as a potential TSG candidate, regardless of which approach has been used for its identification, it must be verified for evidence of disease association. Because tumorigenesis results from inactivation of TSGs, it is common to test whether the candidate gene is functional in normal cells but inactivated in tumor cells. TSGs are generally inactivated by deletions or mutations. In some cases, TSGs are found to be inactivated by transcriptional silencing due to methylation at their 5′ ends.

As mentioned previously (*see* Deletion Mapping), large deletions are detectable by cytogenetic analysis. Deletions also can be identified by LOH analysis using polymorphic markers located within or flanking the candidate gene. Southern blot analysis is a useful tool for analyzing hemizygous or homozygous deletions. In addition, PCR is frequently used to quickly screen tumor specimens for homozygous deletions, as illustrated in Figure 1-30. Primer pairs usually are designed to amplify individual exons from genomic DNA. In the experiment shown in Figure 1-30, three primer pairs were used to amplify each of the three exons of *p16* in a panel of malignant mesothelioma cell lines. *p16* was selected as a candidate TSG in this study through a positional candidate approach; the gene is located at chromosome 9p21-22, a region frequently deleted in mesothelioma, and its protein product is capable of binding to and inhibiting CDK4, one of the several cyclin-dependent kinases that drives the cell through the cell cycle and into cell division. PCR products can

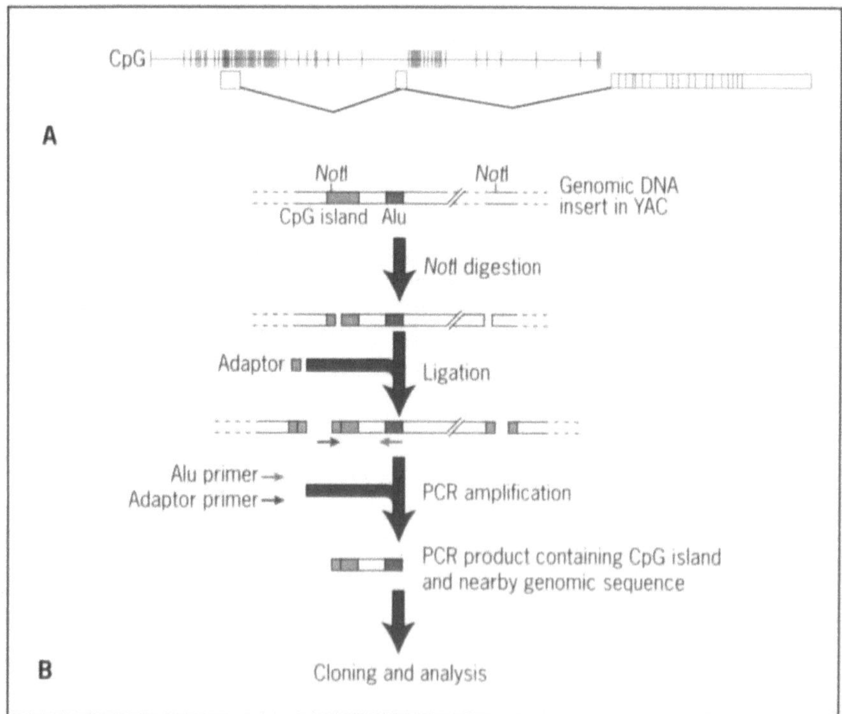

Figure 1-29. CpG island rescue polymerase chain reaction (PCR). **A,** The CpG island structure of the retinoblastoma gene (*RB*). Vertical lines represent the positions of the CpG dinucleotide in the 5′, 10-kb sequence of this 177-kb gene. *Boxes* represent exons, with splicing pattern shown for the exons located within the 10-kb sequence. **B,** The island rescue PCR technique. Yeast artificial chromosome (YAC) is digested with the rare cutting restriction enzyme *NotI*, ligated to an adaptor, and PCR is amplified with an adaptor-specific primer and an *Alu*-specific primer. The PCR product, which contains the CpG island and nearby genomic sequences, then can be cloned and analyzed.

be visualized easily by agarose gel electrophoresis and ethidium bromide staining. Absence of the expected PCR product indicates that all or part of the exon has been homozygously deleted from the cell line.

The inactivation of both alleles of a TSG is required to start or contribute to the tumorigenic process. Even if one allele of a candidate gene has been verified to be deleted in the tumor cells, it is still necessary to confirm that the remaining allele is inactivated. If no deletion is found, both alleles of the candidate gene could be inactivated by other mechanisms, such as point mutations and small insertions or deletions involving only a few nucleotides. These small changes can be detected clearly by comparing gene sequences of the potential candidate in normal and tumor cells. DNA sequences are determined manually or by machine, using enzymatic DNA synthesis in the presence of base-specific dideoxynucleotide triphosphate (ddNTP) chain terminators (Fig. 1-31). Traditionally, the DNA fragment to be sequenced was cloned into a plasmid to prepare a template for sequencing, but currently, PCR products are being used more frequently as sequencing templates. The first step in a sequencing reaction is to heat denature the DNA template and allow it to bind a sequencing primer that contains a sequence complementary to one of the two template DNA strands, at a region adjacent to the region to be sequenced. Next, four parallel DNA synthesis reactions are carried out with DNA polymerase in the presence of all four deoxynucleotides (dNTPs) and one of the four ddNTP chain terminators. ddNTPs are analogues of normal dNTPs that lack a hydroxyl group at the 3′ carbon position. With the same triphosphate group as normal dNTPs at the 5′ carbon position, these ddNTPs can incorporate into the growing DNA chain. However, without a hydrox-

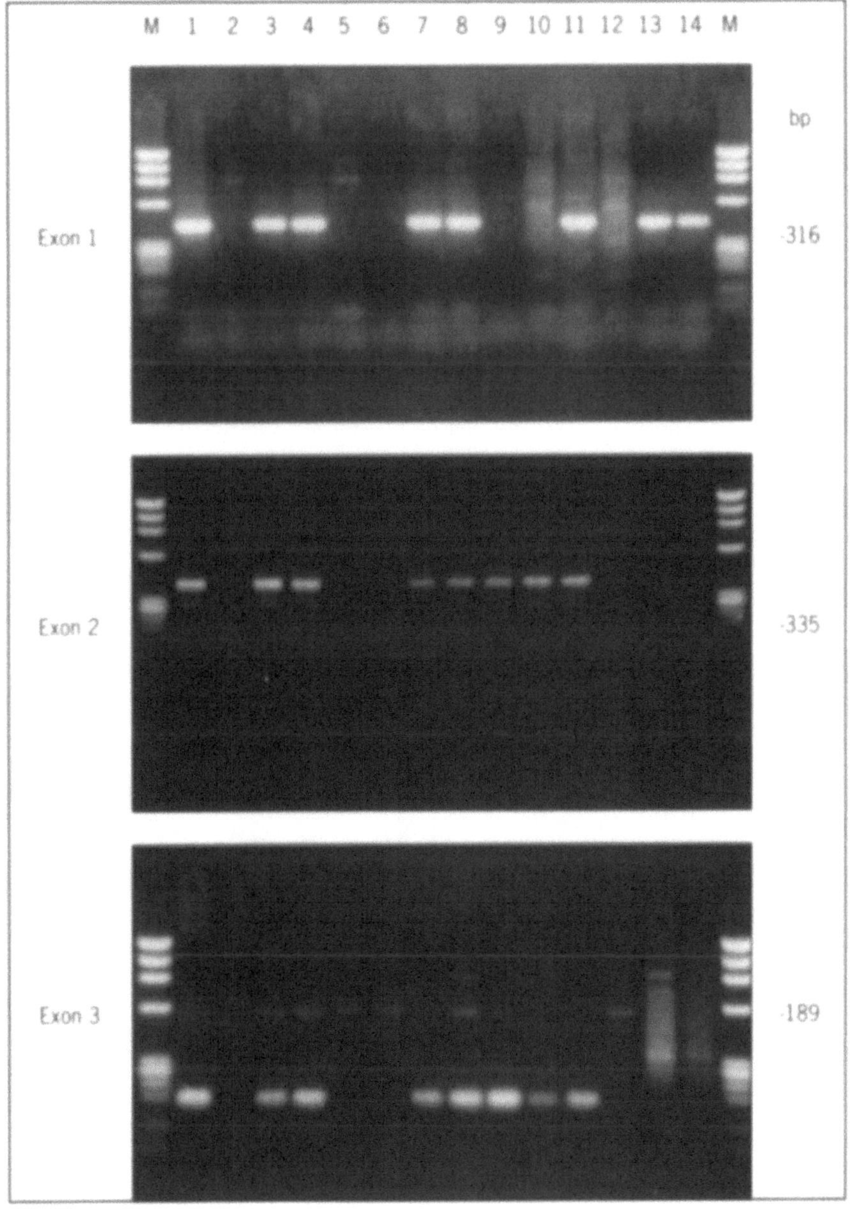

Figure 1-30. Homozygous deletions of *P16* in malignant mesothelioma cell lines detected by polymerase chain reaction (PCR). Ethidium bromide–stained gels of PCR products amplified using primer pairs for each of the three *P16* exons; identical cell lines are shown in each gel. Marker (M) DNA is run in the outer lanes to estimate the size of the PCR products. Deletions of only exon 1 occur in cases 9 and 10, whereas deletions are confined to exons 2 and 3 in cases 13 and 14.

yl group at the 3′ carbon position, the incorporated ddNTP prevents any new nucleotide from being added to its 3′ end and thus terminates the DNA synthesis reaction. In each of the four DNA synthesis reactions, chain termination occurs at a different base, dictated by the ddNTP added. By setting the concentration of the ddNTP much lower than that of its normal dNTP analogue in the reaction, the ddNTP is incorporated only occasionally into a growing strand, so that eventually a collection of newly synthesized DNA is obtained that is comprised of strands of different sizes, each of which results from termination at one of the many positions into which the specific ddNTP can possibly incorporate. This collection can be analyzed by denaturing polyacrylamide gel electropheresis, which is capable of separating single-

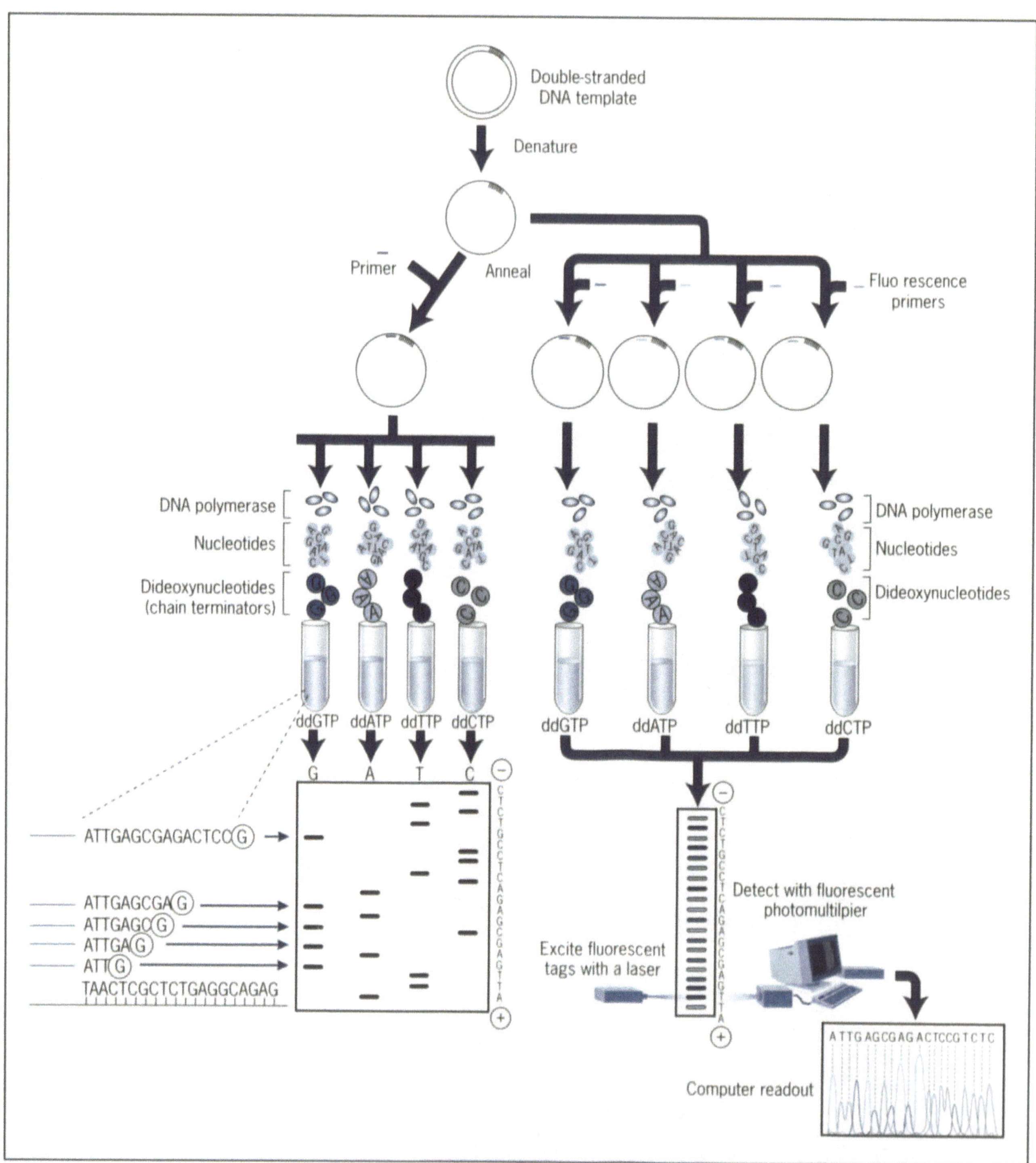

Figure 1-31. DNA sequencing by enzymatic DNA synthesis in the presence of base-specific dideoxynucleotide chain terminators. This process can be carried out manually (*left*) or by machines (*right panel*).

stranded DNA fragments that differ in size by even a single nucleotide. In the manual sequencing procedure, these newly synthesized fragments usually are detected by including radiolabeled nucleotides in the DNA synthesis reaction or by using a sequencing primer that previously has been labeled with a radioactive isotope. The reaction products are loaded into separate lanes, and the sequence can be obtained by reading from the bottom of the gel toward the top. In the automated sequencing procedure, four different fluorescent dyes are used to label the primers or the ddNTPs added to each of the four DNA synthesis reactions, and the products from all four reactions are pooled and loaded into a single lane. During electrophoresis, a laser beam focused at a fixed position of the gel excites the dye in the DNA fragments as they migrate through this position. Products from individual reactions can be distinguished by the specific wavelength of fluorescence emitted by the four different dyes. The fluorescent signals are detected with a photomultiplier and translated by computer into a nucleotide sequence that is then stored in a database.

When screening for mutations in tumor cells, only cDNA and exon-coding regions of the candidate gene are typically sequenced, because sequence variations in the noncoding intervening regions are common and usually do not affect gene function. Figure 1-32 demonstrates several types of mutations that can be detected by sequencing exon regions and exon-intron boundaries of genomic DNA (Fig. 1-32*A, B*), or cDNA (Fig. 1-32*C*). Figure 1-32*A* shows a portion of a sequencing gel identifying an A→G transition in tumor cell line M159. This point mutation is located at the second nucleotide of the intron that is adjacent to the splice donor site of the second exon of *p16*. Because this position is highly conserved among splice donor sites, this mutation is expected to result in abnormal splice products. Figure 1-32*B* shows sections of density tracings of automated sequencing gels. When compared with the sequence of the *NF2* gene from normal cells, an intragenic 1-bp deletion was detected in DNA from tumor cell line 6-53. This deletion is predicted to cause a frameshift in protein translation leading to a truncated protein. In Figure 1-32*C*, an exon-skipping alteration was identified in tumor cell line 222 when comparing the cDNA sequences of the *NF2* gene in normal and tumor cells. In this case, exon 10 is absent from the transcript of the tumor cells; translation of an aberrant protein is predicted lacking amino acids 296 to333.

Although routinely performed in molecular biology laboratories, the manual sequencing procedure is a very labor-intensive and time-consuming process. Thus, techniques have been developed to rapidly screen a sizable panel of samples for any deviation from the normal sequence; only the variants detected are further characterized by DNA sequencing. One method frequently used to screen tumor specimens for mutations in candidate TSGs is the single-strand conformation polymorphism (SSCP) technique. Single-stranded DNA has a tendency to fold up and form a complex structure that is stabilized by weak intramolecular interactions, such as base-pairing hydrogen bonds. When a single-stranded DNA fragment is subjected to electrophoresis in a nondenaturing gel, the mobility of this DNA fragment depends not only on its length, but also on the conformation determined by its sequence. To perform SSCP, specific PCR primers are used to amplify segments of the coding sequence of the candidate gene from genomic DNA samples if the sequences of the exon–intron boundaries are known, or from cDNA generated from mRNA by reverse transcription. The amplified products are denatured into single strands and separated on a polyacrylamide gel under nondenaturing conditions. One of the PCR primers is usually radiolabeled so that the amplified fragments can be visualized using autoradiography (Fig. 1-33). A control sample is usually included in the same gel so that any variation from the wild-type pattern can be identified. The aberrant bands can be excised from the gel and the variant SSCP conformers can be eluted, re-amplified, and sequenced to identify the mutations.

If an antibody capable of specifically recognizing the protein product of a candidate gene is available, Western blot analysis can be used to rapidly screen a large panel of specimens for mutations, such as frameshift, splice site, and nonsense mutations that result in protein truncation. Figure 1-34 demonstrates such a screening using a monoclonal antibody specific for the APC protein. Germline mutations in the *APC* gene account for most, if not all, cases of familial adenomatous polyposis. Somatic *APC* mutations also are found in many sporadic colorectal tumors. In the examples shown in Figure 1-34, only truncated proteins are present in the colorectal cancer cell lines, indicating that no wild-type *APC* allele is retained in these cells. Conversely, only full-length proteins are observed in the prostatic and pancreatic carcinoma cell lines, suggesting that no *APC* mutation occurred in these tumors.

The protein truncation test (Fig. 1-35) is frequently used to screen large transcripts for protein-truncating mutations. In this procedure, a cDNA of the candidate gene is prepared from RNA isolated from tumor cells. The coding region of the cDNA is then PCR-amplified with a forward primer that contains a T7 promoter at the 5′ end of the gene-specific sequence, and a reverse primer. The PCR products then are used to produce polypeptides in a coupled transcription-translation system. ^{35}S-methionine is usually included in the reaction so that the in vitro synthesized polypeptides can be visualized after being separated on an SDS polyacrylamide gel. A protein with a mobility faster than that of the wild-type protein would indicate a stop codon in the amplified coding sequence. If there is no full-length protein produced from the tumor specimen, it would suggest that no functional product of the gene under investigation is present in the tumor cells, possibly due to inactivation of both alleles of the gene.

In addition to deletions and mutations, some TSGs can be inactivated in tumors by methylation of the CpG islands located at the 5′ regulatory region of the genes. This methylation leads to transcriptional repression and thus, deprives the cell of the gene product. Figure 1-36 illustrates a method commonly used to detect CpG island methylation, and the correlation between such methylation and the expression of the TSG *p16*. Methylation-sensitive rare base-cutting restriction enzymes such as *Sma*I (used in this study) are frequently used for detecting methylation in CpG islands. The 5′ CpG island of the *p16* gene is located within a 4.3-kb *Eco*RI restriction fragment containing three *Sma*I sites. If the CpG island is unmethylated, the probe PE1 should recognize the 0.4- and 0.65-kb fragments on Southern blot analysis of genomic DNA samples digested with *Eco*RI and *Sma*I, as seen in several of the small cell lung cancer (SCLC) cell lines tested (Fig. 1-36*B*, lanes 3 through 7). Conversely, methylation of the CpG island would protect these sites from *Sma*I digestion, and the probe PE1 should hybridize to the 4.3-kb *Eco*RI fragment on the same Southern blot, as detected in most non–small cell lung cancer (NSCLC) cell lines (Fig. 1-36*B*, lanes 8 through 10) and one SCLC cell line (Fig. 1-36*B*, lane 11). The expression of *p16* in these cells was examined by reverse transcription of total RNA

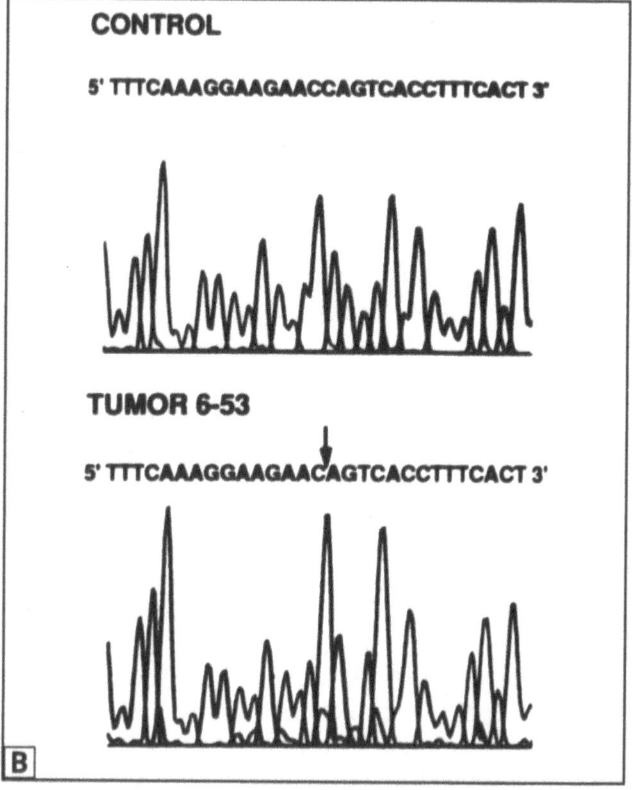

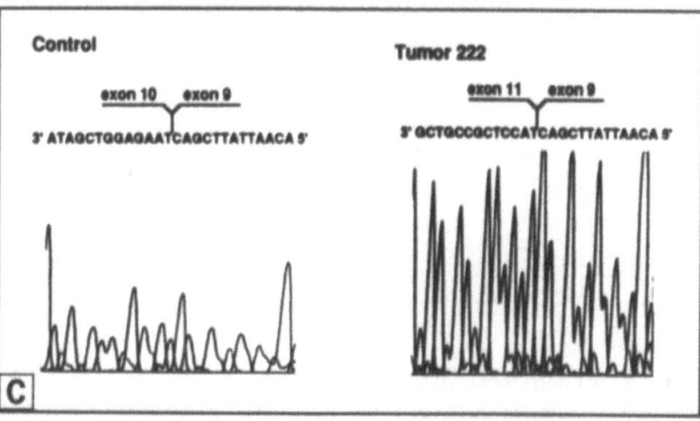

Figure 1-32. Mutations identified by sequence analysis. **A,** An A→G transition in the mesothelioma cell line M159 was identified by manual sequencing. This point mutation is located at the second nucleotide of the intron adjacent to the splice donor site of the second exon of *P16*. (*From* Cheng *et al.* [12]; with permission.) **B,** An intragenic 1-bp deletion was detected in exon 3 of the *NF2* gene of mesothelioma cell line 6-53 by automated sequencing. This deletion would cause frameshift, leading to a truncated protein. **C,** An exon-skipping alteration of the *NF2* transcript was identified in mesothelioma cell line 222 by automated sequencing. (*B* and *C from* Bianchi *et al.* [13]; with permission.)

extracted from the cell lines, followed by PCR amplification of the 428-bp cDNA stretch corresponding to the first and second exons of *p16* (Fig. 1-36C). A 321-bp fragment of the *TP53* gene was amplified simultaneously to serve as an internal control for RNA integrity. A clear pattern is observed when comparing 5′ CpG methylation and the expression of *p16*; none of the methylated cell lines expressed *p16*, whereas all of the unmethylated cell lines did, suggesting that CpG island methylation is an alternative way to inactivate *p16*.

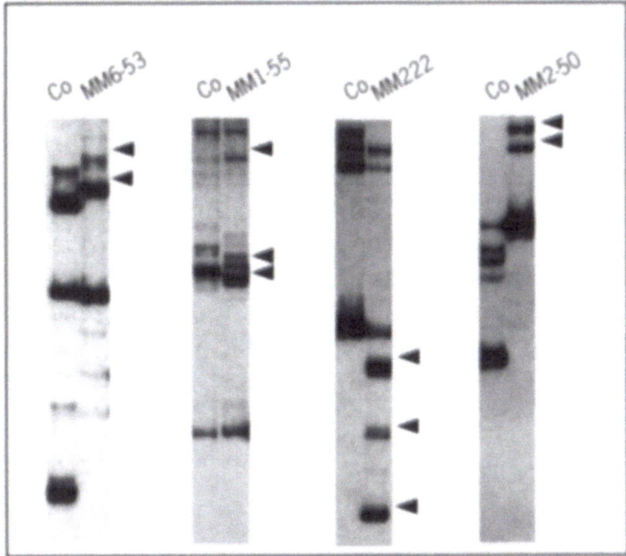

Figure 1-33. Single-strand confirmation polymorphism (SSCP) analysis of various regions of the *NF2* gene in malignant mesotheliomas. Specific primer pairs were used to amplify various portions of the *NF2* complementary DNA reverse transcribed from RNA isolated from normal mesothelial control cells (Co) and mesothelioma cell lines as indicated. Polymerase chain reaction products were separated on a nondenaturing polyacrylamide gel. *Arrowheads* indicate the variant SSCP conformers. (*From* Bianchi *et al.* [13]; with permission).

DIFFERENTIAL CLONING

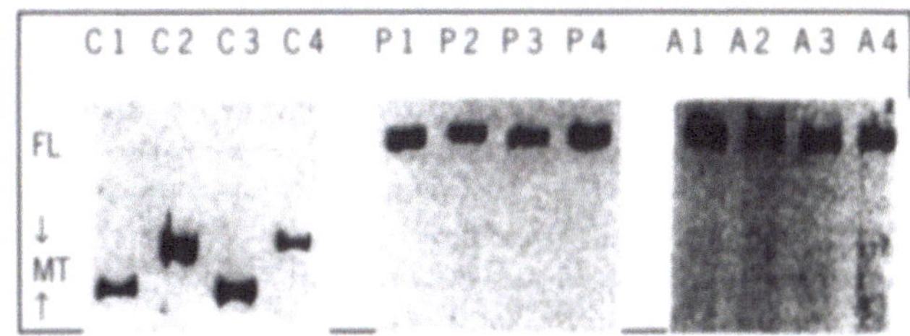

Figure 1-34. Protein truncation identified by Western blot analysis. A monoclonal antibody specific to the APC protein was used to analyze total protein lysates isolated from colon cancer (C1), colon adenoma (C2–C4), prostate cancer (P1–P4), and pancreatic cancer (A1–A4) cell lines. Truncated proteins were identified in the colon cancer and colon adenoma cell lines. FL—full-length protein; MT—mutant truncated protein. (*From* Smith *et al.* [14]; with permission.)

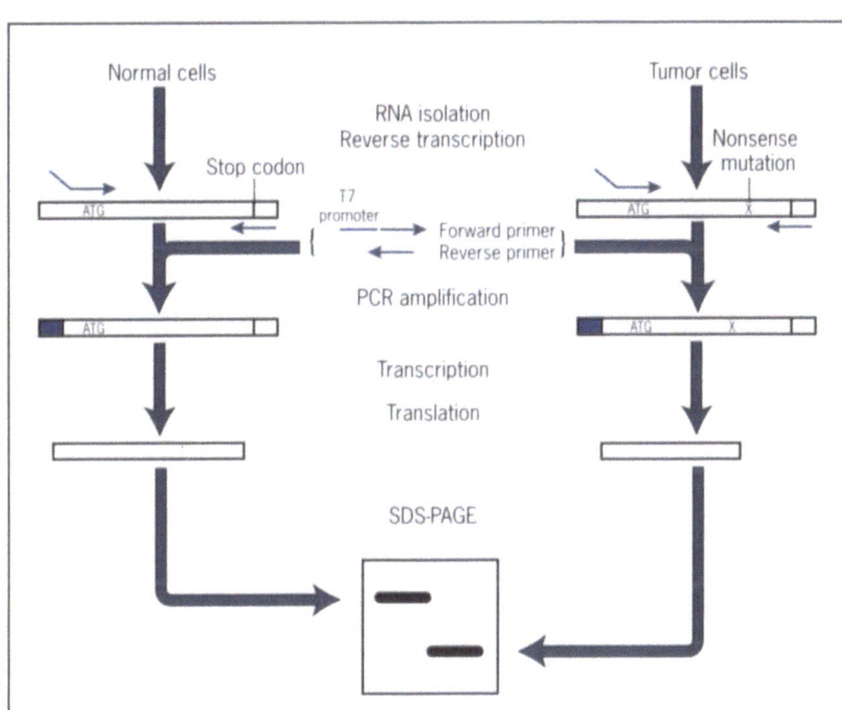

Figure 1-35. Protein truncation test. The coding sequence of the complementary DNA prepared from extracted RNA is amplified by polymerase chain reaction (PCR) using a specific set of primers to attach a T7 promoter at its 5′ end. A coupled transcription-translation system is then used to produce polypeptide from the amplified products. In the scenario depicted, a nonsense mutation within the coding region in the tumor cells leads to a truncated protein that can be detected as a faster mobility band in the sodium dodecyl sulfate–polyacrylamide gel electrophoresis (SDS-PAGE).

of subtractive hybridization is illustrated in Figure 1-37. DNA fragments prepared from two sources (tester and driver) are mixed, denatured, and then allowed to re-anneal. By having a large excess of the driver DNA, the single-stranded tester DNA is much more likely to find and hybridize to a complementary strand from the driver DNA and form a heteroduplex. However, certain tester fragments (the target sequences, such as fragment C in this case) cannot find their complementary sequences in the driver DNA sample and thus reassociate with their complimentary sequences within the tester DNA to form homoduplexes. Homoduplexes also form within the driver DNA fragments because they are in vast excess. After reassociation, homoduplexes of tester DNA are separated from the DNA population containing driver fragments to enrich the target sequences. One frequently used method for distinguishing the tester fragments from the driver fragments is to prepare the tester and driver fragments with different ends so that only tester homoduplexes contain the correct "sticky" ends that can be ligated into the complementary cloning site in a vector. Another method used is to biotinylate the driver DNA prior to mixing it with the tester so that after reassociation, the driver DNA and heteroduplexes can be removed by biotin-avidin chromatography.

This basic subtraction scheme has many applications in cancer research. Both genomic DNA and cDNA have been used in these types of experiments to identify cancer-related genes. For example, homozygously deleted regions of the tumor genome can be cloned by using normal genomic DNA as the tester and tumor DNA as the driver. Oncogenes that are overexpressed in tumor cells also can be detected by using cDNA prepared from the tumor cells as the tester and that from normal cells as the driver.

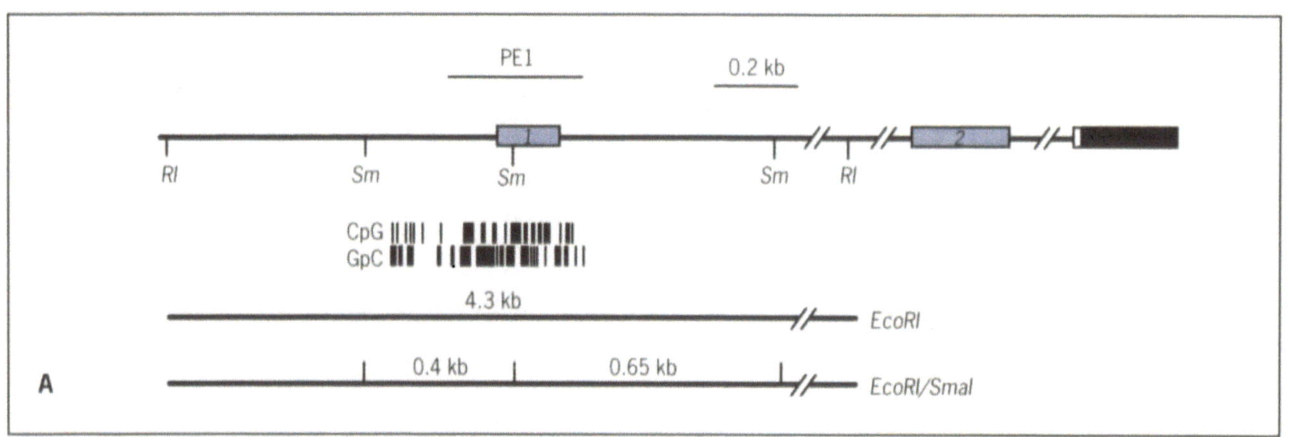

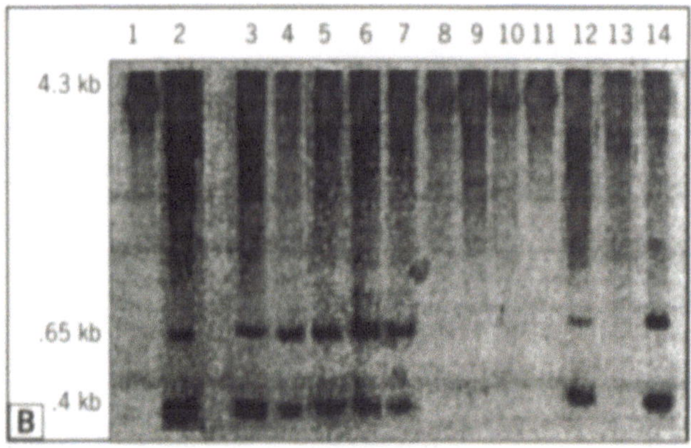

C 428 bp 321 bp

Figure 1-36. Expression of *p16* and methylation of the 5′ CpG island. **A,** Restriction map and CG dinucleotide density of *p16*. *Open boxes* indicate the three coding exons, and the *shaded area* represents a 3′untranslated region. RI indicates an *Eco*RI site; Sm indicates an *Sma*I site. The densities of CG and GC dinucleotides are represented by vertical bars. PE1 indicates the location of the probe used for the Southern blot shown in *panel B*. Also shown are the expected fragment sizes recognized by the PE1 probe when genomic DNA in the normally unmethylated state is digested with the indicated restriction enzymes. **B,** Methylation of the 5′ CpG island of *p16* examined by Southern blot analysis with the PE1 probe. The 4.3-kb fragment generated with *Eco*RI digestion is shown in lane 1. Digestion of DNA isolated from normal tissue with *Sma*I alone yields 0.65- and 0.4-kb fragments, indicating that all sites are unmethylated (lane 2). Genomic DNA from small cell lung cancer cell lines (lanes 3–7 and 11) and non–small cell lung cancer cell lines (lanes 8–10, 12, and 14) were digested with *Eco*RI and *Sma*I. Methylation is indicated clearly in cell lines of lanes 8 through 11 by the absence of the 0.65 and 0.4-kb fragments. Lane 13 demonstrates a homozygous deletion of *P16*. **C,** The expression of *p16* in the same cell lines as in *panel B* was examined by reverse transcription of total RNA and polymerase chain reaction amplification of a 428-bp complementary DNA stretch corresponding to the first and second exons of *p16*. The 321-bp fragment was amplified simultaneously from the *TP53* gene to serve as an internal control for RNA integrity. Note that all the methylated cell lines and the homozygously deleted cell line lack the 428-bp p16 product, whereas all the unmethylated cell lines express p16. (*From* Merlo *et al.* [15]; with permission.)

Representational Difference Analysis

The total enrichment of the target sequences by subtractive hybridization, even with repeated subtractive steps, is only about 100-fold within the human genome because its high complexity prevents effective and complete hybridization. An enrichment of 10^5-fold or greater is necessary to identify the small differences frequently encountered in human cancers. The method of representational difference analysis (RDA; Fig. 1-38) was developed to greatly improve the efficiency of subtractive hybridization by adding two additional elements: representation and kinetic enrichment.

Representation refers to the fact that only a representative portion of the genome is used as the tester and driver for subtractive hybridization. This is achieved by digestion of genomic DNA with a relatively infrequent cutting restriction endonuclease, ligation of oligonucleotide adaptors to the restriction fragments, and PCR amplification to produce "amplicons." Because only DNA fragments smaller than 1 kb can be PCR amplified effectively under standard PCR conditions, most of the restriction fragments are too long to be amplified. Hence, the tester and driver DNA samples have reduced sequence complexity, which allows greater completeness of hybridization, leading to more efficient subtractive enrichment. Although only a subset of the genome is represented in each hybridization experiment, the whole genome can be scanned using sets of amplicons prepared with different restriction endonucleases.

In representational difference analysis, the subtractive hybridization and kinetic enrichment are combined into a single hybridization–amplification step. The adaptors are first removed from the tester and driver amplicons by restriction cleavage. The tester fragments are ligated to new oligonucleotide adaptors at their 5′ ends and then are mixed with a large excess of the driver amplicons. After denaturation and reassociation, the mixture is treated with *Taq* DNA polymerase to fill in the cohesive ends and then PCR amplified with the same oligonucleotides ligated to the tester as to the primers. Homoduplexes of the tester have oligonucleotides at the 5′ ends of each strand, so both 3′ ends can be filled in to provide the primer binding sites for exponential amplification. The tester–driver heteroduplexes have primer sequence on one end only and thus are amplified at a linear rate. Homoduplexes of the driver, having no primer sequence, are not amplified. Therefore, without physically separating the homoduplexes from the mixture as in the traditional subtractive hybridization methods, the target sequences are selectively enriched after amplification. The hybridization–amplification step can be repeated after replacing the adaptors of the amplified products with another oligonucleotide and mixing with fresh driver. Two different adaptors are used in alternate rounds of hybridization and amplification so that the enrichment is not affected by the efficiency of restriction digestion. In the second round, the target sequences that have already been enriched re-anneal to form homoduplexes much faster than the

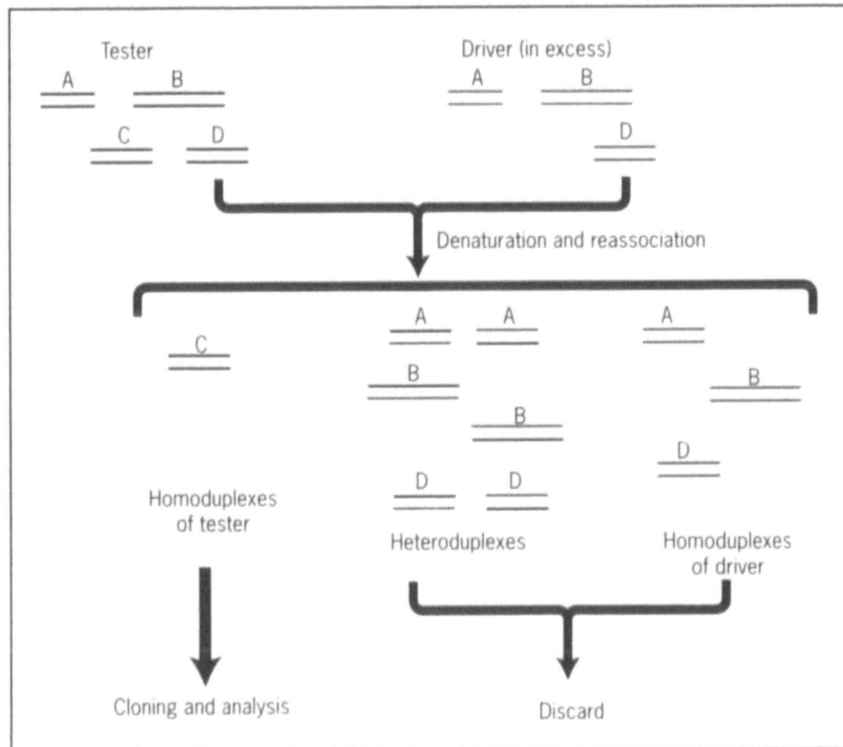

Figure 1-37. Subtractive hybridization. To identify sequences present in one DNA sample (tester) but not the other (driver), the tester and driver fragments are mixed, denatured, and then allowed to re-anneal. Three types of duplexes are formed: homoduplex of the tester, homoduplex of the driver, and heteroduplexes of tester-driver hybrids. Because of the large excess of driver DNA, a single-stranded tester fragment is much more likely to form a heteroduplex. However, some tester fragments (*eg*, fragment C) form homoduplexes because no complementary sequences are present in the driver. The homoduplexes of the tester DNA can be separated from the DNA population containing the driver fragments for additional studies.

nontarget tester fragments because they are present at a much higher concentration. This kinetic enrichment, adding to the power of selective amplification of homoduplexes, can achieve more than 10^7-fold enrichment in target sequences after three rounds.

Representational difference analysis has been applied successfully to detect DNA deletion and amplification in cancer cells. Although originally designed to clone differences between two complex genomes, RDA also can be adapted to identify genes whose expression is changed during tumorigenesis by using cDNA prepared from normal and tumor cells.

Differential Display

Differential display was devised to identify differences in gene expression in comparative studies. In this technique, cellular mRNAs are divided into subsets so that manageable numbers of transcripts can be displayed on a single gel for side-by-side comparison, *eg*, between normal and tumor cells of the same cell type (Fig. 1-39). One of a set of oligo-dT primers is used to prime total RNA isolated from cells for cDNA synthesis by reverse transcriptase. Each of these oligo-dT primers contains a stretch of thymidine nucleotides followed by a diverse combination of two bases at the 3′ end and thus is expected to preferentially anneal to a selective portion of mRNAs. For example, a primer with the T_{12}GA sequence would bind primarily to the poly(A) tails of mRNAs whose 5′ sequence ends with UC. After reverse transcription, a subset of the cDNA is amplified with the original oligo-dT primer and an arbitrary 10mer, and the amplified products are separated using a DNA sequencing gel. Radioactive nucleotides, such as ^{32}P or ^{35}S-dATP, are included in the PCR reaction mixtures so that the products can be visualized using autoradiography. Because each pair of oligo-dT primers in combination with the 10mer is able to amplify only certain mRNA species, a specific pattern of bands is produced.

Differential display is frequently used to detect genes whose expression is altered in tumor cells. RNAs isolated from corresponding normal and tumor cells (*eg*, normal lung and lung tumor cells) are amplified with the same pair of primers, and the products are displayed side by side on the same gel so that differences can be readily identified, as demonstrated in Figure 1-40. Typically, various combinations of oligo-dT 3′ primers and 5′ oligonucleotide primers are included in a single study to get sufficient coverage of mRNA repertoires. Genes that are differentially expressed can be cloned by isolating specific bands from the gel for re-amplification with the same primers.

Serial Analysis of Gene Expression

Serial analysis of gene expression (SAGE) was developed to simultaneously analyze thousands of transcripts so that the expression levels of a large number of genes in a particular tissue or cell type can be quantitated. SAGE is based on the observation that a 9-bp sequence tag, located at a defined position within a transcript, contains sufficient information to uniquely identify more than 95% of human genes. Figure 1-41 depicts how sequence tags are gathered from the transcripts for sequence analysis. A biotinylated oligo-dT primer is annealed to mRNA for cDNA synthesis. The resulting double-stranded cDNA is then restriction digested with the anchoring enzyme. Typically, restriction endonucleases with 4-bp recognition sites are used because they cleave, on average, every 256 bp and are expected to cut most cDNA molecules at least once. The most 3′ portion of the cleaved cDNA is captured with streptavidin beads, divided in half, and ligated to one of two linkers containing a recognition site for the tagging enzyme. The tagging enzyme is one of the type IIS restriction endonucleases that cleave at a defined distance up to 20 bp away from their asymmetric recognition site. The linkers

Figure 1-38. (*On next page*) Representational difference analysis. Restriction fragments from two sources (tester and driver) are ligated to adaptors so that they have a long oligonucleotide at their 5′ ends. A short oligonucleotide raises the efficiency of the ligation but does not become covalently attached. At elevated temperatures, the short oligonucleotide dissociates from the DNA fragments; thus, DNA polymerase can fill in the 3′ ends at each strand. Polymerase chain reaction (PCR) with the oligonucleotide as the primer selectively amplifies short fragments (average length, 600 bp) so that only a portion of the whole genome is represented in the subsequent hybridization-amplification step. The tester amplicons are ligated to new oligonucleotide adaptors at their 5′ ends and mixed with a large excess of the driver amplicons. After denaturation and reassociation, the mixture is treated with Taq DNA polymerase to fill in the cohesive ends and then PCR amplified with the same oligonucleotides ligated to the tester as the primers. The tester fragment containing the target sequences absent in the driver predominantly self–re-anneal to form homoduplexes. With the adaptor sequence at both ends, the tester homoduplexes are amplified at an exponential rate. Conversely, as a result of the vast excess of driver amplicons, the nontarget tester fragments tend to form heteroduplexes with driver fragments and are amplified only at a linear rate. Therefore, the target sequences are selectively enriched in the amplified products, which then can be cloned and analyzed or further enriched by repeating the hybridization-amplification step.

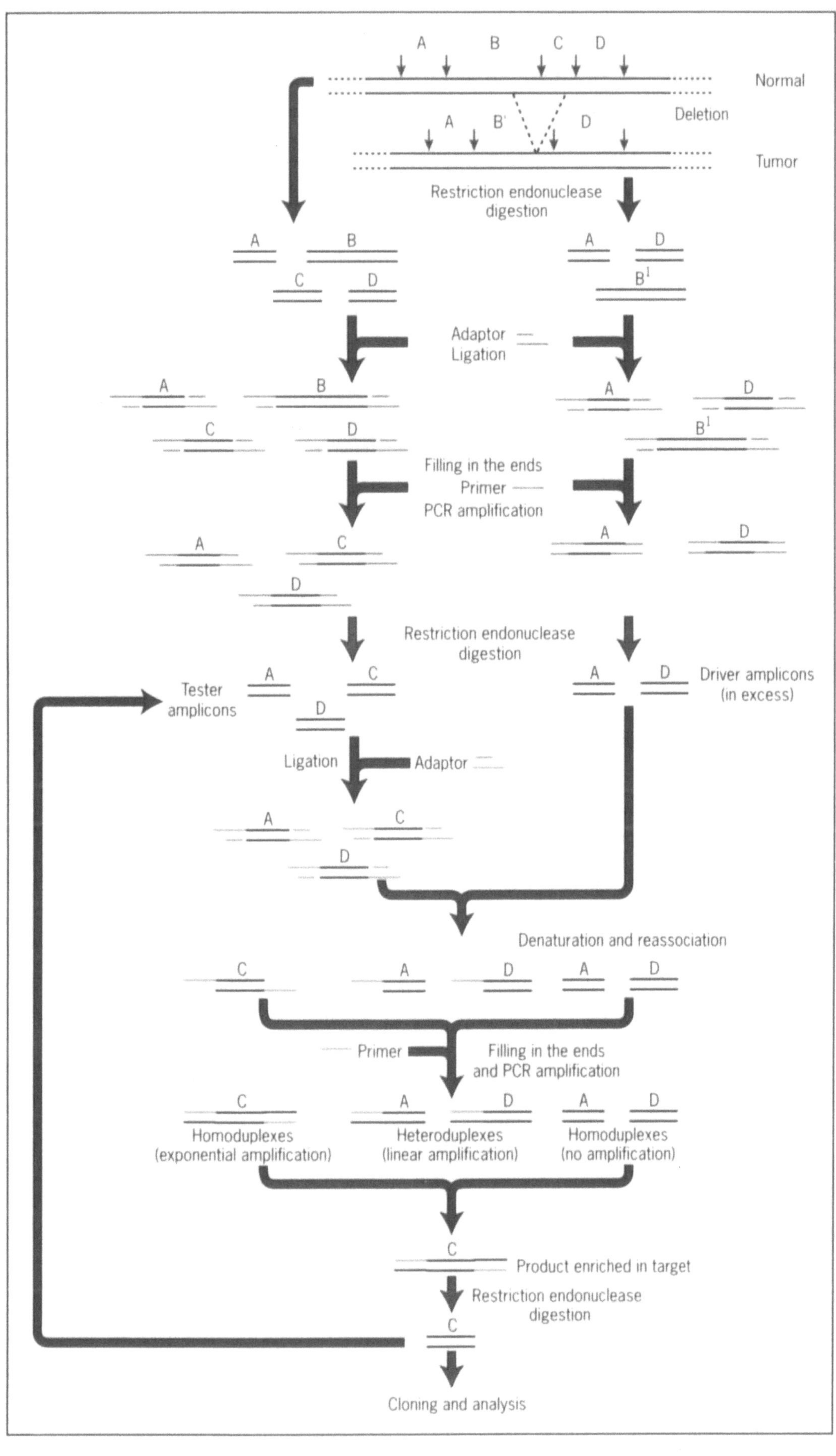
A
B
C
D
Normal
Deletion
A
B'
D
Tumor
Restriction endonuclease digestion
Adaptor
Ligation
Filling in the ends
Primer
PCR amplification
Restriction endonuclease digestion
Tester amplicons
Driver amplicons (in excess)
Ligation
Adaptor
Denaturation and reassociation
Primer
Filling in the ends and PCR amplification
Homoduplexes (exponential amplification)
Heteroduplexes (linear amplification)
Homoduplexes (no amplification)
Product enriched in target
Restriction endonuclease digestion
Cloning and analysis

are designed so that a short stretch of the cDNA containing at least 9 bp, together with the ligated linker, can be released from the beads after digestion with the tagging enzyme. After the cohesive ends created by the tagging enzyme are filled in, the two pools of released tags are ligated to each other; then PCR primers specific to each linker are used to amplify the ligated ditags. The amplified products are cleaved with the anchoring enzyme, and fragments containing the ditags are isolated, concatenated by ligation, cloned, and sequenced. In the final sequencing template, which contains multiple tags, sequences of individual tags can be readily determined because every ditag, composed of two tags linked tail to tail, is flanked by the 4-bp anchoring enzyme sites. Although the SAGE method includes an amplification step, distortions produced by PCR can be detected through the analysis of ditags. Because of the huge number of transcripts involved, the probability of any two tags, even for abundant transcripts, to be coupled into a ditag is small. Repeated ditags potentially produced by biased PCR are excluded from the analysis. Thus, the frequencies of the tags can provide quantitative measurements of the levels of gene expression.

With an automated sequencer, more than 1000 SAGE tags can be analyzed in a single 3-hour run. Therefore, it is feasible to use SAGE to simultaneously compare the expression patterns of thousands of genes in two different cell types, such as in corresponding normal and tumor cells. Variations in the abundance of the tags can lead to the identification of differentially expressed genes. The identity of a tag can be obtained by matching its 9-bp sequence with sequences of all known transcripts found in genetic databases. However, if no such match can be found, each SAGE tag, which defines a 13-bp sequence in the transcript (the 4-bp restriction sites of the anchoring enzyme plus the 9-bp tag), can be used to identify

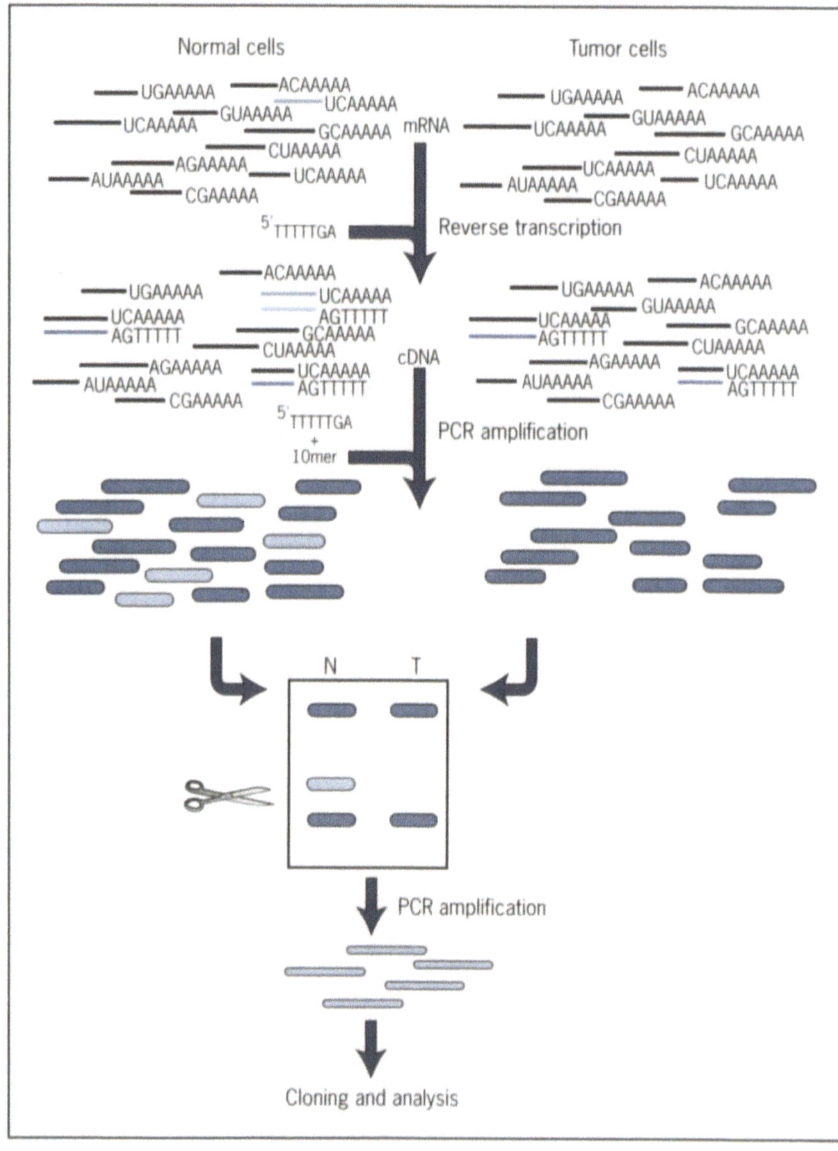

Figure 1-39. Differential display. A subset of mRNAs isolated from normal and tumor cells is selectively annealed to one of a set of oligo-dT primers. Each primer contains the same thymidine stretch, but a diverse two base combination at the 3′ end. After reverse transcription, an arbitrary 10-mer and the original oligo-dT primer are used to amplify a portion of the complementary DNA (cDNA) by polymerase chain reaction (PCR). Amplified DNA fragments are separated on a DNA sequencing gel and analyzed. Genes that are differentially expressed can be cloned by isolating specific bands from the gel for reamplification with the same primers.

novel expressed genes. Multiple cDNA clones for a tag can be isolated by screening a cDNA library with the 13-bp oligonucleotide as the hybridization probe.

NEW TECHNOLOGY

DNA Microarray Technology

Microarrays, or "DNA chips," are miniature, parallel analytic devices produced by arraying defined cDNAs or oligonucleotides on a solid support in a high-density configuration. The basic element of microarray analysis is hybridization. However, unlike Southern or Northern blot analysis, in which a single probe is hybridized to its target sequence on a blot, multiple probes located in the microarray are analyzed simultaneously by hybridizing with fluorescently labeled target nucleic acids, such as cDNA prepared from isolated mRNA or genomic DNA. Currently, the hybridization signals are detected with advanced optical systems based on CCD cameras or scanning confocal microscopes. Computers equipped with image analysis software are required to collect and interpret the vast amount of data produced by microarrays.

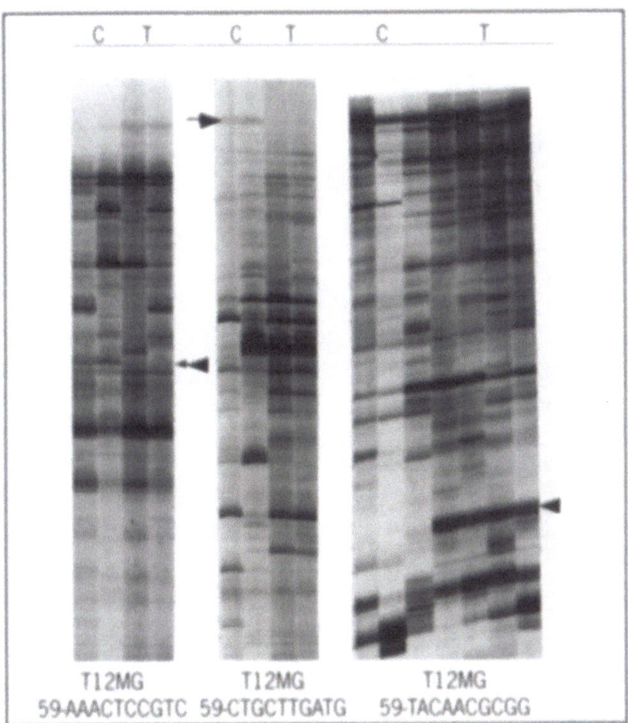

Figure 1-40. Differential display of mRNA from normal control (C) versus mesothelioma tumor (T) cell lines. Poly(A)$^+$ RNAs isolated from cell lines were reverse transcribed with an oligo-dT primer (*bottom*) to prepare complementary DNAs (c DNAs; M = AGC). The resulting complementary DNAs were polymerase chain reaction (PCR)-amplified using the same oligo-dT primer and a 10-mer (*bottom*) in the presence of α-^{35}S-dATP. The PCR products were separated on a sequencing gel. Examples of RNA species present in control cell lines and absent in mesothelioma cell lines, and vice versa, are indicated by *arrows*.

Typically, cDNA probes are generated by PCR and then printed robotically onto glass microscope slides. With the current resolution of 200–250μ center-to-center spacing between adjacent spots, more than 40,000 spots can be printed on a standard microscope slide. Oligonucleotide probes can be synthesized in situ on the solid support, or they can be attached to the solid support by postsynthetic coupling. By adapting the photolithographic methods used in the semiconductor industry, developmental instrumentation has demonstrated successful in situ synthesis of oligonucleotides at a 10 μ resolution, which allows 1 million synthesis sites per square centimeter. This extraordinary parallel analytic power of the microarray analysis revolutionizes not only the methodology but also the fundamental approaches in many areas of biologic study. Tens of thousands of gels and hybridizations can be substituted by a single microarray on a glass slide. Questions that were too enormous to imagine studying manually now may be answered in a single experiment using microarray analysis.

Figure 1-42 shows an example of how an oligonucleotide array designed to match specific sequences is used to determine the identity of a target sequence. An array can be designed so that each position in the target sequence is queried by a set of four probes that are identical except at a single position. One probe in each set is complementary to a consensus sequence, and the central positions of the other three probes are replaced with one of the alternative bases. This type of allele-specific oligonucleotide scanning array is generated with a light-directed chemical synthesis process using nucleotide precursors with a photocleavable protecting group. A specific pattern can be deprotected at each synthetic cycle by shining light through a mask. Thus, a probe of any sequence can be synthesized at any discrete, specific location in the array. In addition, any set of probes composed of the four nucleotides only requires a maximum of 4N synthetic cycles, where N is the length of the longest probe in the array.

In each set of four probes, the perfect complement of the labeled target sequence will hybridize much more strongly than mismatched probes, leading to the highest signal intensity; thus, the identity at each position of the target sequence and variations from the consensus sequence can be determined. Both genomic DNA and cDNA generated from mRNA can be used to hybridize with the DNA chips, making this type of scanning array a powerful tool for screening mutations in a very long sequence as well as for detecting single nucleotide polymorphisms in large panels of samples.

cDNA microarrays have also been applied to the study of complex changes in patterns of gene expression during the development and progression of cancer. For example, tens of thousands of elements, which are usually cDNAs prepared by PCR, can be printed with an arraying robot in an area of about 1 cm^2 on a glass microscope slide. This array can then be used to study the differences in gene expression between normal and tumor cells. Fluorescent cDNAs can be prepared by reverse transcription of the total poly(A)$^+$ mRNAs isolated from normal and tumor cells in the presence of red or green fluorochrome-labeled nucleotide analogues, respectively. These two pools of labeled cDNAs are mixed in equal proportions, hybridized to a single DNA microarray, and scanned separately for each fluorochrome with the appropriate

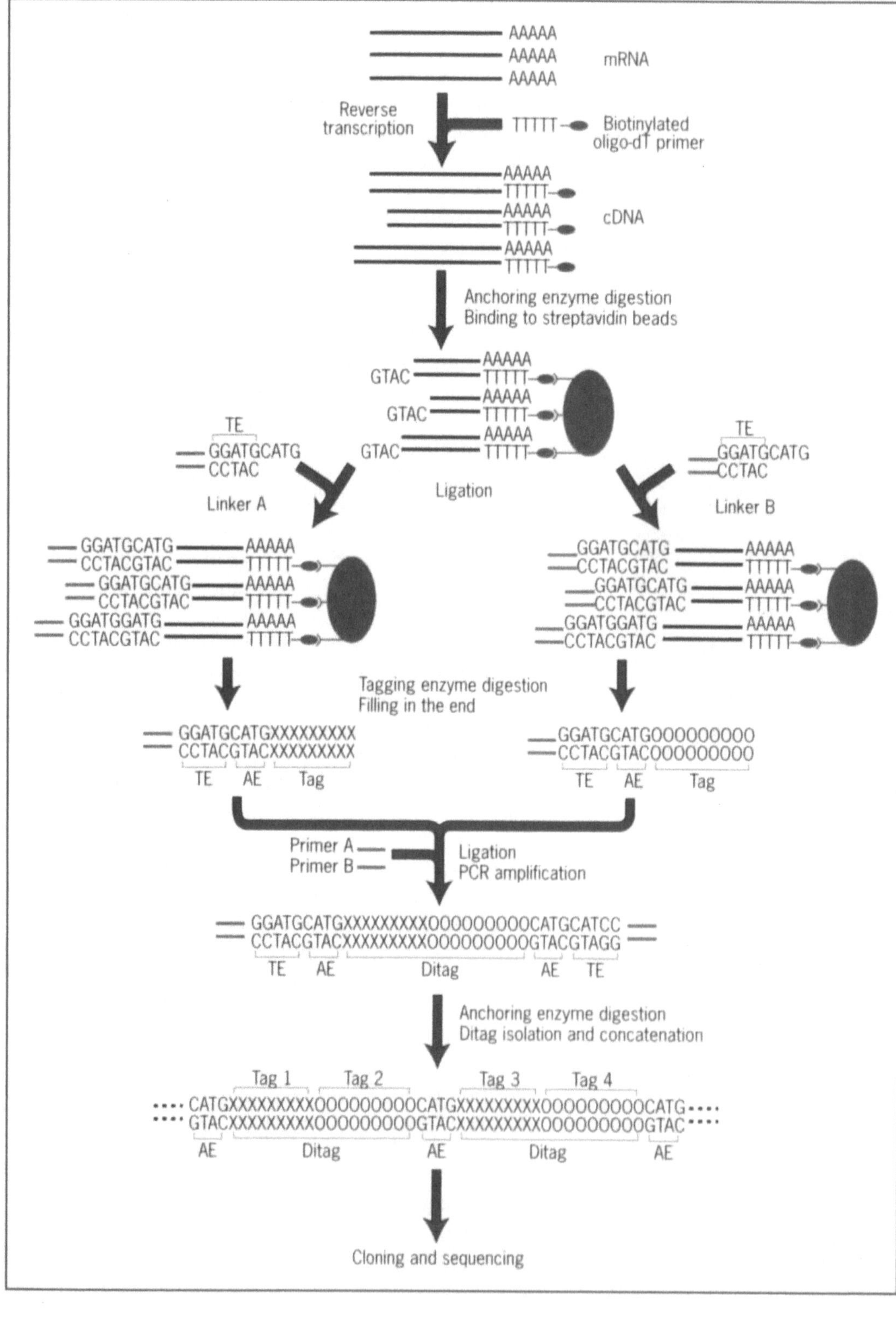

Figure 1-41. Serial analysis of gene expression. Short sequence tags are isolated from complementary DNA (cDNA) by digestion with the anchoring enzyme (*Nla*III), ligation of a linker, and digestion with the tagging enzyme (*Fok*I). Ditags, containing two tags linked tail to tail, are concatenated, cloned, and sequenced. AE and TE indicate recognition sites for anchoring and tagging enzymes, respectively. PCR—polymerase chain reaction.

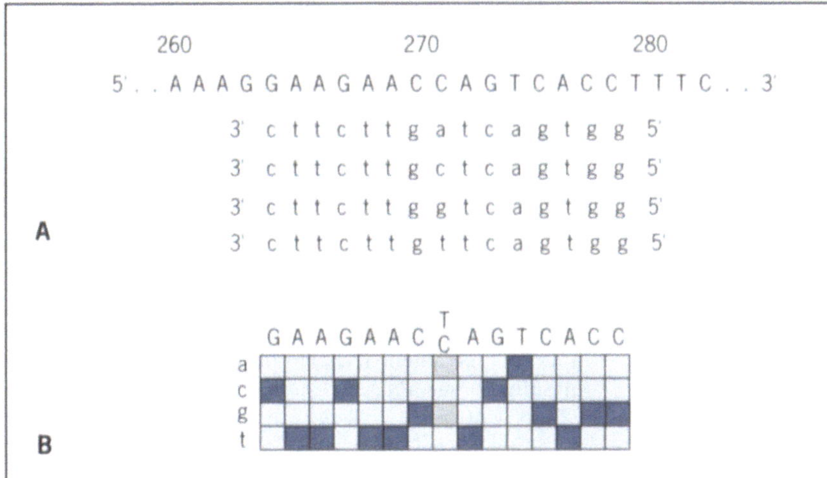

Figure 1-42. Allele-specific oligonucleotide scanning array. **A,** Each position of the *NF2* complementary DNA (*upper-case letters*) is queried by a set of four probes (*lower-case letters*) on the chips. Sequences of probes for nucleotide 271 are shown. **B,** The expected pattern of hybridization (*blue boxes*) of the array for an individual who has a wild-type *NF2* allele and one mutant allele with a C→T transition at position 271.

excitation line. The two scanned images are then combined into a ratio image, in which green spots correspond to genes preferentially expressed in the tumor cells and red spots correspond to genes preferentially expressed in the normal cells. Genes expressed at similar levels in the two cell lines appear as yellow or brown. With the current capacity of more than 40,000 spots per microscope slide and availability of partial transcript sequences from more than 60,000 different human genes in public databases, cDNA microarrays hold great promise as an effective device for the initial identification of potential candidate genes whose altered expression is associated with tumorigenesis.

Multicolor Spectral Karyotyping

Multicolor spectral karyotyping (SKY) was devised to simultaneously and unequivocally identify all human chromosomes in a metaphase spread with a single FISH experiment. Chromosome-specific painting probes are generated by PCR from flow-sorted chromosomes with fluorochrome-conjugated nucleotide analogues. Only five different fluorochromes are used to label all 24 human chromosomes. By combining differentially labeled chromosome painting probes, a specific combinatorial fluorescence can be produced for each chromosome. After a composite probe set containing all 24 chromosomes has been hybridized to metaphase chromosomes, the emission spectra are measured through a custom-designed filter set and an interferometer, and the spectral image is captured with a cooled CCD camera. All pixels of the same spectrum are assigned the same pseudocolor, such that individual chromosomes can be identified by their specific pseudocolors. A related technical innovation, multiplex fluorescence in situ hybridization (M-FISH) uses multiple epifluorescence filter sets and computer software for the detection and discrimination of the individual DNA probes hybridized simultaneously to tumor metaphase spreads.

Cytogenetic analysis is commonly used to provide critical diagnostic and prognostic information that is used in the treatment of hematologic malignancies as well as to detect recurrent chromosomal alterations for the identification of oncogenes and TSGs in both hematologic and solid tumors. However, karyotypic analysis based on conventional chromosome banding techniques is frequently hampered by low mitotic index, poor quality of metaphase spreads, and the presence of highly rearranged marker chromosomes. SKY and M-FISH can be used to detect subtle chromosomal translocations, clarify complex chromosomal rearrangements, and identify marker chromosomes. With currently available painting probes, the sensitivity of the SKY technique for metaphase chromosome analysis is between 500 and 1500 kb. Thus, this technique can be used as a screening method for identifying chromosomal aberrations in clinical samples. In addition, by combining SKY and the standard banding techniques, chromosomal alterations can be characterized with unprecedented accuracy.

Acknowledgment

The authors thank Drs. Jin Quan Cheng, Binaifer Balsara, and Zemin Liu for providing photographs.

References

1. Taguchi T, Cheng GZ, Bell DW, *et al.*: Combined chromosome microdissection and comparative genomic hybridization detect multiple sites of amplified DNA in a human lung carcinoma cell line. *Genes Chromosomes Cancer* 1997, 20:208–212.

2. Testa JR, Liu Z, Feder M, *et al.*: Advances in the analysis of chromosome alterations in human lung carcinomas. *Cancer Genet Cytogenet* 1997, 95:20–32.
3. Cheng JQ, Godwin AK, Bellacosa A, *et al.*: *AKT2*, a putative oncogene encoding a member of a subfamily of protein-serine/threonine kinases, is amplified in human ovarian carcinomas. *Proc Natl Acad Sci USA* 1992, 89:9267–9271.
4. Cheng JQ, Ruggeri B, Klein WM, *et al.*: Amplification of *AKT2* in human pancreatic cancer cells and inhibition of *AKT2* expression and tumorigenicity by antisense RNA. *Proc Natl Acad Sci USA* 1996, 93:3636–3641.
5. Cheng JQ, Altomare DA, Klein MA, *et al.*: Transforming activity and mitosis-related expression of the *AKT2* oncogene. *Oncogene* 1997, 14:2793–2801.
6. Ruggeri B, Huang L, Wood M, *et al.*: Amplification and overexpression of the *AKT2* oncogene in a subset of human pancreatic ductal adenocarcinomas. *Mol Carcinog* 1998, 21:81–86.
7. Bishop JM, Hanafusa H: Proto-oncogenes in normal and neoplastic cells. In *Molecular Oncology*. Edited by Bishop RA. New York: Scientific American; 1996.
8. Taguchi T, Jhanwar SC, Siegfried JM, *et al.*: Recurrent deletions of specific chromosomal sites in 1p, 3p, 6q, and 9p in human malignant mesothelioma. *Cancer Res* 1993, 53:4349–4355.
9. Lee W-C, Balsara B, Liu Z, *et al.*: Loss of heterozygosity analysis defines a critical region in chromosome 1p22 commonly deleted in human malignant mesothelioma. *Cancer Res* 1993, 53:4349–4355.
10. Micklos DA, Freyer GA: DNA Science: a first course in recombinant DNA technology. Cold Spring Harbor, NY: Cold Spring Harbor Laboratory Press; 1990, p 155.
11. Claudio JO, Marineau C, Rouleau G: The mouse homologue of the neurofibromatosis type 2 gene is highly conserved. *Hum Mol Genet* 1994, 3:185–190.
12. Cheng JQ, Jhanwar SC, Klein WM, *et al.*: *p16* Alterations and deletion mapping of 9p21-p22 in malignant mesothelioma. *Cancer Res* 1994, 54:5547–5551.
13. Bianchi AB, Mitsunaga SI, Cheng JQ, *et al.*: High frequency of inactivating mutations in the neurofibromatosis type 2 gene (*NF2*) in primary malignant mesotheliomas. *Proc Natl Acad Sci USA* 1995, 92:10854–10858.
14. Smith KJ, Johnson KA, Bryan TM, *et al.*: The *APC* gene product in normal and tumor cells. *Proc Natl Acad Sci USA* 1993, 90:2846–2850.
15. Merlo A, Herman JB, Mao L, *et al.*: 5′ CpG island methylation is associated with transcriptional silencing of the tumor suppressor *p16/CDKN2/MTS1* in human cancers. *Nat Med* 1995, 1:686–692.
16. DeRisi J, Penland L, Brown PO, *et al.*: Use of a cDNA microarray to analyse gene expression patterns in human cancer. *Nat Genet* 1996, 14:457–460.
17. Schrock E, du Manoir S, Veldman T, *et al.*: Multicolor spectral karyotyping of human chromosomes. *Science* 1996, 273:494–497.
18. Veldman T, Vignon C, Schrock E, *et al.*: Hidden chromosome abnormalities in haematological malignancies detected by multicolor spectral karyotyping. *Nat Genet* 1997, 15:406–410.

CHAPTER

2

Oncogenes

Matthias H. Kraus

Cancer arises from the progressive accumulation of genetic lesions that are somatically acquired or, in certain instances, present in the germline. Two major categories of genes including proto-oncogenes and suppressor genes, are affected. They can be distinguished according to positive or negative regulatory properties exerted on cell growth by their corresponding gene products. Genetic changes converting proto-oncogenes to oncogenes result in constitutive gain of function of the gene product and consequently exert a dominant effect on phenotype. Mutations resulting in loss of function of suppressor genes determine phenotype usually in a recessive manner but can sometimes gain dominant properties. Proto-oncogene activation and inactivation of suppressor gene function both contribute to the lack of growth control and unrestrained proliferation characteristic of tumor cells [1,2]. Direct corroboration of the genetic basis of cancer originated from observations emerging from studies of acute transforming retroviruses, which led to the identification of oncogenes. The normal counterparts of oncogenes comprise a limited number of evolutionarily conserved molecules (*ie*, proto-oncogenes) that are frequently activated as cellular oncogenes (c-*onc*) independent of retroviruses in spontaneous human cancer. Proto-oncogenes encode proteins residing at decisive checkpoints within a complex cellular signaling network controlling growth and proliferation. Under physiologic conditions, they integrate growth programs of a cell in response to extracellular signals and thereby exert control on the homeostasis of metazoan organisms. Subversion of their physiologic control function by activation to cellular oncogenes represents an intricate component in the pathogenesis of cancer [3].

GENETIC BASIS OF CANCER

The genome of a metazoan organism contains coding information for pleiotropic biologic phenotypes, including proliferation, differentiation, and apoptosis (Fig. 2-1). Determination of a cell to proliferate, differentiate, or undergo apoptosis is controlled by transcriptional regulation of distinct gene cassettes. Because these phenotypes are, for the most part, mutually exclusive, gene products of diverse functional properties have been identified. Proto-oncogenes promote cell growth and are counterbalanced by the activity of suppressor genes, which induce growth arrest. In addition, genetic pathways effecting differentiation or apoptosis have been discovered. Physiologic homeostasis depends on the regulated balance of activities of such gene products in response to extracellular signals. Extracellular signals provide a mechanism for integrating individual cell fate within its cellular environment. Based on the dominant nature of proto-oncogene function, their activity must be tightly controlled in normal cells. Their constitutive activation to oncogenes defined the first category of genes implicated in neoplastic growth, establishing incontrovertible evidence for the genetic basis of cancer [2].

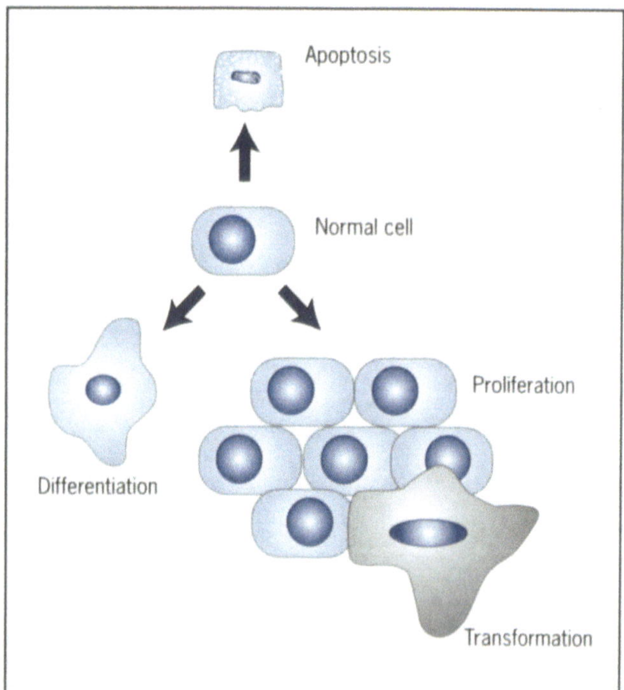

Figure 2-1. Cell fate in multicellular organisms. Destiny of normal cells, including apoptosis, differentiation, and proliferation, is physiologically regulated by discrete sets of gene products, whereas neoplastic transformation results from subversion of normal growth control.

ACUTE TRANSFORMING RETROVIRUSES

The extraordinary importance of acute transforming retroviruses is reflected in their ability to transduce from the complexity of the mammalian genome (≈10^5 genes) a limited number of cellular proto-oncogenes (<10^2 genes) that are conserved in evolution and can confer potent transforming ability upon appropriate activation. Induction of tumors in vivo and neoplastic transformation in vitro established the causative relation between acute transforming retroviruses and neoplastic growth. Following cell-free inoculation, acute transforming retroviruses produce tumors in animals and effect primary transformation of cells in culture (Fig. 2-2). Based on high penetrance and short latency of tumor development, the principle of direct genetic transmission of the neoplastic phenotype has been established by these agents. They originate from nontransforming counterparts following retroviral transduction in host cells [4].

Molecular dissection of the viral genomes of acute transforming retroviruses (Fig. 2-3) demonstrated that cellular sequences that were incorporated during retroviral transduction and substituted viral sequences necessary for replication contained the genetic information responsible for the malignant phenotype. Acquisition of new genetic information was facilitated by their recombination with the host genome. These genes, termed *viral oncogenes* (v-*onc*) are frequently expressed as fusion proteins between residual viral and acquired cellular coding sequences (gag-onc) [5]. The designation v-*onc* signifies activation of a cellular proto-oncogene by viral transduction, as distinguished from oncogenes arising by cellular mechanisms (c-*onc*) independent of retroviral involvement [6]. At the same time, it became clear that viral oncogenes had frequently undergone structural alterations conferring activation of protein function and distinguishing them from their normal cellular ancestors, designated proto-oncogenes. The heterogeneity in subcellular localization and intrinsic protein activity of many retroviral oncogenes provided early clues to the functional diversity of oncogenic proteins. Although the majority of human malignancies do not involve retroviruses as etiologic agents, they were instrumental in the identification of cellular genes capable of producing the neoplastic phenotype [7].

Oncogenes and Growth Regulation

Based on the ability of oncogenes to cause neoplastic growth, a function of their normal cellular counterparts (*ie*, proto-oncogenes) in growth regulation was anticipated. This assumption was confirmed by the discovery of normal functions of proto-oncogene products. Initial observations that the *SIS* oncogene encodes platelet-derived growth factor (PDGF) and the *ERBB* oncogene encodes a structurally activated version of the epidermal growth factor (EGF) receptor directly linked oncogene function to growth factor signaling. More recently, complex cytoplasmic signaling cascades have been delineated that relay signals from activated growth factor receptors to the nucleus. There, by virtue of specific transcription factors, expression of early response genes is induced, culminating in cell cycle entry, DNA synthesis, and mitosis (Fig. 2-4). Integration of hierarchical control systems, including receptor activation, recruitment of cytosolic signal pathways, nuclear translocation of transcription factors, gene expression regulation by DNA-binding proteins, and activation of cell cycle regulatory machinery, under physiologic conditions is executed as a highly regulated process that allows a cell to respond to extracellular signals by initiation of defined and coordinated biologic programs. Growth factor receptor–mediated signaling cascades are a frequent target for oncogenic conversion of proto-oncogenes conferring constitutive activation of protein function and withdrawal from regulatory constraints in tumors (Fig. 2-4). Consistent with the heterogeneity of human malignancies, cellular oncogenes have been identified at all levels of receptor-mediated signal pathways [2,8]. Genes for secreted proteins that represent growth factors include *SIS*, which encodes the B chain of PDGF, and *INT2*, which is a fibroblast growth factor (FGF) family member. The majority of oncogenic transmembrane proteins identified are

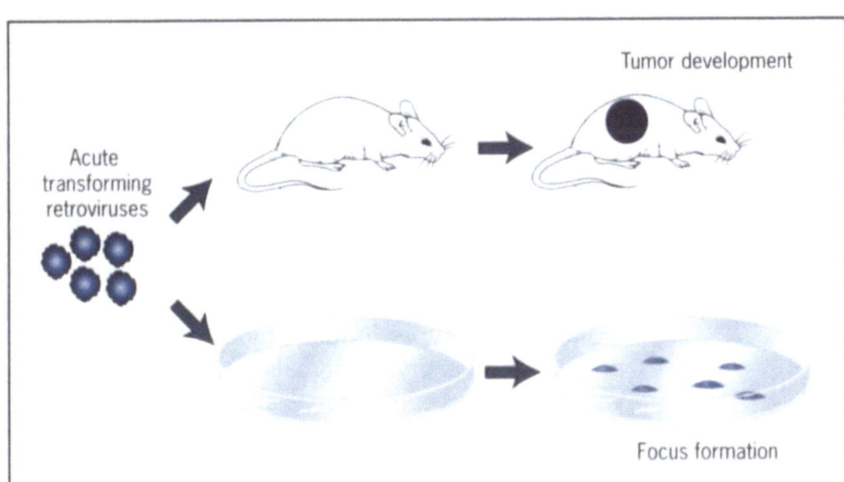

Figure 2-2. Acute transforming retroviruses. Short-latency tumor induction in animals and transformation in vitro established these type C retroviruses as genetic vehicles for neoplastic growth.

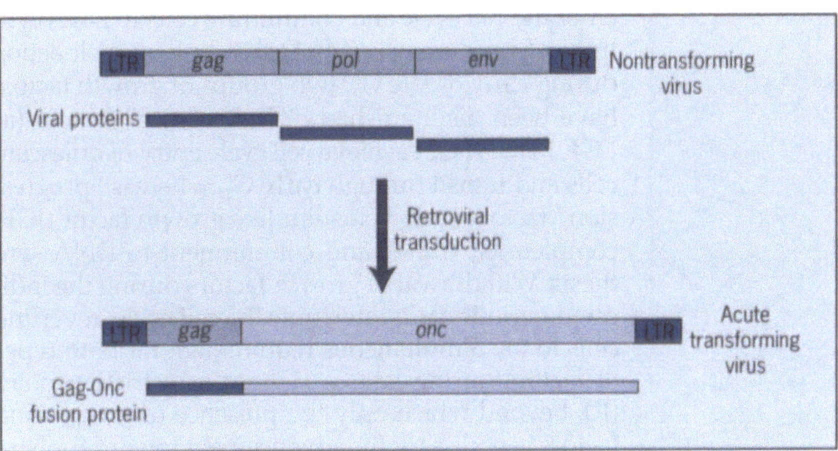

Figure 2-3. Cellular origin of oncogenes. Comparison of the molecular structure and encoded proteins of a nontransforming retrovirus (*top*) and its derivative transforming progeny (*bottom*). Retroviral long terminal repeats (LTRs) provide signals for integration, replication, and expression of the provirus. The *gag*, *pol*, and *env* viral genes are essential for viral structure and replication. The *onc* gene represents a transforming gene of cellular origin captured by the retrovirus from the host cell's genome.

receptor tyrosine kinases (RTKs). As bifunctional molecular switches, they specifically bind ligands and initiate regulated stimulation of intracellular signaling networks, resulting in mitogenicity upon ligand binding. Secondary cytoplasmic signal transducers include cytosolic tyrosine kinases (Src, Abl) or serine/threonine kinases (Raf, Mos), small GTPases (Ras) or heterotrimeric G proteins (Gsp), guanine nucleotide exchange factors (GEFs; Dbl,Vav) for small guanine nucleotide (G)-binding proteins, and adapters containing modular protein-binding domains (SH2, SH3) that recruit substrates to activated receptors (Crk). Nuclear oncogenes encode DNA-binding proteins acting as transcription factors in the regulation of gene expression [2,7].

Pleiotropic biologic responses induced by activation of growth factor RTKs are paralleled by a complex network of intracellular signal transduction pathways propagating signals from the cytoplasmic membrane to the nucleus, where transcriptional activation of distinct sets of genes ensues (Fig. 2-5). One major pathway involved in transformation transduces signals from activated growth factor receptors through the Ras protein and the mitogen-activated protein kinase (MAPK) cascade to the nucleus. Based on biochemical and genetic elucidation of this pathway, a link was established in transduction of signals from activated receptors to transcription of early response genes. Activation of RTKs by ligand results in receptor and substrate phosphorylation on tyrosine. Protein adapter molecules (*eg*, Grb2) with dual binding ability for tyrosine phosphorylated receptors and the GEF, Sos, recruit active Ras to the receptor. Activated Ras, in turn, propagates the signal through a cytoplasmic cascade of serine/threonine kinases (*ie*, MAPK cascade), a process associated with Raf recruitment to the membrane by active Ras. MAPK, on activation, translocates to the nucleus, where it phosphorylates the transcription factor ELK, inducing transcription of the early response gene *FOS*. Elucidation of this pathway has established the central role of small G-binding proteins of the Ras family in downstream signal transmission from activated receptors. The general importance of this cytoplasmic signaling pathway for cell proliferation and differentiation is underscored by findings that the majority of growth factor RTKs use this pathway for intracellular signal propagation. Moreover, multiple components of this cascade represent frequent targets for oncogenic conversion in human cancer; RTKs and Ras proteins are some of the most frequent oncogenic abnormalities in human cancer. Activation of parallel cytoplasmic G protein cascades by Ras is required for complete representation of biologic phenotypes induced by activated Ras. Other pathways diversifying signals emanating from activated RTKs are operational and subjected to oncogenic activation in cancer, as indicated by Src, Myc, PI3K, Abl, Jun, and Bcl2 [3,9].

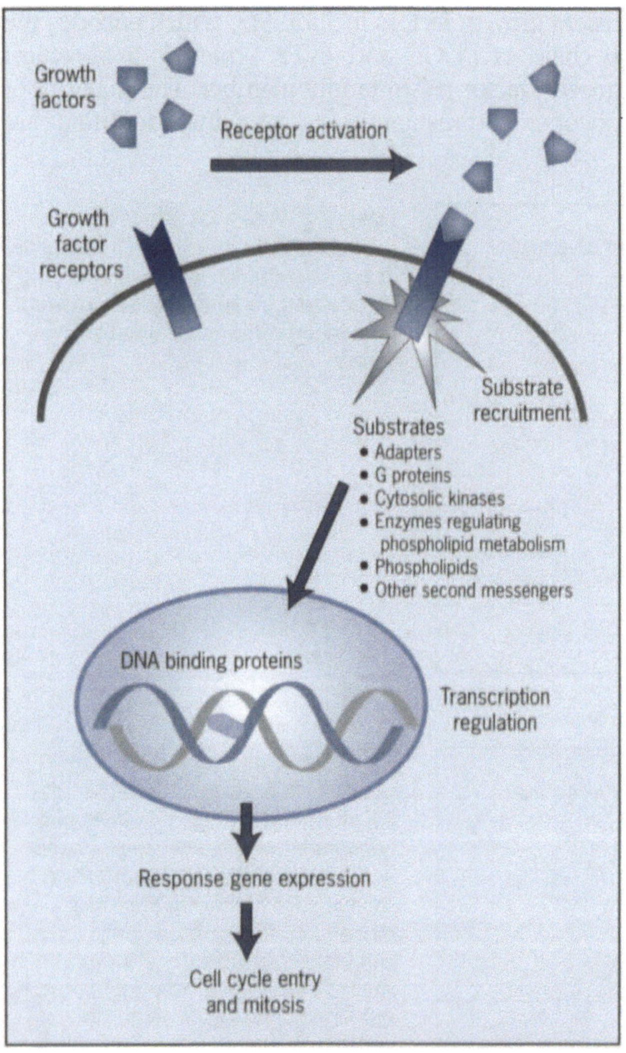

Figure 2-4. Physiologic proto-oncogene function. Oncogenes are activated versions of normal genes that encode regulatory components of mitogenic signaling pathways.

Mitogens activate growth factor receptor–mediated signaling pathways causing quiescent cells (G_0) to enter the cell cycle and committing cells to DNA synthesis (S) and mitosis (M). Depending on their action during early or late G_1, two groups of growth factors have been distinguished. "Competence" factors (*ie*, EGF, PDGF, FGF) achieve cell cycle entry of quiescent cells and transit through early G_1, whereas "progression" factors such as insulin-like growth factor (IGF) complete G_1 transit and commitment to DNA synthesis. Withdrawal of growth factors during the indicated periods of G_1 interrupts the cell cycle, reverting cells to G_0. Simultaneous requirement for both types of factors during late G_1 defines a restriction point (R), beyond which only the presence of progression factors is necessary for advancement toward S-phase

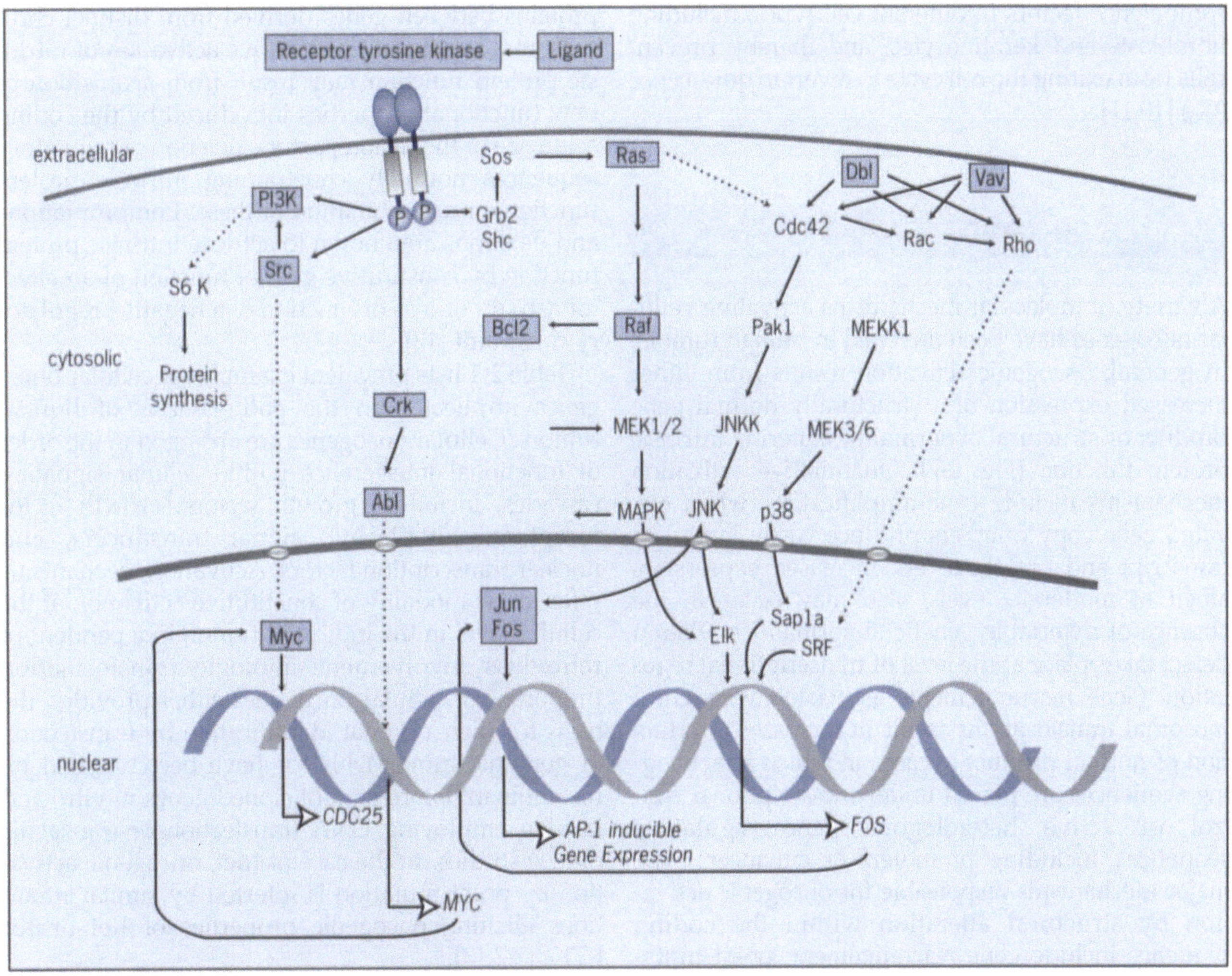

Figure 2-5. Subversion of signaling pathways by oncogenes. Selected signaling pathways pertaining to oncogenic function. Proteins that can acquire oncogenic properties are depicted in *solid boxes. Hyphenated arrows* indicate functional interactions that are indirect. P—phosphorylation; PI3K—phosphatidylinositol 3-kinase; SRF—serum response factor.

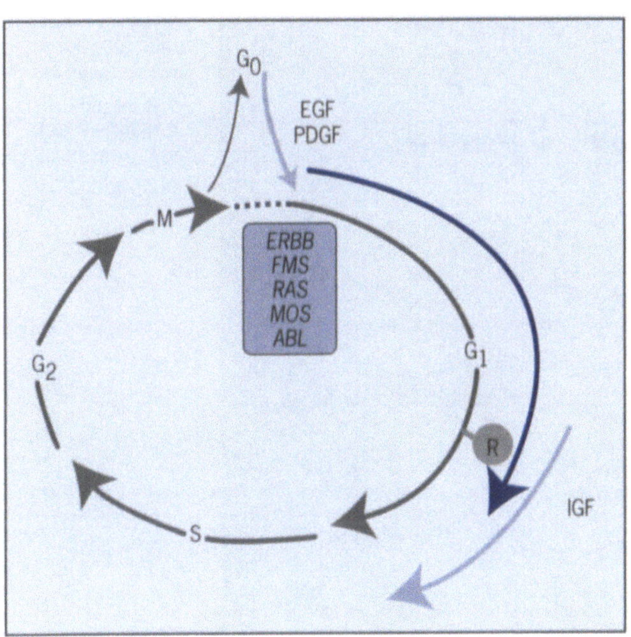

Figure 2-6. Oncogenes and mitogenesis. Activation of the cell division cycle by competence and progression factors, whose continuous presence is required for G_1 progression as indicated. R denotes the restriction point during late G_1. Oncogene activity (*dashed line*) can substitute for competence factors. EGF—epidermal growth factor; IGF—insulin-like growth factor; M—mitosis; PDGF—plate-let-derived growth factor; S—S-phase.

(Fig. 2-6). Activated oncogenes can substitute for competence factors in different cell types, including fibroblasts and keratinocytes, and thereby prevent cells from exiting the cell cycle to revert to quiescence (G_0) [10,11].

CELLULAR ONCOGENES

A variety of molecular mechanisms activating cellular oncogenes have been unveiled in human tumors. In general, oncogenic activation results from either increased expression of a structurally normal gene product or structural abnormalities altering intrinsic protein function (Fig. 2-7). Quantitative activation mechanisms include gene amplification, when elevated gene copy numbers produce vastly increased transcript and protein levels. Increased expression, albeit at moderate levels, also may occur in the absence of detectable genetic abnormalities when a defect takes place at the level of transcriptional regulation. Gene rearrangements associated with chromosomal translocations result in increased production of normal product in cases in which intact coding sequences are placed under transcriptional control of active heterologous gene regulatory sequences, including promoters or enhancers. The major mechanisms responsible for oncogenic activation by structural alteration within the coding sequence include gene rearrangement, point mutation, and deletion. Translocations produce fusion proteins between genes derived from distinct chromosomal locations. Constitutive activation of intrinsic protein function may result from acquisition of new functional properties introduced by the coding sequence of the fusion partner, deletion of regulatory sequences normally constraining intrinsic protein function, or a combination of these. Point mutations and deletions are known to activate intrinsic protein function by constitutive gain of function of an effector activity or loss of function of a negative regulatory constraint [12].

Table 2-1 lists prevalent examples of cellular oncogenes implicated in the pathogenesis of human tumors. Cellular oncogenes are arranged in the order of functional interference within cellular signaling cascades, including growth factors, growth factor receptors, cytoplasmic signal transducers, and nuclear transcription factors. Activation mechanisms refer to the modality of constitutive activation at the cellular level in the indicated tumor, independent of retrovirus involvement. Biologic transformation properties of cellular oncogenes either provided the basis for their original identification by transfection of genomic tumor DNA or have been verified by recombinant expression of cloned genes in vitro and in vivo employing DNA transfection or transgenic mouse studies. In the case of Met, oncogenic activation by point mutation is inferred by similar mutations eliciting oncogenic properties of Ret or Kit RTKs [2,7,13].

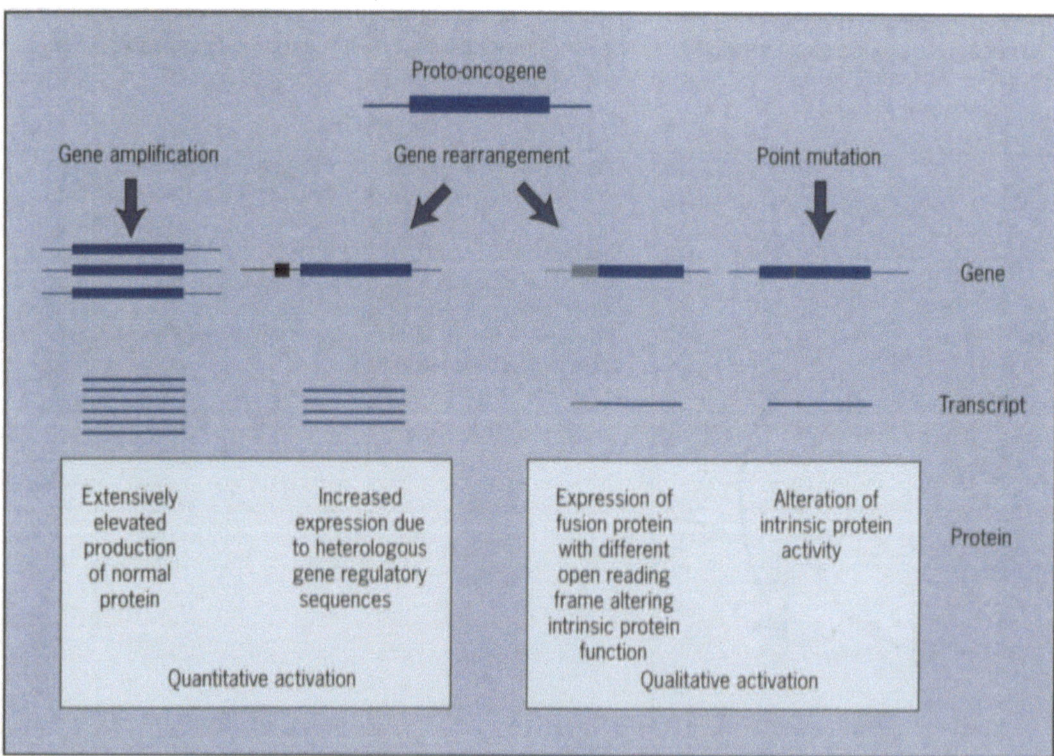

Figure 2-7. Mechanisms activating cellular oncogenes. Different molecular mechanisms lead to quantitative or qualitative activation of cellular oncogenes.

Ligands and Receptors

Ligands (*ie,* cytokines, growth factors, and hormones) are physiologic means of signal transmission between different cells; this action is made possible by their ability to specifically bind and activate cell surface receptors. Typically, a ligand and its corresponding receptor are expressed by distinct cell types (Fig. 2-8). Because ligands are frequently secreted, the source for ligand production and the target cell can be distant from each other. Endocrine action is typical for hormones such as insulin, in which hematogenic dispersion can reach ubiquitous target cells expressing the corresponding receptor within the entire organism.

Table 2-1. Cellular oncogenes in human tumors

Oncogene	Activation mechanism	Tumor	Gene product	Gene discovery	v-*onc*
SIS	Autocrine expression	Glioblastoma, meningioma	Growth factor (PDGFB)	v-*onc*	v-*sis*
ERBB	Gene amplification, gene rearrangement	Squamous cell carcinoma (cervix, lung), glioblastoma, adenocarcinoma (mammary gland, pancreas)	Receptor tyrosine kinase, epidermal growth factor receptor (EGFR, HER)	v-*onc*	v-*erb*B
ERBB2 (*NEU*)	Gene amplification	Adenocarcinoma (mammary gland, stomach, ovary, colon, pancreas, lung, kidney, salivary gland)	Receptor tyrosine kinase (ErbB2, Neu, HER2)	DNA transfection and gene amplification of c-*onc*	—
TRK	Gene rearrangement	Colon carcinoma, thyroid carcinoma	Receptor tyrosine kinase, nerve growth factor receptor	DNA transfection of c-*onc*	—
RET	Gene rearrangement	Thyroid carcinoma, multiple endocrine neoplasia types 2A and 2B	Receptor tyrosine kinase, GDNF receptor	DNA transfection of c-*onc*	—
MET	Gene rearrangement, point mutation	Gastric and renal carcinoma	Receptor tyrosine kinase, HGF receptor	DNA transfection of c-onc	—
H-*RAS*	Point mutation	Carcinoma (bladder, kidney, lung, colon, mammary gland)	G-binding protein	v-*onc*	H-*ras*
K-*RAS*	Point mutation	Carcinoma (lung, colon, ovary)	G-binding protein	v-*onc*	K-*ras*
N-*RAS*	Point mutation	Leukemia and lymphoma, neuroblastoma, lung carcinoma, melanoma, sarcoma	G-binding protein	DNA transfection of c-*onc*	—
ABL	Gene rearrangement	Chronic myelogenous leukemia	Cytosolic tyrosine kinase	v-*onc*	v-*abl*
MYC	Gene amplification, gene rearrangement	Lymphoma, carcinoma (lung, mammary gland, cervix)	Nuclear transcription factor	v-*onc*	v-*myc*
N-*MYC*	Gene amplification	Neuroblastoma, retinoblastoma	Nuclear transcription factor	Gene amplification	—
L-*MYC*	Gene amplification	Small cell lung carcinoma	Nuclear transcription factor	Gene amplification	—

Paracrine action of growth factors is spatially restricted, resulting in stimulation of receptors on cells residing in close proximity to the expressor, such as that occurring during wound healing. Even tighter control is gained by growth factors that are membrane-anchored, triggering receptors on adjacent cells—a condition encountered during development. The potent mitogenic capacity of growth factors necessitates tight regulation of their expression in physiologic conditions. Uncontrolled and sustained expression might entail oncogenic activation of a growth factor pending activity of its corresponding receptor. One example is autocrine signaling (Fig. 2-8), which occurs when the same cell produces growth factor and its corresponding receptor. Autocrine loops are the basis for the transforming action of Sis, an oncogenic growth factor implicated in human neoplasia. Int2 represents a member of the FGF family whose ectopic expression induced by retroviral promoter insertion leads to mammary tumors in animals. Other examples of autocrine loops in human cancer include EGFR activation by coexpressed transforming growth factor α (TGF-α) in epithelial malignancies. Whether an autocrine loop will result in transformation or other disease conditions depends on the signaling properties of the corresponding cell surface receptor that effects growth factor–mediated signals within the cell [10,14].

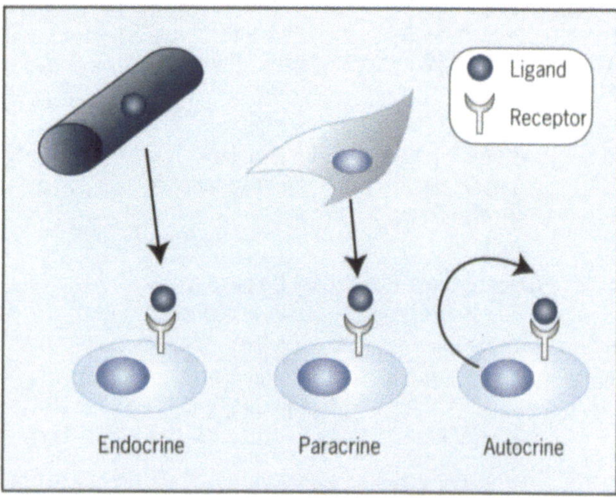

Figure 2-8. Cytokines as oncogenes. Examples of ligand–growth factor receptor interactions in multicellular organisms.

Receptor tyrosine kinases reside as inactive monomers on the cell surface. Binding of specific ligands (*ie,* growth factors and hormones) to the extracellular domain of the receptor induces receptor oligomerization, which encompasses conformational changes in the receptor structure activating its intrinsic tyrosine kinase located within the intracellular domain of the receptor (Fig. 2-9). Constituent polypeptide chains of the receptor oligomer become mutually transphosphorylated on tyrosine, creating specific binding sites for substrates with Src homology 2 (SH2) and phosphotyrosine-binding (PTB) domains. Substrates recruited to the receptor are then phosphorylated on tyrosine, routing signals from active receptors through cytoplasmic signaling cascades to the nucleus. Accumulating evidence suggests that biochemical and biologic properties of activated receptors, including receptor phosphorylation, substrate recruitment, and mitogenic activity, require receptor oligomerization, a process inducible by specific ligands. These processes trigger physiologic growth of a cell in response to signals from its environment. The growth response is transient and controlled. Oncogenic conversion of tyrosine kinase receptors is invariantly associated with constitutive receptor activity by various mechanisms. In theory, any tyrosine kinase receptor promoting growth could become subverted as an oncogene. Based on complex regulation of receptor activity, it appears that the like-

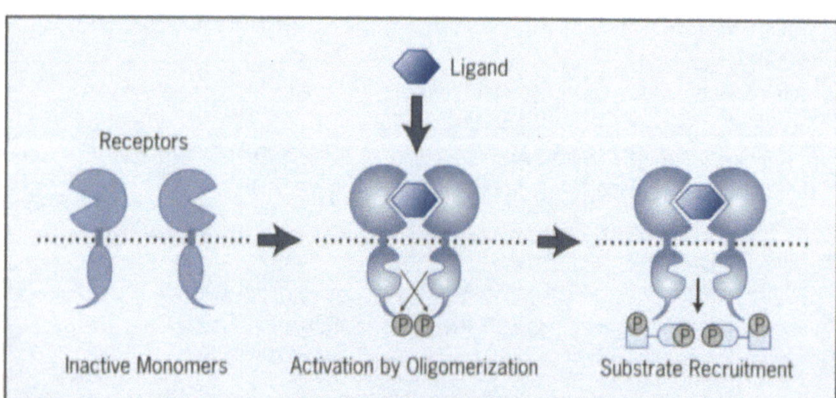

Figure 2-9. Allosteric receptor activation by oligomerization. Ligand binding induces receptor oligomerization, resulting in activation of receptor tyrosine kinase (RTK) catalytic activity, RTK phosphorylation (P), and substrate recruitment and phosphorylation. Active RTK kinase domains are represented as bilobar structures in this schematic. Substrates (*green*) are recruited to specific phosphotyrosine-containing regions of the receptor by Src homology 2 (SH2) or phosphotyrosine-binding (PTB) domains (*boxes*) and become phosphorylated by the activated receptor.

lihood of an RTK to acquire oncogenic properties depends on its propensity to dimerize or undergo mutation, the abundance of specific ligands in the organism, and its inherent activity [15,16].

During evolution of metazoan organisms, ligands, as well as their receptors, segregated into families of related molecules sharing structural and functional properties. In general, members of a ligand subfamily activate molecules of a corresponding receptor subfamily (Fig. 2-10). As might be expected during the hierarchical diversification of biologic signals, most ligands trigger only subsets of receptor families. Certain ligands are capable of activating heterodimers between related receptors of a subfamily; this capability has been established for members of the epidermal growth factor receptor (EGFR) and platelet-derived growth factor receptor (PDGFR) family. Although the majority trigger growth signals, several unique aspects of ligand-receptor interactions reflect their functional heterogeneity. Insulin receptor (IR) signals metabolic responses, whereas the related IGF1 receptor transmits mitogenic signals. The growth arrest–specific gene 6 (*GAS6*), which encodes a product with G domain structure, binds all three known members of the UFO receptor family [17]. Glial cell–derived neurotrophic factor (GDNF) recruits complexes consisting of Ret and a high-affinity glycosyl phosphatidylinositol (GPI)-anchored cell surface receptor [18]. The fast expanding LERK family of EPH receptor ligands is unique in providing predominantly cell-associated ligand molecules, creating positional signals for axon guidance during neuronal development. These ligands are immobilized on the cell surface either by a transmembrane domain or a GPI-anchor [19]. Other ligands such as neuregulins (NRG) of the EGF superfamily or nerve growth factor (NGF) have the ability to trigger both growth and differentiation. Ligands of the PDGF family are, thus far, the only growth factors known to form covalently linked dimers [14,20].

Likewise, RTKs constitute families of structurally related molecules (Fig. 2-10). Sequence conservation between multiple members identified in most families, is highest in their tyrosine kinase domain and less pronounced in their extracellular domain, which is responsible for ligand binding. PDGFR and FGFR family members have insert regions of relatively low homology in their kinase domain, and insulin receptor family members assemble into a heterotetrameric receptor structure. Individual members within one family share overall structural homology, including their ligand-binding domain, which has diverged among different receptor families. Similarity of extracellular domains within receptor families provides the basis for specific recognition of molecules of a corresponding ligand family (Fig. 2-10). Sequence regions of least homology include carboxyl-terminal and interkinase coding sequences, which serve as specific substrate association sites due to tyrosine phosphorylation sites targeted by SH2- or PTB-binding domains of substrates [20].

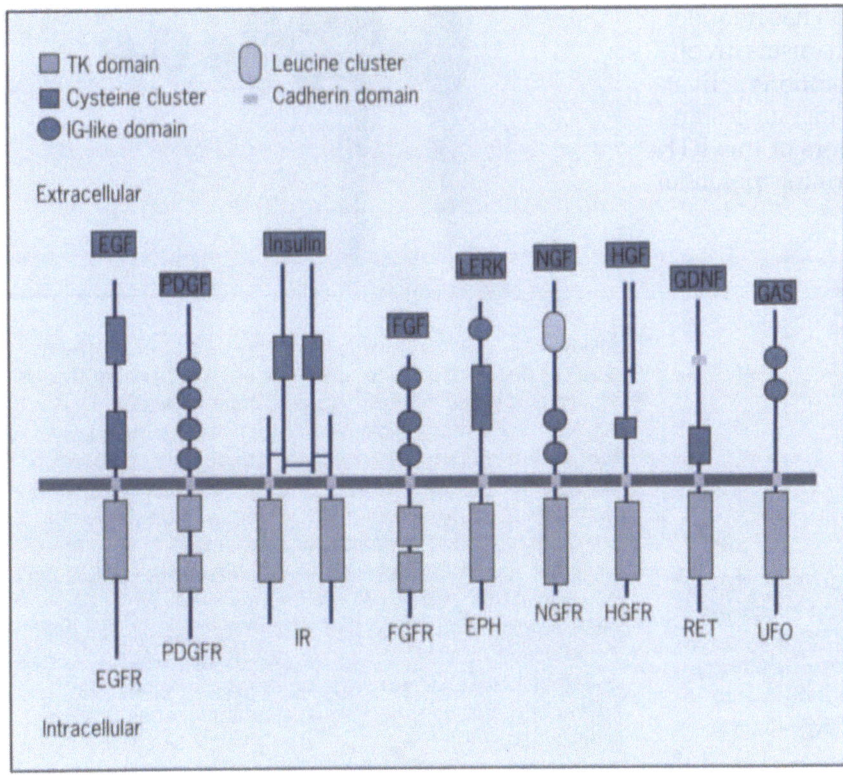

Figure 2-10. Evolutionary divergence of families of receptor tyrosine kinases and specific ligands. RTK subfamilies are depicted and identified by their prototypic family member. EGF—epidermal growth factor; PDGF—platelet-derived growth factor; FGF—fibroblast growth factor; LERK—ligands for EPH receptor kinases; NGF—nerve growth factor; HGF—hepatocyte growth factor; GDNF—glial cell-derived neurotrophic factor; GAS—growth arrest-specific gene; IR—insulin receptor; TK—tyrosine kinase domain; IG—immunoglobulin-like domain.

Oncogenic activation affecting cytoplasmic signaling pathways frequently occurs at the receptor level. Gene amplification of an intact transcription unit represents a quantitative activation mechanism that can result in increased transcript and protein expression. An example is shown for *ERBB2* gene amplification (Fig. 2-11), which is known to be associated with 20% to 30 % of primary human breast cancer and adenocarcinoma of other organs. In these cases, gene amplification results in high-level overexpression of structurally normal transcript (Fig. 2-12) and protein (Fig. 2-13). In addition, *ERBB2* overexpression at moderate levels can be observed in the absence of gene amplification (Fig. 2-12). These observations indicate that amplified gene copies are functional and imply that additional mechanisms at the level of transcription regulation might be operative to augment *ERBB2* overexpression in breast cancer. RTKs frequently implicated in human cancer by these mechanisms belong to the EGFR subfamily. In addition to *ERBB2,* also *EGFR* gene amplification has been found in adenocarcinoma but appears more prevalent in squamous cell carcinoma and glioblastoma. Gene amplification also has been reported for other RTKs, including *K-SAM* (*FGFR2*) and *HGFR* (*MET*) in human stomach cancer and *PDGFRα* in glioblastoma [7]. Oncogenicity of elevated receptor levels is conditioned by intrinsic functional properties of the normal product. High-level overexpression of ERBB2 has proven oncogenic in model systems; this could be due to its comparably high kinase activity in vivo or its propensity to oligomerize in the absence of mutations. Conversely, EGFR overexpression has frequently been associated with autocrine mechanisms involving its ligand TGF-α or structural alterations activating its kinase activity in epithelial malignancies and glioblastoma [21]. Intriguingly, receptors of this RTK subfamily synergize in their transforming potential by heterodimerization, thus lowering the threshold of normal protein levels required for oncogenicity. Coexpression of *ERBB3,* a third member in this receptor subfamily, can elicit transformation by *ERBB2* at moderate expression levels of the latter and enhance its transforming activity at high expression levels (Fig. 2-14). Cooperation in transformation by heterodimer formation also has been demonstrated for ErbB2 and EGFR [16,40].

In physiologic conditions, transient activation of RTK activity is regulated by ligand exposure inducing dimerization and conformation change. In malignancy, chronic ligand-independent activation results from gene mutations of the RTK coding structure, including DNA rearrangement and point mutation. DNA rearrangement of RTK coding sequences associated with human tumors involves substitution of extracellular ligand-binding and transmembrane domain sequences (Fig. 2-15). Fusion of receptor cytoplasmic domains with oligomerization domains typical for genes encoding transcription factors leads to constitutive dimer formation and kinase activation. In addition, substitution of receptor extracellular and transmembrane domains may encompass altered subcellular distribution of rearranged fusion proteins. DNA rearrangements of RTKs by chromosomal aber-

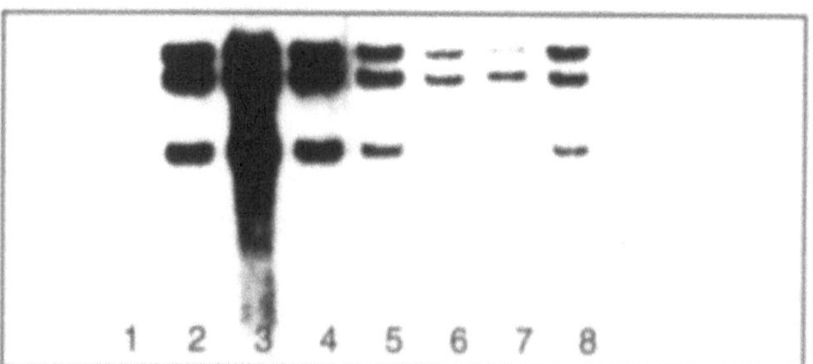

Figure 2-11. Receptor gene amplification. Southern blot analysis of genomic DNA cleaved by *Xba*I and hybridized with the entire coding sequence of human *ERBB2* as a probe. Gene amplification involving the entire *ERBB2* coding sequence is shown in tumor cells (lanes 2–5) in contrast to control (lane 1) and tumor cell lines lacking gene amplification (lanes 6–8) [36].

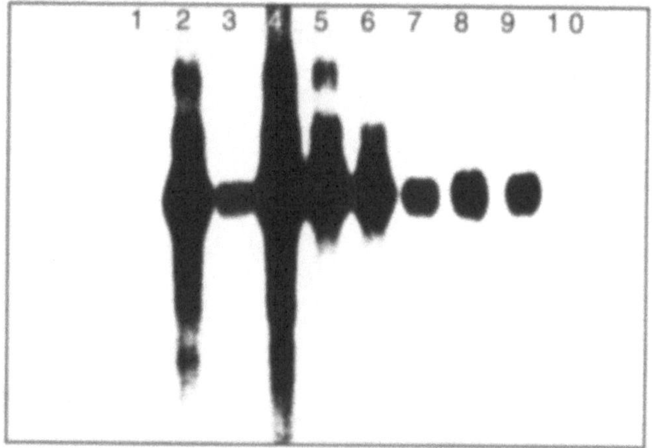

Figure 2-12. Receptor mRNA overexpression in the presence or absence of gene amplification. Northern blot analysis using a human *ERBB2*-specific complementary DNA (cDNA) probe for hybridization of total cellular RNA from human breast tumor cell lines and controls. In comparison with control samples (lanes 1 and 10), normal-sized *ERBB2* transcript is overexpressed at high levels in breast tumor cell lines harboring gene amplification (lanes 2, 4, 5, and 6). In addition, *ERBB2* overexpression at moderate levels can be seen in four additional breast tumor cell lines lacking gene amplification (lanes 3, 7, 8, and 9). Quantitative estimates following standardization with a reference probe indicate that *ERBB2* overexpression ranges from one to two orders of magnitude, depending on the presence of gene amplification [36].

rations have been described in a variety of human tumors. Some genes, including *TEL* and *TRP*, are common targets for rearrangement with different RTKs (Table 2-2). *TEL*, which encodes a transcription factor of the Ets family, also undergoes rearrangements with the cytosolic tyrosine kinase gene *ABL* in acute myeloid leukemia [3]. Another mechanism for ligand-independent activation of RTK function in neoplasia is represented by point mutations in RTK coding sequences (Fig. 2-16). In general, mutations in extracellular, transmembrane, and juxtamembrane domains result in constitutive receptor oligomerization, whereas mutation of tyrosine kinase domain residues activates the catalytic function of the receptor by an intramolecular mechanism (Table 2-3). Common mutations affecting the *RET* and *MET* RTKs are of particular importance, because they have been identified as germline mutations associated with autosomal dominant disease pre-

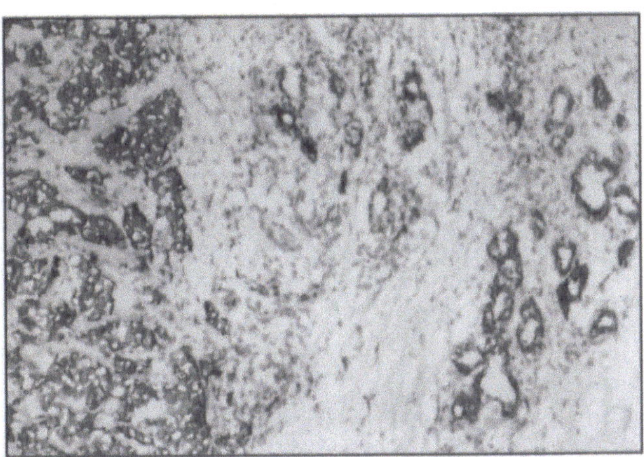

Figure 2-13. Receptor overexpression. Immunohistochemical staining of a frozen section from a primary human mammary carcinoma using an ErbB2-specific monoclonal antibody. Intense staining of virtually all tumor cells (*left*) in comparison with nonmalignant epithelial ducts (*right*) reflects high-level ErbB2 protein overexpression in a representative primary breast carcinoma with *ERBB2* gene amplification and mRNA overexpression.

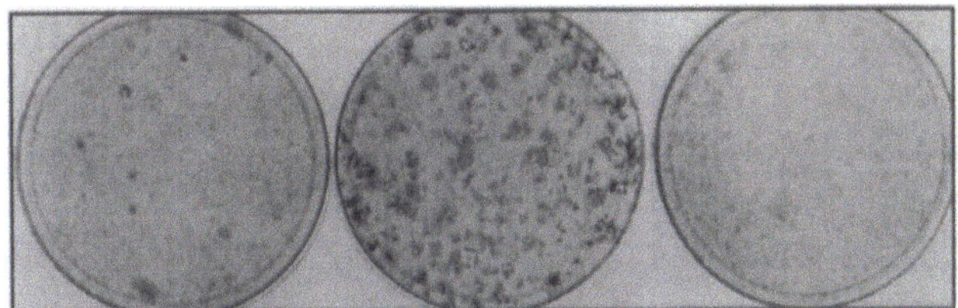

Figure 2-14. Receptor synergy in oncogenicity. Heterologous expression of normal ErbB2 and ErbB3 coding sequences in immortal NIH 3T3 fibroblasts by transfection of eukaryotic long terminal repeat–driven expression vectors. Overexpression of ErbB2 protein at high levels causes transformation (left), whereas ErbB3 does not induce foci (right). Coexpression of ErbB2 and ErbB3 (center) at comparable receptor levels as in the individual transfectants shows evidence of cooperation between ErbB2 and ErbB3 in oncogenic transformation, exceeding ErbB2 transformation by one order of magnitude. Synergistic transformation is accompanied by ErbB3-ErbB2 heterodimerization in vivo [37].

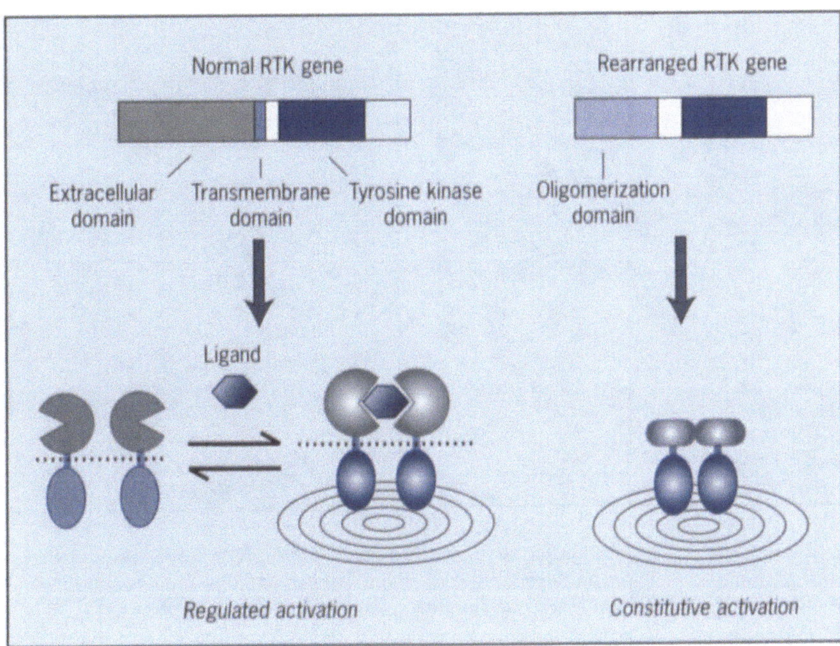

Figure 2-15. Constitutive receptor tyrosine kinase (RTK) activation by gene rearrangement. The tyrosine kinase domain is shown in dark blue, the extracellular domain is shown in grey, and the oligomerization domain is shown in light blue.

disposition in familial cancer syndromes including familial medullary thyroid carcinoma (FMTC) and multiple endocrine neoplasia types 2A (MEN2A) and 2B (MEN2B) in the case of *RET* and hereditary papillary renal carcinoma in the case of *MET* [22,13]. In addition to diagnostic or therapeutic potential, these examples illustrate that oncogenic mutations can precede tumor onset in humans. A transmembrane mutation activating the rat homologue of *ERBB2* in chemically induced rat neuroblastoma has thus far not been described in human tumors [3].

Cytoplasmic Oncogenes

Neoplastic transformation of immortalized NIH 3T3 fibroblasts by transfection of high-molecular-weight genomic tumor DNA provided the basis for direct identification and molecular characterization of cellular oncogenes from human tumors (Fig. 2-17). The majority of oncogenes detected in this manner are members of the *RAS* family and include *HRAS, KRAS*, and *NRAS*. *RAS* oncogenes are activated by single point mutations in two confined areas of the protein

Table 2-2. Receptor tyrosine kinase activation by gene rearrangement

Oncogene	Cytogenetics	Tumor	RTK gene	Fusion gene	Dimerization domain
PTC-RET	inv10(q11.2;q21)	Papillary thyroid carcinoma	*RET*	*PTC*	—
TEL-PDGFRβ	t(5;12)(q33;p13)	Chronic myelomonocytic leukemia	*PDGFRβ*	*TEL*	Helix-loop-helix
TPM3-TRK	Intrachromosomal 1	Thyroid carcinoma	*TRKA (NGFR)*	*TPM3*	—
TPR-TRK				*TPR*	Leucine zipper
TFG-TRK				*TFG*	Coiled coil
TPR-MET	t(1;7)	Gastric carcinoma	*MET (HGFR)*	*TPR*	Leucine zipper
NPM-ALK	*t(2;5)(2p23;q35)*	Non-Hodgkin's lymphoma	*ALK*	*Nucleophosmin*	N-terminal

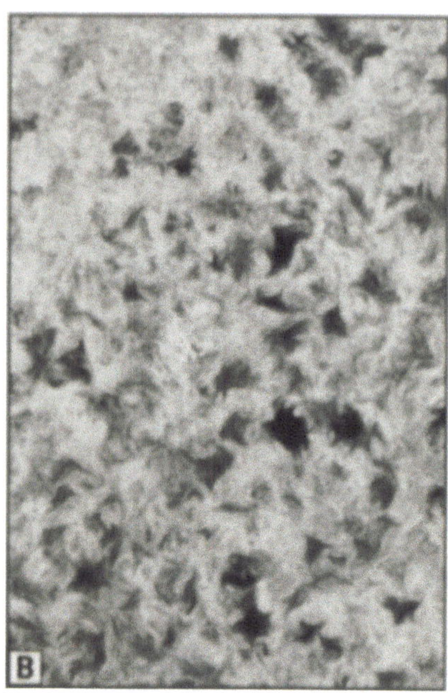

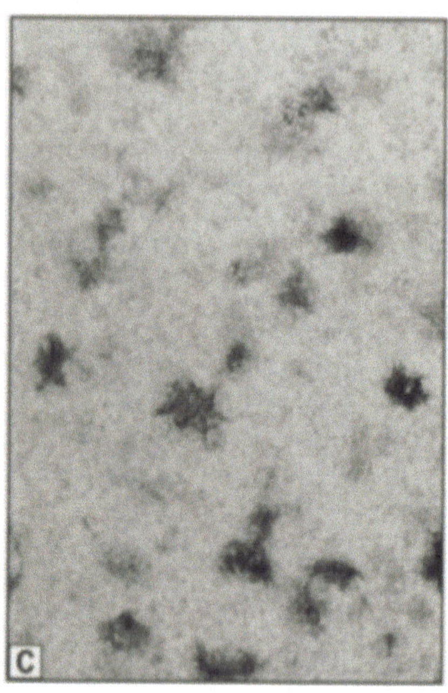

Figure 2-16. Oncogenic activation of receptor tyrosine kinases (RTKs) by point mutation. Induction of primary focus formation in NIH 3T3 cells by RET MEN2A (RET C634Y) (**B**) and RET MEN2B (RET M918T) (**C**) mutants but not by normal RET (**A**) reflects ligand-independent oncogenic activation by point mutation in the extracellular or tyrosine kinase domain. Transformation is associated with increased kinase activity in vivo and in vitro due to covalent dimer formation in MEN2A and direct alteration of catalytic function in MEN2B [38].

around codon 12 or codon 61. Somatic mutations of *RAS* oncogenes are not restricted to a particular tumor type and are estimated to occur in 5% to 15% of all human malignancies, thus representing one of the most prevalent oncogenic alterations detected in human cancer. Certain tumor types show a higher incidence of *RAS* activation (*eg*, lung and colon carcinoma, acute myelogenous leukemia), whereas prevalence is low in others (*eg*, mammary carcinoma) [7]. Normal Ras proteins function as binary switches in receptor-mediated signaling pathways. They are small monomeric GDP/GTP-binding proteins harboring intrinsic GTPase activity. Several functional domains have been identified that are responsible for G binding, effector function, and membrane association of RAS (Fig. 2-18). G-binding domains (aa 5–22 and aa 109–120) are conserved with other G-binding proteins. Some oncogenic mutations (*ie*, codons 12 and 13) reside in these regions. Effector (aa 30–40) and membrane attachment domains are essential for oncogenic Ras properties. Their normal function depends on the ability to cycle between an active and inactive state, represented by GTP-bound Ras and GDP-bound Ras, respectively (Fig. 2-19). GEFs such as Sos catalyze the conversion of Ras from the inactive (GDP-bound) to the active (GTP-bound) form, whereas GTPase-activating proteins (GAPs) accelerate the intrinsically slow GTPase activity of Ras, returning it to its inactive state. The basis for Ras oncogenic function is a reduction in its ability to hydrolyze GTP, a process associat-

Table 2-3. Receptor tyrosine kinase activation by point mutation

Oncogene	Mutation	Domain	Tumor	Occurence	Mechanism
RET	Cys609→ Cys611→ Cys618→ Cys620→ Cys634→	Extracellular domain	Familial medullary thyroid carcinoma Multiple endocrine neoplasia type 2A	Germline Germline	Covalent dimerization inducing kinase activation
RET	Glu768→Asp Leu804→Val	Tyrosine kinase domain	Familial medullary thyroid carcinoma Sporadic medullary thyroid carcinoma	Germline Somatic	Kinase activation?
RET	Met918→Thr	Tyrosine kinase domain	Multiple endocrine neoplasia type 2B Sporadic medullary thyroid carcinoma Sporadic pheochromocytoma	Germline Somatic Somatic	Intramolecular kinase activation
MET (HGF-R)	Met1149→Thr Val1206→Leu Val1238→Ile Asp1246→Asn Tyr1248→Cys	Tyrosine kinase domain	Hereditary papillary renal carcinoma (HPRC)	Germline	Kinase activation ?
MET (HGF-R)	Leu1213→Val Asp1246→His Tyr1248→His Mel1268→Thr	Tyrosine kinase domain	Sporadic papillary renal carcinoma	Somatic	Kinase activation ?
NEU (*ERBB2*)	Val664→Glu	Transmembrane domain	Chemically induced rat neuroblastoma	—	Dimerization enhancing kinase activity
FMS (CSF-1R)	Leu301→Ser	Extracellular domain	Retroviral activation	—	Dimerization
KIT (SCFR)	Val559→Gly	Juxtamembrane domain	Mast cell leukemia cell lines	—	Dimerization
KIT (SCFR)	Asp814→Val	Tyrosine kinase domain	Mast cell leukemia cell lines	—	Intramolecular kinase activation

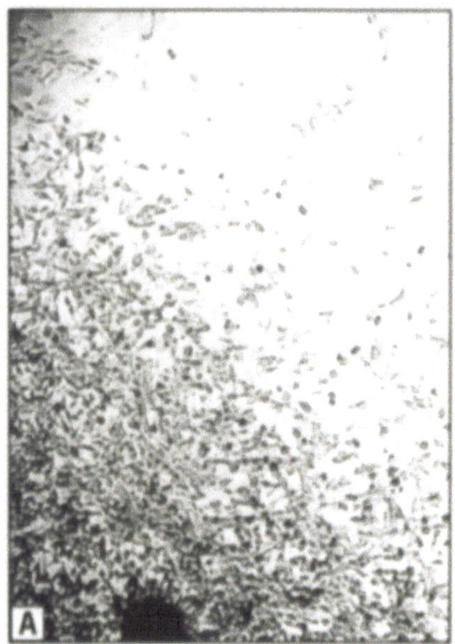

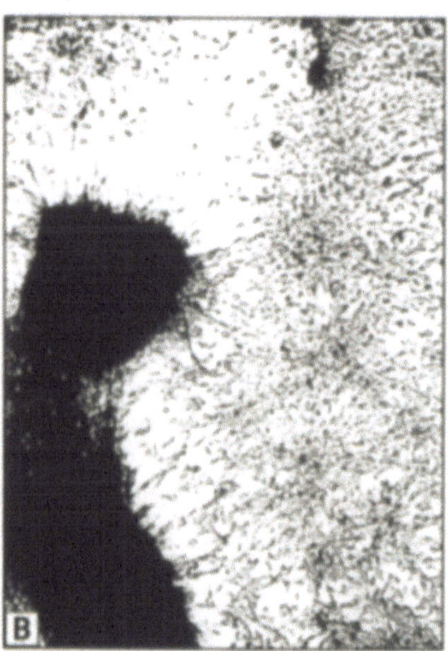

Figure 2-17. *RAS* oncogene activation in human tumors by point mutation. Primary focus formation is induced by transfection of human genomic tumor DNA harboring a somatic codon 12 mutation of *HRAS* (Val12→Asp) [39]. The border (**A**) and center (**B**) of a primary focus consisting of highly refractile transformed cells lacking contact inhibition are visible against the background of a flat monolayer of untransformed NIH 3T3 fibroblasts.

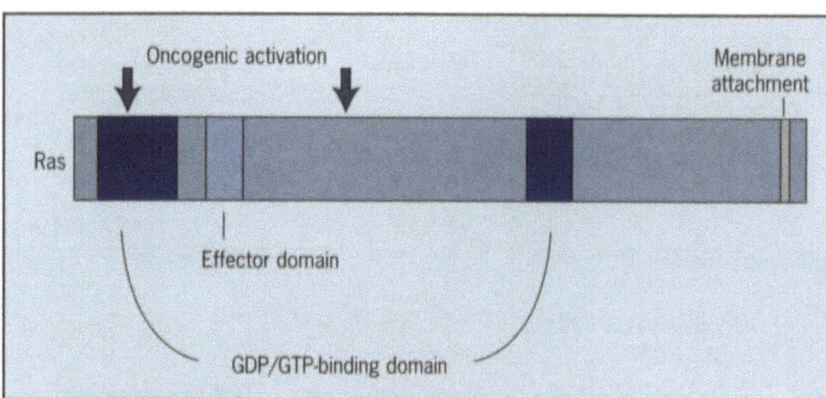

Figure 2-18. Ras protein structure. GDP/GTP-binding domain blue regions are essential for guanidine diphosphate/guanidine triphosphate binding. *Arrows* denote positions frequently undergoing mutation in human malignancy. The effector domain and membrane attachment domain is essential for Ras activity. GDP—guanidine diphosphate; GTP—guanidine triphosphate.

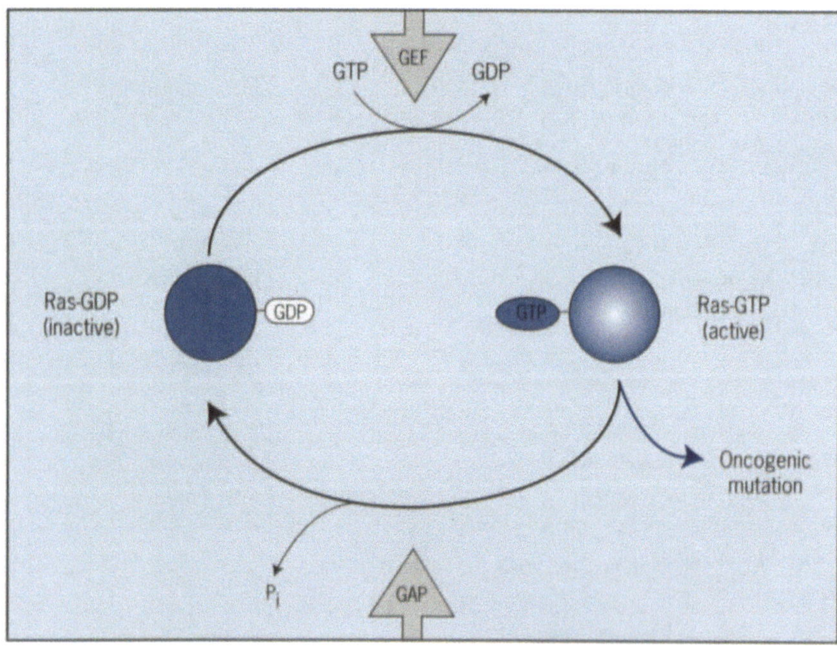

Figure 2-19. Oncogenic Ras protein function. GAP—GTPase-activating protein; GEF—guanine nucleotide exchange factor; P_i—phosphate.

ed with a conformational change in normal Ras proteins. Mutations around codon 12 directly affect GTP binding, whereas mutations near codon 61 prevent conformational changes necessary for inactivation. Therefore, oncogenic mutations constitutively lock Ras in its active GTP-bound configuration, preventing GAP-catalyzed conversion to its inactive state. Thus, the ratio of GDP/GTP-bound Ras is shifted toward the active form, which chronically triggers downstream signaling pathways [23].

Cytoplasmic tyrosine kinases serve as signal transducers downstream of transmembrane receptors. The cytosolic tyrosine kinase Abl is the target of oncogenic activation in a variety of human leukemias associated with chromosomal translocation (Fig. 2-20). In chronic myelogenous leukemia, gene rearrangement involving chromosomes 9 and 22 (t[9;22]; the Philadelphia chromosome) results in fusion of the amino terminal half of *BCR* with the *ABL* coding sequence lacking its first exon. Another t(9;22) translocation associated with acute lymphocytic leukemia produces a fusion protein encoded by the first exon of *BCR* and *ABL* devoid of its first exon. A t(9;12) translocation in acute myeloid leukemia generates gene rearrangement between the Ets-related transcription factor *TEL* and *ABL*. Oncogenicity of all three fusion proteins results from constitutive activation of Abl catalytic function associated with oligomerization of the fusion protein. The fusion partner of the Abl kinase contributes a dimerization interface, which in the case of Bcr contains a coiled coil domain at its amino-terminus and in the case of Tel contains a helix-loop-helix motif [3,24]. Src was the first oncogenic tyrosine kinase identified as a viral oncogene. Extensive structure-function analysis of the transforming properties of *SRC* and the recently resolved crystal structure of the normal protein indicate active self-regulatory containment of its activity by intramolecular mechanisms in physiologic conditions. Src and related cytoplasmic tyrosine kinases possess, in addition to the catalytic domain, modular binding regions (including SH2 and SH3) which bind specific phosphotyrosine residues and polyproline target sequences, respectively. Normal Src is phosphorylated by C-terminal Src kinase (Csk) on Tyr_{527}, which provides a binding target for its own SH2 domain (Fig. 2-21). This event results in a three-dimensional configuration of SH2 kinase linker and N-terminal kinase lobe resembling a polyproline II helix serving as target for intramolecular binding of its own SH3 domain. The folded (*ie*, closed) structure attenuates kinase activity of normal Src. Dephosphorylation of Tyr_{527} disrupts the intramolecular bond between SH2 and Tyr_{527}, followed by dissociation of intramolecular SH3 binding. Unfolding results in activation of intrinsic Src catalytic and biologic function, which is enhanced by phosphorylation of Tyr_{416}. Accordingly, substitution of the carboxyl-terminal Tyr_{527} is responsible for oncogenic properties of v-*src*. To date, genetic alterations activating Src have not been described in human tumors. Based on the ability of Src and related cytoplasmic kinases to associate with RTKs or receptors lacking intrinsic kinase activity, it is conceivable that Src activation in human tumors may occur at the post-translational level by binding of its SH2 or SH3 domain to heterologous proteins, thereby releasing intramolecular constraints on its tyrosine kinase activity. Evidence for Src activation in receptor-mediated signaling, for example, has been established for EGF and PDGF [25].

Members of the Bcl2 family of proteins share the propensity of homodimer and heterodimer forma-

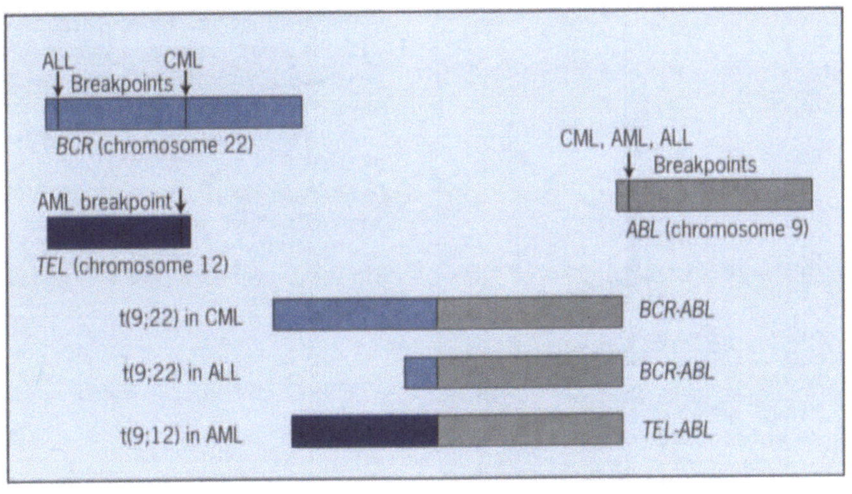

Figure 2-20. Oncogenic conversion of *ABL* by chromosomal translocation: *ABL* (Chromosome 9), *BCR* (Chromosome 22), and *TEL* (Chromosome 12). *Arrows* denote breakpoints. ALL—acute lymphoid leukemia; AML—acute myeloid leukemia; CML—chronic myeloid leukemia; t—translocation.

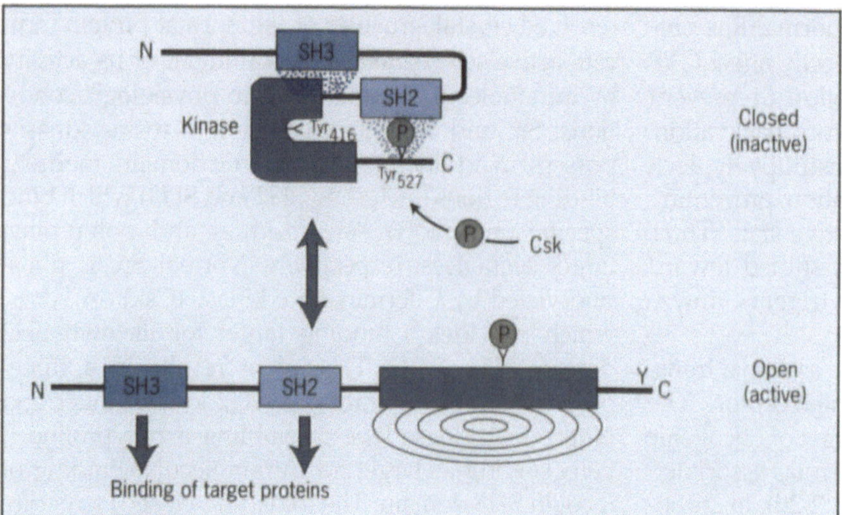

Figure 2-21. Autoregulatory properties of Src. Src homology domains: tyrosine kinase (SH1), Src homology 2 (SH2) domain, Src homology 3 (SH3) domain. Intramolecular bonds are stippled. C—carboxy terminus; Csk—C-terminal Src kinase; N—amino terminus; Y—Tyr; P—phosphate.

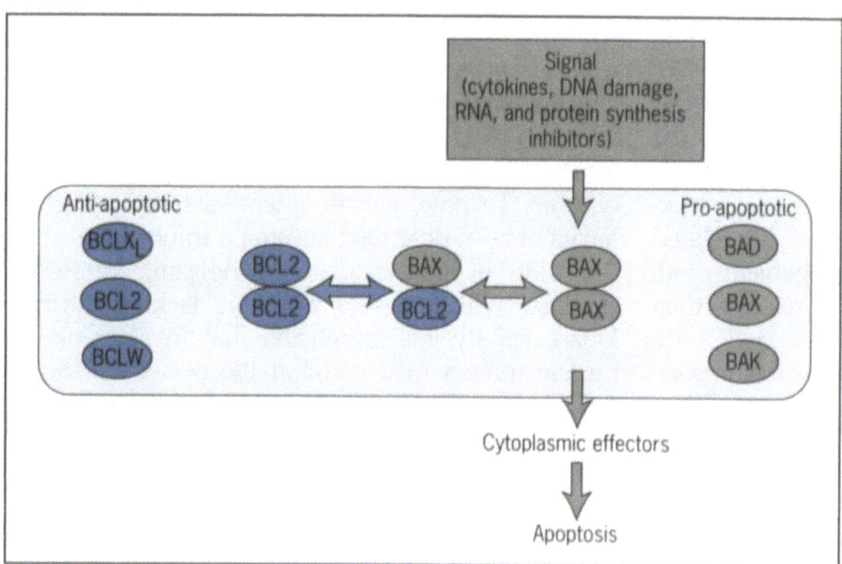

Figure 2-22. Oncogenic properties of *BCL2* by inhibition of apoptosis. Oncogenic *BCL2* inhibits apoptosis by disturbing the balance between pro-apoptotic (*grey*) and anti-apoptotic (*blue*) proteins in the cytoplasm.

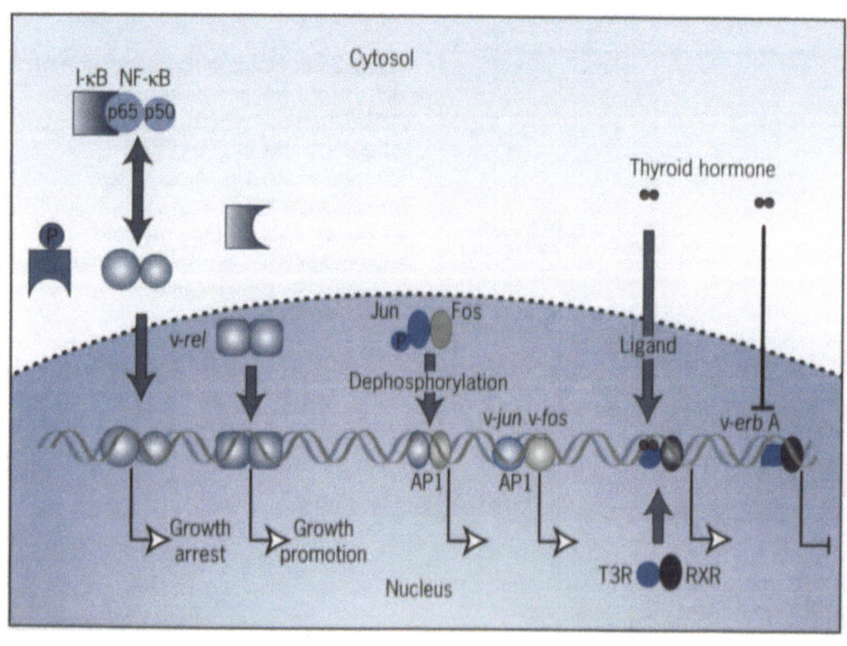

Figure 2-23. Oncogenic conversion of transcription factors. Oncogenic activation of three transcription factor complexes subjected to distinct mechanisms of physiologic regulation is shown. Normally, NFκB is activated by release of the inhibitor IκB on phosphorylation, Jun-Fos complexes are activated following dephosphorylation, and thyroid hormone receptor ErbA-RxR complexes are activated by ligand binding.

tion. They can be distinguished by functional criteria as inducers (Bax, Bad, Bak) or inhibitors (Bcl2, Bcl-x_L, Bcl-w) of apoptosis. An oncogenic effect of Bcl2 that is activated by chromosomal rearrangement in follicular lymphoma is based on the ability of Bcl2 overexpression to block apoptosis (Fig. 2-22). Because Bax induces apoptosis and Bcl2 blocks it, Bax homodimers provide effector signals for apoptosis. Bcl2 overexpression is thought to compete for binding with Bax and to shift the dimer equilibrium toward the left, eliminating apoptotic signals that emanate from Bax homodimers [26].

Nuclear Oncogenes

Nuclear oncogenes are characterized by their ability to bind DNA and regulate transcription. Mutations converting transcription factors to oncogenes involve changes in their regulatory properties on gene expression. Mutations can have activating effects (*eg*, v-*jun*, v-*fos*) or inactivating effects (*eg*, v-*erb*A), or they may shift the pattern of gene expression (*eg*, v-*rel*). Transcription factors normally function as oligomers activated by different mechanisms (Fig. 2-23). Members of the Rel family, including NF-κB, consist of oligomers formed between 65-kD and 50-kD subunits, which represent the active form. A cytosolic inhibitor, I-κB suppresses the heteromeric complex by binding and retaining it in the cytoplasm. Phosphorylation of I-κB releases the inhibitor from the active complex, which translocates to the nucleus and induces promoters with κB target sites. One known effect of oncogenic conversion of Rel is loss in ability to bind the inhibitor, explaining its retention in the nucleus. However, oncogenic conversion of v-*rel* must involve alteration of additional functional properties for full oncogenic potential, which may result from alteration in the pattern of genes induced. Jun-Fos heterodimers are part of the AP1 transcription complex whose activity is regulated by post-translational mechanisms involving Jun dephosphorylation in transcription activation. Oncogenic versions of either Jun or Fos, which are structurally altered, induce constitutive transcription from AP1–controlled promoters. Transcription regulation by thyroid hormone is exerted by nuclear receptors triiodothyronine receptor (T3R) (ErbA) complexed with retinoid X receptor (RXR). The dimer is constitutively bound to DNA, and transcription is induced by binding of the ligand (*ie*, thyroid hormone) to its receptor (*ie*, T3R). Oncogenic alteration of the latter in v-*erb*A abolishes ligand-binding ability also suppressing transcriptional activity of its dimerization partner, RXR. This implies that genes normally induced by ErbA may suppress transformation and probably control differentiation [27].

The nuclear oncogenes most frequently implicated in human cancer belong to the *MYC* gene family. Activation occurs by gene rearrangement or gene amplification. Both mechanisms give rise to deregulated overexpression (Fig. 2-7). Certain leukemias and lymphomas etiologically involve the *MYC* gene in chromosomal translocation (Table 2-4). Gene

Table 2-4. Nuclear oncogenes in human cancer

Tumor	Oncogene	Activation	Protein function	Rearranging gene	Cytogenetics
Burkitt's lymphoma	*MYC*	Gene rearrangement	bHLH transcription factor	IgH, IgL	t(8;14)(q24;q32)
Burkitt's lymphoma–acute lymphocytic leukemia					t(2;8)(p12;q24) t(8;22)(q24;q11)
Acute lymphocytic leukemia	*MYC*	Gene rearrangement	bHLH transcription factor	TCR-α	t(8;14)(q24;q11)
Chronic lymphocytic leukemia, acute lymphocytic leukemia	*MYC*	Gene rearrangement	bHLH transcription factor	—	t(8;12)(q24;q22)
Neuroblastoma, retinoblastoma	N-*MYC*	Gene amplification	Transcription factor	—	HSR, DM
Small cell lung carcinoma	L-*MYC* N-*MYC* *MYC*	Gene amplification	Transcription factor	—	—

bHLH—basic helix-loop-helix; DM—double minutes; IgH—immunoglobulin heavy chain; IgL—immunoglobulin light chain; TCR—T-cell receptor; HSR—heterogeneous staining region.

rearrangements place *MYC* under the regulatory sequences of immunoglobulin heavy chains (IgHs), immunoglobulin light chains (IgLs), or T-cell receptors (TCRs), resulting in overexpression of *MYC*, which encodes a basic helix-loop-helix (bHLH) transcription factor. Other genes structurally related to *MYC*, including *NMYC* and *LMYC*, have been implicated by gene amplification at high frequency in neuroblastoma and small cell lung cancer, respectively. Gene amplification of *NMYC* in neuroblastomas is accompanied by double-minute (DM) chromosomes or homogeneous staining regions (HSRs) [7,24]. *MYC* gene rearrangement is found in virtually 100% of cases of Burkitt's lymphoma, a B-cell malignancy associated with one of three reciprocal translocations between the *MYC* gene locus on chromosome 8 and IgH, κ light chain, or λ light chain on chromosome 14, 2, or 22, respectively (Fig. 2-24). In the most common translocation [t(8;14)(q24;q32)], *MYC*, along with the distal portion of chromosome 8, is relocated to chromosome 14 and joined in a head-to-head transcriptional orientation with heavy chain constant region exons; heavy

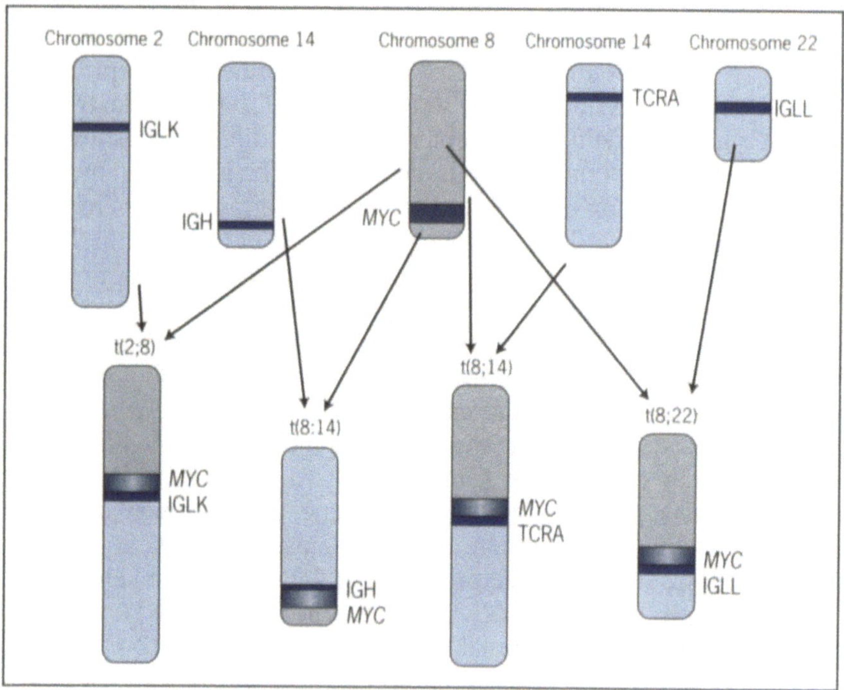

Figure 2-24. *MYC* activation by gene rearrangement. The *MYC* gene becomes activated in hematopoietic malignancies that involve specific chromosomal translocations. Normal (*top*) and rearranged (*bottom*) human chromosomes involving *MYC* in human cancer are shown. Although these translocations are balanced (*ie*, without loss of chromosomal material) only the rearranged chromosomes harboring *MYC* are shown. Rearrangements with immunoglobulin heavy- (*IGH*) or light- (*IGL*) chain loci are associated with B-cell malignancies, whereas translocations with T-cell receptor α loci (*TCRA*) occur in T-cell malignancies (see Table 2-4). Rearrangement results in constitutive *MYC* expression induced by regulatory elements of immunoglobulin or *TCR* genes.

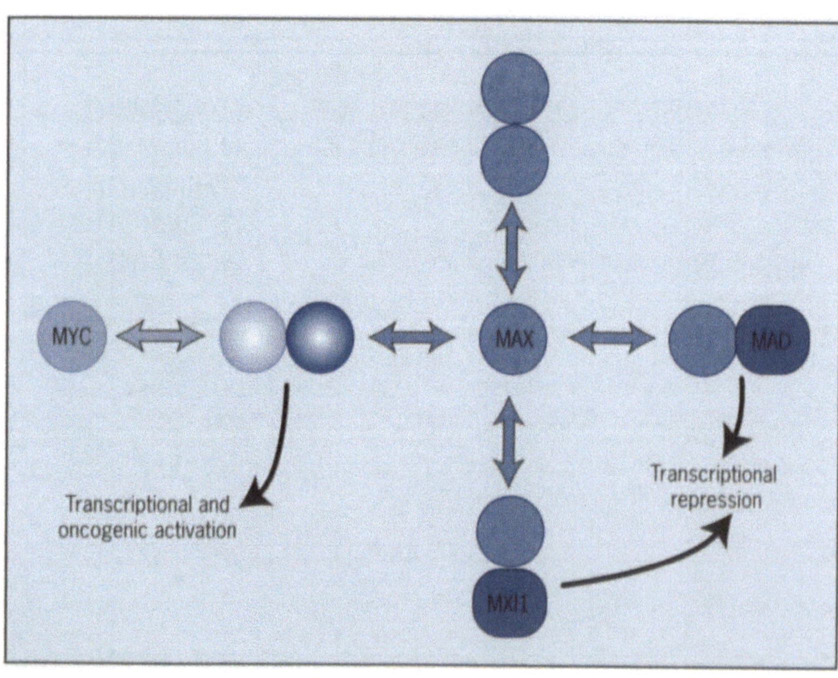

Figure 2-25. Functional consequence of constitutive *MYC* activation.

chain variable gene segments, along with the distal portion of chromosome 14, move in the reciprocal exchange to chromosome 8. The breakpoint on chromosome 14 is typically within the diversity or joining regions interspersed between the variable and constant regions of the IgH chain locus. In the other translocations illustrated, *MYC* remains on chromosome 8, with the breakpoint residing at the 3′ end of the gene to which IgL sequences from chromosome 2 or 22 translocate in the same transcriptional orientation as the *MYC* gene. Similarly, t(8;14)(q24;q11) associated with T-cell acute lymphocytic leukemia involves transfer of *TCR* gene segments in the vicinity of the *MYC* gene locus on chromosome 8 [24].

The Myc protein contains sequence motifs characteristic of transcription factors, including a basic region for DNA binding as well as helix-loop-helix and leucine zipper dimerization interfaces. It directly or indirectly affects at least three other factors with bHLH and ZIP domains, including Max, Mad, and Mxi1 (Fig. 2-25). Myc dimerizes with Max, which itself can bind DNA and form homodimers or heterodimers with Mad or Mxi1. Myc-Max dimers are transcriptionally active and necessary for oncogenic activity, whereas Max-Mad and Max-Mxi1 dimers repress transcription. Considering equilibrium between the monomers and various dimers, chronic *MYC* overexpression due to gene rearrangement or amplification in human tumors would shift the balance toward transcriptionally active Myc-Max heterodimers, resulting in deregulated induction of target gene expression. *MYC*, along with *FOS*, *JUN*, and *REL*, belong to a class of so-called "immediate early genes," indicating rapid induction of their expression on mitogen stimulation. This property functionally implicates *MYC* and other immediate early genes in cell cycle entry. The ability of Myc to induce expression of Cdc25 (Fig. 2-5), a dual-specificity phosphatase activating cyclin-dependent kinases, establishes a direct link between an oncogene and control of the cell cycle. Consistent with this function, overexpression of Myc resulting from oncogenic conversion causes activation of cyclin D-Cdk4 and cyclin E-Cdk2 complexes in quiescent cells [3,24].

MULTISTEP ETIOLOGY OF CANCER

At least three major biologic characteristics distinguish malignant tumor cells from their normal progenitors in a metazoan organism (Fig. 2-26). Immortalization relates to the property of indefinite survival of cells due to functional defects in programmed pathways that limit the life span of any normal cell by apoptosis or senescence. Sustained proliferation is a consequence of immortalization. Immortalized and proliferating cells may still share normal morphology and grow within the confines of their physiologic boundaries. Furthermore, they still are susceptible to regulation by extracellular signals. Transformation defines features of malignant cells to possess altered morphology and to grow autonomously and aggressively, transgressing the physiologic boundaries genetically imprinted on their normal progenitors. Molecular dissection of these biologic stages indicates that several genetic lesions must accumulate in a normal cell to generate the full malignant phenotype of a tumor cell. In this process, immortalization may precede transformation in tumor development. An example is the step-

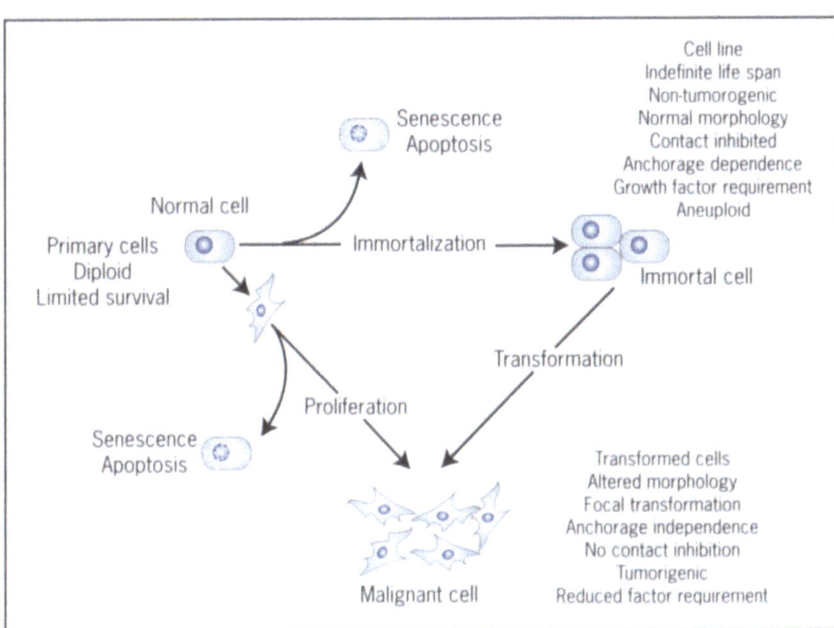

Figure 2-26. Neoplastic conversion of a normal cell. Biologic characteristics of normal, immortal, and malignant cells are listed. Established cell lines, even those that are nonmalignant, (*ie*, NIH 3T3) are already immortalized. Conversion to malignancy requires only a single oncogenic hit, which explains the utility of established cell lines in functional assessment of oncogenic properties for individual oncogenes.

wise progression in the development of colon cancer or preneoplastic lesions preceding other cancers. Recent observations indicate that expression of an activated *RAS* oncogene, which causes transformation in immortal cells, induces senescence in normal cells, a process linked to induced expression of the suppressor genes $P16^{INK4A}$ and *P53*. Active resistance to oncogenic transformation by induction of senescence or apoptosis might reflect a potent defense mechanism of normal cells in averting tumorigenesis [28]. At the same time, it is conceivable that transformation can precede proliferation if the signal triggering senescence fails due to successive mutation or conditions in which growth cues ablate senescence. The latter situation may arise under certain conditions of an organism when tumor development is conditioned by physiologic hormone or growth factor activity.

Oncogene Cooperation

Early evidence for multiple genetic steps in transformation derived from the analysis of DNA tumor viruses. In contrast to single-stranded RNA retroviruses, which transduce transforming sequences (*ie*, oncogenes) from the host genome, DNA tumor viruses encode multiple transforming proteins by production of alternatively spliced mRNAs. Several of these proteins have immortalizing function, whereas others induce phenotypic transformation. For example, both the middle T (MT) and large T (LT) oncogenes of polyomavirus are required to induce a fully tumorigenic phenotype in normal cells. Polyoma MT transforms immortalized cells, whereas polyoma LT immortalizes normal cells. This observation biochemically discerned immortalization and transformation as discrete steps in tumor development. Several of these viruses have been etiologically implicated in human cancer, including Epstein-Barr virus (EBV) in nasopharyngeal carcinoma and Burkitt's lymphoma or human papillomavirus (HPV) in cervical carcinoma [12,29].

The paradigm of cooperation between cellular oncogenes was established by demonstration that *RAS* and *MYC* cooperate in the complete transformation of primary rat embryo fibroblasts, whereas neither gene transforms by itself. *RAS* appeared to confer phenotypic transformation properties, whereas *MYC* caused immortalization. Functional cooperation between transformation- and immortalization-competent oncogenes was confirmed in multiple cell backgrounds in vitro, and synergy in transformation was supported by in vivo evidence generated in transgenic mouse studies. Other oncogenes were found to substitute either for *RAS* or *MYC* function (Fig. 2-27). Oncoproteins inducing immortalization typically localize to the nucleus, whereas those conferring morphologic transformation properties represent cytosolic or membrane proteins. The category of nuclear proteins comprises transcription factors or molecules directly affecting the cell cycle regulatory machinery. Oncogenes competent for morphologic transformation encode proteins controlling receptor-mediated signaling cascades. Cooperation between *RAS* and mutant *P53* unwittingly provided early mechanistic evidence for synergy in neoplastic transformation of an activated oncogene and an inactivated suppressor, as expression of the *P53* mutant gene mimicked a loss of function of normal *P53* [8,29].

Chemical carcinogens in experimental animal models cause activation of proto-oncogenes. The type of mutation observed is consistent with the known mutagenic effect of the chemical compound. Although oncogene activation represents the initiating mutagenic event, it is clearly not sufficient for tumor development. This has been experimentally verified in the two-step mouse skin carcinogenesis model, in which tumor progression is effected by phorbol ester treatment following initiation by the

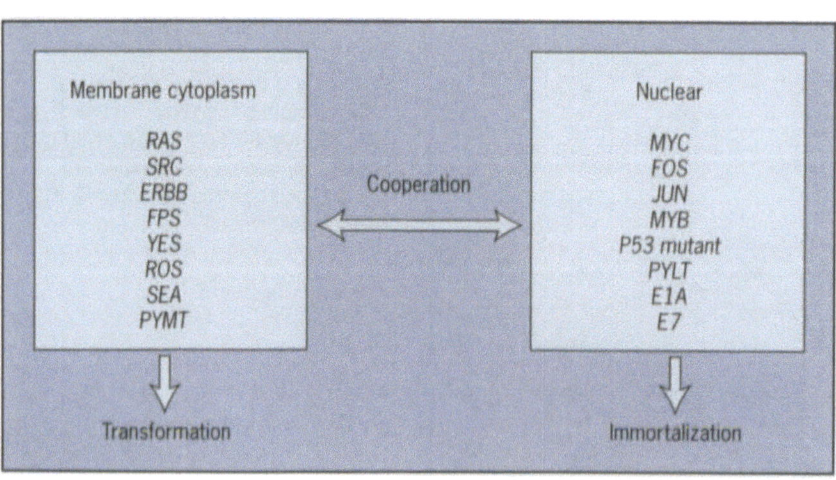

Figure 2-27. Cooperation of cellular oncogenes. Genes with transforming and immortalizing properties are shown. PYMT—polyoma middle T; PYLT—polyoma large T.

mutagen. In other models, it is reflected by particular physiologic conditions of the organism coinciding with tumor induction by single chemical carcinogens. Tumor promotion in NMU-induced rat mammary carcinomas has been attributed to the effect of endogenous estrogens, whereas progression of ENU-induced neuroblastoma or 3-MC-induced thymic lymphoma in rodents may depend on specific developmental condition of neural or thymus tissue, respectively, at the time of tumor growth [8].

Oncogenes and Tumor Suppressors

Cyclin–cyclin-dependent kinase complexes are the engines driving the cell cycle, whereas retinoblastoma protein (Rb) and transcription factor E2F exert integration and control function. Cyclin-dependent-kinase inhibitors and p53 tune the regulatory machinery by direct or indirect inhibition of cell cycle progression, ascertaining fidelity of DNA replication (Fig. 2-28). During G_1, normal cells respond to extracellular signals and, pending mitogenic or antiproliferative cues, advance toward mitosis or revert to quiescence (G_0). After passing a restriction point (R) late in G_1, the cells become refractory to extracellular signals and complete an autonomous program resulting in cell division. During G_1, cyclin D-Cdk activation by specific dephosphorylation leads to Rb inactivation by phosphorylation. Active Rb in hypophosphorylated state sequesters the transcription factor E2F. Hyperphosphorylation in late G_1 inactivates Rb, releasing E2F which activates cyclin E-Cdk2 complexes. These events are essential for passing checkpoint control, G_1 completion, and S-phase entry, committing the cell to mitosis. Different cyclin-Cdk combinations ensure progression toward mitosis. Rb remains phosphorylated and inactive until cycle completion. It becomes dephosphorylated at the end of M-phase, resetting the replication machinery, at which point cells regain sensitivity to extracellular signals. Cyclin D-Cdk4,6 complexes regulating Rb activity upstream are the "sensors" connecting afferent mitogen and oncogene signals to the cell cycle machinery. Moreover, some oncogenes have been shown to directly interact with cell cycle regulatory proteins. Expression of the dual-specificity phosphatase Cdc25, which activates Cdks by specific dephosphorylation, is induced by the transcription factor Myc. Functionally, *CDC25* has been shown to cooperate with *RAS*, substituting for oncogenic *MYC* function. Furthermore, the overexpression and gene amplification of cyclin D and E have been associated with certain human cancers. Several oncogenic viral proteins sequester the hypophosphorylated form of Rb or block the cyclin-dependent kinase inhibitor p27, facilitating constitutive cycling. Upregulated expression of cell cycle inhibitory molecules, including p53 and p16, by oncogenic *RAS* in normal cells may represent an important cellular defense mechanism against transformation [3,11,28,30].

Activation of oncogenes and inactivation of suppressor genes are co-selected in the majority of human tumors. Furthermore, elucidation of cellular signaling networks produces accumulating evidence for close functional interaction of both categories of molecules. The neurofibromatosis (*NF1*) suppressor gene encodes a GAP that regulates Ras function by accelerating GTP release and GDP loading (Fig. 2-19). Lack of NF1 product due to mutation in Recklinghausen's disease is associated with elevated

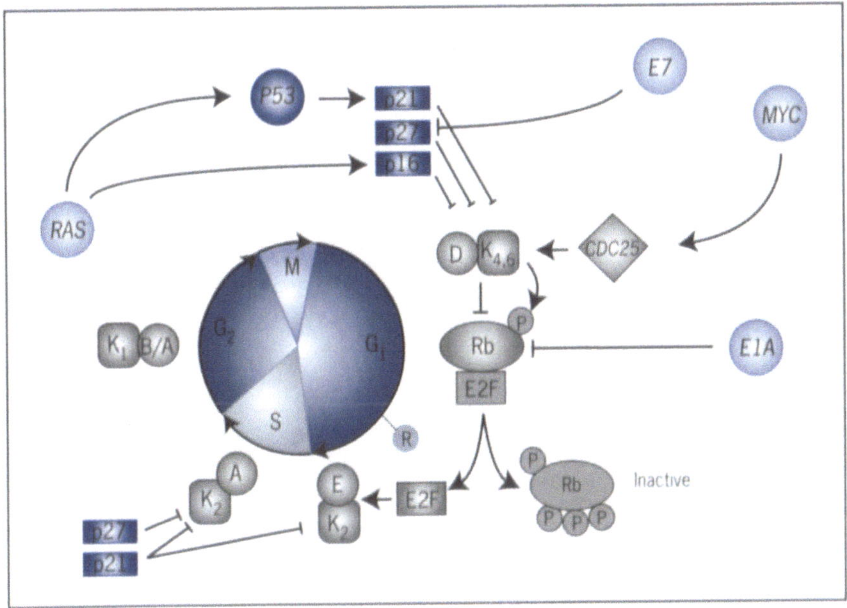

Figure 2-28. Oncogenes and cell cycle regulators. Immediate effects of oncogenes (*light blue*) on cell cycle regulatory (*grey*) and tuning (*dark blue*) molecules. A, B, D, and E are cyclins. *Arrows* indicate activation, and *lines ending in a crosshatch* indicate inhibition. K—cyclin-dependent kinase (Cdk); M—mitosis; Rb—retinoblastoma protein; S—S-phase.

levels of active Ras-GTP in NF1-derived schwannomas consistent with a GAP function of normal NF1 (Fig. 2-19). *VHL* is mutated in von Hippel-Lindau syndrome, predisposing to renal carcinoma and pheochromocytoma. Based on normal protein function as a competitive inhibitory subunit of a transcription elongation cofactor, its lack due to mutation may result in overexpression of specific proteins, including positive growth regulators. Mutational inactivation of APC expression in adenomatous polyposis coli activates the proto-oncogene β-catenin, which transactivates gene expression and is normally sequestered by APC in the cytoplasm. Viral oncoproteins such as E1A and E7 or cellular *MDM2* oncogene product exert their proliferative function by inhibiting suppressor gene products Rb, p27, or p53. All of these examples are compatible with proto-oncogene activation as a result of suppressor inactivation or suppressor inactivation as a consequence of oncogene activation. However, evidence is emerging for a more complex functional capacity of oncogenes and suppressor genes. Induction of senescence by expression of oncogenic *RAS*, which is associated with p53 and p16 expression, has already been mentioned. In addition to its oncogenic and immortalizing properties, Myc has been described to induce apoptosis under certain conditions, an effect that can be abrogated by IGF1. Finally, the normal *P53* suppressor gene induces expression of the *MDM2* proto-oncogene, which would be predicted to give rise to proliferative signals. Mutual regulation of *MDM2* and *P53* may indeed constitute an autoregulatory loop between a proto-oncogene and a suppressor gene. Such examples raise the possibility that heterogeneity of oncogene and suppressor gene function within a cell might be more diversified, either due to intrinsic functional properties or indirectly by interaction with other regulatory molecules [3,30–32].

The pleiotropism of malignant phenotypes is reflective of the heterogeneity of genetic changes acquired during cancer development. The number of genetic hits activating oncogenes or inactivating suppressor genes required for a tumor to arise from a normal cell varies among different tumors but can be projected within the first order of magnitude. Such estimates correlate with projected mutation probability of oncogenes or suppressor genes and age-dependent cancer incidence. Thereby, cumulative acquisition of mutations appears to be more crucial than a specific sequence of events to defeat an organism's natural protective barriers against cancer. A stepwise progression toward cancer has long been perceived by morphologic criteria as hyperplasia, metaplasia, and neoplasia describe incremental stages of deviation from normal tissue. In a genetic model for colorectal tumorigenesis, the stepwise accumulation of genetic lesions involved has been correlated with clinical and histopathologic progression towards colon cancer by Fearon and Vogelstein [33]. Deletions on 5q, 18q, and 17p reflect loss-of-function mutation of suppressor genes, whereas mutation of *KRAS* represents activation of an oncogene (Fig. 2-29). Hypomethylation is thought to contribute to chromosomal instability and may indirectly enhance loss of genetic material [1,2,33].

CLINICAL PERSPECTIVE

A selection of putative or exercised applications of oncogenic abnormalities associated with human cancer feature aspects of diagnostic and prognostic value (Table 2-5). Some of these, including detection of specific translocation breakpoints involving onco-

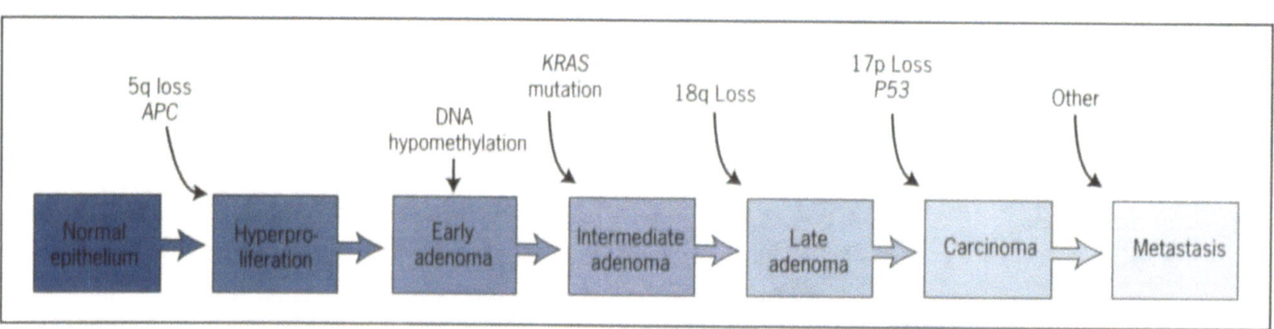

Figure 2-29. Multistep genetic process of tumorigenesis. The stepwise transition from normal epithelium to metastatic cancer in human colon carcinoma is paralleled by the cumulative acquisition of genetic lesions. (*Adapted from* Fearon and Vogelstein [33].)

Table 2-5. Clinical applicability of oncogene alterations

Tumor	Oncogene	Feature	Technique	Test	Application
Multiple endocrine neoplasia type 2A	*RET*	Point mutation	PCR sequence	Detection of germline mutations in PBL of presymptomatic carriers	Cancer risk assessment
Multiple endocrine neoplasia type 2B	*RET*	Point mutation	PCR sequence	Detection of germline mutations in PBL of presymptomatic carriers	Cancer risk assessment
Familial medullary thyroid carcinoma	*RET*	Point mutation	PCR sequence	Detection of germline mutations in PBL of presymptomatic carriers	Cancer risk assessment
Mammary carcinoma	*ERBB2*	Gene amplification, overexpression	Southern blot, quantitative PCR, immuno-blot, immunohistochemistry	Detection of elevated gene copy number or expression in tumor	Prognosis and adjuvant therapy, tumor imaging
Adenocarcinoma of lung and colon	K-*RAS*	Point mutation	PCR sequence	Detection of point mutation in tumor	Prognosis
Myelodysplasia	N-*RAS* K-*RAS*	Point mutation	PCR sequence	Detection of point mutation	Prognosis
Chronic myelogenous leukemia	*BCR-ABL*	Rearrangement	FISH, Southern blot, RT-PCR	Detection of break-point at DNA or RNA level	Diagnosis and monitoring of residual disease
Acute lymphocytic leukemia	*BCR-ABL*	Rearrangement	FISH, Southern blot, RT-PCR	Detection of break-point at DNA or RNA level	Diagnosis and monitoring of residual disease
Follicular B-cell lymphoma	*BCL-2*	Rearrangement	FISH, Southern blot, PCR	Breakpoint detection	Monitoring of residual disease
Burkitt's lymphoma	*MYC*	Translocation	FISH	Detection of translocation	Diagnosis
Neuroblastoma	N-*MYC*	Gene amplification	Southern blot, quantitative PCR	Assessment of gene copy number	Prognosis and therapy selection

genes in certain human leukemias or determination of *NMYC* gene amplification in neuroblastoma, have already entered clinical practice. Specific *RET* point mutations associated with cancer susceptibility in MEN2A, MEN2B, and FMTC represent examples of hereditary cancer in which autosomal dominant predisposition to disease has been linked to germline mutation of an oncogene as opposed to suppressor genes. Applicability of *RET* point mutations for cancer predisposition testing in MEN2A and MEN2B has been considered by the American Society of Clinical Oncology under class I criteria, along with testing of *RB1* in retinoblastoma, *VHL* in von Hippel-Lindau syndrome, and *APC* in familial adenomatous polyposis coli [34]. In addition to diagnostic applications, future therapeutic value can be envisioned in conditions in which oncogenic abnormalities can be targeted in a tumor-specific manner to interfere with the oncogenic alteration or to deliver cytotoxic compounds. In this context, *ERBB2* abnormalities in human breast and other epithelial cancer, as well as expression of specific fusion proteins by hematopoietic malignancies, hold the potential for future therapeutic applicability. Likewise, a treatment regimen ablating selectively the function of mutated RAS without interfering with the normal RAS proteins could have considerable therapeutic benefit [7,35].

REFERENCES

1. Knudson AG: Antioncogenes and human cancer. *Proc Natl Acad Sci USA* 1993, 90:10914–10921.
2. Weinberg RA: Oncogenes and tumor suppressor genes. *CA Cancer J Clin* 1994, 44:160–170.
3. Hunter T: Oncoprotein networks. *Cell* 1997, 88:333–346.
4. Weiss R, Teich N, Varmus H, Coffin J: *RNA Tumor Viruses.* Cold Spring Harbor, NY: Cold Spring Harbor Laboratory Press; 1985.
5. Weiss RA, Teich N, Varmus H, Coffin J: *Molecular Biology of Tumor Viruses.* Cold Spring Harbor, NY: Cold Spring Harbor Laboratory Press; 1984.
6. Lewin B: *Genes V.* New York: Oxford University Press; 1994.
7. Bishop JM: Molecular themes in oncogenesis. *Cell* 1991, 64:235–248.
8. Hunter T: Cooperation between oncogenes. *Cell* 1991, 64:249–270.
9. McCormick F: Signal transduction: how receptors turn Ras on. *Nature* 1993, 363:15–16.
10. Aaronson SA: Growth factors and cancer. *Science* 1991, 254:1146–1153.
11. Sherr CJ: Cancer cell cycles. *Science* 1996, 274:1672–1677.
12. Alberts B, Bray D, Lewis J, *et al.*: *Molecular Biology of the Cell.* New York: Garland Publishing; 1994.
13. Schmidt L, Duh FM, Chen F, *et al.*: Germline and somatic mutations in the tyrosine kinase domain of the MET proto-oncogene in papillary renal carcinomas. *Nat Genet* 1997, 16:68–73.
14. Cross M, Dexter TM: Growth factors in development, transformation, and tumorigenesis. *Cell* 1991, 64:271–280.
15. Schlessinger J: Signal transduction by allosteric receptor oligomerization. *Trends Biochem Sci* 1988, 13:443–447.
16. Heldin CH: Dimerization of cell surface receptors in signal transduction. *Cell* 1995, 80:213–223.
17. Nagata K, Ohashi K, Nakano T, *et al.*: Identification of the product of growth arrest-specific gene 6 as a common ligand for Axl, Sky, and Mer receptor tyrosine kinases. *J Biol Chem* 1996, 271:30022–30027.
18. Treanor JJ, Goodman L, de Sauvage F, *et al.*: Characterization of a multicomponent receptor for GDNF [comments]. *Nature* 1996, 382:80–83.
19. Tessier-Lavigne M: Eph receptor tyrosine kinases, axon repulsion, and the development of topographic maps. *Cell* 1995, 82:345–348.
20. van der Geer P, Hunter T, Lindberg RA: Receptor protein-tyrosine kinases and their signal transduction pathways. *Annu Rev Cell Biol* 1994, 10:251–337.
21. Di Fiore PP, Kraus MH: Mechanisms involving an expanding erbB/EGF receptor family of tyrosine kinases in human neoplasia. In *Genes, Oncogenes, and Hormones: Advances in Cellular and Molecular Biology of Breast Cancer.* Edited by Dickson RB, Lippman ME. Boston: Kluwer Academic Publishers; 1991:139–160.
22. Mak YF, Ponder BA: RET oncogene. *Curr Opin Genet Dev* 1996, 6:82–86.
23. Boguski MS, McCormick F: Proteins regulating Ras and its relatives. *Nature* 1993, 366:643–654.
24. Rabbitts TH: Chromosomal translocations in human cancer. *Nature* 1994, 372:143–149.
25. Pawson T: New impressions of Src and Hck [news; comment]. *Nature* 1997, 385:582–583, 585.
26. Farrow SN, Brown R: New members of the Bcl 2 family and their protein partners. *Curr Opin Genet Dev* 1996, 6:45–49.
27. Lewin B: Oncogenic conversion by regulatory changes in transcription factors. *Cell* 1991, 64:303–312.
28. Weinberg RA: The cat and mouse games that genes, viruses, and cells play. *Cell* 1997, 88:573–575.
29. Weinberg RA: Oncogenes, antioncogenes, and the molecular basis of multistep carcinogenesis. *Cancer Res* 1989, 49:3713–3721.
30. Levine AJ: p53, the cellular gatekeeper for growth and division. *Cell* 1997, 88:323–331.
31. Marshall CJ: Tumor suppressor genes. *Cell* 1991, 64:313–326.
32. Peifer M: Beta-catenin as oncogene: the smoking gun [comment]. *Science* 1997, 275:1752–1753.
33. Fearon ER, Vogelstein B: A genetic model for colorectal tumorigenesis. *Cell* 1990, 61:759–767.
34. Statement of the American Society of Clinical Oncology: Genetic testing for cancer susceptibility, Adopted on February 20, 1996. *J Clin Oncol* 14:1730–1740.
35. Sklar J: Principles of molecular cell biology of cancer: molecular approaches to cancer diagnosis. In *Cancer: Principles and Practice of Oncology.* Edited by De Vita VT, Hellman S, Rosenberg SA. Philadelphia: JB Lippincott; 1993:92–113.
36. Kraus MH, Popescu NC, Amsbaugh SC, King CR: Overexpression of the EGF receptor-related proto-oncogene erbB-2 in human mammary tumor cell lines by different molecular mechanisms. *EMBO J* 1987, 6:605–610.
37. Alimandi M, Romano A, Curia MC, *et al.*: Cooperative signaling of ErbB3 and ErbB2 in neoplastic transformation and human mammary carcinomas. *Oncogene* 1995, 10:1813–1821.
38. Santoro M, Carlomagno F, Romano A, *et al.*: Activation of RET as a dominant transforming gene by germline mutations of MEN2A and MEN2B. *Science* 1995, 267:381–383.
39. Kraus MH, Yuasa Y, Aaronson SA: A position 12-activated H-ras oncogene in all HS578T mammary carcinosarcoma cells but not normal mammary cells of the same patient. *Proc Natl Acad Sci USA* 1984, 81:5384–5388.
40. Graus-Porta D, Beerli RR, Daly JM, Hynes NE: ErbB-2, the preferred heterodimerization partner of all ErbB receptors, is a mediator of lateral signaling. *Embo J* 1997, 16:1647–1655.

CHAPTER

3

Tumor Suppressor Genes

Tracey L. Plank
Elizabeth Petri Henske

Tumor suppressor genes (TSGs) are genes whose protein products function in the control of cellular proliferation. In contrast to oncogenes, which are activated in cancer, TSGs are functionally inactivated in cancer. In general, TSGs are characterized by loss-of-function mutations in human tumors. These loss-of-function mutations can be missense mutations that alter critical amino acid residues, mutations that cause premature protein truncation resulting in the loss of functional domains or unstable products, or deletion of the entire gene. Loss-of-function mutations are often accompanied by loss of heterozygosity (LOH) at the TSG locus; LOH can be detected by comparing the pattern of a polymorphic DNA marker in tumor versus normal DNA (*see* Chapter 1).

According to the Knudson "two-hit" TSG model, which was initially proposed to explain the occurrence of familial and sporadic retinoblastoma [1], inactivating mutations in both alleles of a TSG are required to give a cell a growth advantage (Fig. 3-1). In an inherited cancer predisposition syndrome, the first inactivating mutation (*ie*, the first hit) occurs in the germline DNA and the mutation in the remaining wild-type copy of the gene (*ie*, the second hit) occurs somatically. Thus, a patient with a cancer predisposition syndrome who develops multiple tumors would be predicted to have different second-hit mutations in each tumor (Fig. 3-2). In cancers arising sporadically, both the first and the second hits occur somatically (Fig. 3-3).

PROPERTIES OF TUMOR SUPPRESSOR GENES

Most TSGs have three properties in common: (1) They are mutated in inherited cancer predisposition syndromes. (2) Somatic mutations are found in spontaneous tumors, often of the same pathologic types that occur in the associated inherited syndrome. (3) They are able to inhibit the growth of transformed cells in vitro. There is, however, no single definition of what constitutes a TSG. Some authors feel that TSGs should meet all three of these criteria [2]. Others prefer more simple definitions such as "genes that sustain loss-of-function mutations in the development of cancer" [3] or "genes whose expression is reduced or lost in cancer cells" [4].

Many TSGs have been identified and cloned because they are mutated in familial cancer syndromes. In many instances, sporadic cancers of similar histologic types are found to have inactivating mutations in the same TSGs involved in the familial syndrome. For example, von Hippel-Lindau disease (VHL) is a rare syndrome characterized by benign and malignant neoplasms of multiple organs [5]. The most frequent tumors include central nervous system hemangioblastomas, clear cell renal carcinomas, and pheochromocytomas. Somatic inactivation of the wild-type copy of *VHL* occurs in tumors of patients with VHL [6]. Consistent with Knudson's model, 85% of clear cell renal carcinomas from patients who do not have VHL, also have inactivation of both copies of the *VHL* gene [7]. In other important examples, however, the genes responsible for inherited cancer syndromes do not appear to play a major role in the pathogenesis of sporadic cancers. For example, *BRCA1* and *BRCA2*, which are mutated in the germline of some families with inherited breast and ovarian cancer syndromes, appear to be rarely mutated in sporadic breast and ovarian cancers.

TUMORIGENESIS AS A MULTISTEP PROCESS

Although inactivating mutations in TSGs appear to be key early events in the development of most cancers, the development of a malignant tumor is a multistep process (Fig. 3-4) that involves mutations in additional TSGs and oncogenes [8]. Many inherited TSG syndromes are characterized by both benign and malignant tumors. This supports the multistep model of tumorigenesis. Because functional loss of both copies of a TSG is predicted to be only the first step in the development of cancer, tumors that sustain a small number of additional inactivating mutations would be expected to remain benign, whereas tumors that sustain a large number of inactivating mutations could become malignant. In some TSG syndromes, such as tuberous sclerosis and neurofibromatosis, the vast majority of tumors remain benign.

GATEKEEPER AND CARETAKER TUMOR SUPPRESSOR GENE MODELS

Kinzler and Vogelstein [9] have proposed a division of TSGs into two categories: gatekeepers and caretakers. Caretakers are genes responsible for maintaining the integrity of the genome, whereas gatekeepers play

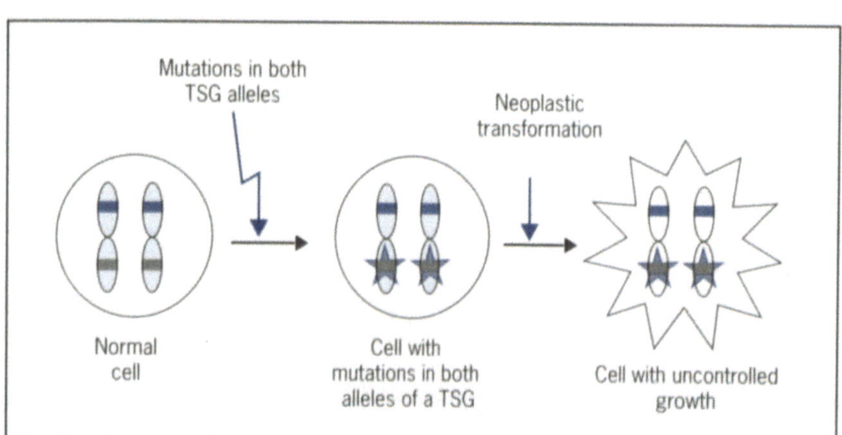

Figure 3-1. Mutations in both alleles of a tumor suppressor gene (TSG) lead to neoplastic transformation and uncontrolled cell growth. A normal cell has two copies of a TSG. After mutation occurs in both alleles, loss of TSG function contributes to unrestrained cell growth.

a direct role in the control of cellular proliferation of specific cell types. In this model, each cell type has only a small number of gatekeepers, and mutations in these gatekeeper genes lead to tumors in only their respective cell types. For example, mutations in the *VHL* gene lead to clear cell renal carcinomas but not to renal tumors of other pathologic types, suggesting that *VHL* is a gatekeeper for a specific type of renal epithelial cell. Similarly, mutations in *RB* lead to retinoblastomas, and mutations in *APC* lead to colonic tumors, suggesting that these genes are gatekeepers for retinal epithelial cells and colonic epithelial cells, respectively.

In contrast, inactivation of caretaker genes does not directly lead to tumor initiation, but to genetic instability with an increased rate of mutation for all genes, including gatekeepers. For a tumor to develop in a patient who has inherited a mutant caretaker gene, such as *MLH1* or *MSH2*, the remaining normal allele of the gene must be mutated, followed by mutations in both alleles of a gatekeeper gene (Fig. 3-5). Based on this model, the frequency of cancer in individuals with an inherited caretaker mutation is predicted to be less than that in individuals with an inherited gatekeeper mutation, because only one additional mutation is required in the gatekeeper model (*eg*, inactivation of the wild-type copy of *VHL*). In the caretaker model, three additional mutations are required (*eg*, inactivation of the wild-type copy of *MLH 1*, followed by inactivation of both copies of another TSG such as *APC*). Similarly, the incidence of caretaker mutations in sporadic cancers

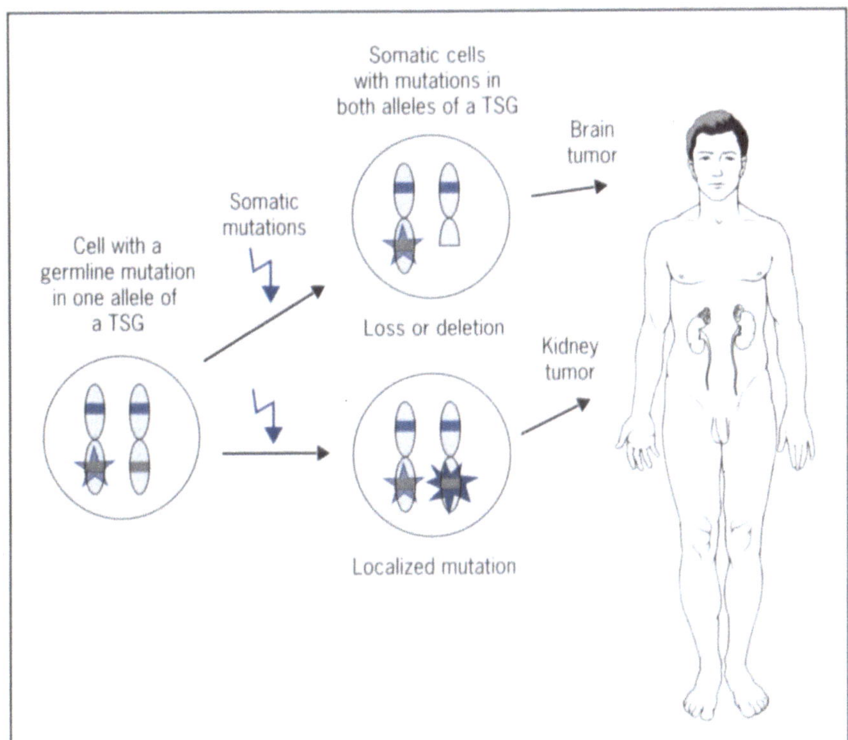

Figure 3-2. Somatic mutation leads to tumorigenesis in an inherited tumor suppressor gene (TSG) syndrome. A germline mutation in one allele of a TSG is transmitted to an individual's offspring (*ie*, the first hit). During a somatic cell event, the remaining normal allele can be mutated (*ie*, the second hit) resulting in loss of both copies of the TSG. This somatic mutation can be a point mutation that inactivates the protein or a deletion that removes part or all of the gene. Different second hits in somatic cells give rise to cancers in their respective organs. If multiple tumors occur in a single organ, each would be predicted to have a different, independently arising second-hit mutation.

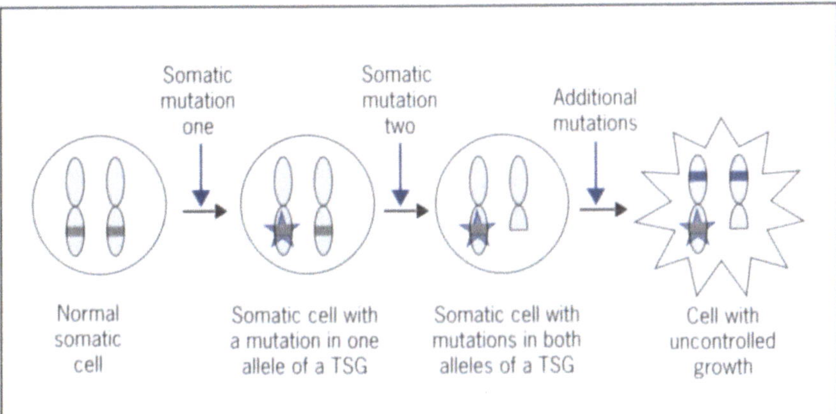

Figure 3-3. The two-hit mechanism for the development of sporadic cancers. The somatic cells of a normal individual will have two wild-type copies of a tumor suppressor gene (TSG). A primary somatic mutation event (*ie*, the first hit) will inactivate one allele of the TSG. A second mutation (*ie*, the second hit) in the remaining copy of the TSG will lead to a loss of functional tumor suppressor protein and uncontrolled cell growth.

might be predicted to be lower than that of gatekeeper mutations, because only one additional mutation is required in the gatekeeper model [9]. Multiple lines of evidence suggest that *BRCA1* and *BRCA2* function as caretakers; this could in part explain the low frequency of mutations in these genes in sporadic breast and ovarian cancers.

von Hippel-Lindau disease is an example of a TSG syndrome whose clinical manifestations fit the gatekeeper model. The penetrance of VHL is high; tumors occur at a young age, with an average age of onset of 30 years for central nervous system hemangioblastomas and pheochromocytomas, and 33 years for renal cell carcinomas; and sporadic tumors of similar histologic type contain inactivating *VHL* mutations. Hereditary nonpolyposis colon carcinoma (HNPCC) is an example of a TSG syndrome fitting the caretaker model. HNPCC is associated with mutations in the mismatch repair genes *MSH2* and *MLH1* that are responsible for the recognition and repair of DNA breaks and mutations. HNPCC is characterized by tumors of multiple organs, including the colon and uterus. Consistent with the caretaker model, the penetrance of HNPCC is lower than that of VHL, the tumors often arise in later adulthood, and the incidence of mutations in sporadic tumors of similar pathologic type [10] is lower than that in VHL.

GENOTYPE–PHENOTYPE CORRELATIONS

In general, the type of inactivating mutations in TSGs tend to be diverse and spread throughout the gene, consistent with the concept that any mutations caus-

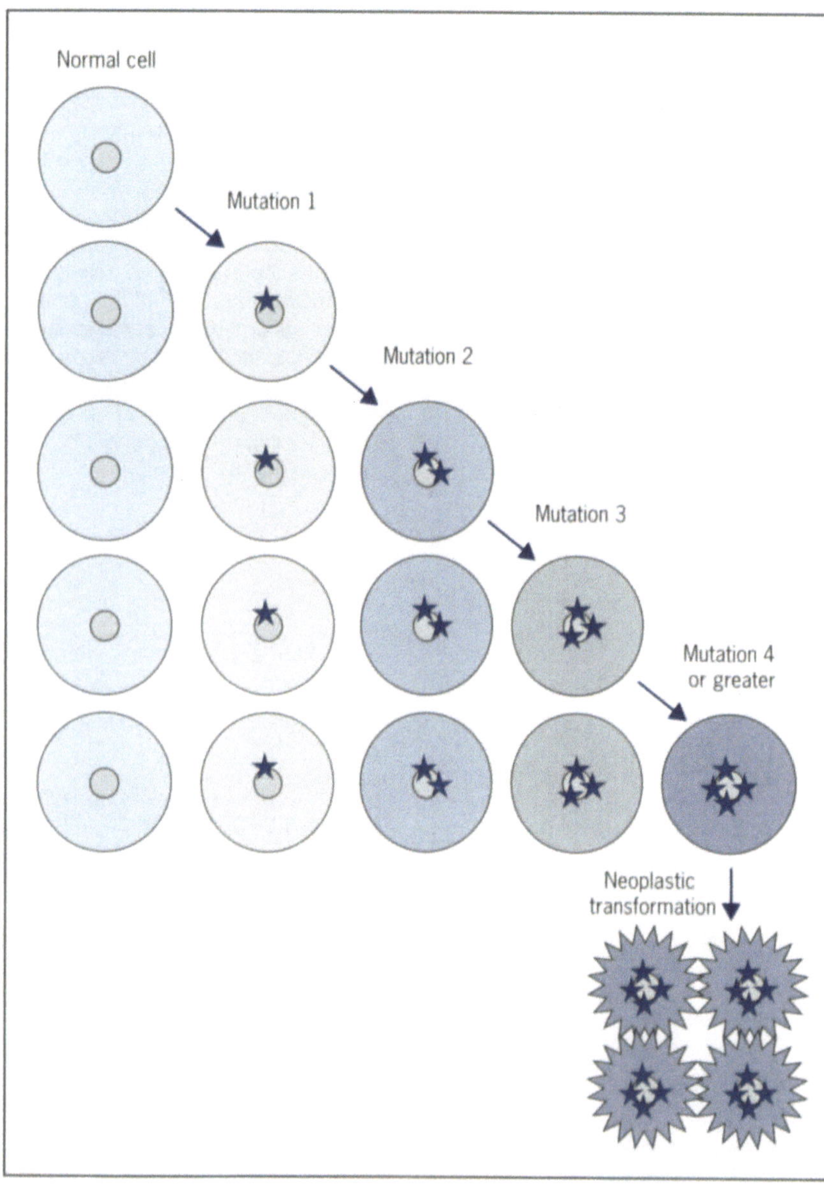

Figure 3-4. Multiple mutations lead to tumor development. Although the exact number of mutations required for the development of a malignant tumor is unknown, neoplastic transformation has been shown to be a multistep process in many cancers. After a primary mutation occurs in an oncogene or tumor suppressor gene, subsequent mutations in other genes may follow during tumorigenesis. The mutations necessary for tumorigenesis can cause an increase in cell proliferation signals and a decrease in apoptotic signals. The accumulation of these various mutations provides a cell with a growth advantage that eventually leads to immortalization and transformation.

ing loss of protein function have the same ultimate effect on cellular proliferation. However, several TSGs exhibit important genotype-phenotype correlations. A genotype-phenotype correlation indicates that specific types of mutations are associated with specific manifestations of the disease. For example, the spectrum of inactivating mutations in VHL families include missense mutations, nonsense mutations, small deletions and insertions, and splice site mutations. However, among the subset of families with adrenal pheochromocytoma, more than 90% have missense mutations [11]. The underlying cellular processes responsible for this have not been elucidated. Other examples of genotype-phenotype correlations include familial adenomatosis polyposis coli, in which mutations in the carboxy-terminus of *APC* are associated with an attenuated form of the disease, with a 90% reduction in the number of colonic polyps [12]; and neurofibromatosis type 2, in which a milder form of the disease is associated with point mutations [13]. As more genotype-phenotype correlations are identified, they may be useful in counseling patients about risk for specific disease complications.

TUMOR SUPPRESSOR GENE FUNCTIONS

Tumor suppressor genes encode a diverse group of proteins that are located in different cellular compartments and function in a wide range of cellular pathways. TSGs are found in the nucleus (*RB1, TP53, WT1*), the Golgi apparatus (*TSC2*) and the cytoplasm (*APC*; Table 3-1). The putative functions of known TSGs include cell cycle regulation (*RB1*), transcriptional regulation (*TP53, WT1*), DNA repair (*MSH2, MLH1, TP53*), signaling through small G proteins including RAS (*NF1*) and RAB5 (*TSC2*), and regulation of cell adhesion (*APC*). To illustrate what is known about TSG functions, four TSG pathways involving *RB1, TP53, P15/P16*, and mismatch repair are discussed in detail in the following sections.

THE RB1 TUMOR SUPPRESSOR GENE

The retinoblastoma TSG, *RB1*, encodes a protein product (RB) that functions at the center of cell cycle regulation [14–17]. RB is a regulatory link between the cell cycle clock and the transcription of genes necessary for progression from G_1 to S-phase. The phosphorylation state of RB regulates progression through the cell cycle (Fig. 3-6). RB contains 12 potential serine and threonine phosphorylation sites, and inhibition of phosphorylation results in growth arrest. RB is hypophosphorylated in quiescent cells in G_0/G_1, hyperphosphorylated at the end of G_1, and dephosphorylated during mitosis. The mitogenic stimulation of cells activates the synthesis of D-type cyclins, which associate to form a binary complex with cyclin-dependent kinases (CDKs). The cyclin D-CDK com-

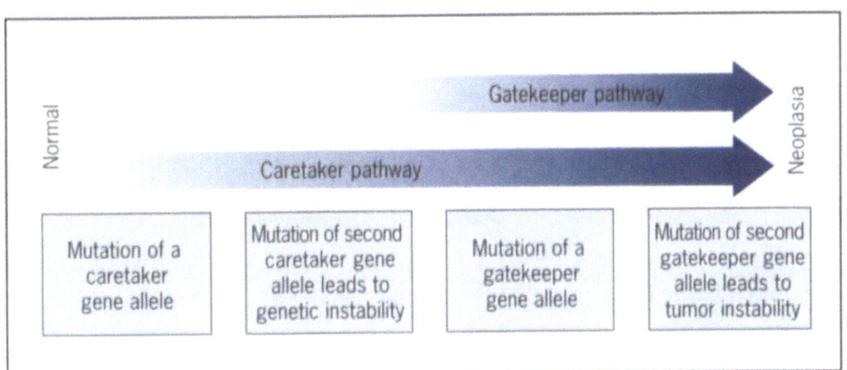

Figure 3-5. The gatekeeper and caretaker models for tumor suppressor genes. Mutations in caretaker and gatekeeper genes are involved in neoplastic transformation. Gatekeeper genes are directly involved in regulating the growth of cells. Mutations in both copies of a gatekeeper gene will lead to neoplasia. Mutations in caretaker genes do not directly initiate tumor formation. However, mutations in both alleles of a caretaker gene promote genetic instability and increase the susceptibility of the cell to mutations in a gatekeeper gene, resulting in neoplastic initiation. In the gatekeeper pathway, only one additional mutation (in the remaining copy of the gatekeeper gene) is required for the initiation of neoplasia. In the caretaker model, three additional mutations are required: mutation of the remaining copy of the caretaker gene, leading to genetic instability, and mutation of both alleles of a gatekeeper gene. (*From* Kinzler and Vogelstein [9]; with permission.)

plexes become catalytically active following phosphorylation by CDK-activating kinase (CAK). The cyclin D-CDK holoenzymes are responsible for the phosphorylation of RB. Hypophosphorylated RB binds to and inhibits the function of the transcription factor E2F, whose function is required for entry into S-phase. This RB-E2F complex arrests the growth of the cell in G_1, providing a checkpoint at which the cell can determine if all the events necessary for entry into S-phase are complete. The growth suppression by RB is

Table 3-1. Chromosomal and cellular locations of selected tumor suppressor genes and gene products

Gene	Chromosomal location	Neoplasm	Cellular location of gene product
APC	5q21	Colorectal cancer	Cytoplasm
P53	17p13.1	Sarcomas, gliomas, carcinomas	Nucleus
RB	13q14	Retinoblastoma, sarcomas, carcinomas	Nuclear matrix
MLH1	3q21.3-p23	Hereditary nonpolyposis colon carcinoma	Nucleus
MSH2	2p22-p21	Hereditary nonpolyposis colon carcinoma	Nucleus
TSC1	9q34.1	Hamartomas	Cytoplasm
TSC2	16p13.3	Hamartomas	Golgi complex
INK4A	9q21	Multiple cancers	Nucleus
INK4B	9p21	Non–small cell lung cancer and others	Nucleus
NF1	17q11.2	Neurofibromatosis type 1	Cytoplasm
WT1	11p12	Wilms' tumor	Nucleus
BRCA1	17q21	Familial breast cancer	Nucleus
BRCA2	13q12-13	Breast and ovarian carcinomas	Nucleus

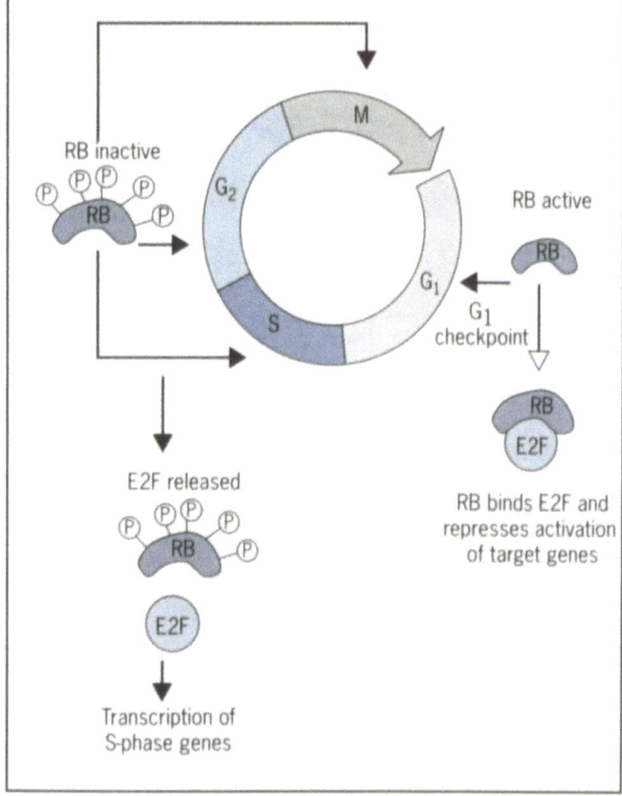

Figure 3-6. The product of the *RB* gene, RB, functions at the center of cell proliferation. The phosphorylation state of RB regulates cell cycle progression. During early G_1, RB is hypophosphorylated and binds to and sequesters the transcription factor E2F. Cell cycle progression arrests at the G_1 checkpoint before entering S-phase (S). After the G_1 checkpoint (late in G_1), RB becomes hyperphosphorylated, releasing E2F, and the cell cycle advances to S-phase. Late in mitosis (M), before entry into G_0/G1, RB is dephosphorylated.

relieved by phosphorylation of RB by cyclin-CDK complexes, resulting in the release of E2F and progression of the cell cycle.

Germline mutations in the *RB1* gene occur in familial retinoblastoma, which is characterized by retinoblastomas that are often bilateral and multifocal. Mutations in *RB1* usually result in the loss of protein product and, because of mutations in both alleles of the TSG in retinoblastoma cells, no RB protein is present. The absence of RB eliminates the G_1 checkpoint (Fig. 3-7) because the regulation by RB of the transcription factor E2F (*see* Fig. 3-6) is relieved, and the cell is free to enter S-phase unrestricted.

THE TP53 TUMOR SUPPRESSOR GENE

Normal cells stop their progression through the cell cycle when nuclear DNA is damaged; damage to DNA can result in the arrest of the cell cycle at checkpoints in the G_1, S, or G_2 phase of the cell cycle. DNA damage induces the expression of p53 protein, which is a critical regulator of cell cycle progression. The p53 protein regulates only the G_1/S checkpoint and induces cell cycle arrest or apoptosis, depending on the phase of the cell cycle at which the DNA damage occurs (Fig. 3-8). When DNA damage occurs early in the G_1 phase of the cell

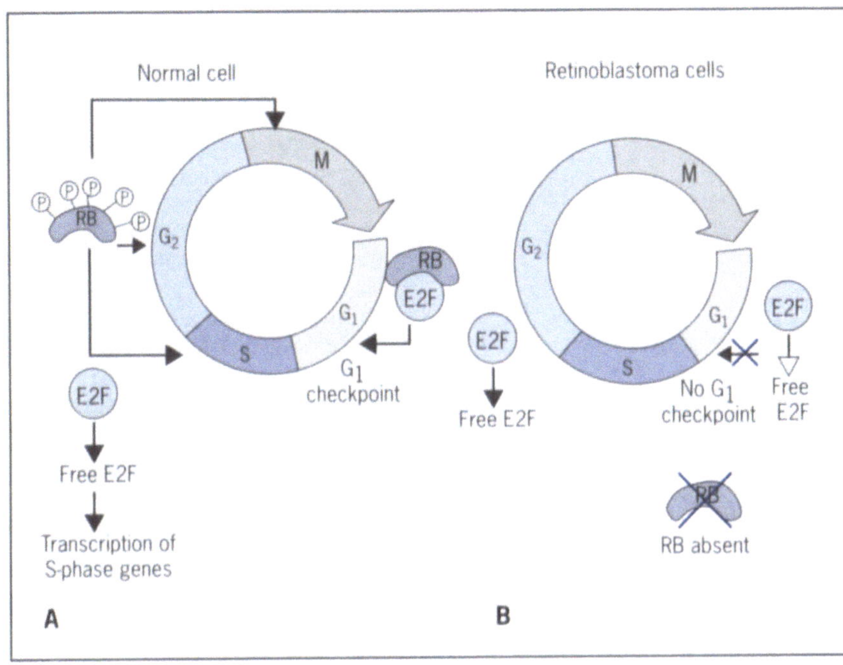

Figure 3-7. Cell proliferation is unregulated in retinoblastoma cells. **A**, In normal cells, RB sequesters E2F in G_1, and growth is arrested at the G_1 checkpoint. After mitogenic stimulation, when the cell is ready to enter S-phase (S), RB is phosphorylated, releasing E2F. **B**, In retinoblastoma cells, RB is absent, so there is no regulation of the cell cycle clock by the transcriptional control mechanisms responsible for the progression from G_1 to S-phase. E2F is free and cell cycle progression is unrestrained, leading to uncontrolled cellular proliferation.

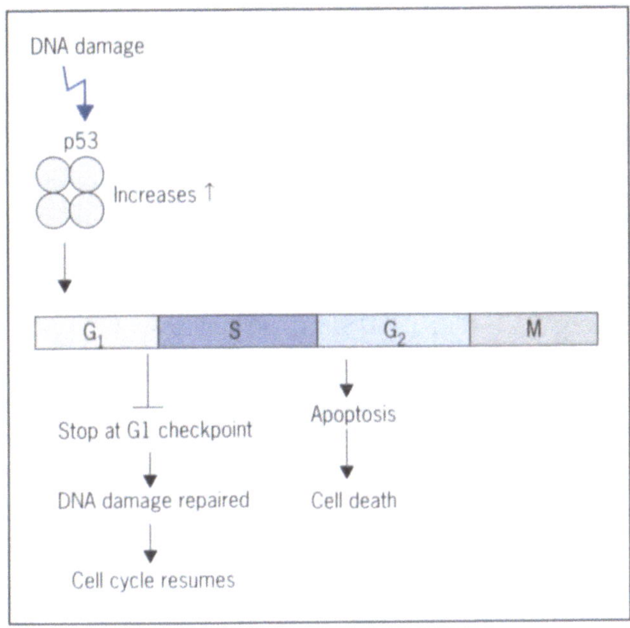

Figure 3-8. Induction of cell cycle arrest or apoptosis by p53. The p53 protein is a critical component of cell cycle regulation that induces cycle arrest at the G_1 checkpoint following DNA damage. In cells with damaged DNA, the levels of p53 protein are upregulated. If the DNA damage occurs early in G_1, the cell cycle will arrest at the G_1 checkpoint until the damage is repaired. After the damage is repaired, the cell will enter S-phase (S). If the damage occurs beyond the G_1 checkpoint, the cells will undergo apoptosis. M—mitosis.

cycle, the level of p53 in a cell increases, resulting in growth arrest at the G_1 checkpoint. Arrest at this checkpoint provides the cell time to repair the damaged DNA before progressing into S-phase. After the damage is repaired, the p53 level declines and the cell cycle progresses. If the damage occurs later in the cell cycle, past the G_1 restriction point, or is too severe for repair, p53 triggers a program of cell death [15–18].

The *TP53* TSG encodes a transcription factor that is a critical component of the cell cycle regulatory network. Following DNA damage, the increased level of p53 protein in the cell induces the transcriptional activation of a CDK-inhibitory protein, $p21^{WAF1/CIP1}$. In proliferating cells, cyclin/cdk complexes are responsible for phosphorylating the tumor suppressor protein RB, which binds to and sequesters the E2F family of transcription factors. When RB is hyperphosphorylated by the cyclin-CDK complexes, E2F is released and is free to bind to regulatory regions of genes responsible for DNA synthesis and entry into S-phase. Before the cyclin-CDK complexes can phosphorylate RB, they must be activated by a CAK. $p21^{WAF1/CIP1}$ sterically inhibits the phosphorylation of the cyclin-CDK complexes by CAK and inhibits the enzymatic activity of any holoenzyme that is already activated. The inactive cyclin-CDK complexes are unable to phosphorylate

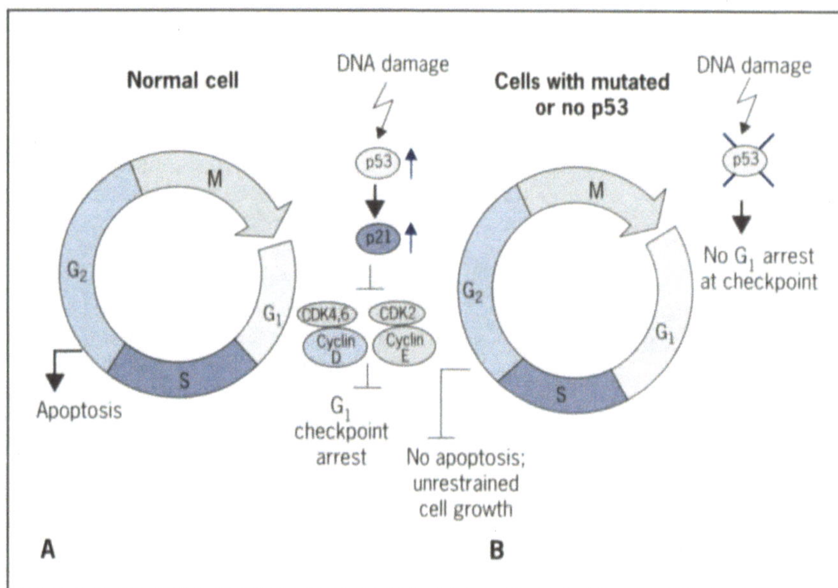

Figure 3-9. Induction of p53 after DNA damage. **A**, After DNA damage, the level of p53 protein in a cell increases, activating the transcription of $p21^{WAF1/CIP1}$, which inhibits the activity of the cyclin-cyclin-dependent kinase (CDK) complexes, cyclin D-CDK4,6 and cyclin E-CDK2. If the DNA damage occurs early in G_1, the cell cycle will arrest at the G_1 checkpoint until the damage is repaired. If the damage occurs later in the cell cycle or is too severe for repair, the cell will undergo apoptosis. **B**, Cells without p53 will fail to undergo the G_1/S checkpoint arrest and p53-induced apoptosis. The cell cycle will progress uncontrolled.

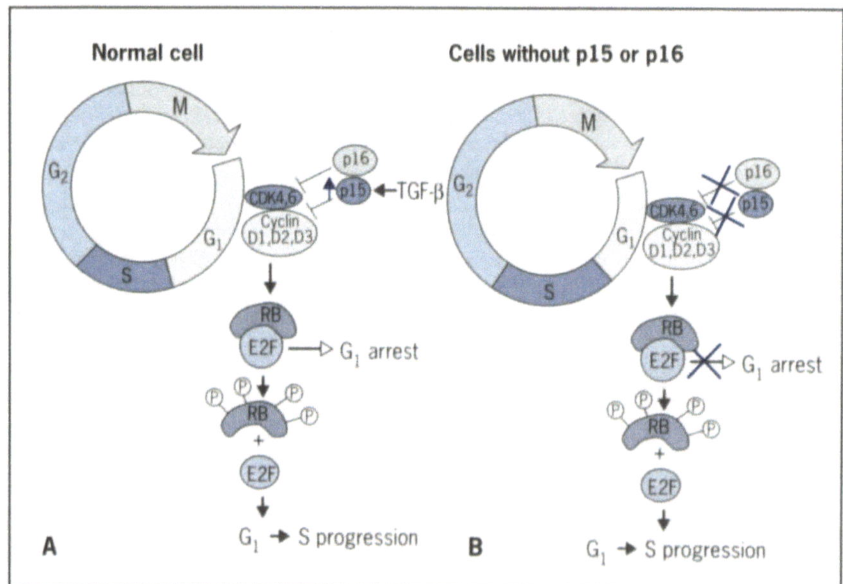

Figure 3-10. The INK4 family of cyclin-dependent kinase inhibitors regulate G_1 progression. **A**, During the G_1 phase of the cell cycle, $p16^{INK4}$ and $p15^{INK4B}$ inhibit the assembly of cyclin D with CDK4 or CDK6. The inactive cyclin D-CDK4,6 holoenzymes are unable to phosphorylate RB, preventing the release of E2F. Cell cycle progression is then arrested at the G_1 checkpoint. **B**, In tumor cells without functional p15 or p16, the cyclin D-CDK4,6 binary complexes are assembled and phosphorylate RB, leading to the release of E2F. The cell cycle progresses through G_1 to S-phase (S) unregulated. M—mitosis.

RB, therefore E2F is not released, and the cell cycle arrests at the G_1 restriction point. If the DNA damage occurs after the G_1 restriction point or is too severe for repair, the cell will arrest transiently in S-phase and may undergo apoptosis in G_2 before undergoing mitosis (Fig. 3-9). In cells that do not express p53 or that have mutations in the *TP53* gene resulting in the loss of p53 protein function, the G_1/S cell cycle checkpoint is absent, leading to unregulated progression of the cell cycle. The inappropriate replication of damaged DNA and failure of cells destined for apoptosis to undergo programmed cell death contributes to malignant transformation.

THE INK4 FAMILY OF TUMOR SUPPRESSOR GENES

One of the families of proteins that inhibit progression of the cell cycle by regulating the activities of cyclin-dependent kinases is the *INK4* family (Fig. 3-10). Cell cycle progression from G_1 to S-phase is negatively regulated by $p16^{INK4}$ and $p15^{INK4B}$. In the mammalian cell cycle, RB is one of the key regulators of progression from G_1 to S-phase. In G_1, RB is present in a hypophosphorylated form that binds the transcription factor E2F and blocks the activation of E2F-responsive genes whose products are required for S-phase entry and DNA synthesis. This G_1 arrest provides the cell a regulatory checkpoint to determine whether all the events necessary for S-phase entry have been completed. Progression to S-phase is accomplished by the inactivation of pRb by phosphorylation and the concurrent release of E2F. The phosphorylation of RB is regulated by cyclin-dependent kinase complexes including cyclin D-CDK4 and cyclin D-CDK6 [17,19], as discussed earlier.

MISMATCH REPAIR GENES

Defects in the genes responsible for mismatch repair have been linked to both inherited and sporadic cancer susceptibility. The mismatch repair genes provide one of the mechanisms involved in the correction of single base mismatches and small insertions and deletions resulting from errors in DNA replication, recombination, or chemical modification. The familial cancer syndrome HNPCC is associated with mutations in three of the mismatch repair genes: *MSH2, MLH1*, and *PMS2*. There is an increased risk for colon, uterine, ovarian, and urothelial cancers in patients with HNPCC. Mutations in the mismatch repair genes lead to microsatellite instability and the accumulation of frameshift and base substitution mutations throughout the genome. Microsatellite instability refers to an unstable pattern of DNA replication at tracts of repetitive DNA sequences [*eg*, dinucleotide repeats such as (GT)n] termed microsatellites.

Mismatches in DNA are recognized and bound by heterodimers of MSH2/MSH6 or MSH2/MSH3 (Fig. 3-11). Single base mismatches are preferentially recognized by MSH2/MSH6 heterodimers, whereas larger insertions or deletions are recognized by both MSH2/MSH6 and MSH2/MSH3. After recognition of the mismatch by the MSH2 heterodimer, a second heterodimer comprised of MLH1 and PMS2 is recruited for repair. The correct DNA sequence is restored by excision of the mismatched bases, synthesis of the correct bases, and re-ligation of the DNA strand [20–25].

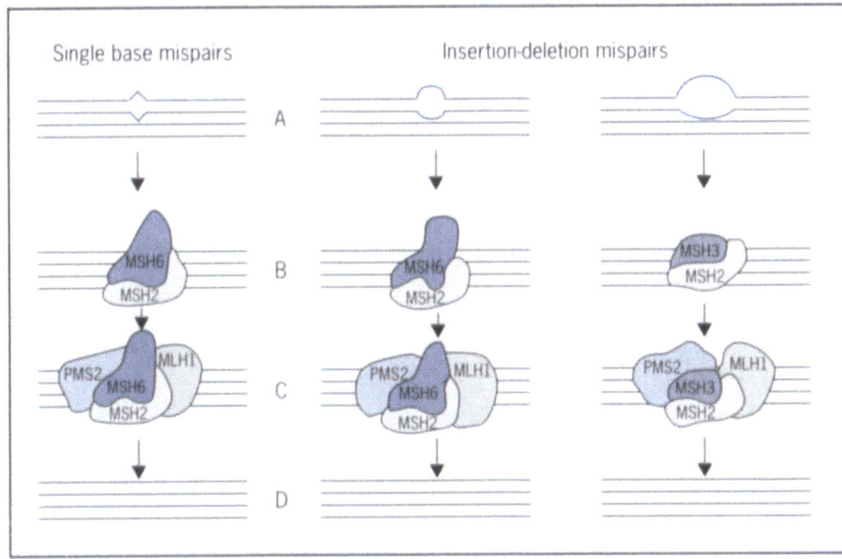

Figure 3-11. Model for the recognition of mismatched bases or insertion and deletion loops in eukaryotes. **A**, Single base mismatches or insertion/deletion loops occur during replication. **B**, Single base mismatches and small insertion/deletion loops are recognized by a heterodimer of MSH2 and MSH6. Larger insertion/deletion loops are bound by a heterodimer of MSH2 and MSH3. **C**, After recognition of the mismatch by these heterodimers, MLH1 and PMS2 are recruited for repair. **D**, The correct DNA sequence is restored after excision of the mismatched bases, resynthesis of the correct DNA sequence, and ligation of the newly synthesized strands. (*Adapted from* Marsischky *et al.* [25]; with permission.)

REFERENCES

1. Knudson A: Mutation and cancer: statistical study of retinoblastoma. *Proc Natl Acad Sci USA* 1971, 68:820–823.
2. Clurman B, Groudine M: Defining tumour-suppressor genes. *Nature* 1997, 389:123.
3. Haber D, Harlow E: Tumour-suppressor genes: evolving definitions in the genomic age. *Nat Genet* 1997, 16:320–322.
4. Knudson A: Antioncogenes and human cancer. *Proc Natl Acad Sci USA* 1993, 90:10914–10921.
5. Neumann H, Lips C, Hsia Y, Zbar B: Von Hippel-Lindau syndrome. *Brain Pathol* 1995, 5:181–193.
6. Prowse A, Webster A, Richards F, *et al.*: Somatic inactivation of the VHL gene in von Hippel-Lindau disease tumors. *Am J Hum Genet* 1997, 60:765–771.
7. Foster K, Prowse A, van den Berg A, *et al.*: Somatic mutations of the von Hippel-Lindau disease TSG in non-familial clear cell renal carcinoma. *Hum Mol Genet* 1994, 3:2169–2173.
8. Fearon E, Vogelstein B: A genetic model for colorectal tumorigenesis. *Cell* 1990, 61:759–767.
9. Kinzler K, Vogelstein B: Gatekeepers and caretakers. *Nature* 1997, 386:761–763.
10. Moslein G, Tester D, Lindor N, *et al.*: Microsatellite instability and mutation analysis of hMSH2 and HMLH1 in patients with sporadic, familial and hereditary colorectal cancer. *Hum Mol Genet* 1996, 5:1245–1252.
11. Neumann H, Bender B: Genotype-phenotype correlations in von Hippel-Lindau disease. *J Intern Med* 1998, 243:541–545.
12. Spirio L, Olschwant S, Groden J, *et al.*: Alleles of the APC gene: an attenuated form of familial polyposis. *Cell* 1993, 75:951–957.
13. Gutmann D, Geist R, Xu H, *et al.*: Defects in neurofibromatosis 2 protein function can arise at multiple levels. *Hum Mol Genet* 1998, 7:335–345.
14. Lin S-C, Skapek S, Lee E-H: Genes in the RB pathway and their knockout in mice. *Semin Cancer Biol* 1996, 7:279–289.
15. Jacks T, Weinberg R: The expanding role of cell cycle regulators. *Science* 1998, 280:1035.
16. Hesketh R: *The Oncogene and Tumor Suppressor Gene Facts Book.* San Diego, CA: Academic Press; 1997.
17. Chin L, Pomerantz J, DePinho R: The INK4a/ARF tumor suppressor: one gene, two products, two pathways. *TIBS* 1998, 23:291.
18. Helin K, Peters G: Tumor suppressors: from genes to function and possible therapies. *Trends Genet* 1998, 14:8–9.
19. Reynisdottir I, Polyak K, Iavarone A, Masague J: Kip/Cip and Ink4 Cdk inhibitors cooperate to induce cell cycle arrest in response to TGF-5. *Genes Dev* 1995, 9:1931–1945.
20. Kolodner R: Mismatch repair: mechanisms and relationship to cancer susceptibility. *TIBS* 1995, 20:397.
21. Kolodner R: Biochemistry and genetics of eukaryotic mismatch repair. *Genes Dev* 1996, 10:1433–1442.
22. Prolla T, Abruin A, Bradley A: DNA mismatch repair deficient mice in cancer research. *Semin Cancer Biol* 1996, 7:241–247.
23. Karran P: Appropriate partners make good matches. *Science* 1995, 268:1857.
24. Kunkel T, Resnick M, Gordenin D: Mutators specificity and disease: looking over the FENce. *Cell* 1997, 88:155–158.
25. Marsischky G, Filosi M, Kane M, Kolodner R: Redundancy of saccharomyces cerevisiae MSH3 and MSH6 in MSH2-dependent mismatch repair. *Genes Dev* 1996, 10:407–429.

CHAPTER

4

Mitogenic Signal Transduction

Jonathan Chernoff

The ability to sense and respond to environmental signals is fundamental to the development and survival of all organisms. At the cellular level, external cues such as temperature, osmotic pressure, presence or absence of nutrients, and presence or absence of specific hormones or growth factors are continuously monitored. The process of perceiving and responding to such signals is termed signal transduction.

This chapter provides an overview of signal transduction mechanisms that affect cell proliferation and morphology. This chapter focuses on mammalian cells, because control of signaling is relevant to the pathogenesis of human malignancies; however, it should be noted that the elements of many signaling pathways are highly conserved in all eukaryotes. The high degree of conservation among signaling pathways has made genetically tractable model organisms such as yeast, fruit flies, and roundworms valuable tools in determining the organization of signaling systems in humans.

Signal transduction entails the reception and transmission of environmental cues, resulting in appropriate biologic responses.

The basic elements of such systems include an external signal, a receptor, one or more signal transducing molecules, and one or more effectors, which ultimately induce the relevant physiologic responses. These responses most often entail changes in gene expression; however, signals may also directly regulate other processes such as the structure of the actin cytoskeleton, which affects cell shape, movement, and adhesion.

IMPORTANCE OF SIGNALING IN CANCER BIOLOGY

In malignant growth, proliferative signal transduction has, by definition, gone awry. The initiation and development of tumors is accompanied by the gradual and progressive loss of a series of key growth control pathways. At the genetic level, loss of growth control is usually initiated by acquired or inherited damage to tumor suppressor genes (*see* Chapter 3), but is also often accompanied by activating mutations or amplifications of proto-oncogenes. The vast majority of tumor suppressor genes and proto-oncogenes encode proteins that play important roles in normal signal transduction. Damage to these genes is thought to lead to dysregulated cell growth, in large part by uncoupling this process from exogenous growth factors (Fig. 4-1).

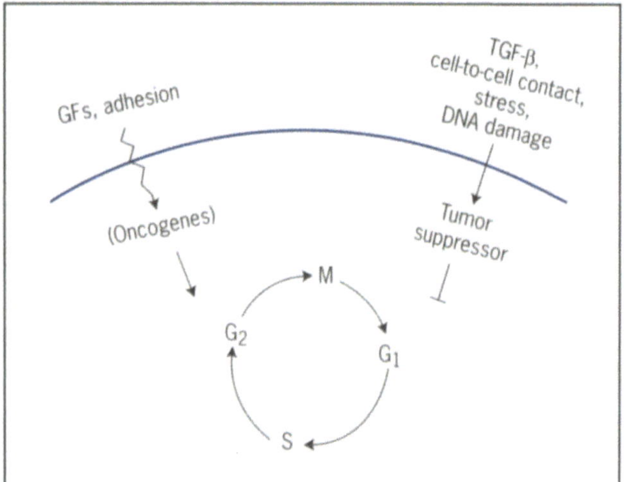

Figure 4-1. Cells respond to both positive and negative growth signals. Cell growth is normally under strict control, responding to a balance of proliferative and growth inhibitory signals. Growth factors (GFs) such as insulin, epidermal growth factor, and platelet derived growth factor provide a stimulatory signal, whereas other factors, such as transforming growth factor beta (TGF-β) and nonhumoral signals provided by cell-to-cell contact stress, or DNA damage, instruct the cell to cease proliferating. Many oncogene products are found among the growth stimulatory machinery, whereas tumor suppressor products often activate growth suppression pathways.

GENERAL STRUCTURE OF SIGNALING PATHWAYS

Transmission of signals for growth control often depends on the ability of one protein to structurally modify a second protein. For example, protein kinases catalyze the addition of phosphate groups to serine, threonine, or tyrosine residues in target proteins. Phosphorylation can induce conformational changes resulting in altered enzymatic activity, location, stability, or ability to associate with other molecules. Other protein modifications important in signal transduction include the addition of guanine nucleotides, lipids, carbohydrates, and ubiquitin moieties to recipient proteins. As with phosphorylation, these modifications can have profound effects on the properties of the target protein.

At the level of the cell, signal transduction begins with the binding of a signaling molecule to its receptor. Binding leads to conformation changes typically associated with oligomerization of the receptor and, in the case of most growth factor (mitogen) receptors, activation of its enzymatic properties. On activation, mitogen receptors attract a variety of intracellular signaling molecules that are required to transmit the signal to the interior of the cell. Such signaling molecules include enzymes, such as protein and lipid kinases and phosphatases, phospholipases, and GTPase accelerating proteins; and adaptor proteins that lack enzyme activity but serve to link additional signaling molecules to the receptor. One key target for these intracellular signaling proteins is the small GTPase, RAS, which acts as a molecular switch (discussed later). When turned on, RAS activates a cascade of protein kinases and other effectors that ultimately link the mitogenic signal to the nucleus (via transcription factors) and to the cytoskeleton (via actin binding proteins; Fig. 4-2).

In addition to soluble mitogens, adherent cells also receive proliferative input from contact with the extracellular matrix, which contains proteins that bind to adhesion receptors. As with growth factor receptors, engagement of these adhesion receptors, termed integrins, activates a cascade of intracellular signaling proteins. For adherent cells, such as epithelial cells and fibroblasts, input from both mitogen and adhesion receptors is critical for proliferation [1,2]. Indeed, in the absence of integrin engagement, many adherent cells not only fail to proliferate, they undergo a form of programmed cell death known as anoikis. Although the dual requirement for growth factor and adhesion signals is not completely understood, it has become clear that cyclin-dependent kinases, which are key regulators of the cell cycle (*see* Chapter 5), represent an important common target for both of these signaling pathways (Fig. 4-3).

GROWTH FACTOR SIGNALING: FROM RECEPTORS TO RAS

Growth factor signaling is initiated by the binding of ligand to receptor. There are many types of receptors for mitogenic signals. In this section, we focus on cell surface receptors rather than cytoplasmic or nuclear receptors, because these are frequently the targets of activating mutations in human malignancies. For proliferative signaling, two types of receptors merit special attention: receptor protein tyrosine kinases [3] and G-coupled receptors [4]. The former contain intrinsic enzymatic activity, whereas the latter lack such activity but instead are closely coupled to GTP-binding proteins within the cell. In the case of receptor protein tyrosine kinases, activation leads to autophosphorylation, dimerization, and the subsequent binding of a host of signaling proteins to the cytoplasmic tail of the receptor. Thus, activation of receptor protein tyrosine kinases leads to the formation of localized clusters of signaling molecules at the interior face of the plasma membrane. Such assemblies are sometimes termed "signalosomes" to denote their large molecular mass and complex composition. In contrast, G-coupled receptors use a completely different strategy, transmitting signals via a heterotrimeric complex of proteins termed Gα, Gβ, and Gγ. Despite these major differences, both receptor protein tyrosine kinases and G-coupled receptors activate many of the same downstream signaling proteins (Fig. 4-4).

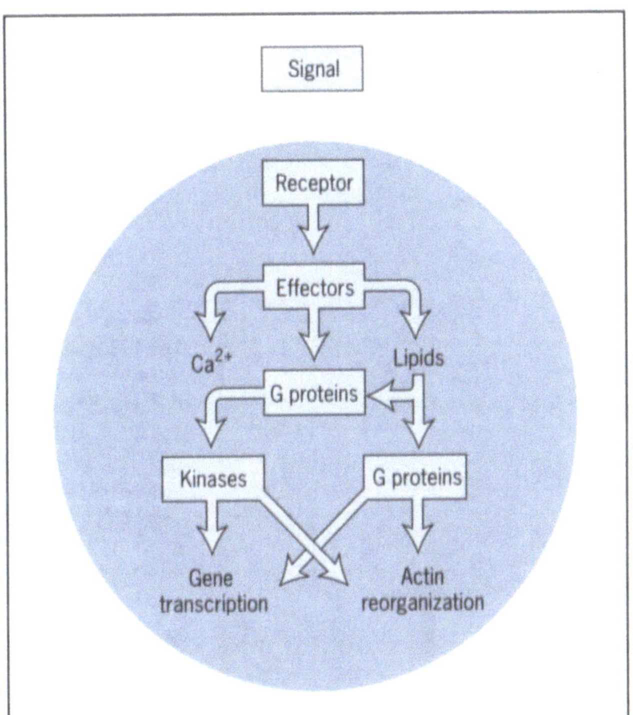

Figure 4-2. Information flow in signal transduction. On ligand engagement, cell surface receptors for growth factors transduce signals through an ordered sequence of events. These events typically include recruitment of effector molecules that induce calcium fluxes, changes in lipid composition, and activation of small GTP binding proteins. In turn, small GTP binding proteins activate numerous signaling pathways, including protein kinases that affect gene transcription in the nucleus, and additional GTPases that affect the organization of the actin cytoskeleton. These changes can result in alterations in cell growth, shape, motility, and adhesion.

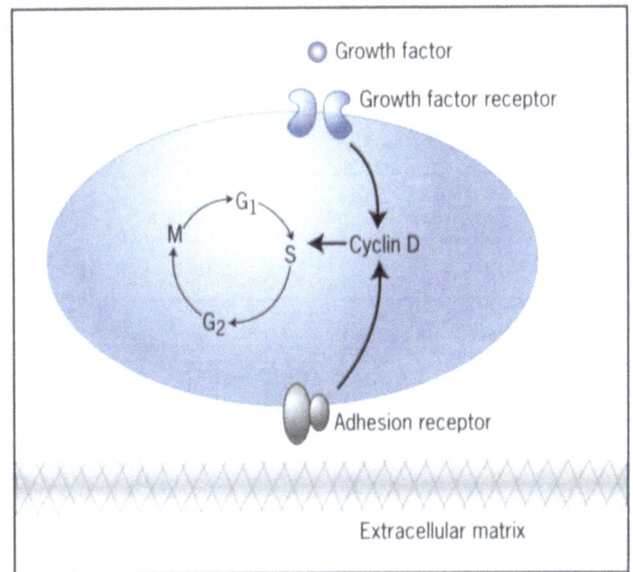

Figure 4-3. Two types of signals stimulate cell proliferation. Both mitogenic growth factors and extracellular matrix affect the expression of G_1 cyclins, which directly regulate the cell cycle. Mitogenic growth factors stimulate G_1-phase cell cycle progression primarily by upregulating expression of cyclin D-CDK4,6 and cyclin E-CDK2. By stimulating the activity of these kinases, growth factors allow for RB phosphorylation, transit through the restriction point, and entry into the mitogen-independent portion of G_1 that correlates with irreversible commitment to cell cycle progression. In addition to regulation by soluble growth factors, cell growth is also influenced by contact with the extracellular matrix. Similar to soluble mitogens, adhesion signals induce increased cyclin D expression. The balance of information from these two signaling systems in large part determine a cell's decision to divide or to remain quiescent.

Receptor protein tyrosine kinases represent a large and diverse group of proteins (Fig. 4-5). On stimulation, they dimerize and autophosphorylate multiple tyrosine residues in the cytoplasmic C-terminal region of the receptor (Fig. 4-6) [5]. Some malignancies are characterized at the molecular level by aberrant activation of receptor protein tyrosine kinases. Such activation may result from gene amplification, point mutation, or fusion of receptor protein tyrosine kinase genes with other genes (Fig. 4-7). In all these cases, receptor protein tyrosine kinase activity is switched on and is likely to contribute to the neoplastic phenotype.

The signaling pathways that are activated by receptor protein tyrosine kinases are organized as a set of modules that are highly conserved throughout evolution. These modules are composed of an activated receptor and its attendant binding proteins, the GTPase RAS and its modulators, one or more mitogen-activated protein kinase modules, and various

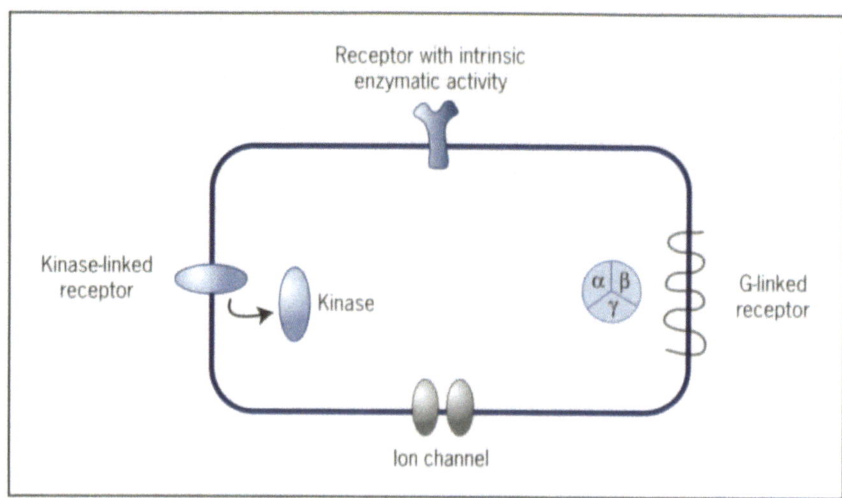

Figure 4-4. Cell surface receptors. Many signals are perceived and transduced by membrane-spanning cell surface receptors. Receptors can be classified into four distinct groups: receptors with intrinsic enzyme activity, such as receptor protein tyrosine kinases (RPTKs) and receptor protein tyrosine phosphatases (RPTPs); receptors that lack intrinsic enzyme activity but are associated with cytoplasmic enzymes; receptors that are associated with heterotrimeric GTP binding proteins (G protein couples [linked]); and ion channels. Receptors with intrinsic tyrosine kinase activity (RPTKs) are critical in transducing many mitogenic stimuli.

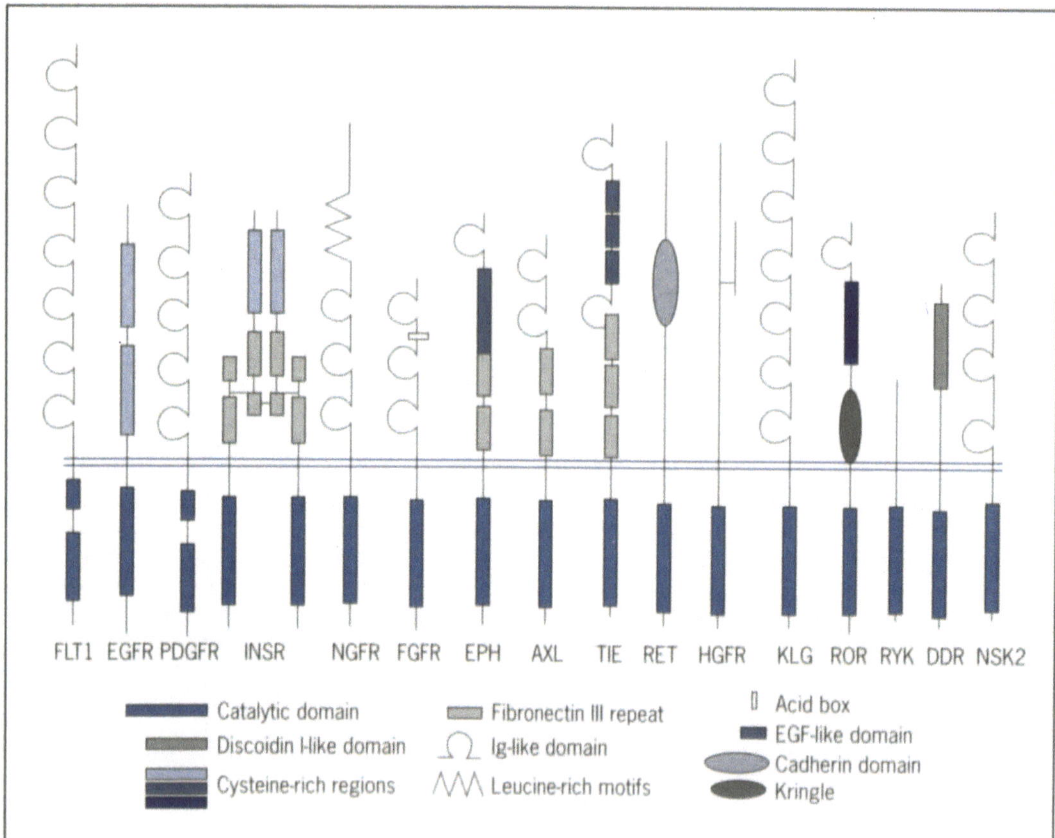

Figure 4-5. Receptor protein tyrosine kinases (RPTKs) represent a diverse group of proteins that can be classified into at least sixteen distinct groups. (*Adapted from* van der Geer *et al.* [3].)

transcription factors that are activated by these kinases (Fig. 4-8). The conservation of these signaling pathways means that genetically tractable organisms such as yeast, fruit flies, and roundworms are useful model systems for studying signal transduction. Indeed, much of our current understanding of proliferative signal transduction is based on data initially obtained from these organisms.

On activation, receptor protein tyrosine kinases autophosphorylate at defined tyrosine residues. These phosphorylated motifs serve as docking sites for signaling molecules (Fig. 4-9). Each receptor protein tyrosine kinase has its own characteristic set of autophosphorylation sites, allowing the assembly of unique ensembles of signaling proteins. These signaling proteins include enzymes and adaptor proteins. Most of the enzymatic signaling proteins are activated as a result of binding to the receptor, and they may also be brought into close proximity to key substrates via this association. In some cases, the activated receptor has a primary target, termed a docking protein, to which signaling molecules

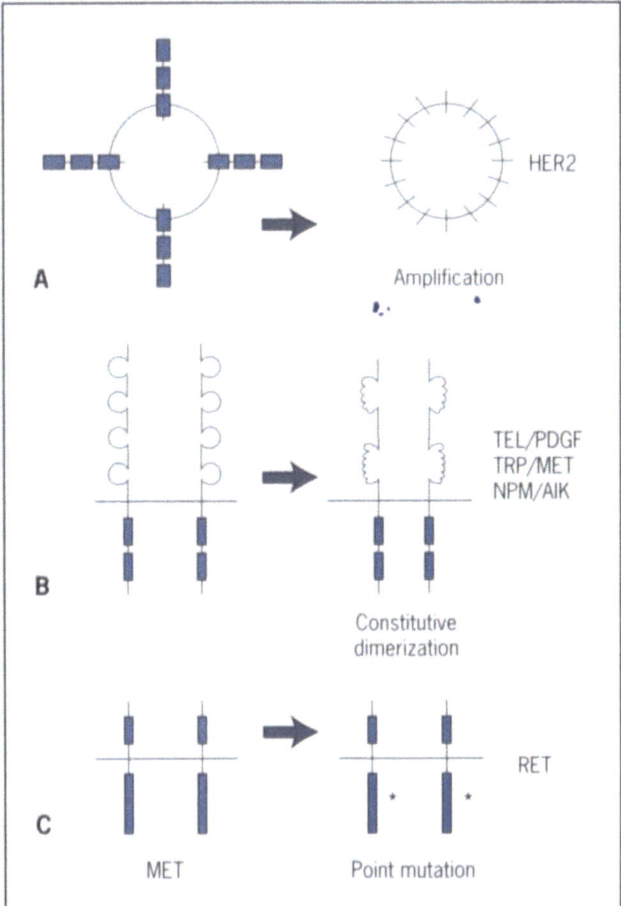

Figure 4-7. Constitutive activation of receptor protein tyrosine kinases (RPTKs) can induce uncontrolled cell proliferation. Such activation can result from overexpression of RPTK genes, from mutations that result in constitutive dimerization, or from mutations that confer ligand-independent activation to the kinase domain. **A**, Overexpression of the HER2 RPTK confers a transformed phenotype to cells in culture. This in vitro behavior correlates well with data from clinical samples. Overexpression of HER2 as a result of gene amplification, increased transcription, or both is seen in up to 30% of breast and ovarian carcinomas. **B**, Oncogenic activation of RPTKs by mutations that lead to constitutive dimerization with subsequent activation of the cytoplasmic catalytic domain. Both point mutations and gene fusions have been shown to result in such constitutively dimerized RPTKs. Examples include the TEL/PDGF fusion protein, which occurs as a result of a translocation between chromosomes 5 and 12, resulting in a fusion protein in which the PDGFR extracellular domain is replaced by a helix-loop-helix structure derived from the TEL transcription factor; and the NEU oncoprotein, which arises are a result of a point mutation within the transmembrane domain of HER2. **C**, N-terminal truncations and mutations within the catalytic domain can also induce ligand-independent activation of RPTKs, changes in substrate specificity, or both. In familial multiple endocrine neoplasia 2B, the RET protein acquires a mutation in the catalytic domain (Met918Thr) that activates RET and confers altered substrate specificity. The protein kinase domain (*hatched box*) and point mutations (*asterisk*) are indicated.

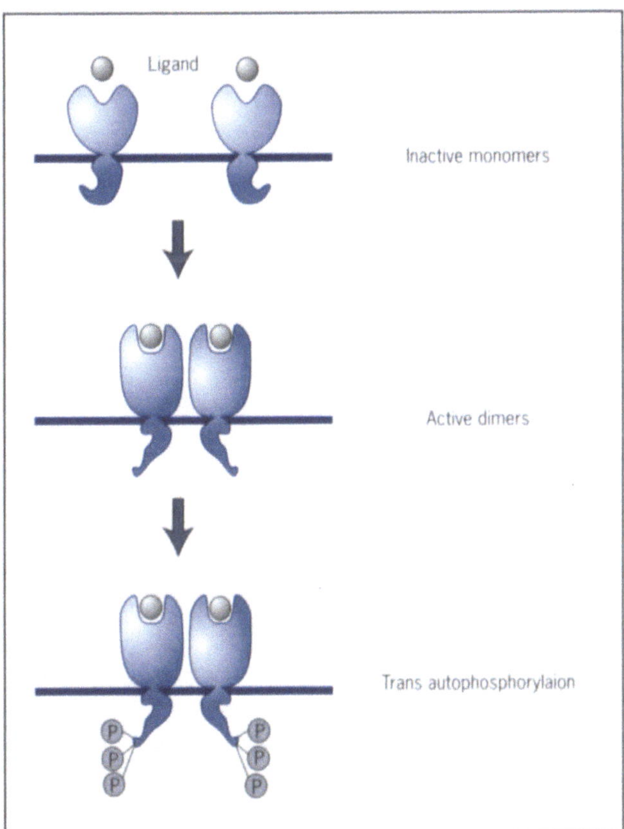

Figure 4-6. Activation of receptor tyrosine kinases by dimerization. On ligand binding, receptor protein tyrosine kinases (RPTKs) undergo a conformational change and dimerize. Dimerization is accompanied by activation of the intracellular tyrosine kinase domain. Activated RPTKs autophosphorylate at multiple tyrosine residues and can also tyrosine phosphorylate exogenous proteins.

bind. Here, the tyrosine-phosphorylated docking protein, rather than the receptor itself, serves as a platform for the assembly of signaling complexes.

The association of signaling proteins to activated receptor protein tyrosine kinases is mediated by specialized phosphotyrosine binding domains such as SRC homology 2 (SH2) and phosphotyrosine binding (PTB) domains [6]. SH2 domains recognize phosphotyrosine residues within a particular sequence context (Fig. 4-10). For example, the SH2 domain of SRC has been shown to prefer phosphorylated tyrosine residues within the motif (phospho)tyrosine-glutamic acid-glutamic acid-isoleucine. Such a motif is present following tyrosine residue 579 in the platelet-derived growth factor receptor, and this has been shown to be the site where SRC docks. SH2 domains in other proteins have different binding preferences, as reflected in their distinct sites of binding to phosphotyrosine residues in activated receptor protein tyrosine kinases. The PTB domain also confers context-specific binding to phosphotyrosine-containing peptides, but with a specificity that is markedly different from that of SH2 domains. In the PTB domain, specificity is conferred mainly by residues N-terminal to the phosphorylated tyrosine. In the case of the adaptor SHC, the PTB domain directs binding to sequences of the type asparagine-proline-X-(phospho)tyrosine.

In addition to SH2 and PTB domains, many of the signaling molecules that associate with activated receptor tyrosine kinases contain other binding domains that have direct association with a wide variety of proteins and lipids (Table 4-1) [7,8]. Two of the best characterized of these are the SRC homology 3 (SH3) and pleckstrin homology (PH) domains. The former binds to proteins containing proline-rich motifs of the type proline-X-X-proline. Such proline-rich motifs adopt a particular helical structure that can serve as a ligand for the SH3 domain. Unlike the other binding domains discussed thus far, it is believed that PH domains usually direct binding to phospholipids rather than to proteins. Curiously, PH domains are structurally related to PTB domains, yet

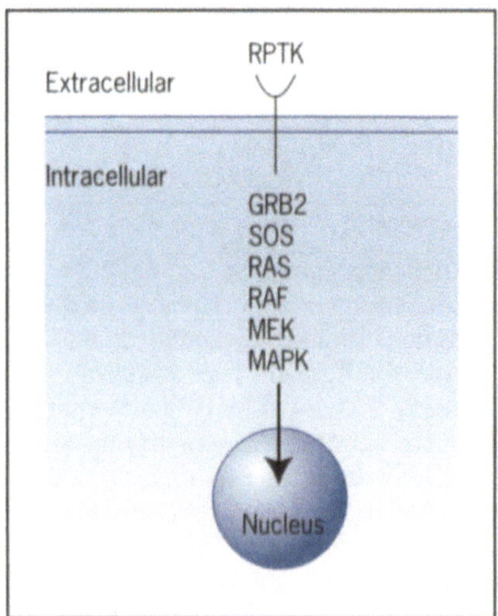

Figure 4-8. Organization of receptor protein tyrosine kinase (RPTK) signaling machinery. Most RPTKs signal through a highly conserved pathway that includes adaptor proteins, the RAS-specific GDP-GTP exchange factors (*eg*, SOS), RAS, and a mitogen-activated protein kinase (MAPK) cascade. This cascade is composed of at least three protein kinases in series: RAF, MAPK kinase (MAPKK), and MAPK. MAPK translocates to the nucleus, where it phosphorylates transcription factors, thus affecting gene expression. The organization of such signaling molecules is similar in organisms as diverse as worms (*Caenorhabditis elegans*), flies (*Drosophila* spp), and humans.

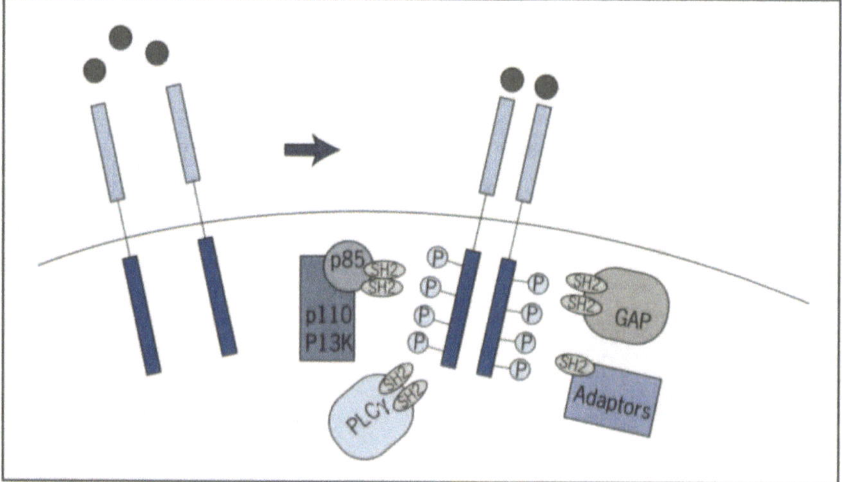

Figure 4-9. Assembly of signaling complexes. Autophosphorylated receptor protein tyrosine kinase (RPTKs) recruit an array of SRC homology 2 (SH2) domain–containing signaling molecules from a common pool. These SH2-containing proteins can include protein tyrosine kinases such as SRC; protein tyrosine phosphatases such as SHP2; enzymes that affect lipid metabolism such as phosphatidylinositol 3-kinase (PI3K) and phospholipase C (PLC); adaptor molecules such as GRB2, CRK, SHC, and NCK; proteins that regulate RAS function such as GTPase-activating protein (GAP); and transcription factors such as STATs. Signaling specificity may be achieved by recruiting specific sets of these signaling molecules.

they do not bind phosphotyrosine-containing peptides. By virtue of its ability to bind phospholipids, the PH domain plays an important role in targeting proteins to the plasma membrane. In addition, some PH domain–containing proteins, such as the protein kinase AKT and its immediate upstream activators, are directly activated by phospholipids. Thus, the PH domain plays a complex and vital role in regulating certain proteins involved in signal transduction.

Both receptor tyrosine kinases and G-coupled receptors recruit enzymes that modulate phospholipid production. These enzymes include phosphatidylinositol 3-kinase (PI3K), which phosphorylates the D3 position of phosphatidylinositol (PI), phosphatidylinositol 4-phosphate (PIP), and phosphatidylinositol 4,5-bisphosphate (PIP_2) [9]; and phospholipase C, which hydrolyzes PIP_2 to inositol 1,4,5-triphosphate (IP_3) and diacylglycerol (DAG) [10]. These phospholipids regulate a host of cellular processes such as calcium homeostasis, activation of protein kinases, and actin organization (Fig. 4-11) [12].

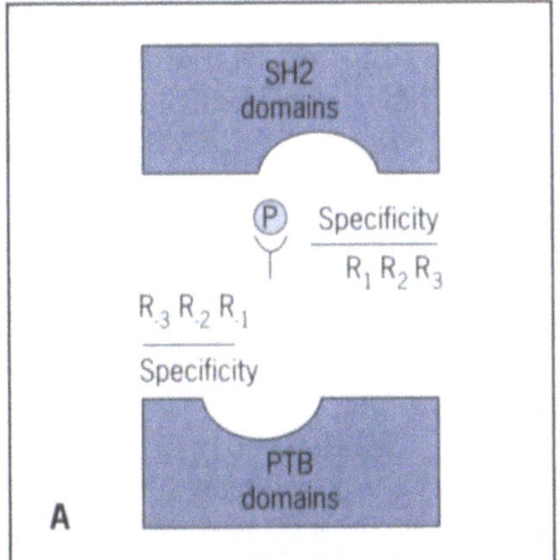

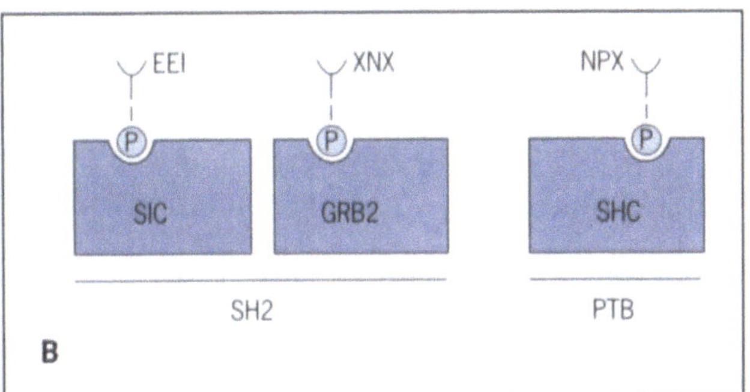

Figure 4-10. Specificity of SRC homology 2 (SH2) and phosphotyrosine binding (PTB) interactions with target peptides. **A**, SH2 domains are short sequences of about 100 amino acids that are found in many proteins implicated in signaling growth. SH2 domains recognize phosphotyrosine residues within specific sequence contexts. The three residues immediately C-terminal to phosphorylated tyrosine (R_3 to R_1) dictate binding specificity, although the N-terminal residues may also have a modest effect. **B**, For example, the SH2 domain from SRC binds sequences of the type Y(P)-E-E-I, whereas the SH2 domain from GRB2 favors sequences Y(P)-X-N-X (where X represents any amino acid). These binding specificities direct SH2-containing proteins to specific sites on autophosphorylated receptor protein tyrosine kinases (RPTKs) and other tyrosine-phosphorylated proteins. Like SH2 domains, PTB domains also recognize phosphotyrosine residues within specific sequence contexts. However, in this case, the amino acids immediately N-terminal to the phosphorylated tyrosine residue dictate binding specificity.

Table 4-1. Protein interaction modules critical for the assembly of signaling complexes

Domain	Binding site
SH2	-(P)Y-X-X-hy-
PTB	-hy-X-N-P-X-(P)Y-
SH3	-P-X-X-P-
WW	-P-P-X-Y-
PH	Phospholipids
PDZ	-E-S/T-V-C-COOH
14-3-3	-R-S-X-(P)S-S-P-

hy—hydrophobic residues; (P)—phosphate group.

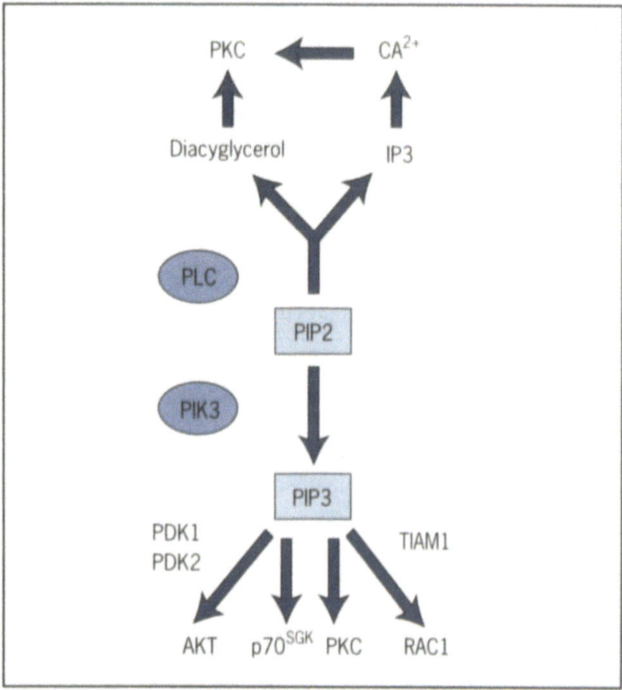

Figure 4-11. Signaling via lipids: phosphatidylinositol kinases. Phosphatidylinositol 3 (PI3) kinases catalyze the phosphorylation of inositol phospholipids in the D-3 position of their inositol ring. There are three recognized classes of PI3Ks in mammalian cells, the first of which is regulated by growth factors. Class 1 PI3 kinases are heterodimeric molecules composed of a p50-101 adaptor subunit and a p110 catalytic subunit. The p85 adaptor unit of PI3K-alpha contains an SH2 domain, providing a link to activated receptor protein tyrosine kinases. Other members of this class, such as PI3K-gamma, are linked to G_I-coupled receptors via a p101 adaptor subunit. Class 1 PI3Ks convert phosphatidylinositol 4,5-bisphosphate (PIP_2) to phosphatidylinositol 3,4,5-triphosphate (PIP_3). PIP_3 is the key activator for a variety of signaling molecules, including protein kinases such as AKT, PDK1, and PDK2 (kinases that assist in the activation of AKT); $p70^{S6K}$; and unconventional isoforms of protein kinase C, as well as guanine-nucleotide exchange factors such as TIAM1 that lead to the activation of the GTPase, RAC. Thus, PI3Ks play a pivotal role in transducing signals from both receptor protein tyrosine kinases and G-coupled receptors via the generation of a biologically active phospholipid.

Signaling via lipids: phospholipase C–mediated cellular responses. Phospholipase C generates second messengers that activate protein kinase C and affect calcium homeostasis. The gamma isoform of phospholipase C (PLC-gamma) associates with activated receptor protein tyrosine kinases (RPTKs) by means of its SRC homology 2 (SH2) domains. This association stimulates the catalytic activity of PLC-gamma. PLC-gamma catalyzes the hydrolysis of phosphatidylinositol 4,5-bisphosphate (PIP_2) to diacylglycerol (DAG) and inositol 1,4,5-triphosphate (IP_3). IP_3 releases calcium from intracellular stores, which in turn activates a variety of calcium-dependent functions. DAG and calcium together activate protein kinase C. A related isoform, PLC-beta, lacks an SH2 domain and is activated by G-protein linked receptors rather than by RPTKs.

Activated receptor tyrosine kinases are linked to guanine-nucleotide exchange factors for the GTPase RAS by adaptor proteins. Adaptor proteins are composed of one or more protein interaction domains such as SH2, SH3, and PTB domains [13]. In the case of the adaptor GRB2, which is composed of a single SH2 domain flanked by two SH3 domains, the SH2 domain binds to phosphotyrosine residues on activated receptor tyrosine kinases, whereas the SH3 domains associate with proline-rich motifs on SOS, a guanine-nucleotide exchange factor for RAS (Fig. 4-12). Other adaptors, such as NCK and CRK, have multiple SH3 domains in addition to an SH2 domain and thus may simultaneously associate with several proteins. Mitogenic compounds that activate G-coupled receptors also signal through RAS, although the mechanisms by which this is achieved differ from those used by receptor protein tyrosine kinases [14]. In the case of G-coupled receptors, the link to RAS may be indirect, mediated by various intracellular protein tyrosine kinases such as SRC or PYK2 (Fig. 4-13).

GROWTH FACTOR SIGNALING: FROM RAS TO THE NUCLEUS

The GTPase RAS represents one of the key molecules in proliferative signal transduction [15]. RAS is highly conserved in eukaryotes from yeast to humans, playing a

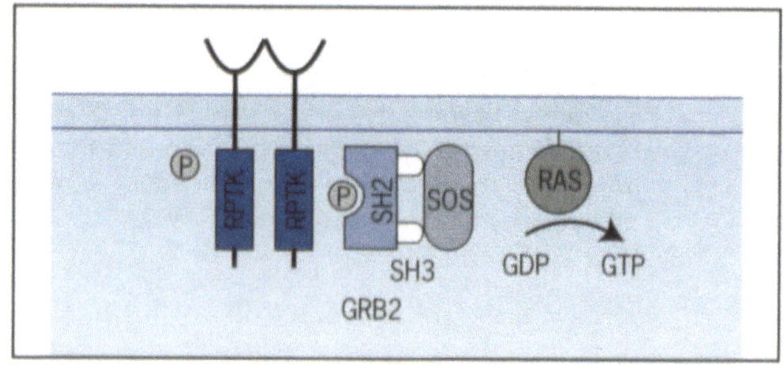

Figure 4-12. Adaptor proteins link receptor protein tyrosine kinases (RPTKs) to activators of Ras. **A**, Adaptor proteins lack intrinsic enzymatic activity but serve to link signaling molecules together. Adaptor proteins consist of one or more SRC homology 2 (SH2), phosphotyrosine binding (PTB), and SRC homology 3 (SH3) domains that can function independently or cooperatively to bind additional proteins. **B**, The SH2 and PTB domains regulate interactions with tyrosine-phosphorylated proteins such as RPTKs, whereas the SH3 domains bind to proteins containing proline-rich sequences of the form P-X-X-P (where X indicates any amino acid). Ras-activating guanine-nucleotide exchange factors such as SOS contain such proline-rich sequences and form complexes with adaptor proteins. This modular design allows adaptor proteins to serve as links between upstream signaling elements and their downstream effectors.

central role in coordinating changes in gene transcription and cytoskeletal structure in response to environmental signals. As might be expected for a molecule that is central to proliferative signaling, activating Ras mutations are frequently found in malignant tissues [16].

Like other GTPases, RAS is activated when complexed with GTP and deactivated on hydrolysis of GTP to GDP (Fig. 4-14). Activation of RAS is stimulated by guanine nucleotide exchange factors (GEFs) such as SOS and RAS guanine nucleotide releasing factor (GRF). As noted previously, in growth factor–treated cells, these GEFs are concentrated at the plasma membrane in the vicinity of receptor protein tyrosine kinases by virtue of their association with adaptor proteins (via SH3/proline interactions) and membrane phospholipids (via lipid/PH domain interactions). RAS activation is antagonized by two sets of regulators: guanine nucleotide dissociation inhibitors (GDIs), which inhibit exchange of GTP for GDP, and GTPase accelerating proteins (GAPs), which hasten the conversion of RAS to the inactive, GDP-bound state.

Another crucial factor in RAS activation is the addition of a farnesyl (lipid) moiety to a cysteine residue near the carboxy-terminus of this protein. Such modification is catalyzed by a specific enzyme (farnesyl transferase) and is required for the proper

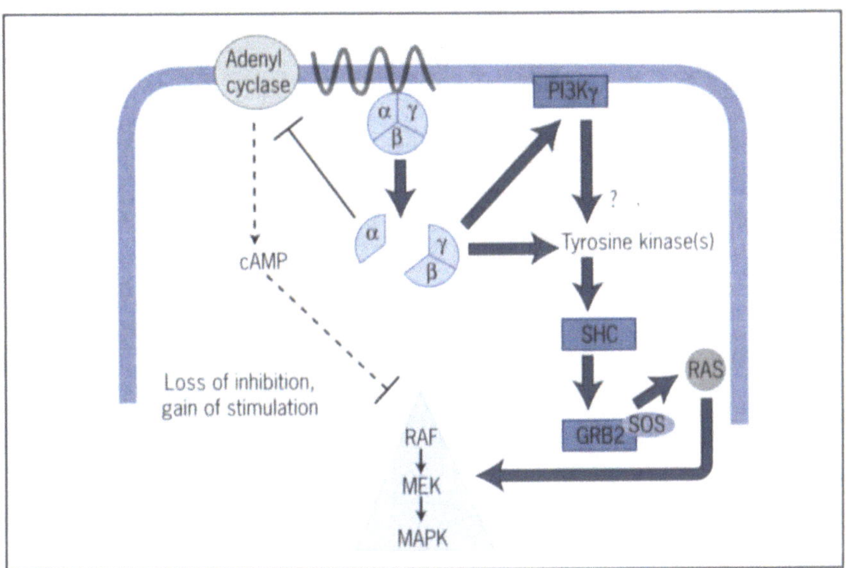

Figure 4-13. Mitogenic signals from G protein–linked receptors also act through RAS. Activation of several kinds of G protein–linked receptors induces a proliferative response. Following ligand-binding, the heterotrimeric alpha beta gamma G protein complex dissociates into two subunits: one composed solely of alpha and the other of a beta gamma dimer. Both of these subunits activate downstream signaling events. For G_i-coupled receptors, the beta gamma dimer is thought to activate tyrosine kinases such as SRC (perhaps through PI3K), which recruits and tyrosine phosphorylates the adaptor protein SHC. SHC then recruits GRB2 and SOS, thus opening a link to RAS and the mitogen-activated protein kinase (MAPK) cascade. In addition, via the α G protein subunit, many G protein–linked receptors inactivate a denyl cyclase, thereby relieving inhibition of the MAPK system.

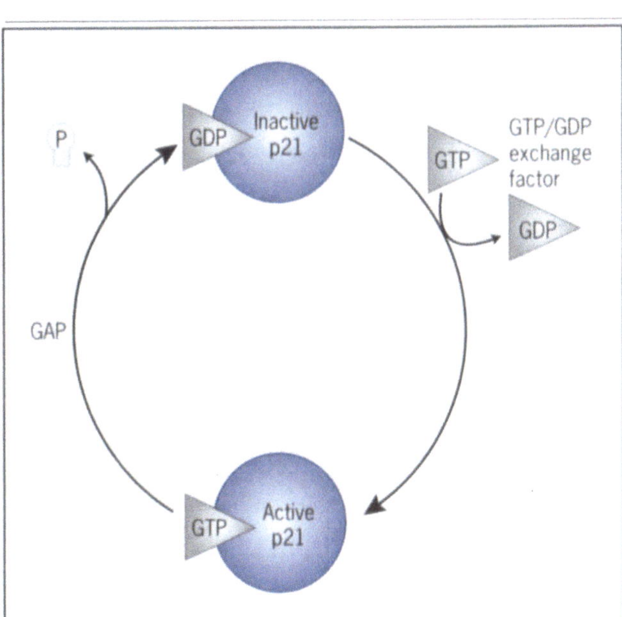

Figure 4-14. RAS is a master molecular switch. Many growth signals induce activation of RAS. In resting cells, RAS exists in an "off" (GDP-bound) state. In stimulated cells, RAS becomes activated by exchanging GDP for GTP. This exchange is accelerated by RAS-specific GDP/GTP exchange factors (GEFs) such as SOS and C3G. On binding GTP, RAS undergoes a conformational change that promotes the binding of multiple effector proteins. Inactivation of RAS is achieved by hydrolysis of GTP to GDP and P_i. RAS itself has a slow intrinsic GTPase activity, but this activity is greatly enhanced by GTPase-activating proteins (GAPs), such as NF1 and $p120^{RASGAP}$. An additional level of control is provided by guanine-nucleotide dissociation inhibitors (GDIs), which regulate the affinity of RAS for GDP and GTP.

membrane localization and biological activity of RAS. Because a limited number of proteins are thought to rely on farnesyl transferases, inhibitors of these enzymes may be therapeutically useful. Farnesyl transferase inhibitors have been shown to induce dramatic tumor regression in mouse models and are currently undergoing clinical trials for efficacy as anticancer agents in humans (Fig. 4-15) [17].

Once activated, RAS undergoes a profound conformation change that permits subsequent binding of a host of effector proteins (Fig. 4-16). These effectors include proteins that affect gene transcription and the

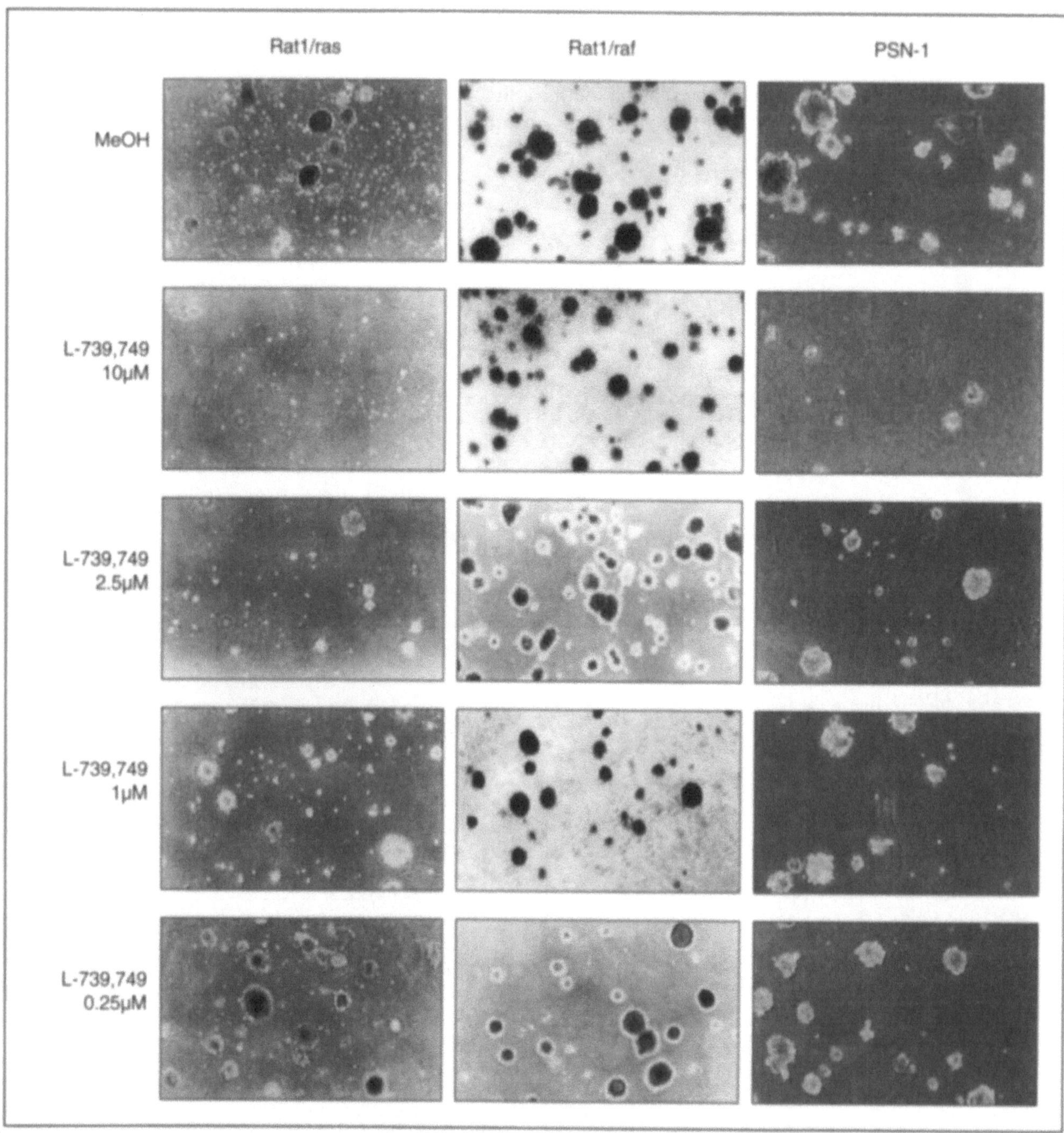

Figure 4-15. Farnesylation of RAS is required for its biological activity. RAS is modified by attachment of farnesyl moieties to a specific cysteine residue in its C-terminus. This modification is catalyzed by the enzyme farnesyl-protein transferase. Unmodified RAS does not localize properly to the plasma membrane and is therefore not capable of transmitting growth signals. For this reason, pharmacologic inhibitors of farnesyl-protein transferases may be useful as anticancer therapeutic agents. Treatment of RAS-transformed cells with a farnesyl-protein transferases inhibitor (L-739,749) causes morphologic reversion. (*From* Kohl *et al.* [17]; with permission.)

actin cytoskeleton, and together regulate cell cycle progression [18,19]. Activation of effector proteins that regulate both of these processes are required for full transformation by RAS [20]. Interestingly, the mitogenic and morphogenic effects of RAS are experimentally separable, suggesting that RAS uses different clusters of effector proteins to regulate cell division and cell shape (Fig. 4-17) [21]. Although the mechanism is not completely understood, RAS activates a related GTPase known as RAC, perhaps via PI3K and an RAC GEF (Fig. 4-18). Like RAS, activated RAC in turn recruits an array of effectors that affect the cytoskeleton, inducing formation of lamellipodia and gene transcription via one or more protein kinase cascades [22]. Two other related GTPases, CDC42 and RHO, also play important roles in regulating cytoskeletal structure and gene transcription, although these two proteins have not been shown to be activated by RAS.

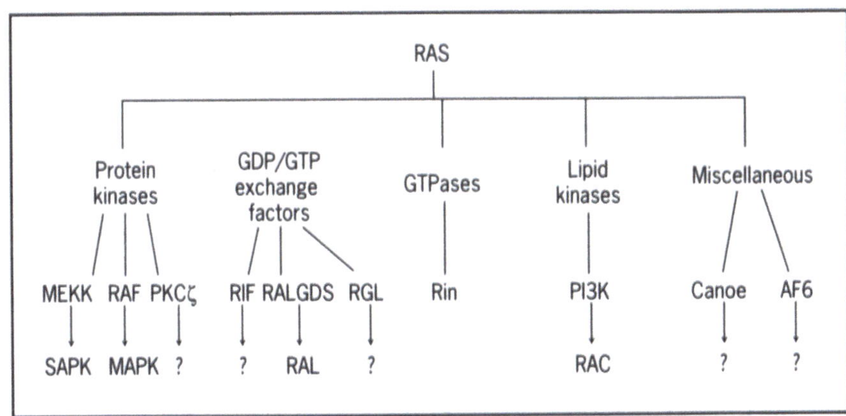

Figure 4-16. RAS activates multiple effector pathways. In its GTP-bound state, RAS binds to and activates a large number of effector proteins. These include serine/threonine-specific protein kinases (RAF, MEKK, and PKC-zeta); GDP/GTP exchange factors (RAL-GDS, RGL, and RIF); GTPases (RIN), lipid-modifying enzymes (PI3K), and proteins of unknown function (AF6 and Canoe). At least two of these effectors, RAF and RAL-GDS, are known to contribute to transformation by oncogenic forms of RAS. A third effector, PI3K, may also contribute to transformation by linking RAS to GTPases of the RHO family (CDC42, RAC, and RHO), which affect the structure of the actin cytoskeleton.

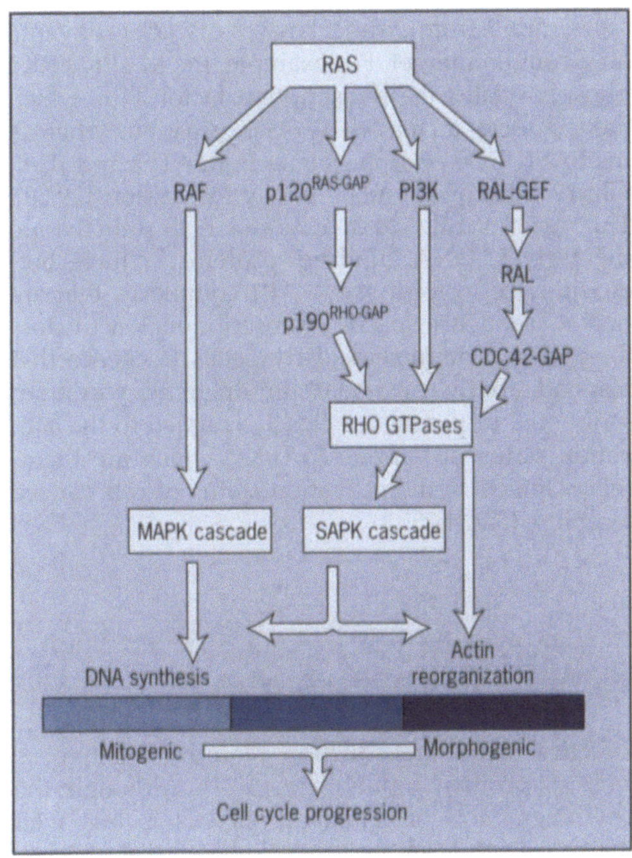

Figure 4-17. RAS controls distinct signaling pathways that affect cell proliferation and cell shape. Many of the effectors of RAS regulate one of two major responses; DNA synthesis or cytoskeletal reorganization. The former response is thought to be mediated in large part by the RAF/MAPK cascade, while the latter is chiefly under the influence of the CDC42/RAC/RHO GTPases that lie downstream of RAS and are distinct from the RAF pathway.

The protein kinase RAF represents another key RAS effector [23]. On binding RAS, RAF becomes associated with the inner face of the plasma membrane, where it is activated by one or more membrane-resident proteins. RAF then phosphorylates another kinase, MEK, which in turn phosphorylates mitogen-activated protein kinases (MAPKs; Fig. 4-19). MEK is an unusual protein kinase, phosphorylating its substrate MAPK at both a threonine and a tyrosine residue. Because phosphorylation of both sites is required for activation of MAPK, this arrangement may contribute to signaling specificity, as it is unlikely that other kinases would be able to activate MAPK directly.

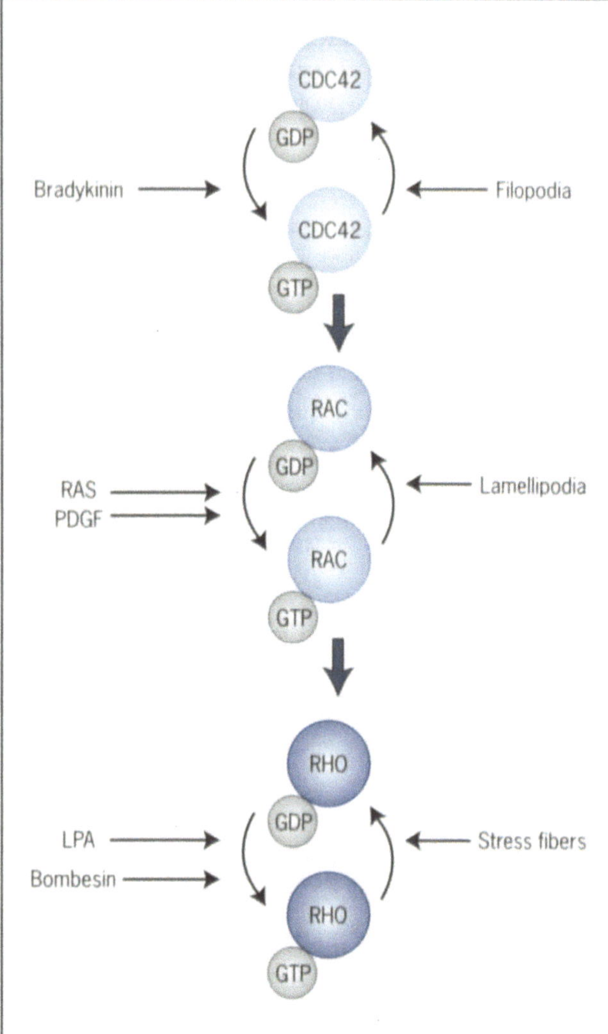

Figure 4-18. Growth factor receptors and RAS activate GTPases that regulate cytoskeletal structure. Stimulation of certain growth factor receptors or RAS activates a group of RAS-related GTPases termed CDC42, RAC, and RHO. Bradykinin stimulates CDC42; platelet-derived growth factor, insulin, and activated forms of RAS stimulate RAC; and lysophosphatidic acid (LPA) and bombesin lead to activation of RHO. The molecular machinery that connects growth factor receptors and RAS to these GTPases is not fully known, but is likely to include PI3K and specific GDP/GTP exchange factors. Like RAS, the GTPases CDC42, RAC, and RHO recruit an array of effector molecules. Among the most important of these are proteins that regulate cytoskeletal structure. Microinjection of activated CDC42 induces the formation of filopodia (actin-based, spike-like structures that protrude from the cell surface). Microinjection of activated RAC induces the formation of lamellipodia (sheet-like structures), whereas microinjection of activated RHO induces formation of actin stress fibers. In some cells, these GTPases may operate in series, with CDC42 stimulating RAC and RAC activating RHO.

Not only are MAPK modules conserved among diverse species of eukaryotic organisms (Table 4-2), but multiple MAPK modules are present within each organism. These modules are insulated from each other by scaffolding proteins that physically interact with multiple members of a given kinase cascade (Fig. 4-20) [24,25]. In humans, such modules can be conceptually divided into two major groups: one that responds to mitogenic stimuli and another that responds to cellular stress. Mitogenic stimuli usually activate the MAPKs ERK1 and ERK2, whereas certain stressful stimuli such as DNA damage, heat shock, or changes in osmolarity activate the JUN-kinase (JNK) and p38 families of stress activated protein kinases (SAPKs) (Fig. 4-21) [26–28].

On activation, both MAPKs and SAPKs translocate to the nucleus (Fig. 4-22) where these kinases phosphorylate various transcription factors, altering their ability to activate gene transcription. In some cases, inputs from distinct kinases cascades converge on a common target. For example, the MAPK ERK1 phosphorylates the transcription factor TCF, which then induces increased *c-FOS* expression, whereas the SAPK JNK phosphorylates both ATF2 and JUN, which together stimulate *c-JUN* expression [29,30]. The newly synthesized JUN and FOS proteins are themselves DNA binding proteins, which heterodimerize to form stable AP1 complexes that are potent, sequence-specific transcriptional activators for a host of immediate-early genes (*ie*, genes that respond rapidly to external stimuli). In this way, transcriptional responses are closely coupled to the activation status of various MAPKs, which are themselves linked to the activation status of cell surface receptors (Fig. 4-23).

DOWNREGULATION OF MITOGENIC SIGNALS

Effective signal transduction requires negative as well as positive inputs (Fig. 4-24). Although the downregulation of mitogenic signals is less well characterized than upregulation, several mechanisms have been identified. Conceptually, these can be divided into negative regulators that work at or near the plasma membrane, those that work in the cytoplasm, and those that work in the nucleus. Receptor protein tyrosine kinase signals may be terminated by endocytosis of the receptor or by dephosphorylation by protein tyrosine phosphatases (PTPs). PTPs may also act on the tyrosine phosphorylated enzymes and adaptors that associate with receptor protein tyrosine kinases. Phospholipid PTPs may also have an important regulatory role, as these may decrease levels of PIP_2 and PIP_3 [31,32]. RAS-GTP levels are decreased by GAPs and mutations; one such negative regulator underlies the pathogenesis of neurofibromatosis [33]. RAF and its downstream targets are thought to be downregulated by protein

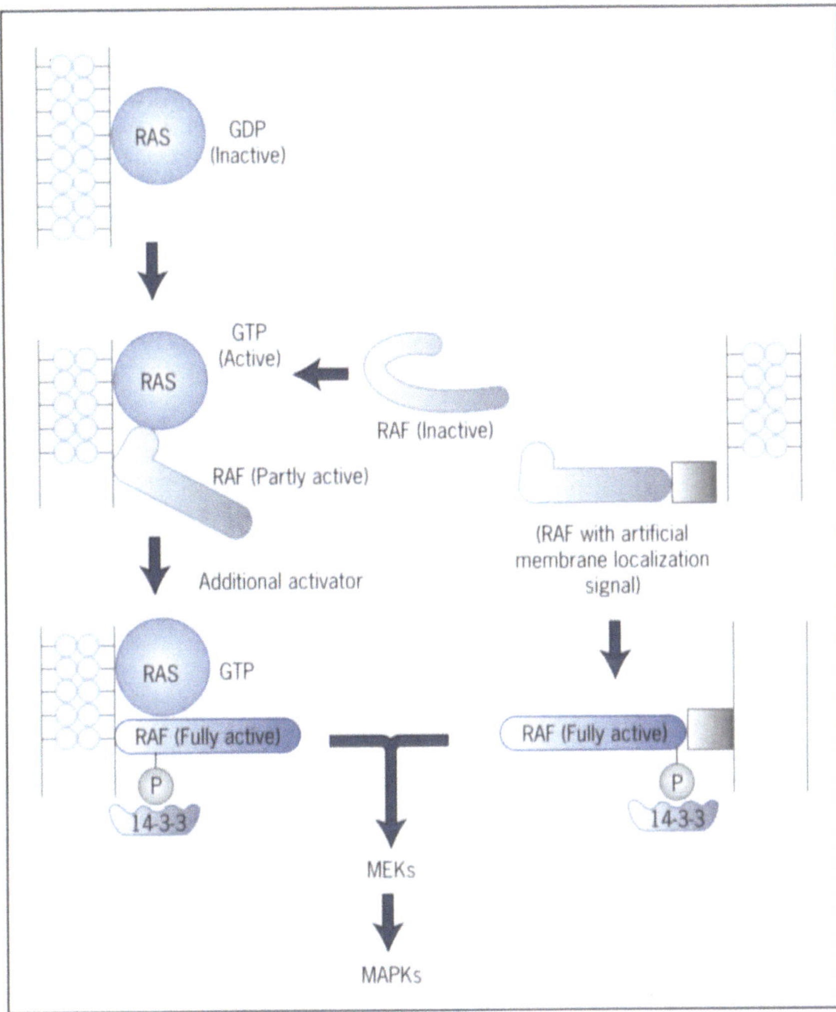

Figure 4-19. RAF and the mitogen-activated protein kinase (MAPK) cascade. RAS recruits the protein kinase RAF to the plasma membrane, where RAF encounters additional activating proteins. RAF that has been artificially engineered to associate constitutively with the plasma membrane is transforming in fibroblasts.

Table 4-2. Highly conserved mitogen-activated protein kinase (MAPK) modules

Mammal	Yeast	Fly	Worm
Ras		Ras-1	LET60
MEKK	STE11		
RAF		DRAF	LIN45
MEK	STE7	DSOR	MEK2
ERK	FUS3/KSS1	Rolled	MPK1 (SUR1)
Myc, ELK1	STE12	YAN, pointed	LIN31, LIN1

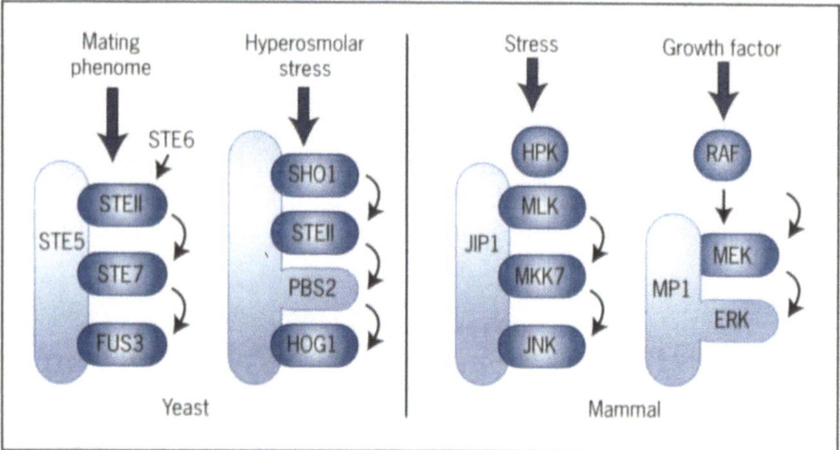

Figure 4-20. Mitogen-activated protein kinase (MAPK) scaffolds. Many, and perhaps all, MAPK modules are held together by scaffolding proteins. The best characterized of these is Ste5 in budding yeast, a mating-specific signaling protein that simultaneously binds Ste11, Ste7, and Fus3. In the hyperosmolar response pathway, the kinase Pbs2 serves not only as an intrinsic member of the kinase module but also as a scaffold, binding Sho1, Ste11, and Hog1. In mammalian cells, similar scaffolds have been found. For example, in the stress-kinase pathway, the JIP1 protein binds MLK, MKK7, and JNK. In the mitogen-activated pathway, MP1 binds MEK and ERK. Such scaffolds increase signaling strength by keeping proteins in physical proximity and may also insulate such modules from inadvertent activation by inappropriate stimuli.

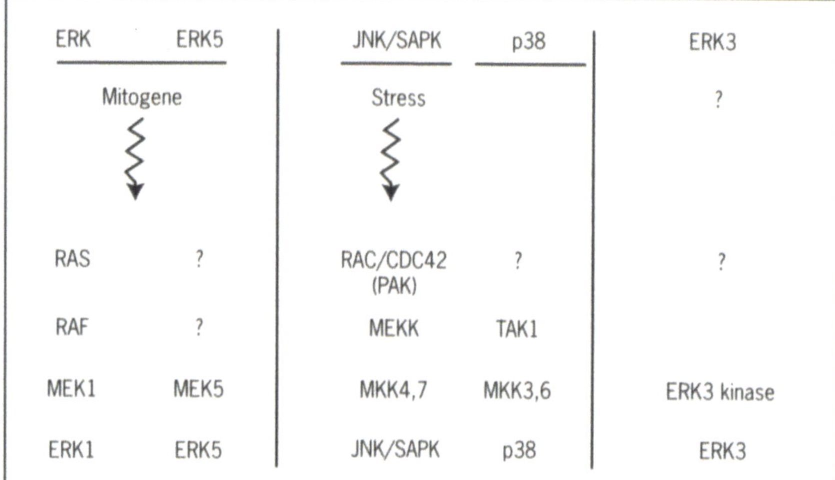

Figure 4-21. Cells possess multiple parallel mitogen-activated protein kinase (MAPK) cascades that serve to integrate a variety of signals. Within a given cell, there are numerous parallel MAPK pathways, each responsive to a particular stimulus, such as mitogens, cytokines, heat shock, DNA damage, and changes in osmolarity.

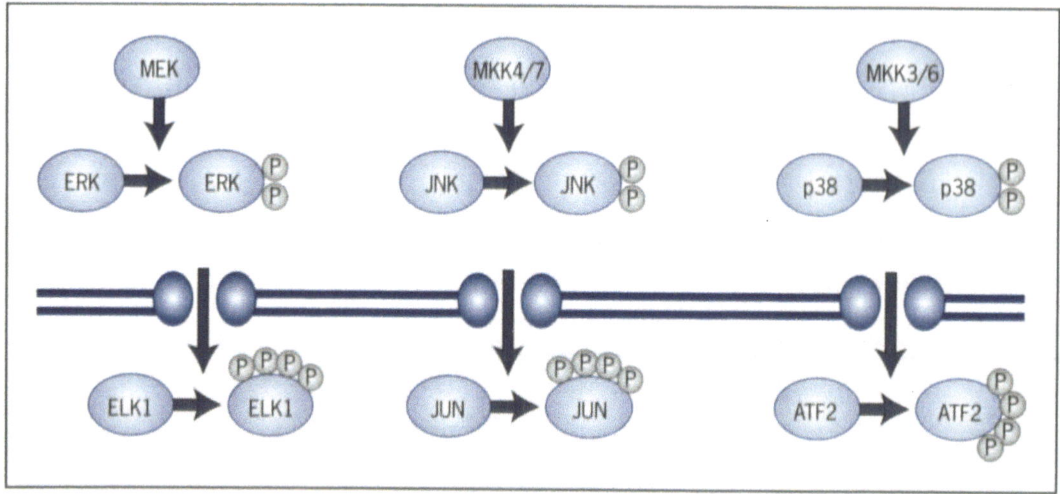

Figure 4-22. Activated mitogen-activated protein kinases (MAPKs) translocate to the nucleus, where they phosphorylate transcription factors. On phosphorylation by MEKs, a portion of the activated MAPK population translocates to the nucleus, where activated MAPKs encounter and phosphorylate a number of transcription factors. Phosphorylation alters the transcriptional activity of these factors.

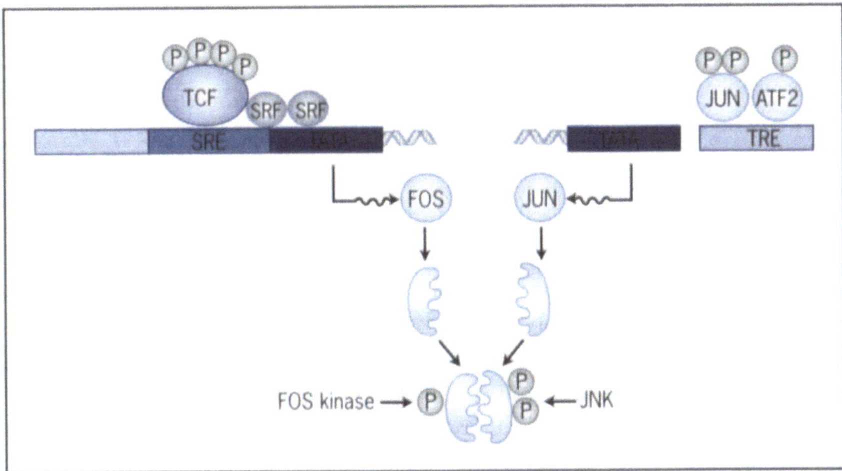

Figure 4-23. Stimulation of AP1 activity by mitogen-activated protein kinases (MAPKs). In the nucleus, ERKs phosphorylate the transcription factor TCF, which is bound together with another factor (known as SRF) to the serum response element of the *FOS* promoter. Phosphorylation of TCF stimulates its transcriptional function, leading to rapid induction of *FOS* transcription. The expression of *JUN* is stimulated by JUN itself, in concert with ATF2, both of which are activated as a result of phosphorylation by JNK. The newly synthesized Jun and Fos can heterodimerize, forming a transcriptional activator known as AP1. Many growth and stress response genes contain AP1 sites within their promoters, and these can be regulated by such stimuli through AP1.

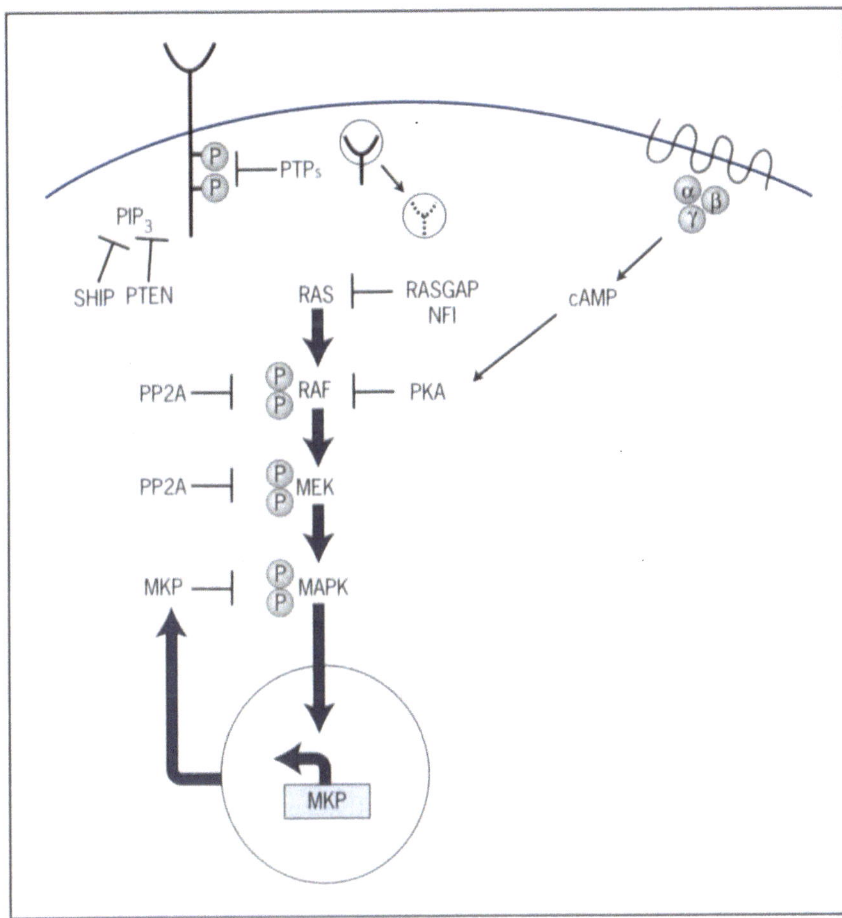

Figure 4-24. Negative regulators of mitogenic signal transduction. Growth signals are tightly regulated by a series of proteins that act at several points along the signaling pathway. At the level of the receptor, activated receptor protein tyrosine kinases (RPTKs) are internalized and degraded by endocytosis, and are also subject to rapid deactivation by protein tyrosine phosphatases (PTPs). In addition, phospholipid messengers such as PIP_3 are dephosphorylated by 5′ and 3′ inositol phosphatases such as SHIP and the tumor suppressor PTEN. At the level of RAS, specific GTPase-activating proteins (RASGAPs) such as NF1 and $p120^{RASGAP}$ convert GTP-bound RAS to its inactive GDP-bound state. Distal to RAS, second messengers such as cyclic AMP (cAMP) are thought to inhibit growth of fibroblasts by activating PKA, which then inactivates RAF via a specific phosphorylation event. Protein serine/threonine specific phosphatases (PSPs) such as PP2A are thought to deactivate key downstream kinases such as RAF and MEK, whereas MAPK phosphatases (MKPs) deactivate MAPKs by simultaneously dephosphorylating critical threonine and tyrosine residues in the activation loop of these kinases. The transcription of some MKPs is increased by activated MAPKs, thus providing feedback control of this pathway.

serine/threonine phosphatases, whereas the MAPKs and SAPKs are subject to inactivation by dual-specificity phosphatases that are able to dephosphorylate both the threonine and tyrosine residues in the activation loop of these kinases [34]. Protein phosphatases also are present in the nucleus, and these may act on nuclear MAPK and SAPKs as well as on phosphorylated transcription factors.

Some extracellular factors have a negative rather than a positive effect on cell proliferation. Among the best known of these is transforming growth factor beta (TGF-beta), which plays an important role in inhibiting cell growth (Fig. 4-25) [35]. The receptor for TGF-beta is a transmembrane, serine/threonine-specific protein kinase which, like receptor protein tyrosine kinases, dimerizes on activation by ligand. In the case of the TGF-beta receptor, activation leads to heterodimerization between two distinct receptor types (termed I and II), both of which are required for signal propagation. The activated type I receptor phosphorylates a number of substrates, including transcription factors known as SMADs, which then translocate to the nucleus. Both the TGF-beta receptor and one of its substrates, SMAD4, are frequently subject to inactivating mutations in human solid tumors. Presumably, these mutations relieve the growth-inhibitory effects of TGF-beta, thus contributing to the neoplastic phenotype.

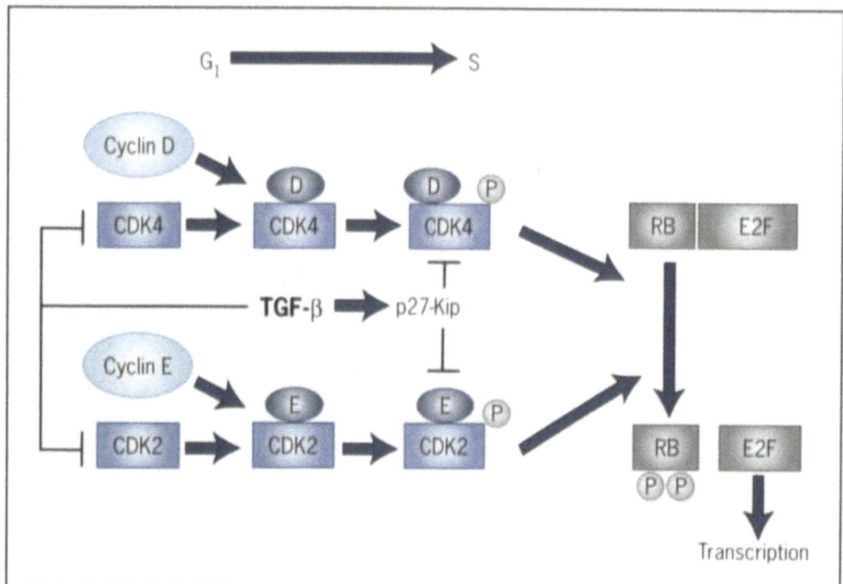

Figure 4-25. The transforming growth factor beta (TGF-beta) pathway. Despite its name, TGF-beta inhibits, rather than enhances, cell growth in many tissues. TGF-beta is the best characterized molecule of the group of growth factors that act primarily to inhibit cell proliferation. The importance of this pathway in regulating cell growth is illustrated by the high frequency of TGF-beta resistance in tumor cells. TGF-beta is thought to inhibit cell cycle progression by inducing increased expression of p27-KIP, a protein that inhibits the activity of cyclin E-CDK2 complexes. Inhibition of these complexes leads to failure to phosphorylate RB, with subsequent cell-cycle arrest at the G_1/S boundary. Mutations in both the TGF-beta receptor and in an effector molecule known as SMAD4 frequently are found in tumor cells derived from colon and pancreatic cancers.

REFERENCES

1. Assoian RK, Zhu X: Cell anchorage and the cytoskeleton as partners in growth factor dependent cell cycle progression. *Curr Opin Cell Biol* 1997, 9:93–98.
2. Giancotti FG: Integrin signaling: specificity and control of cell survival and cell cycle progression. *Curr Opin Cell Biol* 1998, 9:691–700.
3. van der Geer P, Hunter T, Lindberg RA: Receptor protein-tyrosine kinases and their signal transduction pathways. *Annu Rev Cell Biol* 1994, 10:251–337.
4. Post GR, Brown JH: G protein-coupled receptors and signaling pathways regulating growth responses. *FASEB J* 1996, 10:741–749.
5. Heldin C-H: Dimerization of cell surface receptors in signal transduction. *Cell* 1995, 80:213–223.
6. Sonyang Z, Shoelson SE, Chaudhuri M, *et al.*: SH2 domains recognize specific phosphopeptide sequences. *Cell* 1993, 72:767–778.
7. Pawson T: Protein modules and signalling networks. *Nature* 1995, 373:573–579.
8. Pawson T, Scott JD: Signaling through scaffold, anchoring, and adaptor proteins. *Science* 1997, 278:2075–2080.
9. Fruman DA, Meyers RE, Cantley LC: Phosphoinositide kinases. *Annu Rev Biochem* 1998, 67:481–507.
10. Kamat A, Carpenter G: Phospholipase C-gamma1: regulation of enzyme function and role in growth factor–dependent signal transduction. *Cytokine Growth Factor Rev* 1997, 8:109–117.
11. Strum JC, Ghosh S, Bell RM: Lipid second messengers: a role in cell growth regulation and cell cycle progression. *Adv Exp Med Biol* 1997, 407:421–431.
12. Li N, Batzer A, Daly R, *et al.*: Guanine-nucleotide-releasing factor hSos1 binds to Grb2 and links receptor tyrosine kinases to Ras signaling. *Nature* 1993, 363:85–88.

13. Schlessinger J: SH2/SH3 signaling proteins. *Curr Opin Genet Dev* 1994, 4:25–30.

14. Gutkind JS: The pathways connecting G protein-coupled receptors to the nucleus through divergent mitogen-activated protein kinase cascades. *J Biol Chem* 1998, 273:1839–1842.

15. Macara IG, Lounsbury KM, Richards SA, *et al.*: The Ras superfamily of GTPases. *FASEB J* 1996, 10:625–630.

16. Bos JL: Ras oncogenesis in human cancer: a review. *Cancer Res* 1989, 49:4682–4689.

17. Kohl NE, Mosser SD, deSolms SJ, *et al.*: Selective inhibition of ras-dependent transformation by a farnesyltransferase inhibitor. *Science* 1993, 260:1934–1937.

18. Katz ME, McCormick F: Signal transduction from multiple Ras effectors. *Curr Opin Genet Dev* 1997, 7:75–79.

19. Vojtek AB, Der CJ: Increasing complexity of the Ras signaling pathway. *J Biol Chem* 1998, 273:19925-19928.

20 White MA, Nicolette C, Minden A, *et al.*: Multiple Ras functions can contribute to mammalian cell transformation. *Cell* 1995, 80:533–541.

21. Joneson T, Bar-Sagi D: Ras effectors and their role in mitogenesis and oncogenesis. *J Mol Med* 1997, 75:587–593.

22. Hall A: Rho GTPases and the actin cytoskeleton. *Science* 1998, 279:509–514.

23. Marshall M: Interactions between Ras and Raf: key regulatory proteins in cellular transformation. *Mol Reprod Dev* 1995, 42:493–499.

24. Whitmarsh AJ, Cavanagh J, Tournier C, *et al.*: A mammalian scaffold complex that selectively mediates MAP kinase activation. *Science* 1998, 281:1671–1674.

25. Schaeffer HJ, Catling AD, Eblen ST, *et al.*: MP1: a MEK binding partner that enhances enzymatic activation of the MAP kinase cascade. *Science* 1998, 281:1668–1671.

26. Robinson MJ, Cobb MH: Mitogen-activated protein kinase pathways. *Curr Opin Cell Biol* 1997, 9:180–186.

27. Brunet A, Pouyssegur J: Mammalian MAP kinase modules: how to transduce specific signals. *Essays Biochem* 1997, 32:1–16.

28. Waskiewicz AJ, Cooper JA: Mitogen and stress response pathways: MAP kinase cascades and phosphatase regulation in mammals and yeast. *Curr Opin Cell Biol* 1995, 7:798–805.

29. Karin M, Hunter T: Transcriptional control by protein phosphorylation: signal transmission from the cell surface to the nucleus. *Curr Biol* 1995, 5:747–757.

30. Karin M: The regulation of AP-1 activity by mitogen-activated protein kinases. *J Biol Chem* 1995, 270:16483–16486.

31. Maehama T, Dixon JE: The tumor suppressor, PTEN/MMAC1, dephosphorylates the lipid second messenger, phosphatidylinositol 3,4,5-triphosphate. *J Biol Chem* 1998, 273:13375–13378.

32. Woscholski R, Parker PJ: Inositol lipid 5-phosphatases: tRaffic signals and signal tRaffic.*Trends Biochem* 1997, 22:427–431.

33. McCormick F: Ras signaling and NF1. *Curr Opin Genet Dev* 1995, 5:51–55.

34. Keyse SM: Protein phosphatases and the regulation of MAP kinase activity. *Semin Cell Dev Biol* 1998, 9:143–152.

35. Massagué J: TGF-beta signal transduction. *Annu Rev Biochem* 1998, 67:753–791.

CHAPTER

5

Cell Cycle Control and Mitosis

Randy Strich

The mitotic cell cycle is designed to produce two cells, each containing a faithfully duplicated nuclear genome and a complete compliment of cytoplasmic organelles such as mitochondria. Given the fundamental importance of this process to the normal growth and development of all organisms, it is not surprising that the basic structure of the cell cycle has been conserved in all eucaryotes from yeast to man. This chapter focuses on the regulatory aspects governing cell cycle progression.

One of the overriding themes emerging from research on this topic is that the cell cycle is controlled by the constant interaction between positive factors that promote cell division and negative activities that function to restrict cell cycle progression. The positive factors respond to nutrients and growth factors, whereas the negative control pathways arrest cell division when activated by a variety of stimuli ranging from that of antimitogens that induce differentiation, to cellular damage. The interplay between these opposing forces, which has been observed at every step in the cell cycle, determines cellular fate and is at the heart of many diseases, including cancer. To provide a comprehensive picture of the molecular details concerning cell cycle control, studies derived from yeast, *Xenopus*, and mammalian systems are discussed.

OVERVIEW OF THE CELL CYCLE

CELL CYCLE ANATOMY

The mitotic cell cycle, as the name implies, consists of cyclic series of events that were first observed more than 100 years ago. The basic cell cycle paradigm (Fig. 5-1) consists of an S-phase, in which DNA synthesis occurs; mitosis or M-phase, during which the chromosomes separate and the cell divides; and two intervening gap phases, G_1 and G_2. Subsequent studies showed that cells do not continually divide. Instead, following mitosis and in response to specific signals (*eg*, nutrient deprivation), the cell may enter a nonproliferative state referred to as G_0. As indicated, entry and exit from the mitotic cell cycle and G_0 occur in the G_1 phase. Although the G_1 and G_2 phases do not contain easily discernible landmark events, research has revealed that it is during these two stages that decisions are made regarding whether to proceed or to arrest cell division. In most cases, commitment to another round of cell division occurs in G_1 at a stage called the restriction point in mammalian cells [1] or START in yeast [2]. START or the restriction point is operationally defined as the point in G_1 after which the cell cycle will continue even if nutrients or growth factors are withdrawn. The execution of the restriction point is controlled by many genes that regulate neoplastic growth; collectively termed oncogenes or tumor suppressor genes. Oncogenes (*eg, RAS, MYC*) push the cell through the restriction point, whereas tumor suppressor genes (*eg, Rb, p53*) provide the brakes for the cell cycle engine. The other critical regulatory juncture occurs at the G_2/M boundary, where an intricate tug of war occurs between a different set of factors that promote or impede the cell cycle. At the center of this molecular battle is an activity termed the maturation-promoting factor (MPF) [3]. MPF may best exemplify the dual nature of cell cycle regulators in that its activity both stimulates G_2 progression and inhibits the exit from mitosis.

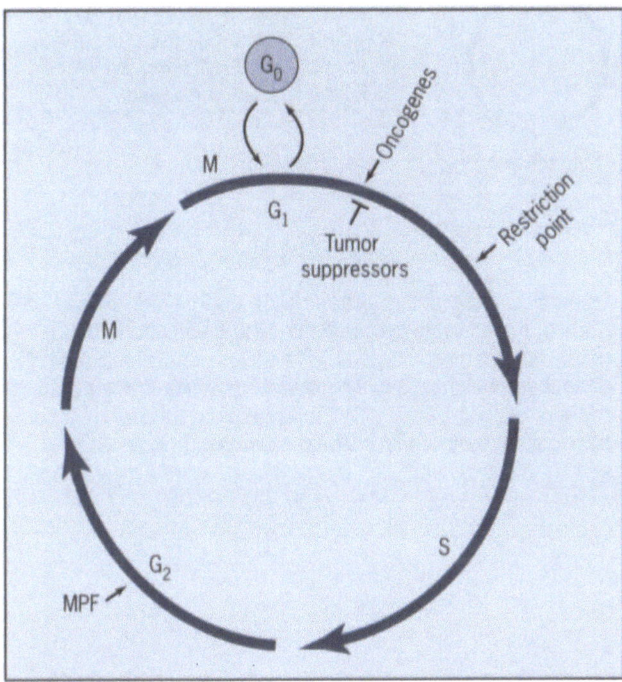

Figure 5-1. The mitotic cell cycle. DNA replication occurs during S-phase. M indicates mitosis, in which the newly replicated chromosomes separate and the cell divides. Two gap phases (G_1 and G_2) occur between S- and M-phase. The restriction point in G_1 defines the regulatory step in which the cell becomes committed to the next cell cycle. In response to nutrient deprivation or developmental cues, the cell will exit the cell cycle in G_1 and enter a nonproliferative state termed G_0. MPF—maturation-promoting factor.

COORDINATION OF THE CELL CYCLE WITH DEVELOPMENT

The cell cycle paradigm described in the previous section is permuted during the embryogenesis of multicellular organisms. During early stages in development, several permutations of the typical cell cycle pattern are observed (Fig. 5-2). Following fertilization, the first 13 cell cycles of *Drosophila* embryos, termed the endocycle, contain only S- and M-phases [4]. Although nuclear divisions occur, the cells do not separate; instead, the nuclear divisions occur within a single cytoplasm, forming a large, multinucleated cell. These divisions occur very rapidly and rely on maternally supplied DNA synthesis precursors and replication proteins. As cellularization commences, a G_2 phase is introduced, and the cell cycle becomes controlled at the G_2/M transition [5]. As different cell lineages develop, a poorly understood switch occurs that results in the introduction of a G_1 phase into the cell cycle. Remarkably, the cell cycle is now controlled during the G_1 phase, and the "complete" cell cycle becomes established [6]. This type of cell cycle allows optimal control over division, because both exogenous factors and intrinsic genetic programs can influence cell cycle progression. The typical G_1-S-G_2-M cell cycle is standard for most ensuing cell divisions for the life of the organism. An exception is observed, however, with the polytene larval cells, which undergo DNA synthesis without chromosome separation. Therefore, by modifying the basic cell cycle machinery, the developing organism is able to rapidly undergo cell division when necessary by streamlining the cell cycle. However, as the cell fates become specified during organogenesis, more control over cell division is exerted by the introduction of G_1 and G_2.

The Cell Cycle Engine

In the past 15 years, it has become clear that cyclin–cyclin-dependent kinase (CDK) activity regulates progression through every stage of the cell cycle (Fig. 5-3). Cyclins are a conserved class of proteins whose association with a specific CDK is required for protein phosphorylation on serine or threonine residues [7]. The task of regulating the cell cycle is divided among the different cyclin-CDKs by their respective point of action. In the case of mammalian cells, progression through G_1 involves the activity of D-type cyclins and several CDKs and the restriction point [8], whereas the G_1/S-phase transition requires cyclin E-CDK2 function [9]. S-phase is driven by cyclin A-CDK2 [10,11] and G_2 by cyclin B-CDC2 [3]. In addition to cyclins and CDKs, other cofactors associate with these kinases and are required for normal activity. In the case of G_1 cyclins, the replication factor PCNA binds to cyclin D-CDK4 [12]. The transcription factor E2F can maximize cyclin E-CDK2 activity [13]. Interestingly, E2F also can function to promote apoptosis and suppress cell growth, depending on the particular cell type [14]. These findings indicate that the

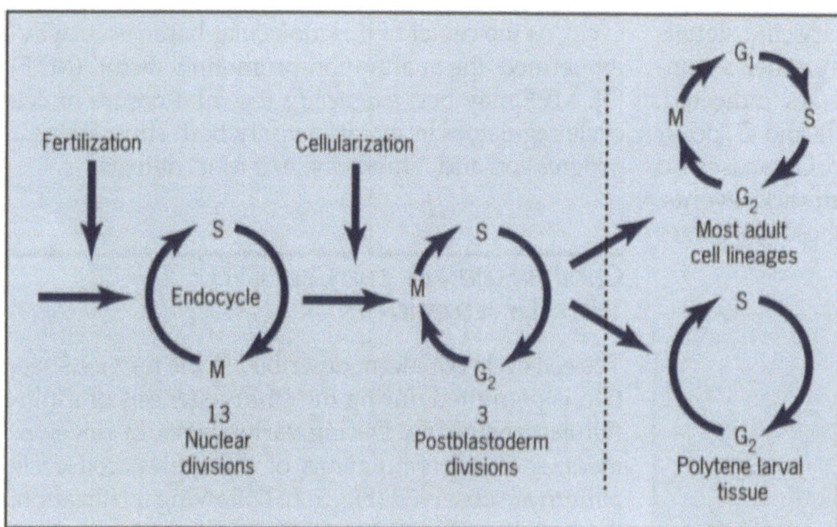

Figure 5-2. Coupling cell cycle control and development. Three cell cycles are observed in *Drosophila* development. The endocycle has DNA replication that is controlled by cyclin E-CDK2 levels, but there is no cell division. The embryonic cycle lacks a G_1 phase and is controlled by oscillation of cyclin A (S-phase) and cyclin B (mitosis). Cyclin E levels remain elevated throughout the cell cycle. The complete mitotic cell cycle (containing G_1) is observed following the first 16 divisions in embryogenesis.

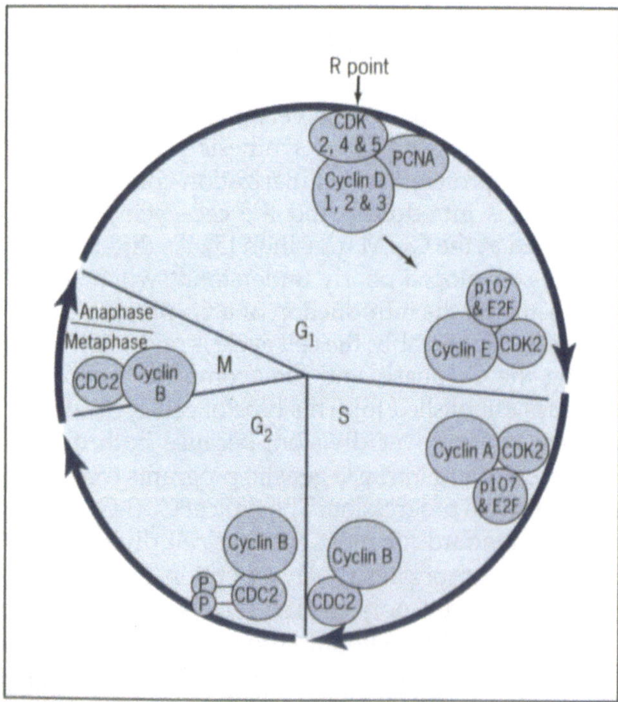

Figure 5-3. Role of cyclin and cyclin dependent kinases (CDKs) in cell cycle progression. The Restriction point (R point) and different stages of the cell cycle are depicted as described in Figure 5-1. The execution point in the cell cycle of various cyclin-CDK complexes are shown. Associating factors involved in maximizing cyclin-CDK activity are indicated with the particular kinase they affect.

molecular context can alter the function of these associating proteins.

Regulation of S-Phase

Early biologists identified two events in the cell cycle, S-phase and M-phase, during which the chromosomes are replicated and segregated into daughter cells, respectively. Most current knowledge regarding the underlying molecular mechanisms governing the regulation of DNA synthesis has been obtained from studies in the budding yeast *Saccharomyces cerevisiae* and the frog *Xenopus laevis*. Studies in yeast have focused on the identification of the first eucaryotic origin of replication, termed the autonomously replicating sequence (ARS) [15]. The origin of replication is bound by a multiprotein complex termed the origin of replication complex (ORC) [16] (Fig. 5-4). The ORC is composed of approximately eight proteins, and for many of these, homologs have been identified in both *Drosophila* and *Xenopus* [17,18]. This observation suggests that the underlying mechanisms and regulation of DNA replication may be conserved among eucaryotes. In yeast, the ORC remains bound to the ARS element throughout the cell cycle (Fig. 5-4). During G_1, a regulatory protein called Cdc6p is synthesized and associates with the ORC on the chromosome [19,20]. Cdc6p is a component of the "licensing factor," an activity required to make an origin competent for DNA replication. Late in G_1, additional regulatory factors known as MCM proteins also associate with the ORC and with sequences flanking the ARS, forming the preinitiation complex (Pre-RC) [21]. The events triggering DNA synthesis remain somewhat of a mystery, although the action of the S-phase cyclin-CDK is essential for this process [22]. As shown in Figure 5-5, phosphorylation of Cdc6p leads to its dissociation from the ORC and the initiation of DNA synthesis [22,23]. Cdc6p is then rapidly destroyed, leaving the origin in a postreplicative state and thus preventing the reinitiation of any competent origins [20]. The association of Cdc6p to the ORC is inhibited by the activity of the G_2 B-type cyclin-CDK complex. Since B-type cyclins are not destroyed until after the commencement of anaphase, this regulatory checkpoint prevents the reinitiation of DNA synthesis until after mitosis.

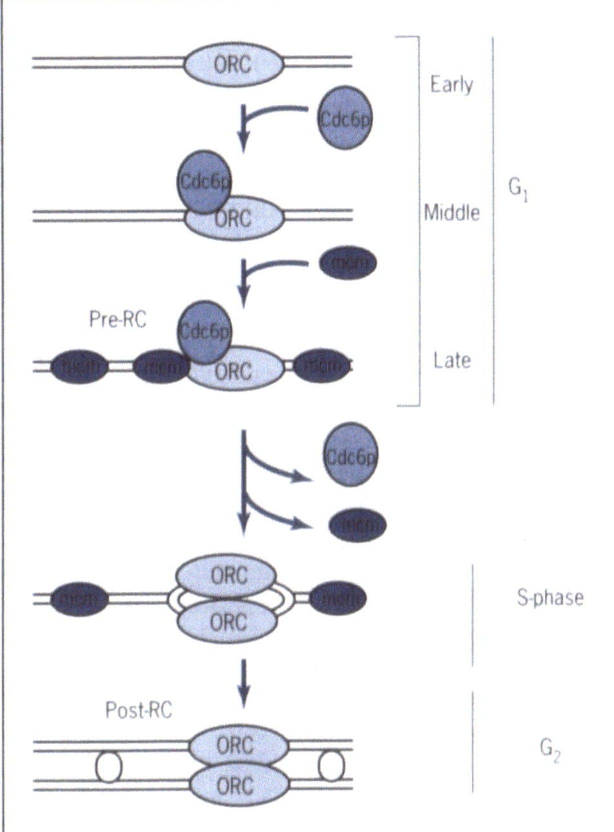

Figure 5-4. Model for regulation of DNA synthesis in yeast. The origin replication complex (ORC) binds the chromosomal origin of replication (ARS) throughout the cell cycle. In middle G_1, prior to the restriction point, a "licensing factor" termed Cdc6p binds the ORC. Subsequent association by auxiliary factors (MCMs) establishes a prereplication complex that is competent to initiate DNA replication. Following initiation, Cdc6p and the MCMs are removed to forbid reinitiation during the same S-phase. Once in G_2, the fully replicated DNA, with an ORC binding both ARS elements, is ready for chromosome separation.

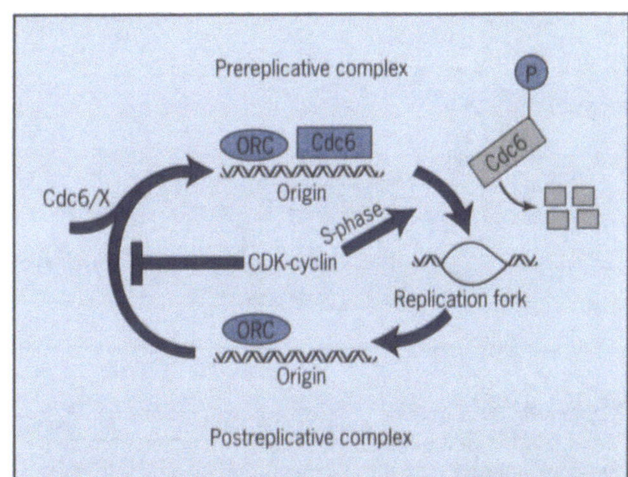

Figure 5-5. Dual role for cyclin-CDK activity in DNA synthesis. Following the establishment of a preinitiation complex including the origin replication complex (ORC) and Cdc6p on the origin of replication, activation of the S-phase cyclin-CDK triggers the transition from an inactive to an actively replicating origin. To prevent reinitiation of the same origin, Cdc6p is degraded in a cyclin-CDK–dependent manner. CDK—cyclin dependent kinase.

Mechanics of Chromosome Separation

Early in S-phase, a complex called the centrosome in mammalian cells or the spindle pole bodies in yeast, duplicates with each product migrating to the opposite sides of the nucleus. Microtubule arrays emanating from the centrosome (polar microtubules) capture and align chromosomes at the metaphase plate (Fig. 5-6), and axial microtubules serve to anchor the centrosome to the cytoskeleton. The polar microtubules attach to the chromosomes at specialized locations called kinetochores or centromeres. Because the newly replicated chromosomes are paired, the kinetochore from each chromosome must be attached to the opposite centrosomes for proper alignment to occur during metaphase. The movements of the centrosomes and chromosomes in this intricate dance are mediated by a class of proteins referred to a kinesins [24]. Members of the kinesin family have been identified in all eucaryotes and serve a variety of functions in the cell. Clues for their respective functions have been obtained from a combination of subcellular localization and mutational/antibody inactivation studies. For example, the *Aspergillus* kinesin BimC is distributed along the length of the microtubules and is involved in spindle pole body movement [25]. The human kinesin CENPE is localized at the kinetochore and is required for chromosome movement away from the metaphase plate [26]. Mutating the consensus cyclin-CDK phosphorylation site in the *Xenopus* Eg5 kinesin prevents normal spindle localization [27]. These findings suggest that the regulation of the various motors is mediated by the oscillating activity of cyclin-CDKs.

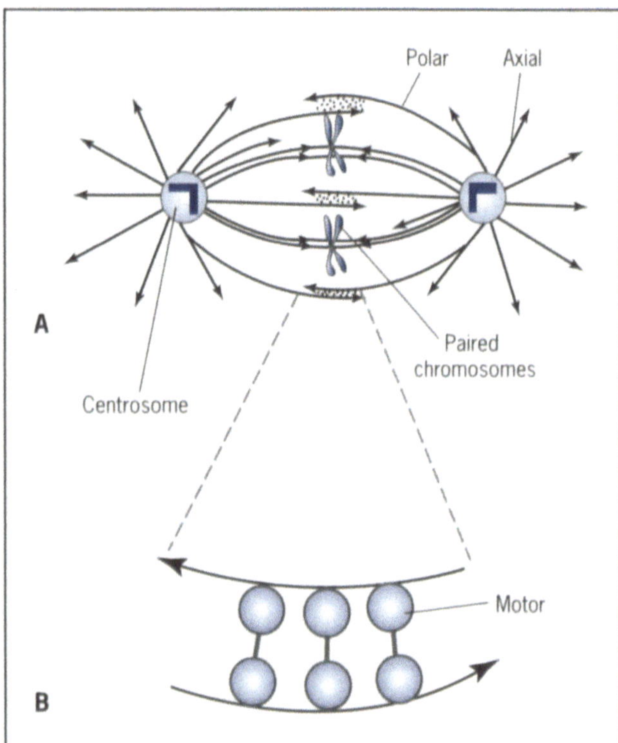

Figure 5-6. Mechanisms of mitotic spindle movement. **A**, Once aligned at the metaphase plate, the action of multiple types of kinesins bound to the polar and kinetochore spindles exert motor force. Anchored by the centrosome and axial microtubules, these forces lead to the separation of the chromosomes toward each pole. **B**, Kinesin-spindle interaction. The kinesin is divided into two domains, and the motor domains at the ends are bridged by a coiled coil structure. This architecture allows two spindles to be bound at the same time.

Regulation of Cyclin–Cyclin-Dependent Kinase Activity

Fitting Cyclins With Their Kinases

The proper execution of cell cycle events requires the activity of cyclin-CDKs that phosphorylate specific substrates within a particular window during the cell cycle. One mechanism for building specificity into this system is the use of the cyclin-CDK two-component protein kinase. Although cyclins are well conserved throughout the eucaryotic kingdom, sequence analysis reveals several classes of proteins based on homology. Moreover, the kinases contain individual "PSTAIRE" motifs (Table 5-1), a domain required for cyclin binding. By combining the binding preferences for both cyclins and CDKs, the number of complexes that can be formed is limited. Because both subunits have been shown to help in substrate selection [28–30], only a subset of proteins with cyclin-CDK consensus phosphorylation sites are actually modified in vivo. For example, histone H1 contains multiple consensus CDK sites and is a substrate in vitro for most of the cyclin-CDKs except cyclin C-CDK8 and cyclin H-CDK7.

Regulation of the Cyclin-Dependent Kinase

Association of the cyclin with the CDK is required for kinase activation. However, cyclin-CDK interaction alone is not sufficient to produce an active kinase. An additional step is required in the form of a modification of the kinase. The CDK must itself be "activated" by phosphorylation of a particular residue (*eg*, threonine 161 for CDC2) [31]. This phosphorylation event is performed by the cyclin H-CDK7 kinase, also referred to as cyclin-activating kinase (CAK) [32] (Fig. 5-7). At present, it is not clear if one of these two events must precede the other or whether they are independent. CAK activity is essential for life in both yeast [33] and *Drosophila* [34], highlighting the importance of its role in cell cycle progression.

In addition to activating phosphorylation, the CDK required for the G_2/M transition (CDC2) also is subjected to inhibitory phosphorylation. This modification occurs at a different part of the protein (tyrosine 14, tyrosine 15, or both) than the activating phosphorylation (Fig. 5-8). The tyrosine kinase *wee1*$^+$ is responsible for this modification [35]. Wee1p is a member of a conserved protein family that has been identified in all eucaryotes examined, including humans [36]. This family was originally discovered in the fission yeast *Schizosaccharomyces pombe* and inactivates cyclin B-Cdc2p activity to allow growth in G_2 prior to mitosis. *wee1*$^+$ received its name due to the phenotype associated with mutations in this kinase. *wee1* mutants fail to remain in G_2 for a sufficient time to permit cell growth. Rather, they rapidly complete cell division, resulting in smaller cells. To alleviate the inactivation associated with this modification, the tyrosine phosphorylation is removed by the Cdc25p phosphatase [37]. Therefore, the activity of Wee1p and Cdc25p on Cdc2p determines whether the cell will proceed through the cell cycle or arrest at G_2. In addition, cyclin B-Cdc2p–directed phosphorylation enhances Cdc25p

Table 5-1. Cyclin-dependent kinases (CDKs)

Kinase	PSTAIRE motif	Cyclin bound	Substrates
CDC2	PSTAIRE	B-type	Nuclear lamins, histone H1
CDK2	PSTAIRE	A-, D-, E-type	Replication protein A, E1A
CDK4	PUSTURE	D-type	pRb, p53
CDK5	PSSALRE	D-type	Unknown
CDK7	NRTALRE	H-type	Other CDKs
CDK8	GMSACRE	C-type	RNA polymerase

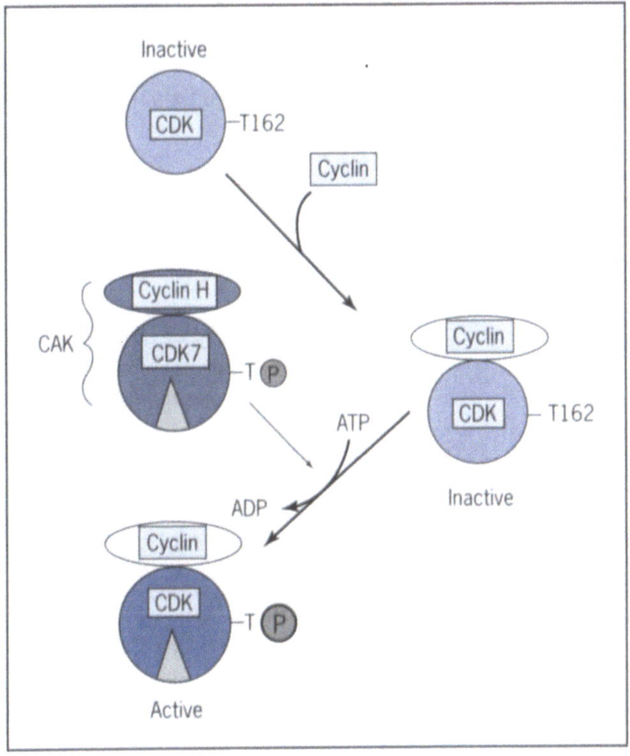

Figure 5-7. Activation of cyclin-CDK kinases by CDK-activating kinase (CAK). An inactive CDK (*top*) containing an unphosphorylated threonine residue (T161 for CDC2 in humans) is bound by a cyclin. This complex remains inactive until the threonine residue is modified by cyclin H-CDK7 or CAK. Once phosphorylated, the cyclin-CDK is active and able carry out its cellular tasks. CDK—cyclin dependent kinase.

phosphatase activity [38] while inhibiting weel kinase [39]. This regulatory strategy initiates a positive feedback loop, resulting in the rapid accumulation of active Cdc2p kinase and the equally rapid inactivation of the mitotic inhibitor Wee1p.

Regulation of Cyclin Levels

An important mechanism for regulating cyclin-CDK activity is through modulating the levels of the cyclin itself. As indicated by its name, cyclin levels oscillate throughout the cell cycle (Fig. 5-9), and cyclin expression closely parallels the point in the cell cycle that it is required. For example, the S-phase cyclin A appears late in G_1 but peaks during S-phase. In addition, the levels of cyclin A are rapidly reduced to basal levels as the cells transit the G_2/M boundary. Cyclin levels are controlled via two pathways. First, their transcription is tightly coupled to the cell cycle. One of the best understood pathways is the control of the budding yeast late G_1 cyclins (Cln1p and Cln2p). The transcription of *CLN1* and *CLN2* require the Swi4p-Swi6p heterodimeric transcription factors. Swi4p-Swi6p will bind the *CLN* promoters only when first modified by the yeast early G_1 cyclin-CDK (Cln3p-Cdc28p) [40]. This regulatory mechanism couples *CLN1* and *CLN2* transcription to one stage in the cell cycle. However, subsequent phosphorylation by Clb2p -Cdc28p G2 kinase inhibits the binding of these transcription factors, thus resetting the promoter for the next cell cycle.

In addition to their periodic transcription, cyclins are also subjected to cell cycle stage–specific proteolysis (Fig. 5-10). This process serves to rapidly inhibit cyclin-CDK activity in a temporal fashion. Because the expression of many cyclins requires the downregulation of the previous set, their precise accumulation and removal is essential for normal cell cycle progression. For example, ectopic overexpression of cyclin D shortens G_1, resulting in smaller cells that no longer respond properly to growth arrest signals [41].

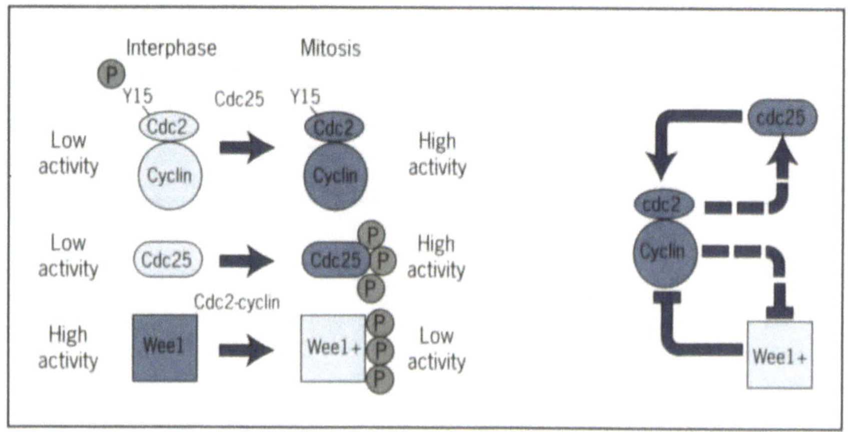

Figure 5-8. Inactivation of cyclin-CDC2 by phosphorylation and dephosphorylation. Following phosphorylation of the CDK on threonine 161 to activate the cyclin-CDK (see Figure 5-7), the kinase can then be inactivated by phosphorylation on tyrosine 15 by the wee1p family of protein kinases. Dephosphorylation of the tyrosine by the dual-specific phosphatase Cdc25p reactivates the kinase to allow cell cycle progression. CDK—cyclin dependent kinase.

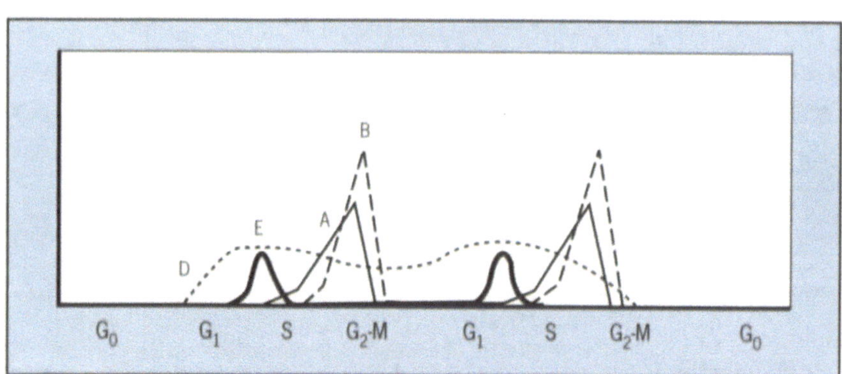

Figure 5-9. Oscillation of cyclin levels through the cell cycle. A typical expression profile of four cyclin subtypes (A, B, D, and E) is depicted with respect to two cell cycles. A-type cyclins are induced late in G_1 and are required for finishing S-phase. B-type cyclins are induced in S-phase and regulate the progression from metaphase to anaphase and mitosis. D-type cyclins respond to early G_1 signals (*eg*, growth factors, hormones) and regulate the cell cycle prior to the restriction point. E-type cyclins are also expressed in G_1 but later than D-type cyclins. E-type cyclins regulate the entry into S-phase and are required for the expression of cyclin A.

More striking is the impact that the constitutive expression of B-type cyclins has on the cell cycle. First observed in yeast and then later found also in mammalian systems, failure to destroy B-type cyclins arrests the cell cycle after anaphase but prior to mitosis [42]. What controls cyclin oscillation? The regulatory system governing cyclin stability has been the topic of intense investigation over the past 10 years. Cyclins are destroyed through a ubiquitin-mediated pathway [43,44] and a proteolysis machine termed the 26S proteasome (Fig. 5-11) [45]. Free ubiquitin is activated by ATP by an enzyme called E1. The activated ubiquitin is transferred to a ubiquitin conjugation enzyme (UBC), or E2. The final substrate for the ubiquitin, in this case a cyclin, is targeted by the combined efforts of the UBC and a specifying enzyme termed E3. After a single ubiquitin moiety has been ligated to the target substrate, additional ubiquitin subunits are rapidly added to the first. This multi-ubiquitinated substrate is then transported to the 26S proteasome, where the ubiquitin is removed and the substrate is reduced to peptides.

Cyclin-Dependent Kinase Inhibitors

The final mechanism for cyclin-CDK regulation discussed in this chapter involves a class of proteins termed cyclin-dependent kinase inhibitors (CDKIs). These proteins directly bind cyclin-CDK complexes and inhibit their activity (Fig. 5-12). Several CDKIs have been identified in yeast and mammals, (Table 5-2) most of which control cyclin-CDK activity in G_1 [47]. The one exception to date is the $p40^{SIC1}$ protein from the budding yeast, which inhibits the activation of S-phase cyclin Clb5p- and Clb6p-CDK activity [48]. By far the largest number of these proteins have been discovered in mammalian cells. This observation makes sense given the complexity of growth signals and developmental cues that must be correctly deciphered in more complex organisms. Each of three well-studied CDKIs—p16, $p21^{CIP1}$ and $p27^{KIP1}$ responds to its own set of signals. $p27^{KIP1}$ is induced in response to antimitogens [49], whereas p21 is activated by intrinsic signals, including DNA damage, through p53-dependent transcriptional activation [50] (Fig. 5-13). Although p16

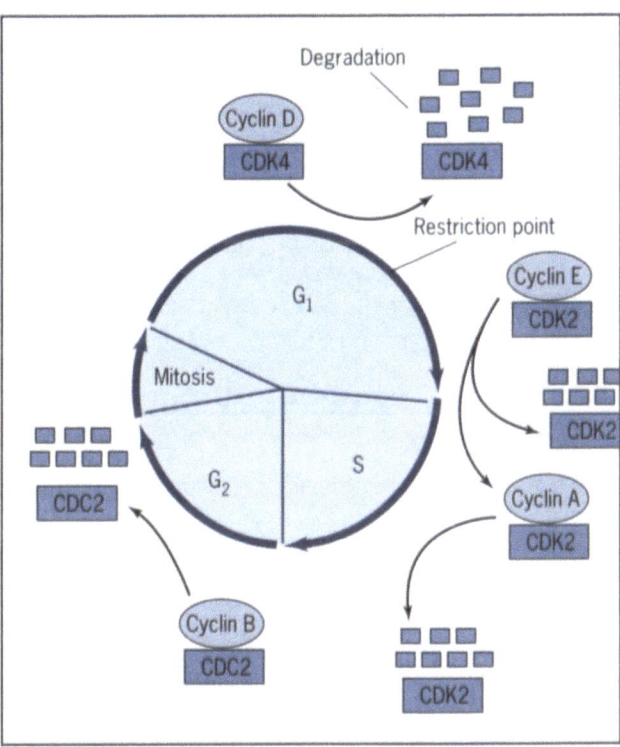

Figure 5-10. Regulation of cyclin-CDK activity by cyclin proteolysis. The regulated destruction of cyclins inactivates the cyclin-CDK complex. Degradation of different cyclins is depicted with respect to cell cycle progression. Even though each cyclin subtype indicated is destroyed at specific times during the cell cycle, only the destruction of B-type cyclins is actually required for cell cycle progression at the G_2/M boundary.

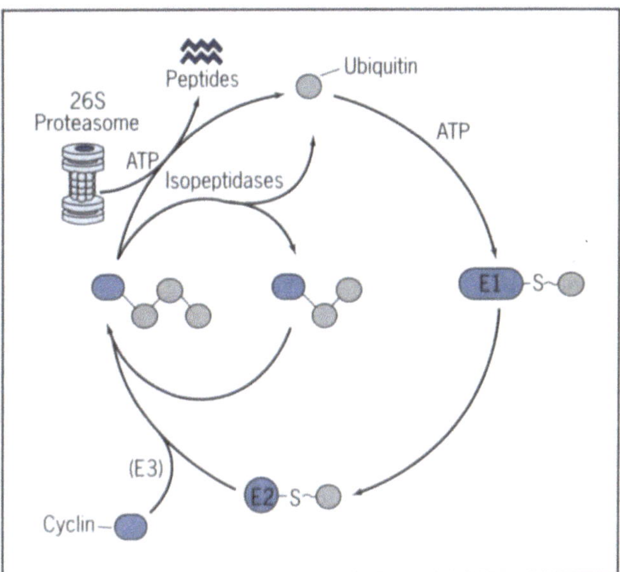

Figure 5-11. Cyclin degradation by the ubiquitin pathway. In a step-wise manner, free ubiquitin is activated by the E1 enzyme in an ATP-dependent reaction. Activated ubiquitin is conjugated to the E2 or ubiquitin conjugating enzyme through a covalent linkage. The E2-ubiquitin conjugate is then targeted to the cyclin by the E3 enzyme at which point the ubiquitin is transferred to the substrate. Additional ubiquitin subunits are rapidly added to the cyclin. The multiubiquitin form is then transported to the 26S proteasome where the ubiquinin is removed and the cyclin destroyed by proteases. The cycle is completed as newly liberated ubiquitin rejoins the free pool.

is also induced in response to cellar damage, its expression appears to be independent of p53 [51]. The importance of these proteins in cancer development was highlighted by the finding that the deletion of p16 is found in many cancer types [52].

REGULATION OF THE RESTRICTION POINT

The classic definition of the restriction point is the stage in G_1 at which the cell becomes irreversibly committed to the execution of another cell cycle regardless of its nutritional status. The restriction point therefore serves as a sensor for both environmental stimuli (*eg*, growth factors; Fig. 5-14) and internal pools of precursors required for DNA, RNA, and protein synthesis. Both internal and external sensing pathways that monitor the availability of nutrients or precursor pool levels affect cell cycle progression in G_1 earlier than the restriction point. Exogenous nutrients and growth factors are sensed by signal transduction pathways that stimulate cell cycle progression through the activation of transcription factors and other regulatory molecules.

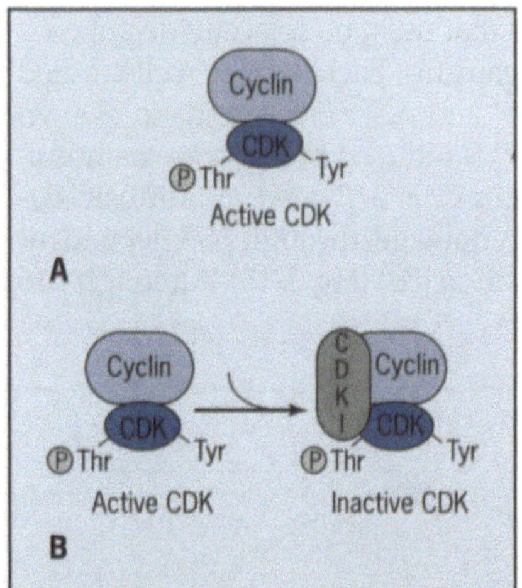

Figure 5-12. Cyclin-dependent kinase inhibitors (CDKIs). **A**, Active CDK requires bound cyclin and phosphorylation on activation threonine. **B**, CDKIs function through direct association to the cyclin-CDK.

Table 5-2. CDK inhibitors and their functions

CDK inhibitor	Organism	Known or possible role
Far1p	Budding yeast	G_1 arrest; activated in response to α factor (antimitogen), inhibitor of G_1 CDK
p27	Mammals	G_1 arrest; activated in response to TGF-β (antimitogen) and cell-cell contact; inactivated by IL2 (mitogen)
p21	Mammals	Checkpoint control; transcriptionally activated by p53
p16	Mammals	G_1/S progression; inactivated in high percentage of tumor cell lines and in familial melanomas
$p40^{SIC1}$	Budding yeast	Cell cycle progression; inhibitor of S-phase CDK; degraded in Cdc34p-dependent manner
p57	Mammals	G1 arrest; not regulated by p53; may be involved in differentiation

CDK—cyclin-dependent kinase.

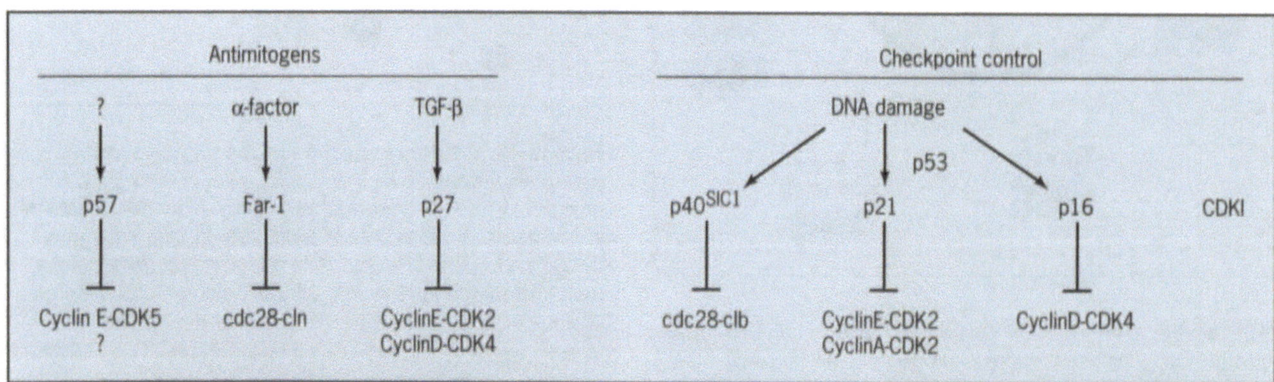

Figure 5-13. Regulation of cyclin-dependent kinase inhibitor (CDKI) activity. Different CDKIs are listed with their proposed regulatory stimulus (*arrows*). The cyclin-CDKs inhibited by each CDKI (*bars*) are indicated. The requirement of p53 for induction of p21 in response to DNA damage is noted. *Far1P* and $p40^{SIC1}$ are yeast genes. The remainder of the genes are mammalian in origin.

Many of the components of these signal transduction pathways [53] or transcription factors [54] were initially described as oncogenes. The mutations in these genes resulted in constitutive activation of their respective pathways and thus allowed unregulated growth.

The control of G_1 represents a continuous battle between growth-promoting factors and those that inhibit cell division. An overview of one such regulatory interplay is described in Figure 5-15. Mitogens induce the expression of members of the D-type cyclin subfamily [55]. The activation of CDK4 by cyclin D leads to activation of the transcription factor E2F (among others in this gene family), which is essential for the transcription of S-phase genes [56]. This pathway is, however, inhibited by tumor suppressor genes and CDKIs at several steps. CDKIs can inhibit cyclin D-CDK4 activity in response to cellular damage, differentiation signals, or lack of growth factors. In addition, the Rb tumor suppressor binds and sequesters the E2F transcription factor early in G_1, thus prohibiting late G_1 or S-phase gene activation. Some of the details surrounding this interplay of positive and negative effectors is shown in Figure 5-16. The increase in cyclin D transcription in response to mitogens increases the formation of cyclin D-CDK4 complexes. This association is inhibited by the p16 family of CDKIs, which compete with the cyclin for binding of CDK4 [51]. Once the cyclin D-CDK4 complex is formed, it must be activated by CAK, a process that can be inhibited by p21 [57] or p27 [58]. Even the CAK-activated cyclin D-CDK4 kinase can be inhibited by these two CDKIs. One target of cyclin D-CDK4 is Rb [13,30]. In its hypophosphorylated state, Rb binds the transcription factor E2F, inhibiting its transcriptional activation ability. When phosphorylated by cyclin D-CDK4, the Rb-E2F association is broken, allowing the activation of S-phase genes by this transcription factor. As cyclin D-CDK4 activity declines following S-phase, Rb returns to its hypophosphorylated form to reset the cell for the next cell cycle [59].

REGULATION OF THE G_2/M-PHASE TRANSITION

Figure 5-17 illustrates the activity of three cyclin-CDKs throughout the cell cycle. As indicated previously, a major regulatory mechanism to control cyclin-CDK activity is the timely destruction of the cyclin. This oscillation of activity correlates with when the particular kinase function is necessary for cell cycle progression. In the case of cyclin B-CDC2, it is required for the G_2/M transition and is historically referred to as mitosis-promoting factor [3]. Similarly, cyclin E-CDK2 complexes are required for S-phase and are sometimes referred to as S-phase–promoting factors. Cyclin A-CDC2 is necessary for the continuation of S-phase, the completion of DNA synthesis, and entry into G_2.

The destruction of B-type cyclins which inactivates MPF and allows the exit from mitosis is mediated by the ubiquitin-dependent pathway and the 26S proteosome. In this system, ubiquitin is targeted to a particular substrate by the E3 enzyme [60]. The destruction of B-type cyclins required for the G_2/M transition is mediated by an E3 enzyme termed the anaphase-promoting complex (APC) [61] (Fig. 5-18). As discussed previously, cyclin B-CDC2 kinase activity is required for cells to enter G_2, but the destruction of cylcin, which leads to inacativation of kinase, is required to exit mitosis and reenter another round of cell division. How does APC fit into this regulatory scheme? Several pieces of data support a model in which APC is activated by cyclin B-CDC2 kinase. Activated APC then

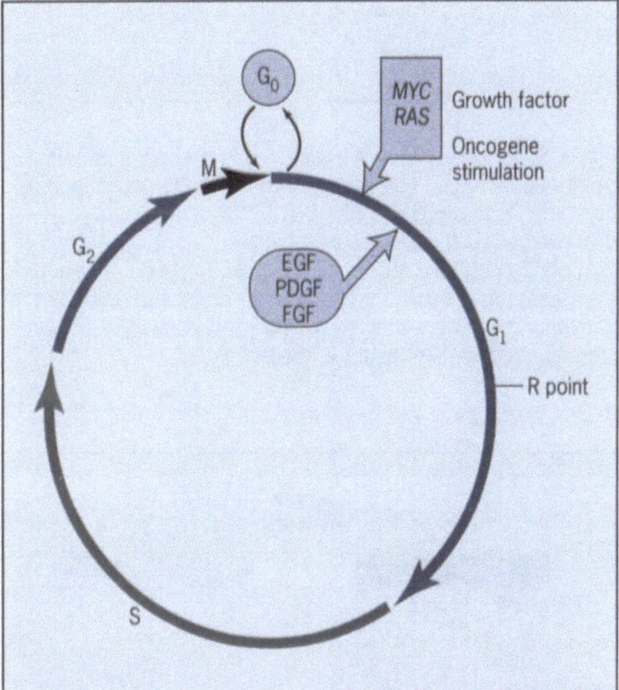

Figure 5-14. Stimulation of the cell cycle by growth factors and oncogenes. Both growth factors (*eg*, EGF, PDGF and FGF) and viral oncogenes (*eg*, v-*ras*, v-*abl*) influence cell division early in G_1, prior to the restriction point (R point). The relative lengths of the different cell cycle phases are indicated by their percentage of the circle. EGF—epidermal growth factor; FGF—fibroblast growth factor; PDGF—platelet-derived growth factor.

triggers the destruction of Pds1p/Cut2p [62], a protein involved in sister chromatid cohesion [63]. APC then directs the destruction of cyclin B [64] that allows exit from M-phase. How is a temporal order established for APC activity? Recent studies have identified components of the APC. One key protein, Cdc20p, is required for the destruction of Pds1p, while a homolog of Cdc20p, Hct1p, directs the destruction of the B-type cyclin Clb2p. Therefore, the timing of events is mediated by different forms of the APC. The finding of APC homologs in higher eucaryotes [65–67] strongly suggests that the basic mechanism controlling the G_2/M transition has been conserved throughout evolution.

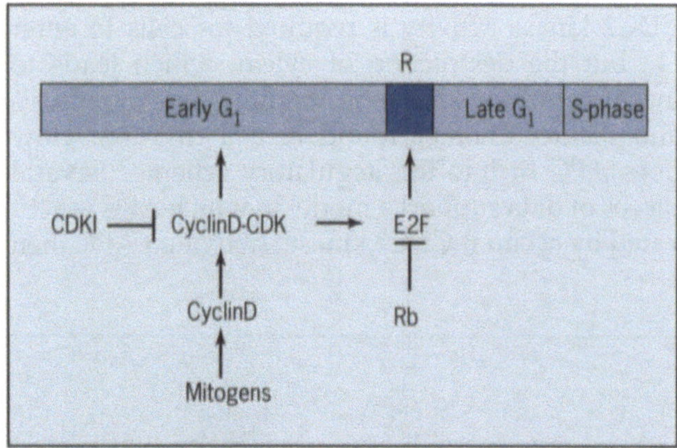

Figure 5-15. Regulation of prerestriction and postrestriction point events in G_1. The restriction point (R) is depicted in a time line illustrating the cell cycle. Positive factors (*arrow*) that promote cell cycle progression are presented. Proteins that play a negative role in growth (also termed tumor suppressors) are indicated. Following the restriction point, the activation of protein kinases (CDK2) and transcription factors required for S-phase are observed.

CHECKPOINT CONTROL

Previous sections of this chapter are dedicated to regulation of the cell cycle under ideal conditions. However, the cell must normally contend with per-

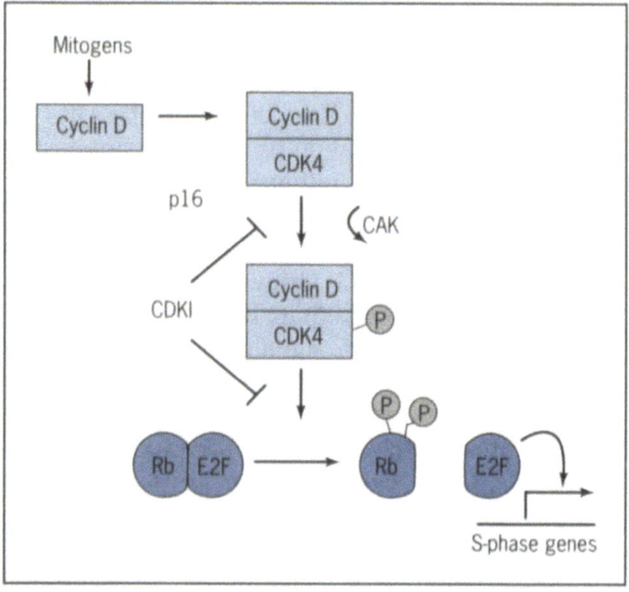

Figure 5-16. Interplay between positive and negative regulators of the restriction point. Mitogens stimulate the transcription of cyclin D, which leads to the formation of cyclin D-CDK4 complexes (*arrows*). This association is inhibited by p16 (*bar*). Activation of cyclin D-CDK4 by CDK-activating kinase (CAK) phosphorylation is indicated, as is the modification of Rb by cyclin D-CDK4. The inhibition of either the CAK or cyclin D-CDK4 step by the p21 or p27 CDK inhibitors is shown. Modification of Rb leads to the disassociation of E2F and the transcription of genes necessary for S-phase.

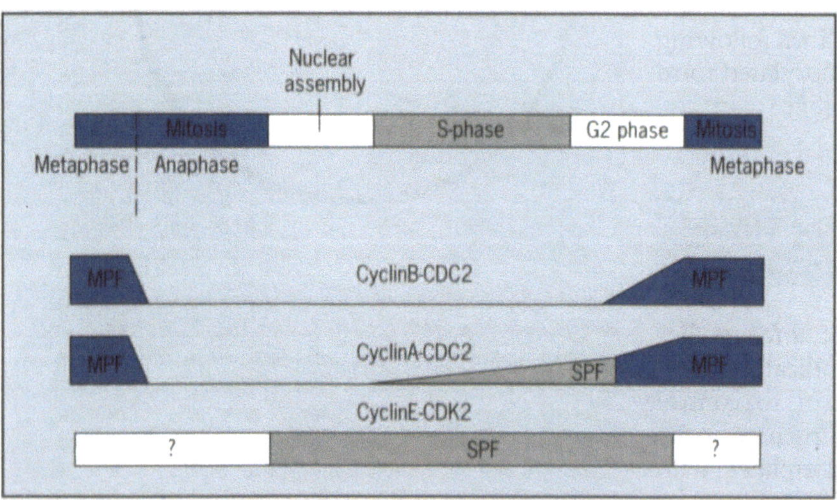

Figure 5-17. Regulation of mitosis by the maturation-promoting factor (MPF). Cyclin B-CDC2, cyclin A-CDC2, and MPF activity are indicated in a single cell cycle time line. MPF activity accumulates in G_2 but is rapidly reduced as the cell transits from metaphase to anaphase. SPF—S-phase promoting factor.

turbations of this cycle due to nutrient limitations, lack of growth factors, or acquired cellular damage. To ensure that the cell is able to faithfully duplicate its genome and partition it correctly to daughter cells, a system of checkpoints is included. The checkpoint system functions on a simple premise; when cellular damage is detected, the cell cycle is halted to allow time for repair [68–70]. Figure 5-19 illustrates the types of stimuli that induce cell cycle checkpoints and their approximate arrest points in the cell cycle. In G_1, the cell must assess its environment, including the availability of growth factors and nutrients. In addition, internal pools of amino acids and nucleotide precursors must be sufficient before another round of cell division is initiated. Mammalian cells also have additional constraints on cell cycle progression in G_1 in the form of contact inhibition and negative growth factors.

The next step monitored by the checkpoint control pathway occurs in DNA synthesis. The cell has two systems that maintain surveillance of DNA integrity. One system monitors unreplicated DNA and is believed to be triggered by the persistence of single-stranded DNA. The second system is activated in the presence of damaged DNA. Damage can be the result of ultraviolet irradiation or other DNA-damaging agents such as alkaloids. When detected, the cell will arrest the cell cycle in G_2 until the proper repairs are made. Several enzymes have been identified that are involved in DNA checkpoint control. The PIK family contains protein kinases that transmit the DNA damage signal [71]. Interestingly,

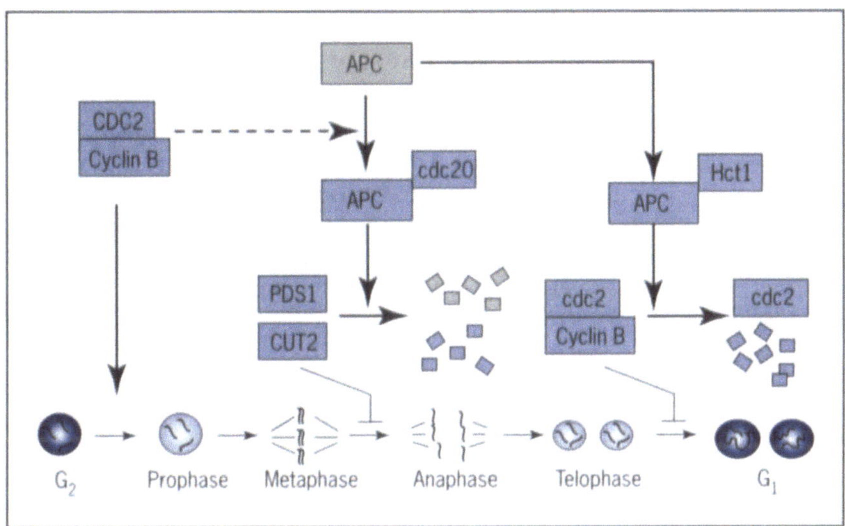

Figure 5-18. Regulation of the metaphase-anaphase transition and mitosis by the anaphase promoting complex (APC). The APC serves as the E3 enzyme to target regulators of mitosis for degradation via the ubiquitin pathway. The APC is activated by cyclin B-CDC2, which leads to the degradation of Pds1p, an inhibitor of the metaphase-anaphase transition. Next, the APC leads to the destruction of cyclin B, thus allowing the cell to exit mitosis.

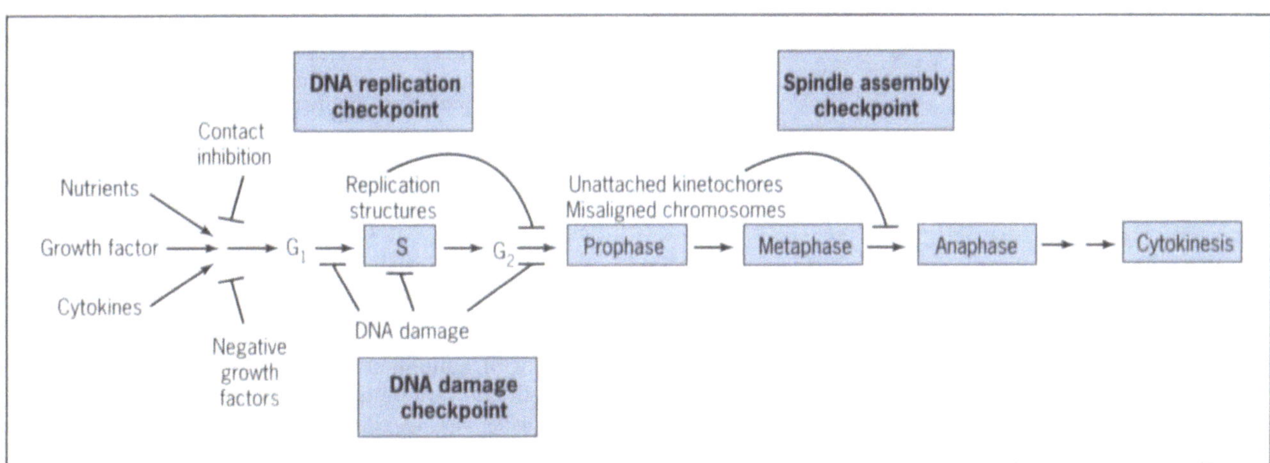

Figure 5-19. Overview of four cell cycle checkpoints. The checkpoint occurring in G_1 senses exogenous signals to determine whether cell division is appropriate. The remainder checkpoint controls monitor internal parameters, including completion of DNA replication, existence of DNA damage, and proper spindle assembly.

their activity is dependent on the presence of DNA, suggesting that these proteins are directly involved in monitoring DNA damage [72]. The importance of these genes in human disease is illustrated by the finding that *ATM* encodes the protein that is mutated in patients with ataxia telangiectasia [73]. The remaining protein classes comprise other important groups that serve a second messenger function. The PI4 and PI3 kinases are responsible for transmitting diverse stimuli, including ligand-bound receptors and stress. Given its important role in many human diseases, including cancer, a significant effort has been made to understand the nature of the DNA damage checkpoint control pathway.

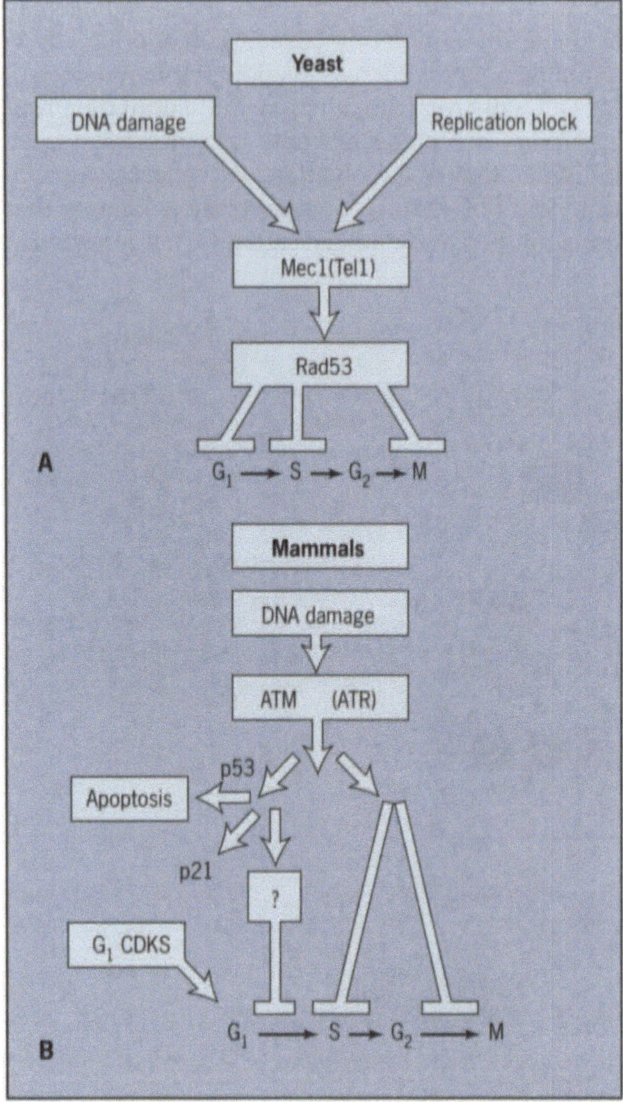

Figure 5-20. Components of the DNA damage and replication checkpoints in yeast and mammals. **A**, DNA damage or unreplicated DNA triggers a kinase cascade that includes *Mec1p* and *Rads53p* in yeast. This pathway mediates cell cycle arrest at various stages in the cell cycle through currently unknown mechanisms. **B**, DNA damage pathway in mammals. DNA damage also initiates a kinase cascade involving ATM, which signals cell cycle arrest through p53-dependent and p53-independent pathways. The p53 pathway can lead to cell cycle arrest through the activation of CDK inhibitors or apoptosis.

In Figure 5-20, the similarities and differences between yeast and human systems are displayed. In yeast, both DNA damage and replication blocks are signaled through the Meclp kinase. The activation of Meclp in turn induces Rad53p activity and can lead to cell cycle arrest at the G_1, S-, or G_2 phase of the cell cycle [71,74]. The most prevalent site of arrest in yeast is G_2. Mammals have more flexibility in their DNA damage response. Similar to yeast, DNA damage is sensed through a PIK family member, ATM [75]. This signal activates the p53 tumor suppressor, which can lead to one of two fates. One branch initiates the apoptotic program that leads to cell death [76]. The other pathway induces the expression of CDKIs. One such CDKI is p21 (Fig. 5-20*B*). In addition to induction of p21, other less well characterized p53-dependent pathways exist that can stop cell cycle progression later in G_1, S-phase, and perhaps at the G_2/M transition.

REFERENCES

1. Pardee AB: G_1 events and regulation of cell proliferation. *Science* 1989, 246:603–608.
2. Hartwell L: Genetic control of cell division cycle in yeast. II. Genes controlling DNA replication and its initiation. *J Mol Biol* 1971, 59:183–194.
3. Masui Y, Markert C: Cytoplasmic control of nuclear behavior during meiotic maturation of frog oocytes. *J Exp Zool* 1971, 177:129–146.
4. Foe VE, Odell GM, Edgar BA: Cell Cycle Reguation in Early Development. In *The Development of Drosophila melanogaster.* Edited by Bate M, Martinez Arias A. Cold Spring Harbor, NY: Cold Spring Harbor Laboratory Press; 1993:149–300.
5. Foe VE: Mitotic domains reveal early commitment of cells in *Drosophila* embryos. *Development* 1989, 107:1–22.
6. Graves BJ, Schubiger G: Cell cycle changes during growth and differentiation of imaginal leg discs in *Drosophila melanogaster. Dev Biol* 1982, 93:104–110.
7. Pines J: Cyclins and cyclin-dependent kinases: take your partners. *TIBS* 1993, 18:195–197.

8. Lew DJ, Dulic V, Reed SI: Isolation of three novel human cyclins by rescue of G_1 cyclin (Cln) function in yeast. *Cell* 1991, 66:1197–1206.
9. Koff A, Cross F, Fisher A, *et al.*: Human cyclin E, a new cyclin that interacts with two members of the *CDC2* gene family. *Cell* 1991, 66:1217–1228.
10. Walker DH, Maller JL: Role for cyclin A in the dependence of mitosis on completion of DNA replication. *Nature* 1991, 354:314–317.
11. Draetta G, Luca F, Westendorf J, *et al.*: Cdc2 protein kinase is complexed with both cyclin A and B: evidence for proteolytic inactivation of MPF. *Cell* 1989, 56:829–838.
12. Xiong Y, Zhang H, Beach D: D-type cyclins associated with multiple protein kinases and the DNA replication and repair factor PCNA. *Cell* 1992, 71:505–514.
13. Hofmann F, Livingston DM: Differential effects of CDK2 and CDK3 on the control of pRb and E2F function during G_1 exit. *Genes Dev* 1996, 10:851–861.
14. Yamasaki L, Jacks T, Bronson R, *et al.*: Tumor induction and tissue atrophy in mice lacking E2F-1. *Cell* 1996, 85:537–548.
15. Stinchcomb D, Mann C, Davis R: Centromeric DNA from *Saccharomcyes cerevisiae. J Mol Biol* 1982, 158:157–179.
16. Bell SP, Stillman B: ATP-dependent recognition of eukaryotic origins of DNA replication by a multiprotein complex. *Nature* 1992, 357:128–134.
17. Rowles A, Chong JP, Brown L, *et al.*: Interaction between the origin recognition complex and the replication licensing system in *Xenopus. Cell* 1996, 87:287–296.
18. Gossen M, Pak DT, Hansen SK, *et al.*: A *Drosophila* homolog of the yeast origin recognition complex. *Science* 1995, 270:1674–1677.
19. Liang C, Weinreich M, Stillman B: ORC and Cdc6p interact and determine the frequency of initiation of DNA replication in the genome. *Cell* 1995, 81:667–676.
20. Piatti S, Lengauer C, Nasmyth K: Cdc6 is an unstable protein whose de novo synthesis in G_1 is important for the onset of S-phase and for preventing a 'reductional' anaphase in the budding yeast *Saccharomyces cerevisiae. EMBO J* 1995, 14:3788–3799.
21. Madine MA, Khoo CY, Mills AD, Laskey RA: MCM3 complex required for cell cycle regulation of DNA replication in vertebrate cells. *Nature* 1995, 375:421–424.
22. Dahmann C, Diffley JF, Nasmyth KA: S-phase-promoting cyclin-dependent kinases prevent re-replication by inhibiting the transition of replication origins to a prereplicative state. *Curr Biol* 1995, 5:1257–1269.
23. Adachi Y, Laemmli UK: Study of the cell cycle-dependent assembly of the DNA pre-replication centres in *Xenopus* egg extracts. *EMBO J* 1994, 13:4153–4164.
24. Vernos I, Karsenti E: Motors involved in spindle assembly and chromosome segregation. *Curr Opin Cell Biol* 1996, 8:4–9.
25. Enos AP, Morris NR: Mutation of a gene that encodes a kinesin-like protein blocks nuclear division in *A. nidulans. Cell* 1990, 60:1019–1027.
26. Yen TJ, Li G, Schaar BT, *et al.*: CENP-E is a putative kinetochore motor that accumulates just before mitosis. *Nature* 1992, 359:536–539.
27. Sawin KE, Mitchison TJ: Mutations in the kinesin-like protein Eg5 disrupting localization to the mitotic spindle. *Proc Natl Acad Sci USA* 1995, 92:4289–4293.
28. Booher RN, Alfa CE, Hyams JS, Beach DH: The fission yeast cdc2/cdc13/suc1 protein kinase: regulation of catalytic activity and nuclear localization. *Cell* 1989, 58:485–497.
29. Kobayashi H, Stewert E, Poon R, *et al.*: Identification of the domains in cyclin A required for binding to, and activation of, $p34^{cdc2}$ and $p32^{CDK2}$ protein kinase subunits. *Mol Biol Cell* 1992, 3:1279–1294.
30. Dowdy SF, Hinds PW, Louie K, *et al.*: Physical interaction of the retinoblastoma protein with human D cyclins. *Cell* 1993, 73:499–511.
31. Solomon MJ, Harper JW, Shuttleworth J: CAK, the $p34^{cdc2}$ activating kinase, contains a protein identical or closely related to $p40^{MO15}$. *EMBO J* 1993, 12:3133–3142.
32. Fisher RP, Morgan DO: A novel cyclin associates with MO15/CDK7 to form the CDK-activating kinase. *Cell* 1994, 78:713–724.
33. Sutton A, Freiman R: The Cak1p protein kinase is required at G_1/S and G_2/M in the budding yeast cell cycle. *Genetics* 1997, 147:57–71.
34. Larochelle S, Pandur J, Fisher RP, *et al.*: CDK7 is essential for mitosis and for I CDK-activating kinase activity. *Genes Dev* 1998, 12:370–381.
35. Russell P, Nurse P: Negative regulation of mitosis by wee1+, a gene encoding a protein kinase homolog. *Cell* 1987, 49:559–567.
36. Igarashi M, Nagata A, Jinno S, *et al.*: Wee1(+)-like gene in human cells. *Nature* 1991, 353:80–83.
37. Russell P, Nurse P: Cdc25+ functions as an inducer in the mitotic control of fission yeast. *Cell* 1986, 45:145–153.
38. Hoffmann I, Clarke PR, Marcote MJ, *et al.*: Phosphorylation and activation of human cdc25-C by cdc2–cyclin B and its involvement in the self-amplification of MPF at mitosis. *EMBO J* 1993, 12:53–63.
39. Tang Z, Coleman TR, Dunphy WG: Two distinct mechanisms for negative regulation of the Wee1 protein kinase. *EMBO J* 1993, 12:3427–3436.
40. Koch C, Schleiffer A, Ammerer G, Nasmyth K: Switching transcription on and off during the yeast cell cycle: Cln/Cdc28 kinases activate bound transcription factor SBF (Swi4/Swi6) at start, whereas Clb/Cdc28 kinases displace it from the promoter in G_2. *Genes Dev* 1996, 10:129–141.

41. Ohtsubo M, Roberts JM: Cyclin-dependent regulation of G_1 in mammalian fibroblasts. *Science* 1993, 259:1908–1912.
42. Ghiara JB, Richardson HE, Sugimoto K, *et al.*: A cyclin B homolog in *S. cerevisiae*: chronic activation of the Cdc28 protein kinase by cyclin prevents exit from mitosis. *Cell* 1991, 65:163–174.
43. Glotzer M, Murray AW, Kirschner MW: Cyclin is degraded by the ubiquitin pathway. *Nature* 1991, 349:132–138.
44. Glotzer M: Cell cycle: the only way out of mitosis. *Curr Biol* 1995, 5:970–972.
45. Hockstrasser M: Ubiquitin, proteosomes, and the regulation of intracellular protein degradation. *Curr Opin Cell Biol* 1995, 7:215–223.
46. Edgar BA, Sprenger F, Duronio RJ, *et al.*: Distinct molecular mechanism regulates cell cycle timing at successive stages of *Drosophila* embryogenesis. *Genes Dev* 1994, 8:440–452.
47. Matthias P, Herskowitz I: Joining the complex: cyclin-dependent kinase inhibitory proteins and the cell cycle. *Cell* 1994, 79:181–184.
48. Mendenhall MD. An inhibitor of $p34^{CDC28}$ protein kinase activity from *Saccharomyces cerevisiae. Science* 1993, 259:216–219.
49. Kato JY, Matsuoka M, Polyak K, *et al.*: Cyclic AMP-induced G_1 phase arrest mediated by an inhibitor (p27Kip1) of cyclin-dependent kinase 4 activation. *Cell* 1994, 79:487–496.
50. el-Deiry WS, Tokino T, Velculescu VE, *et al.*: WAF1, a potential mediator of p53 tumor suppression. *Cell* 1993, 75:817–825.
51. Serrano M, Hannon GJ, Beach D: A new regulatory motif in cell-cycle control causing specific inhibition of cyclin D/CDK4. *Nature* 1993, 366:704–707.
52. Kamb A, Guris NA, Weaver-Feldhaus J, *et al.*: A cell cycle regulator potentially involved in genesis of many tumor types. *Science* 1994, 264:436–440.
53. Ellis R, DeFeo D, Shih T, *et al.*: The p21 src genes of Harvey and Kirsten sarcoma viruses originate from divergent members of the family of normal vertebrate genes. *Nature* 1981, 292:506–511.
54. Alitalo K, Ramsay G, Bishop JM, *et al.*: Identification of nuclear proteins encoded by viral and cellular myc oncogenes. *Nature* 1983, 306:274–277.
55. Lukas J, Barkova J, Bartek J: Convergence of mitogenic signalling cascades from diverse classes of receptors on the cyclin D-CDK-pRb-controlled G_1 checkpoint. *Mol Cell Biol* 1996, 16:6917–6925.
56. Matsushime H, Ewen ME, Strom DK, *et al.*: Identification and properties of an atypical catalytic subunit (p34PSK-J3/CDK4) for mammalian D type G_1 cyclins. *Cell* 1992, 71:323–334.
57. Polyak K, Lee MH, Erdjument-Bromage H, *et al.*: Cloning of p27Kip1, a cyclin-dependent kinase inhibitor and a potential mediator of extracellular antimitogenic signals. *Cell* 1994, 78:59–66.
58. Toyoshima H, Hunter T: P27, a novel inhibitor of G_1 cyclin-CDK protein kinase activity, is related to p21. *Cell* 1994, 78:67–74.
59. Chen PL, Scully P, Shew JY, *et al.*: Phosphorylation of the retinoblastoma gene product is modulated during the cell cycle and cellular differentiation. *Cell* 1989, 58:1193–1198.
60. Hershko A: Roles of ubiquitin-mediated proteolysis in cell cycle control. *Curr Opin Cell Biol* 1997, 9:788–799.
61. Irniger S, Piatti S, Michaelis C, Nasmyth K: Genes involved in sister chromatid separation are needed for B-type cyclin proteolysis in budding yeast. *Cell* 1995, 81:269–278.
62. Visintin R, Prinz S, Amon A: *CDC20* and *CDH1:* a family of substrate-specific activators of APC-dependent proteolysis. *Science* 1997, 278:460–463.
63. Yamamoto A, Guacci V, Koshland D: Pds1p is required for faithful execution of anaphase in the yeast, *Saccharomyces cerevisiae. J Cell Biol* 1996, 133:85–97.
64. Schwab M, Schulze Lutum A, Seufert W: Yeast Hct1 is a regulator of Clb2 cyclin proteolysis. *Cell* 1997, 90:683–693.
65. Weinstein J, Jacobsen FW, Hsu-Chen J, *et al.*: A novel mammalian protein, p55CDC, present in dividing cells is associated with protein kinase activity and has homology to the *Saccharomyces cerevisiae* cell division cycle proteins Cdc20 and Cdc4. *Mol Cell Biol* 1994, 14:3350–3363.
66. Dawson IA, Roth S, Artavanis-Tsakonas S: The *Drosophila* cell cycle gene fizzy is required for normal degradation of cyclins A and B during mitosis and has homology to the *CDC20* gene of *Saccharomyces cerevisiae. J Cell Biol* 1995, 129:725–737.
67. Shirayama M, Zachariae W, Ciosk R, Nasmyth K: The Polo-like kinase Cdc5p and the WD-repeat protein Cdc20p/fizzy are regulators and substrates of the anaphase promoting complex in *Saccharomyces cerevisiae. EMBO J* 1998, 17:1336–1349.
68. Weinert TA, Hartwell LH: The *RAD9* gene controls the cell cycle response to DNA damage in *Saccharomyces cerevisiae. Science* 1988, 241:317–322.
69. Weinert TA, Hartwell LH: Cell cycle arrest of cdc mutants and specificity of the *RAD9* checkpoint. *Genetics* 1993, 134:63–80.
70. Hartwell LH, Weinert TA: Checkpoints: controls that ensure the order of cell cycle events. *Science* 1989, 246:629–634.

71. Weinert TA, Kiser GL, Hartwell LH: Mitotic checkpoint genes in budding yeast and the dependence of mitosis on DNA replication and repair. *Genes Dev* 1994, 8:652–665.

72. Paulovich AG, Hartwell LH: A checkpoint regulates the rate of progression through S phase in *S. cerevisiae* in response to DNA damage. *Cell* 1995, 82:841–847.

73. Savitsky K, Bar-Shira A, Gilad S, *et al.*: A single ataxia telangiectasia gene with a product similar to PI-3 kinase. *Science* 1995, 268:1749–1753.

74. Allen JB, Zhou Z, Siede W, *et al.*: The SAD1/RAD53 protein kinase controls multiple checkpoints and DNA damage-induced transcription in yeast. *Genes Dev* 1994, 8:2401–2415.

75. Painter RB, Young BR: Radiosensitivity in ataxia-telangiectasia: a new explanation. *Proc Natl Acad Sci USA* 1980, 77:7315–7317.

76 Yin Y, Tainsky MA, Bischoff FZ, *et al.*: Wild-type p53 restores cell cycle control and inhibits gene amplification in cells with mutant p53 alleles. *Cell* 1992, 70:937–948.

CHAPTER

6

Transcriptional Regulation

Kathleen W. Scotto
Tan A. Ince

The eukaryotic cell is remarkably versatile. Whether it is destined to spend its existence producing antibodies for immune response or moving mucus over the epithelial sheets of the colon is determined by the myriad of proteins that it manufactures. Some processes are shared by all cells. Therefore, most cells contain a subset of common proteins, including proteins involved in forming the cytoskeleton, proteins intrinsic to the membranes of the golgi and endoplasmic reticulum, ribosomal proteins, and other "housekeeping proteins." In contrast, subsets of proteins are expressed only in specialized cells, where they serve specific and often unique functions. Cellular specialization is controlled by gene expression, in which groups of genes are activated or repressed in response to internal and external stimuli. Moreover, the integrity with which gene expression is controlled can determine whether a cell performs its function in harmony and collaboration with its surroundings or defies the controls of growth and proliferation and invades territories normally reserved for other cells, resulting in malignancy.

The regulation of gene expression can occur at a variety of levels, beginning with the initial synthesis of the RNA molecule from its DNA template, through the processing and transport of mRNA to the cytoplasm, to the translation, modification, and degradation of the protein product (Fig. 6-1).

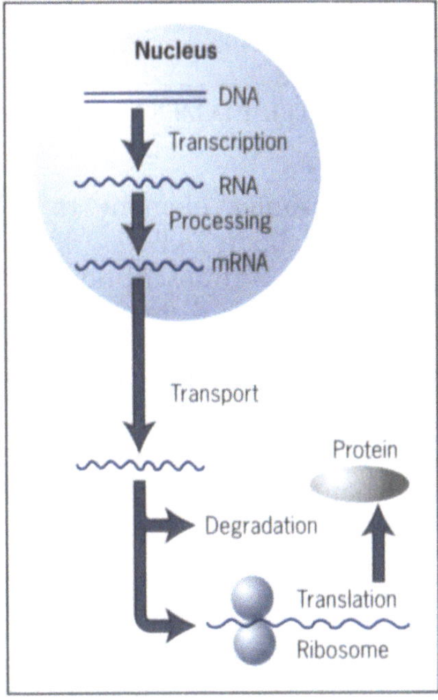

Figure 6-1. Regulation of gene expression can occur at multiple levels, beginning with alterations of the chromatin template through changes in post-translational modifications.

In principle, control imposed at all these levels can determine cell fate. Nevertheless, for most genes, regulation at the level of transcription is paramount. To insure coordinated regulation of the genome in response to both the intracellular and extracellular environment, cells must be able to rapidly up-regulate and down-regulate transcription of particular subsets of protein-coding genes. Transcriptional regulation and its alteration in the disease process are the subjects of this chapter.

BIOCHEMISTRY OF TRANSCRIPTION

Transcription is the synthesis of RNA from DNA templates and is carried out by enzymes collectively referred to as RNA polymerases [1,2]. In eukaryotes, three polymerases undertake this function: RNA polymerase I (RNAPI) transcribes ribosomal (class I) genes, RNA polymerase II (RNAPII) transcribes protein-coding (class II) genes and some small nuclear RNAs, and RNA polymerase III (RNAPIII) transcribes tRNAs and most small nuclear RNA (class III) genes. Although differing with respect to their DNA

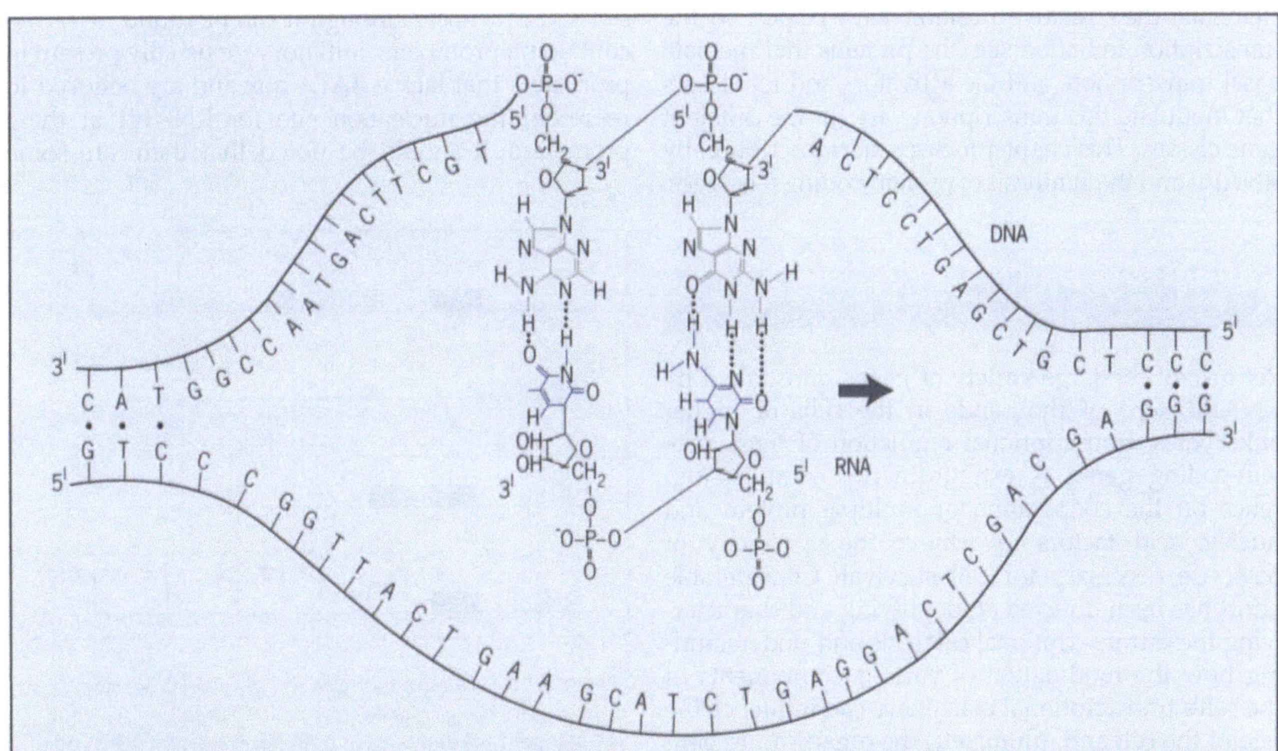

Figure 6-2. Transcription begins when the preinitiation complex binds to a promoter element and unwinds the DNA to expose the template strand. The DNA strand is read in a 3' to 5' direction and complementary ribonucleotide triphosphates are added in a 5' to 3' direction. This process continues until a termination signal is detected, at which point the complex is released and at least some components are recycled for future transcription events.

template and mechanisms of regulation, the three eukaryotic polymerases have similar structures and catalyze the synthesis of RNA in the same manner. Nucleation of the polymerase at a gene template is mediated by DNA sequences within a region referred to as the "promoter" and requires the interaction of other nuclear proteins referred to as basal or general transcription factors (GTFs). On binding to a defined region within the promoter, the polymerase-transcription factor complex unwinds the double helix to expose two short fragments of DNA, one of which will act as a transcription template (Fig. 6-2). The first two ribonucleoside triphosphates complementary to the DNA template are joined by the polymerase, then additional complementary ribonucleotides are sequentially added through the interaction of their 5′ phosphate with the 3′-OH end of the growing RNA chain. This is accompanied by a release of pyrophosphate, the hydrolysis of which helps to drive the reaction. Because synthesis occurs in this 5′-to-3′ direction, convention dictates that the RNA molecule and its nontemplate DNA strand are written in a 5′-to-3′ orientation. The process of unwinding and polymerization continues until a termination signal is detected, and the nascent RNA chain is released and the RNA polymerase is recycled.

Although this general scheme of RNA synthesis applies to all transcription, the nature of the promoter elements, their relative position with respect to the transcription initiation site, the proteins that mediate basal transcription, and the activators and repressors that modulate this transcription vary for the different gene classes. This chapter focuses on transcription by RNAPII and the synthesis of protein-coding messages.

TRANSCRIPTION BY RNAPII

Because of the large variety of genes transcribed by RNAPII, tens of thousands in the cells of higher eukaryotes, transcriptional regulation of these protein-coding genes is extraordinarily complex and relies on the cooperation of multiple protein and nucleic acid factors to achieve the specificity of response necessary for cell survival. Considerable effort has been directed at identifying and characterizing these transcriptional catalysts and understanding how the modulation of various components of the cell's transcriptional machinery can influence the fate of the cell and, ultimately, the organism. In general, these determinants can be divided into three classes: those that direct initiation of basal transcription, those that are involved in the activation or repression of basal expression, and those that are involved in regulation by chromatin. A schematic representation of typical RNAPII gene promotors is shown in Figure 6-3. The majority of RNAPII genes are transcribed from a single site, referred to as the transcription start site or initiation site (+1). In general, most DNA promoter sequences and control elements (enhancer or repressor elements) lie upstream (5′) of the +1 site.

COMMON RNAPII PROMOTER ELEMENTS

TATA Box

The first eukaryotic promoter element to be described was the hexanucleotide TATAAA, located upstream of the start site of transcription and commonly referred to as a TATA box. In promoters that contain this element, the first event is the recognition and binding of the TATA box by the general transcription factor TFIID. Through protein-protein interactions, RNAPII is recruited to the TATA element and initiates transcription 25 to 30 nucleotides downstream.

Initiator

A second common RNAPII promoter element is the initiator. This element was so named because it encompasses the transcription initiation site. Unlike the TATA box, the initiator element has no clear consensus sequence. Although it can be found in TATA-containing promoters, initiators are usually present in promoters that lack a TATA box and are believed to represent the nucleation site for RNAPII in these promoters. It should be noted that there are some

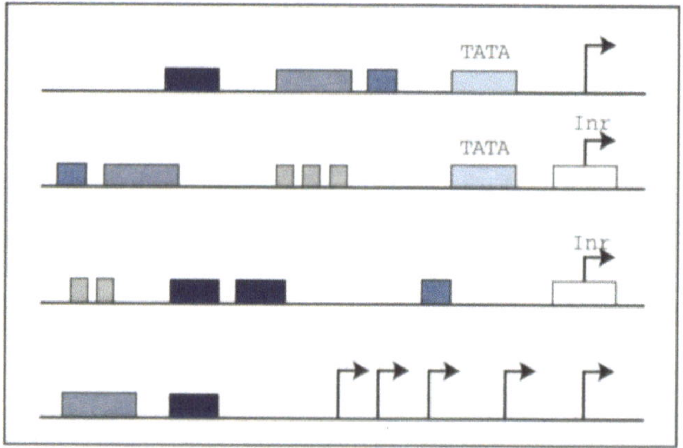

Figure 6-3. There are four classes of RNAPII promoters: single start site promoters can include either a TATA box, an initiator (Inr) element, or both. Multiple start site promoters lack a TATA box, may or may not contain Inr elements, and often contain a downstream element referred to as MED-1. *Arrows* indicate start sites and direction of transcription. *Colored boxes* indicate generic activator/repressor binding sites.

promoters that apparently contain neither a TATA motif nor an initiator; how the preinitiation complex is directed to the accurate transcription start site in these promoters is as yet unknown.

Enhancer, Activator, and Repressor Elements

In addition to the core promoter elements responsible for the correct positioning of RNAPII at the transcription start site, additional elements function as binding sites for activator and repressor proteins. The complement and positioning of these elements define the promoter architecture, which in turn determines how a given promoter responds to the many transcription factors in the cell. Although promoters that respond to the same stimuli often share many of the same regulatory elements, it is unlikely that any two eukaryotic genes will share an identical promoter architecture.

Preinitiation Complex Formation and Transcription Initiation

Transcription by RNAPII can be divided functionally into five stages: formation of the preinitiation complex, initiation, promoter clearance, elongation, and termination. Transcription initiation is defined as the series of events leading to the formation of the first phosphodiester bond in the nascent RNA transcript. Most information regarding the events leading up to transcription initiation has come from in vitro studies in which RNA synthesis by RNAPII can be recapitulated in a cell-free system. When these studies were first initiated two decades ago, it became immediately clear that, in addition to the polymerase, accurate initiation of transcription required other protein factors as well as specific promoter sequences that direct RNAPII to the precise start site of transcription [3–6].

RNA polymerase II cannot interact directly with promoter sequences; rather, it is recruited to the promoter by interacting with the GTFs, forming a complex referred to as the preinitiation complex (Fig. 6-4). During the past decade, tremendous effort has been directed at the purification and characterization of the GTFs required for basal transcription from RNAPII promoters. All of these factors have now been purified and cloned. Collectively, the GTFs comprise more than 30 subunits and include TFIIA, TFIIB, TFIID, TFIIE, TFIIF, and TFIIH. Based on early in vitro studies, the GTFs were believed to assemble at the promoter in a sequential pattern. However, there is growing evidence to suggest that at least a subset of RNAPII may exist in a large complex in vivo as the RNAPII holoenzyme, which includes many of the GTFs in addition to other transcription factors. Nevertheless, because the majority of information regarding the role of the GTFs has come from the sequential order of addition model, assembly of the preinitiation complex is discussed in the context of that model.

In promoters that contain a TATA motif, the first event in the formation of the preinitiation complex is the recognition of this motif by TFIID, a multi-subunit complex that includes the DNA-binding protein TBP and a number of TBP-associated factors referred to collectively as TAFs. TFIID, or more specifically, its TBP subunit, is the only member of the preinitiation complex that possesses sequence-specific DNA binding activity. Binding of TBP to the minor groove leads to a severe distortion of the DNA; it has been suggested that this distortion stabilizes interaction of other GTFs or proximal proteins, and prevents the packaging of TATA elements into nucleosomes. The interaction of TFIID with the TATA element nucleates assembly of the remaining GTFs in the preinitiation complex. The next GTFs to enter the complex are TFIIA and TFIIB, both of which can interact directly with TFIID. TFIIB has two critical roles in transcription initiation. First, it acts as a "bridging factor" and

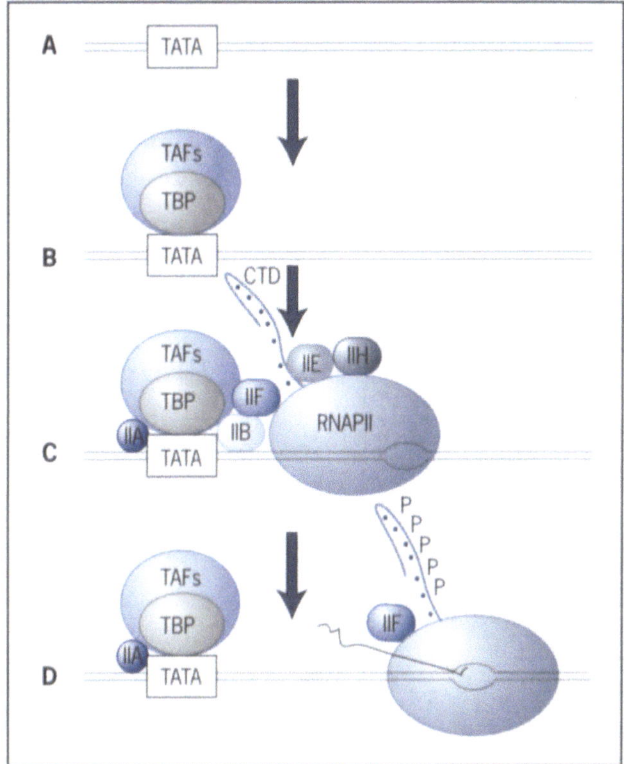

Figure 6-4. Initiation of transcription requires the assembly of a large multiprotein complex on the promoter that includes RNAPII. Initial in vitro studies suggested that the general transcription factors assembled in a sequential manner, beginning with the direct binding of TFIID to a promoter element. More recent evidence indicates that RNAPII, along with the GTFs, may preexist in the form of a holoenzyme. See text for more information on the function of the GTFs.

recruits TFIIF/RNAPII to the promoter. Second, studies of TFIIB mutants in yeast have indicated that this factor aids in the selection of the transcription start site. TFIIB interacts with TFIID-DNA asymmetrically and contacts the phosphodiester backbone of DNA both upstream and downstream of the TATA element. Interestingly, the position of the amino terminus of TFIIB in the DNA-IID-IIB complex places it at or near the transcription start site, and it has been suggested that TFIIB may stabilize the melting of the promoter that precedes RNA synthesis. Although the requirement for TFIIB in complex assembly is clear, the need for TFIIA is somewhat controversial, although it has been shown to stabilize the TBP-DNA interaction and appears to play a role in derepression.

Following assembly of the DNA-TFIID-(TFIIA)-TFIIB complex, RNAPII is recruited to the promoter by TFIIF. TFIIF has been shown to weaken or prevent the interaction of RNAPII with nonspecific promoter sites. It also has been implicated in start site selection, because photo–cross-linking studies have shown that, like TFIIB, TFIIF makes contact with DNA downstream of the TATA box, immediately upstream of the initiation site. RNAPII is comprised of 10 subunits, many of which share homology to the subunits of other polymerases (Fig. 6-5). However, one subunit unique to RNAPII is the carboxy-terminal domain (CTD), which is a substrate for phosphorylation. Only the hypophosphorylated form of RNAPII can be recruited to the pre-initiation complex (PIC) subsequent phosphorylation of the carboxy terminal domain is required for transcription initiation and promoter clearance.

Through interactions with the GTFs and RNAPII, TFIIE joins the complex and recruits TFIIH. TFIIH is the last GTF to join the preinitiation complex. This factor exhibits various ATP-dependent catalytic activities, including CTD kinase, DNA-dependent ATPase, and DNA helicase activities; it also plays a role in nucleotide excision repair and cell cycle regulation. The recruitment of TFIIE and TFIIH completes preinitiation complex assembly, but the interaction of this massive (approximately 1000 kD) preinitiation complex with the core promoter is not sufficient to initiate transcription. First, the CTD of RNAPII must be phosphorylated by TFIIF, and ATP hydrolyzed. Then, in the presence of nucleotide triphosphates, DNA melting, initiation of synthesis, and promoter clearance can occur.

Although the majority of information on RNAPII transcription has come from the study of TATA-containing promoters, an equal number of human RNAPII promoters lack this core element. Many TATA-less promoters direct transcription from a single start site or cluster of start sites, whereas some transcribe from multiple start sites spanning dozens of nucleotides (Fig. 6-3). Relative to TATA-driven transcription, transcription of TATA-less promoters is less

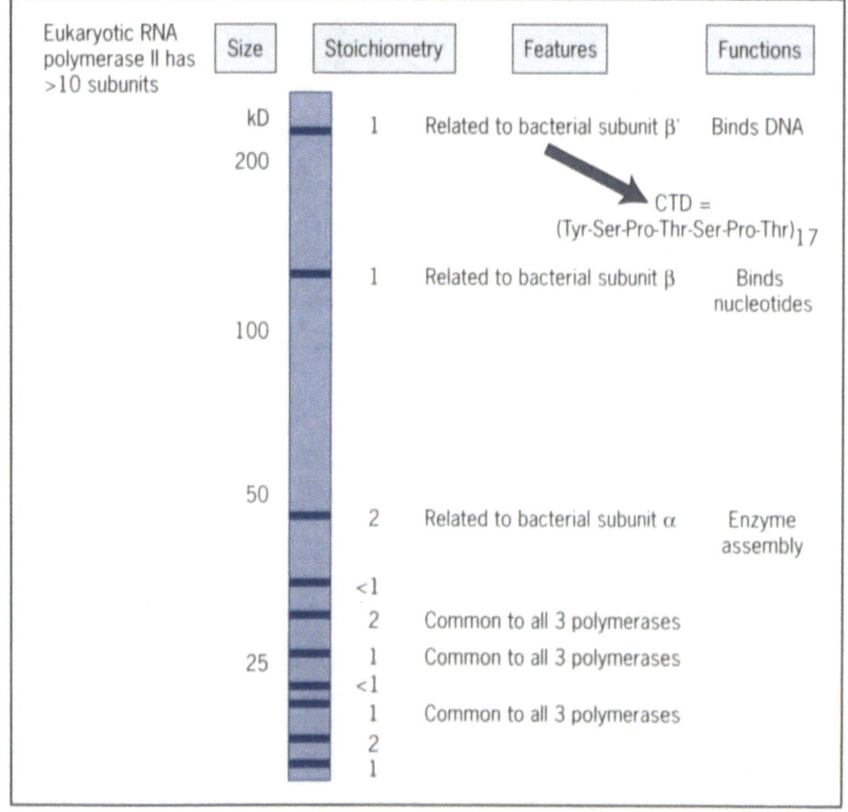

Figure 6-5. RNAPII is a large (≈ 500 kD) protein that contains more than 10 subunits. Many of these subunits are shared with RNAPI and PNAPIII, and some have homology to bacterial polymerase. (*Adapted from* Lewin [1].)

well understood. Analysis of the TATA-less mouse terminal deoxynucleotidyl transferase promoter identified a second core element, the initiator, which encompasses the transcription start site and is sufficient to position the basal machinery in the absence of a TATA motif. (Although initiators were later found also to be components of many TATA-containing promoters, due to space constriction they are discussed in this chapter only in relation to TATA-less transcription.) By random mutagenesis, computational analysis, and functional assays, a consensus initiator sequence, PyPyA(+1)NT/APyPy, was identified. One unresolved issue is the nature of the protein factor or factors that interact with the initiator; several models for recruitment of RNAPII to the initiator have been proposed. Among the transcription factors that have been proposed to play this role are TFII I, a factor which was initially identified as the protein interacting with the initiator element in the TATA-containing adenovirus major late promoter; the ubiquitous transcription factors YY1 and SP1; the TAFs of TFIID, particularly TAF150; and RNAPII itself. Although the myriad of models for TATA-less transcription seem confusing and sometimes contradictory, it should be kept in mind that, to date, a very limited number of TATA-less promoters have been analyzed. Additionally, regardless of the sequence-specific DNA binding protein implicated in these different models, it is clear that TFIID plays a major role in directing the formation of the PIC on all class II promoters.

Transcription Elongation and Termination

For RNAPII transcription to proceed, additional protein factors are required [5,7,8]. To date, several "elongation factors" have been identified: TFIIF, SII, SIII (elongin), ELL, and P-TEFb. TFIIF is unique among the RNAPII GTFs in that it plays a dual role in initiation and elongation. Although the elongation factors work through different mechanisms, their overall function is to suppress or prevent premature pausing of RNAPII as it traverses the DNA template. In effect, by expediting the passage of RNAPII through the long stretches of DNA commonly comprising a class II eukaryotic gene, the elongation factors promote a higher overall rate of productive mRNA synthesis.

Little is known about the mechanisms governing termination of RNAPII transcription, because precise "termination signals" have not yet been mapped. However, the 3′ end of the mRNA molecule is determined not by the site of termination but rather by the site of cleavage of the terminated transcript, because RNAPII transcripts are cleaved during maturation at a site precisely localized by a polyadenylation signal 11 to 30 bp upstream. Following termination, RNAPII is released from the DNA template and nascent transcript, dephosphorylated, and recycled for use in future transcription initiation.

Regulation of Transcription

The basal transcription complex, containing RNAPII and the GTFs, is sufficient to initiate transcription of protein-coding genes. However, the efficiency with which these genes are expressed is determined by other factors, collectively referred to as activators and repressors. These factors function through direct interaction with DNA elements within the promoter and via protein-protein interactions with other transcription factors or the basal machinery. A myriad of DNA binding elements are located within a promoter; however, the mere presence of a transcription factor binding site within a promoter does not predict whether or how the promoter will be regulated by the cognate binding protein. Rather, the activation or repression of a gene in a given cell type or under different physiologic conditions is determined by the presence, complexity, arrangement, and accessibility of DNA response elements within the promoter, as well as by the complement of transcription factors that interact with these elements.

Regulatory Transcription Factors

In general, transcription factors fall into two classes: those that activate basal transcription and those that repress or silence transcription. These two classes can be further subdivided into factors that exert their activity by direct interaction with promoter sequences and factors that function via protein-protein interactions without direct interaction with DNA. The latter category includes a group of proteins referred to as co-activators and co-repressors, many of which appear to act as a "bridge" between transcriptional activators and repressors, respectively, and the basal machinery; others mediate changes in chromatin structure. Most transcription factors contain at least two domains; one allows for the recognition of specific promoters, either by direct DNA binding or protein-protein interactions, and the other mediates regulation of that promoter by affecting DNA structure or basal machinery. Additional domains may be present in different activator classes (Fig. 6-6*A*). In recent years it has become apparent that most transcription factors can be classified according to shared common motifs of DNA binding or activation. Less is known about repression (discussed later).

Transcription Factor Motifs and DNA Binding Domains

The recognition of specific DNA sequences is mediated by defined structural motifs within DNA binding proteins. There are at least five classes of DNA binding motifs that have been extensively characterized [1,2,9–12] (Fig. 6-6*B*). All of these motifs are fairly short, representing only a small portion of the transcription factor, and most have been named according to the protein structure that is critical for DNA binding. They include the zinc finger motif, the steroid hormone binding motif, the helix-loop-helix (HLH) motif, the helix-turn-helix (HTH) motif, and the leucine zipper. These are described in more detail later in this chapter.

Zinc finger motif. First identified in the RNAPIII transcription factor TFIIIA, the zinc finger motif can exist in several forms. The classic zinc finger consists of about 30 amino acids that fold to form a minidomain with a single zinc ion coordinated by two cysteines and two histidines (Cys_2-His_2); the resulting structure links an α-helix to a β-sheet such that the

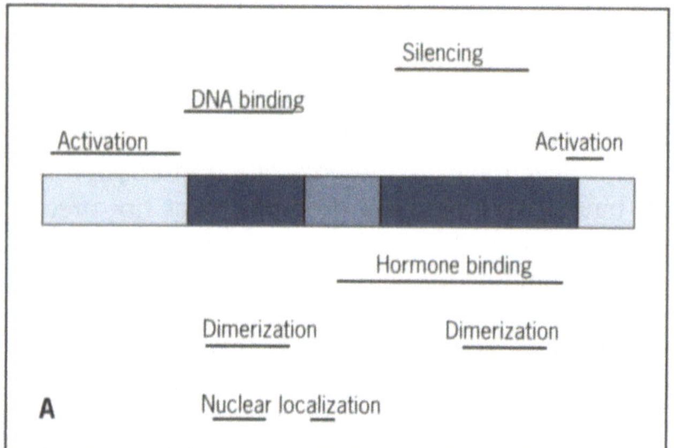

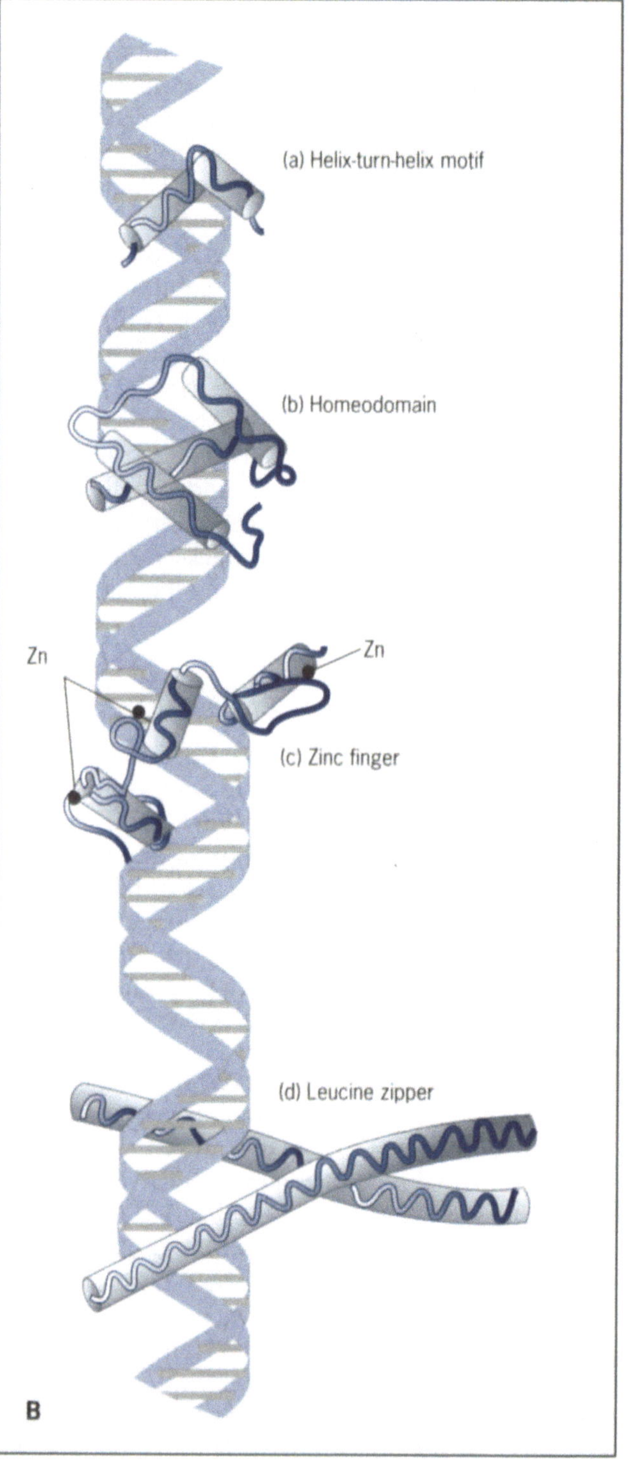

Figure 6-6. **A**, Transcription factors comprise multiple functional domains and can often be classified according to the complement of domains that they contain. For example, hormone receptors share similar domains for DNA binding, ligand binding, protein-protein interaction, nuclear localization, and activation. **B**, Most transcription factors bind to bases within the major groove, although a few, like TBP and NF-Y, are minor-groove binding proteins. Specificity of binding is regulated by the recognition of specific sequences within the promoter by structural motifs, such as the zinc finger and helix-turn-helix. See text for details. (*Adapted from* Raven and Johnson [2].)

helical segment fits into the major groove of DNA. Several variations of this general motif have been identified, including the "ring finger," in which two zinc ions are coordinated by four ligands. Classic zinc fingers exist in multiples ranging from 2 to 27; in general, the more fingers in the cluster, the higher its affinity for DNA.

Helix-turn-helix motif. As the name implies, the helix-turn-helix (HTH) motif consists of two α-helices separated by a nonhelical turn. It is generally comprised of approximately 20 amino acids, with the two helices separated by a 4–amino acid turn. The second helix, referred to as the recognition helix, interacts with specific base pairs in the major groove, whereas the first helix lies at an angle across the DNA. The HTH DNA binding family can be further subdivided based on the presence and positioning of other structural elements such as α-helices, β-strands, and hairpins. One of the best studied classes of HTH proteins is the homeodomain family of transcription factors, initially found in the promoters of *Drosophila* genes that are regulated during early development. The homeodomain is usually approximately 60 amino acids long and contains three α-helices, including the HTH domain. It appears that all homeodomains bind DNA in the same manner, with the N- and C-termini of the homeodomain responsible for DNA contact.

Basic helix-loop-helix domain.The basic helix-loop-helix (bHLH) domain is one of the most common transcription factor motifs involved in dimerization and DNA binding in eukaryotes. It is characterized by a stretch of 40 to 50 amino acids containing two amphipathic α-helices separated by a loop of 5 to 24 amino acids. The amphipathic helices confer the ability to form the homodimers and heterodimers necessary for DNA binding. The ability to heterodimerize also affects the activity of the HLH protein, because the choice of partners influences the affinity of the dimer for DNA. In some cases, an HLH partner may function as a dominant negative regulator of transcription (discussed later). Adjacent to most HLH motifs is a highly basic domain, and many HLH proteins contain an additional motif referred to as the leucine zipper (ZIP; discussed later), which forms a continuous helix with the second helix of the HLH. In HLH-ZIP proteins, the zipper region appears to confer the specificity of dimerization. Examples of bHLH proteins include MYO-D and E47; examples of the bHLH-ZIP class include MAX and USF.

Leucine Zipper.The leucine zipper (ZIP) class of transcription factors is identified by the presence of a coiled coil motif that includes a stretch of amino acids with a leucine occurring every seventh residue. Leucine zippers are often found in conjunction with other DNA binding motifs, where they are directly linked to the motif (bHLH-ZIP and homeodomain-ZIP proteins) or are connected to the DNA binding domain by a short linker (yeast GAL4 and PPR1 transcription factors). The leucine zipper promotes formation of dimers, because it forms an amphipathic helix in which the leucines of the zipper on one protein can interdigitate with the leucines on the zipper of another protein, forming a coiled coil. The region adjacent to each zipper is highly basic and forms the DNA binding domain. Two interacting zippers form a Y shape in which the zippers are the stem and the highly charged basic residues are the arms that bind the DNA. Among the well-studied members of the zipper family of transcription factors are the AP1 components FOS and JUN and their related family members and the C/EBP family of transcription factors. Formation of homodimers and heterodimers within these protein families regulates their transcriptional activity.

Other DNA binding motifs. Although the previously mentioned classes of DNA binding proteins include the majority of transcription factors, there are other motifs that are not as common. The MADS box is a conserved motif found within the DNA binding domain of several transcription factors from a diverse range of organisms, including the human serum response factor and muscle-specific MEF2 proteins. The MADS motif is a contiguous sequence of 56 amino acids in which the N-terminal half is involved in DNA binding and the C-terminal half is required for dimerization. Therefore, like the ZIP-containing proteins, heterodimerization of MADS box proteins regulates their transcriptional activity by allowing for the formation of proteins with subtly different DNA specificities.

The REL family of transcription factors, which includes NFAT and NF-κB, share similarities in their DNA binding domain, which is comprised of two β-barrel structures that grip DNA in the major groove. The folds of these domains are related to immunoglobulin-like modules, and both domains contact the DNA backbone. Although this region is similar in both proteins, NFAT lacks the C-terminal dimerization domain found in NF-κB; this results in profound differences in their regulatory properties.

TRANSCRIPTIONAL ACTIVATION

In contrast to the DNA-binding motifs, the protein domains required for transcriptional activation are less well defined. Transcriptional activation domains have been experimentally defined as regions of a transcription factor that, when linked to a heterologous DNA binding domain, are able to enhance transcription from a promoter containing a cognate DNA binding sequence. Using these criteria, most transcriptional activators contain one or more of three distinct domains that are defined on the basis of their amino acid content: the acidic domain, the glutamine-rich domain, and the proline-rich domain. The activation domains of other classes of transcription factors, including the steroid hormone receptors, do not conform to these recognizable motifs, and the sequences involved in activation by these molecules have only been grossly defined.

Considerable progress has been made in the past few years in defining the mechanism or mechanisms by which these activator domains facilitate the increased transcription of a promoter. Most activators appear to function by interacting with some component of the basal transcriptional machinery. The consequences of this interaction may be an enhanced recruitment of RNAPII to the promoter or stabilization of the basal initiation complex bound to the promoter. The interaction of activators with the basal machinery can occur either directly or indirectly (Fig. 6-7). A breakthrough in our understanding of the communication between activator molecules and the basal machinery came with the discovery that although TBP was sufficient to nucleate formation of the preinitiation complex, it was not sufficient to mediate activation. Rather, other proteins mediate the function of activators and are referred to as coactivators [6,13–16]. Among the first class of coactivators to be identified were the TAFs, which are components of the TFIID complex that interact with both transcriptional activators and the basal machinery [17–20]. Therefore, TAFs serve as a bridge between activator proteins and the basal factors. Although TAFs do not appear to be required for the function of all activators, they are a critical component in the regulation mediated by many transcription factors. Recently, the role of chromatin in the regulation of transcription has received considerable attention, and many of the known transcriptional activators and coactivators function through the modification of chromatin structure. This is discussed in more detail later in this chapter.

Most if not all promoters of higher eukaryotes have evolved to contain multiple binding sites for transcriptional activators. An array of promoter-bound activators, each of which contains one or more activation domains, functions in concert and often synergistically to regulate transcription (Fig. 6-8). Thus, regulation of a given promoter in response to a particular set of signals is achieved by the precise assembly of multiprotein complexes; the exact nature of the multiprotein complex, although grossly dictated by the promoter architecture, can differ subtly in response to different signals, leading to profound regulatory switches. Adding to this complexity is the presence of repressor proteins, which negatively regulate transcription.

TRANSCRIPTIONAL REPRESSION

Most of the studies of transcriptional regulation have focused on factors that activate transcription. However, another class of transcription factors are involved in repression, or gene silencing [21]. Like transcriptional activators, these proteins function either by direct DNA binding or protein-protein interactions (Fig. 6-9). Repressors can act through a variety

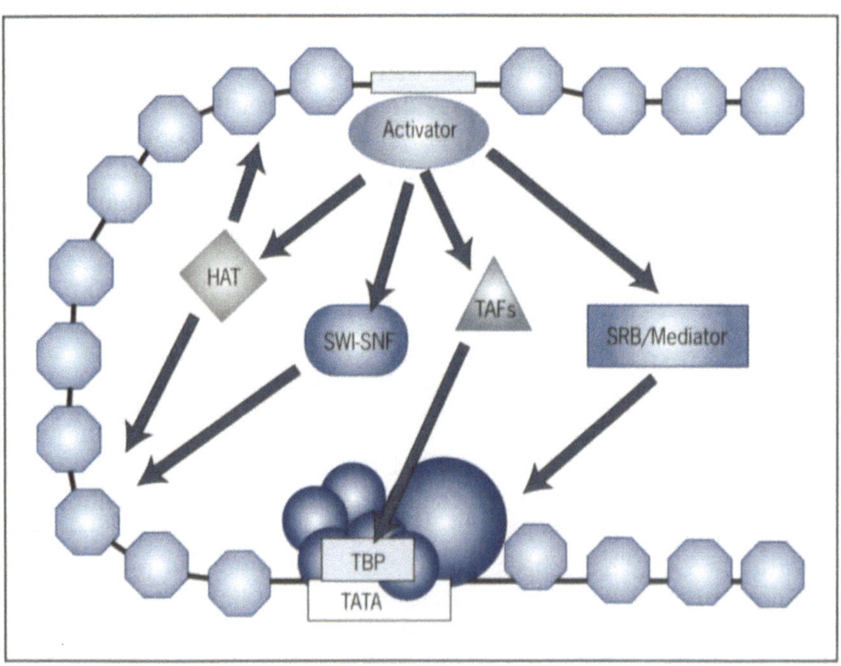

Figure 6-7. Multiple transcriptional activators interact with coactivators—including histone acetyltransferases (HATs), TFIID-associated factors (TAFs), chromatin remodeling proteins (SWI/SNF), and other complexes (mediator, SRB and others)—to regulate transcriptional output.

of mechanisms. Many repressor proteins, more accurately referred to as deactivator proteins, exert their influence by interfering with the function of a transcriptional activator. This can be achieved by interfering with the interaction of the activator with the promoter, either by binding to and obstructing the activator binding element or by perturbing the activator protein in such a fashion as to alter its DNA binding domain. Alternatively, a repressor can interact with the activator and block the function of its activation domain, resulting in a phenomenon known as transcriptional quenching. Another class of repressor proteins exerts its effect in the absence of activators and, like many of the activator proteins, appears to function via direct interaction with the basal machinery. This class possesses specific domains that, when linked to a heterologous DNA binding domain, are able to repress a promoter containing a cognate DNA binding site. Therefore, this class of repressors is the converse of the typical activator protein. Finally, additional protein factors, referred to as co-repressors, lack DNA binding activity but aid in transcriptional repression by interacting with DNA-bound repressor molecules [16]. Many transcriptional co-repressors act through the catalytic modification of chromatin structure and are discussed later in this chapter.

Regulation of Transcription Factor Activity

A higher order of transcriptional regulation is achieved by the regulation of the transcription factors

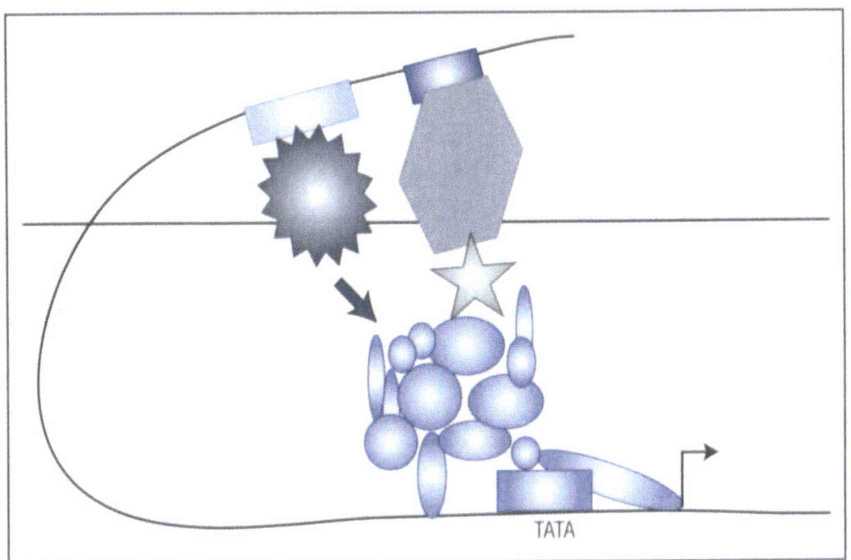

Figure 6-8. Multiple activators and coactivators function in concert to regulate transcription from a given promoter.

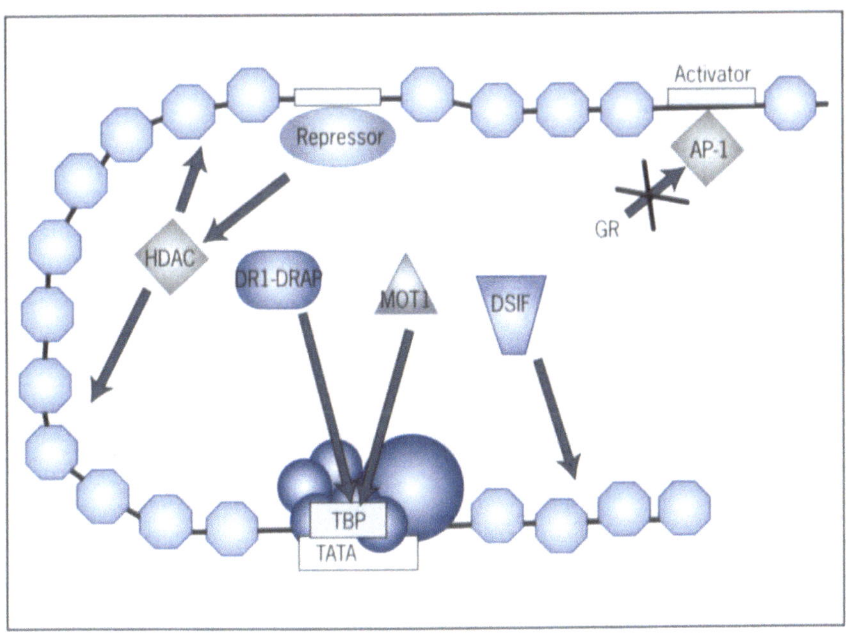

Figure 6-9. Like transcriptional activators, transcriptional repressors function with co-repressors to silence transcription in response to environmental cues. Some repressors work directly on the basal machinery, others suppress the activity of activator proteins, and others inhibit transcription by modifying chromatin structure.

themselves. This can be effected at two levels: regulation of factor synthesis and regulation of factor activity (Fig. 6-10) [1,2,10,22]. The synthesis of several transcription factors can be regulated in a tissue-specific or cell-cycle specific fashion or in response to specific stimuli. An example of a tissue-specific factor is MyoD, which is synthesized only in skeletal muscle cells where it is involved in the activation of genes required for muscle differentiation.

There are a number of mechanisms by which the activity of a transcription factor can be regulated. Post-translational modification, particularly phosphorylation, plays a major role in the regulation of some transcription factors. For example, HSTF is activated by phosphorylation, whereas the AP1 component Jun is activated by dephosphorylation. The binding of a ligand can also regulate factor activity. For example, nuclear hormone receptors are in a repressed state in the absence of ligand due to their interaction with a repressor protein complex; binding of ligand releases the repressor complex and allows for the recruitment of an activator complex to the promoter. An interesting variation of this phenomenon is seen with the steroid hormone receptors. In the absence of ligand, the glucocorticoid receptor (GR) is complexed with heat shock and other proteins and sequestered in the cytoplasm. Following ligand binding, GR is released from this complex and transported to the nucleus, where it is able to interact with its target promoters. Control of nuclear protein import is a means of regulating the NF-κB transcription factor. In this scenario, NF-κB is stored in the cytoplasm complexed to its specific inhibitor IκB; in response to certain stimuli, IκB is phosphorylated, allowing for

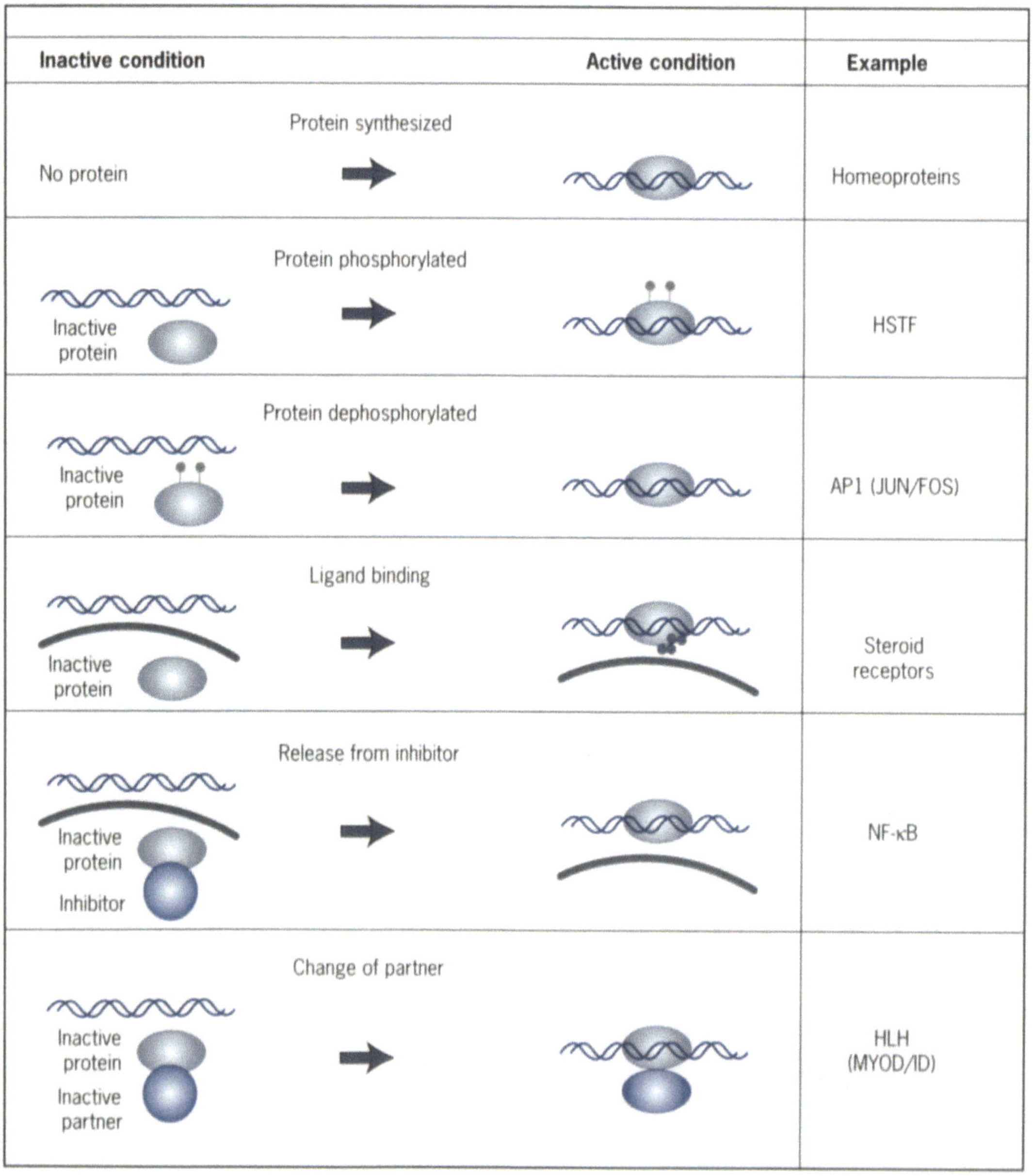

Inactive condition		Active condition	Example
No protein	Protein synthesized →		Homeoproteins
Inactive protein	Protein phosphorylated →		HSTF
Inactive protein	Protein dephosphorylated →		AP1 (JUN/FOS)
Inactive protein	Ligand binding →		Steroid receptors
Inactive protein Inhibitor	Release from inhibitor →		NF-κB
Inactive protein Inactive partner	Change of partner →		HLH (MYOD/ID)

Figure 6-10. Transcription factors can themselves be regulated by several mechanisms, including changes in synthesis (transcriptional, translational), post-translational modifications (phosphorylation), ligands, binding partners, and nuclear localization. (*Adapted from* Lewin [1].)

the release and subsequent transport of NF-κB into the nucleus.

Keeping with the theme of dimerization, some transcription factors have multiple potential binding partners that share similar dimerization motifs; depending on the partnership achieved, the resulting heterodimer may vary with respect to binding target and transcriptional activity. For example, when the AP1 family member JUN dimerizes with a CRE/ATF family member, the resulting heterodimer has preference for the CRE/ATF binding site, thereby conferring TPA inducibility (a property of AP1 proteins) on CRE/ATF site–containing promoters. Dimerization of transcription factors with unrelated DNA binding domains also can occur. An example of this can be seen with the bZIP family member JUN and the zinc-finger family member GR. When JUN and GR interact through their DNA binding domains, each represses the DNA binding activity of the other, resulting in loss of transcriptional activation.

CHROMATIN AND TRANSCRIPTION

We have discussed transcription as the interaction of transcription factors with their cognate DNA binding sites and with each other. However, superimposed on the regulation mediated by those interactions is the role of chromatin in permitting this interplay to occur. The basic transcriptional state of chromatin is inactive; the DNA wrapped in a nucleosomal complex, which consists of octamers of the core histones, is generally inaccessible to transcription factors (Fig. 6-11). For many years, elucidation of the mechanism by which this innate transcriptional repression is overcome to activate transcription remained elusive; however, a breakthrough in understanding the role of chromatin in transcriptional regulation has come from the recognition that chromatin is a dynamic structure and that signals from the environment trigger changes in chromosomal architecture. Moreover, the recent identification of protein factors whose primary function is to alter chromatin in such a way as to regulate the accessibility of the DNA sequence to the transcriptional apparatus has paved the way for a more detailed analysis of chromatin's role in transcriptional control. These proteins fall into two classes: chromatin-modifying enzymes and ATP-dependent chromatin-remodeling factors.

CHROMATIN-MODIFYING ENZYMES

The role of chromatin-modifying enzymes in trascription is reviewed elsewhere [23–26]. More than 30 years ago, Allfrey [27] proposed that acetylation of the lysine-rich tails of core histones could result in a destabilization or opening of chromatin structure. Biochemical and immunohistochemical studies indicated that hyperacetylated histones were associated with active genes, whereas hypoacetylated chromatin corresponded to regions of gene silencing. Although the specific role of histone acetylation in transcriptional regulation is still under active investigation, the recent cloning of enzymes involved in maintaining the acetylated state of histones in chromatin has begun the elucidation of their mechanism of action.

In 1996, the first histone acetylase (HAT) was isolated from *Tetrahymena* [28], sparking a renewed interest in the role that chromatin modifications play in gene regulation. Although the precise function of these acetylases remains to be determined, it is clear that acetylation can neutralize the positive charge of the lysine-rich histone tails, thereby weakening the interaction of histones with the negative-

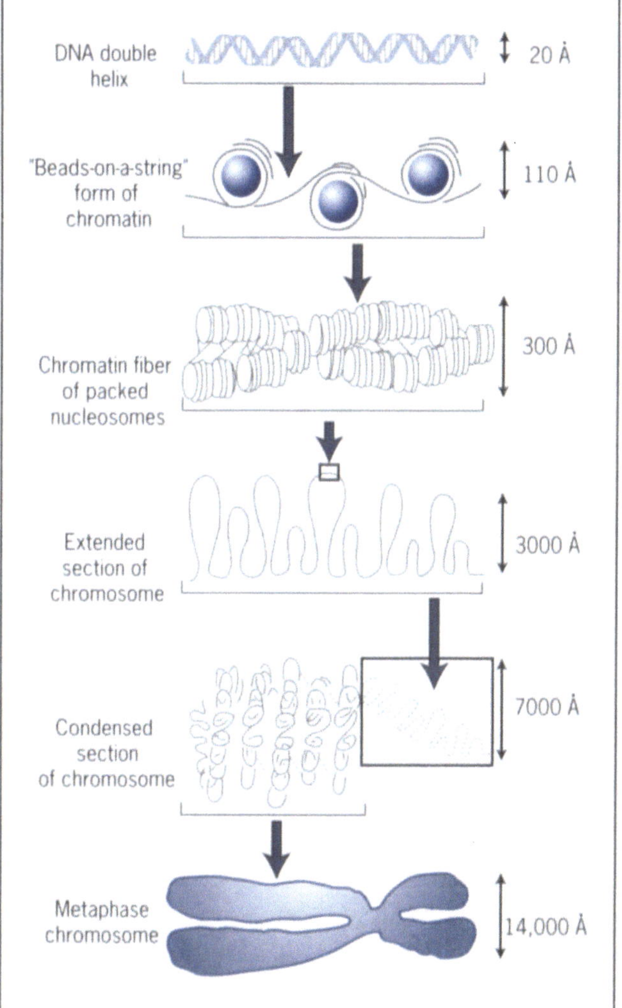

Figure 6-11. Schematic representing the packing of DNA into ordered chromatin and chromosomes.

ly-charged DNA molecule and leading to an "open" chromatin conformation. A second, less studied theory is that acetylation of chromatin acts as a signal for the interaction of histones with other transcription factors, resulting in nucleosome disruption. More recently, it has been shown that HATs can also acetylate certain transcription factors, adding an additional layer of complexity to the story. A critical turning point in our understanding of the mechanism of action of transcriptional activators and coactivators came with the observation that many of these proteins contain intrinsic HAT activity, suggesting that they may activate transcription via chromatin disruption.

Because histone acetylation is a dynamic process, the activity of the HATs must be reversible. This is accomplished by the histone deacetylase (HDAC) family of chromatin-modifying enzymes. To date, eight mammalian HDACs have been identified. In the current model, HDACs are recruited to the promoter by sequence-specific repressor proteins, thereby maintaining the gene in a hypoacetylated, inactive state (Fig. 6-12). In response to specific stimuli, transcriptional activators recruit HATs, which acetylate histones, resulting in conformational changes within the nucleosomal array. Although this is an attractive model, the majority of studies that have led to this theory were performed in yeast systems or on artificial promoter constructs . However, we have recently shown that activation of the human MDR1 promoter is mediated by the HAT protein P/CAF, which is recruited to the promoter via its interaction with the transcriptional activator NF-Y [29].

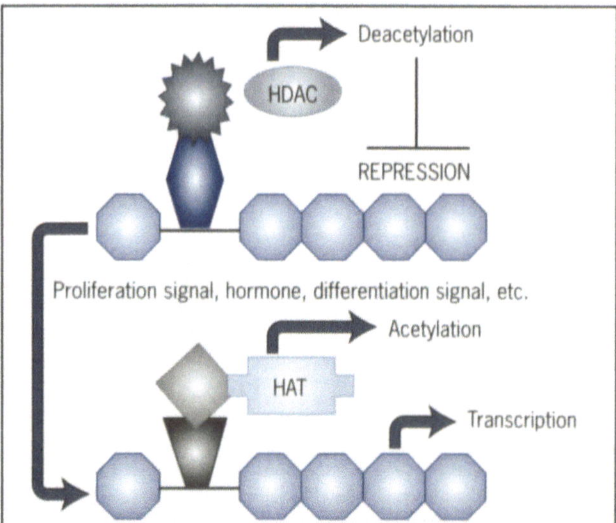

Figure 6-12. Regulation of transcription by histone acetylation involves an equilibrium between enzymes that add acetyl groups to histone tail (histone acetyltransferases [HATs]) and enzymes that remove acetyl groups (histone deacetylases [HDACs]). This equilibrium can be altered in response to environmental triggers. In the simplest model, the equilibrium between these opposing enzymes maintains a steady-state level of transcription.

Chromatin-Remodeling Complexes

In addition to the histone-modifying enzymes, additional protein complexes have been identified that are able to alter nucleosome structure in an ATP-dependent manner [25]. Although the precise mechanism by which these chromatin-remodeling complexes affect transcription is still under investigation, it appears that they can increase accessibility of transcription factors to DNA without removing histones. Instead, they "remodel" preexisting nucleosomes, thereby altering local promoter architecture. The prototype of these remodeling factors are the yeast Swi/Snf proteins, which contain both ATPase and DNA helicase activity; human homologs of these yeast proteins have recently been identified [30]. One of the critical questions concerning the role of these remodeling complexes in vivo is how they are targeted to specific promoters. In that regard, it has recently been shown that the human SWI/SNF complex can interact with the GR, suggesting that the targeting of a remodeling complex may be one of the critical functions of GR in transcriptional activation.

DNA Methylation and Gene Expression

The role of DNA methylation in transcriptional silencing is probably best known with respect to X chromosome inactivation. However, an increasing body of evidence indicates that DNA methylation may significantly contribute to the activation and repression of many different genes [31–34], including genes encoding tumor suppressor and drug resistance proteins. In general, the mammalian genome is bimodal with respect to methylation; the CpG islands of housekeeping genes are generally hypomethylated, whereas those of tissue-specific genes are hypermethylated in tissues in which they are not expressed. Although it is not yet clear how the methylation status of a gene influences transcriptional output, it has been shown that methyl groups on transfected promoter sequences prevent access of transcription factors to the chromatin-imbedded promoter. A link between DNA methylation and histone acetylation has been established; it has been shown that the methyl-DNA binding protein MeCP2 interacts with histone deacetylases [35]. Therefore, the prevailing hypothesis is that methylation status helps to define the acetylation state of local chromatin, where hypomethylated DNA is transcriptionally active and hypermethylated and deacetylated chromatin provides a barricade to the transcriptional machinery. Aberrant methylation has been associated with transcriptional dysregulation in many diseases [36]. In cancer, hypomethylation can lead to the activation of oncogenes, whereas hypermethylation has been found to be associated with the silencing of tumor suppressor genes. In the following section, the effect of aberrant transcription and mutant transcription factors on carcinogenesis is described in more detail.

TRANSCRIPTION FACTORS AND CANCER

It is now widely accepted that tumorigenesis is a multistep process by which several genetic lesions accumulate until the cell acquires the ability to override normal proliferative controls and circumvent cell death. At the molecular level, many of these genetic lesions impair the cell's ability to regulate transcription. Notably, many proto-oncogene and tumor suppressor genes encode transcription factors, and their aberrant activation or mutation and silencing, respectively, leads to malignancy. A large number of transcription factors have been implicated in tumorigenesis; these include components of the basal machinery, elongation factors, transcriptional activators, transcriptional repressors, and factors involved in modifying chromatin proteins. For the purpose of this review, only a few of the best studied transcriptional alterations associated with the malignant phenotype are described.

ALTERED EXPRESSION OF TUMOR SUPPRESSORS AND ONCOGENES

p53

The *p53* tumor suppressor gene is a transcription factor that was initially identified by virtue of its association with a viral gene product, T-antigen, in virally transformed cells [37,38]. Early studies showed that cells lacking p53 were unable to control proliferation, implying that normal cells have a capacity for uncontrolled growth that is somehow inhibited by the presence of the wild-type protein. More refined studies indicated that p53 acts at a specific point in the cell cycle (G_1) and suggest that the role of p53 in cell cycle arrest is to prevent the proliferation of cells carrying damaged DNA. Therefore, p53 acts as a "guardian" of the genetic information that is passed on to daughter cells, by either transiently halting the cell cycle to allow damaged DNA to be repaired or by driving the damaged cell down an irreversible apoptotic pathway of cellular suicide. The ability of p53 to exert its downstream effects is dependent on its interaction with other cellular proteins as well as its ability to negatively or positively regulate the promoters of many genes involved in growth control. In the absence of functional p53, monitoring of DNA integrity is lost, leading to the accumulation of genetically damaged cells with marked genomic instability. Perhaps it is not surprising that at least 50% of all human tumors carry *p53* mutations, making *p53* the most common change in human cancer. *p53* is therefore referred to as a tumor suppressor gene because it plays a role in the prevention of uncontrolled growth and transformation.

Retinoblastoma Gene

The retinoblastoma gene product (Rb) is a transcription factor that, like p53, is involved in the regulation of the cell cycle [39,40]. The function of Rb in the normal cell cycle is regulated by phosphorylation. In the unphosphorylated state, Rb binds to another transcription factor, E2F, and prevents this factor from activating genes involved in cell cycle regulation and DNA synthesis. When Rb is phosphorylated during the cell cycle, E2F is released from the inhibitory complex and is able to turn on the genes necessary for progression. Deletion or mutation of Rb allows the activation of proliferative genes by E2F to go unchecked, resulting in uncontrolled growth. Rb was first identified as a tumor suppressor gene that is lost or mutated in all cases of retinoblastoma, a malignant tumor of the retina. More recently, it has been found to be missing in several common mesenchymal and epithelial malignancies, including carcinoma of the lung, breast, and bladder.

Wilms' Tumor Gene

The Wilms' tumor (*WT1*) gene was first identified as a deletion in the 11p13 locus in Wilms' tumor, a pediatric kidney cancer [42–44]. It encodes a zinc-finger transcription factor that represses the activity of many genes involved in growth and differentiation, including the colony-stimulating factor-1 (*CSF1*) gene, insulin-like growth factor receptor (*IGFR*) gene, early growth response gene *Egr*, transforming growth factor β (TGF-β), and the apoptosis gene *BCL2*. In addition to its association with Wilms' tumor, aberrant expression of *WT1* has been described in some leukemias, mesotheliomas, Leydig cell tumors, and ovarian cancers, although its role in the pathogenesis of these tumors is not clear. WT1 also has been found as a chimeric protein with EWS, a member of the ETS family of transcription factors. The EWS-WT1 fusion protein contains the activation domain of EWS and the DNA binding domain of WT1, which results in a protein that can bind to WT1 promoters and activate, rather than repress, their transcription. Chromosomal translocations resulting in the synthesis of chimeric transcription factors is a common theme in malignancies.

myc Proteins

c-myc was first identified as an oncogene involved in the pathogenesis of avian lymphoma and is a key transforming agent in the etiology of Burkitt's lymphoma [45]. It has since been found to be dysregulated in a number of human tumors, including breast cancer, colon cancer, cervical carcinomas, small cell lung cancer, osteosarcoma, glioblastoma, and myeloid leukemia. N-*myc*, a related family member, is overexpressed in a large number of childhood neuroblastomas. The myc proteins are sequence-specific DNA-binding transcription factors that can activate and repress transcription of target genes. The c-*myc* gene product is involved in cell cycle regulation, inhibition of terminal differentiation, and potentiation of apoptosis, and although the mechanism by which overexpression of myc leads to malignancy is unclear, it appears that it is myc's role as a transcriptional repressor, rather than transcriptional activator, that best correlates with its tumorigenic potential.

Rel/NF-κB

The Rel/NF-κB transcription factors play a major role in immune and inflammatory responses as well as in proliferation and apoptosis [46]. Many of these family members have been associated with transformation as a result of overexpression, gene amplification, gene rearrangement, and translocation in a variety of tumor types. For example, c-*rel* maps to locus 2p14-15, a region that is amplified in nearly 25% of extranodal diffuse large-cell lymphomas and primary mediastinal B-cell lymphomas and in 50% of non–small cell lung cancers analyzed to date. Similarly, overexpression of NF-κB subunits has been detected in 80% of non–small cell lung cancers and in some colon, prostate, breast, bone, and brain tumor specimens. Although the exact consequence of the overexpression of this family of transcription factors has not been adequately defined, the current model, based on considerable experimental evidence, is that this overexpression results in inappropriate activation of transcription.

Elongin and the von Hippel-Lindau Gene

von Hippel-Lindau (VHL) disease is a rare disorder that predisposes patients to a variety of cancers. The *VHL* gene is mutated in families that carry this disease, indicating that VHL is a tumor suppressor protein. In normal cells, VHL tightly binds to elongin (SIII), a factor that increases the overall transcription rate by decreasing the frequency or duration of pausing during elongation, and it has been suggested that VHL regulates elongin activity [5]. A subset of VHL mutants has reduced affinity for elongin, and this may play a role in tumorigenesis.

CBP/P300

Core binding protein (CBP) and P300 are multifunctional transcription factor proteins that modulate the activity of a number of protein partners [25,26]. They interact with transcriptional activators and repressors, acting as a bridge between these regulators and the basal machinery. Moreover, they have intrinsic histone acetyltransferase activity that functions in chromatin remodeling, they interact with P53 and are involved in apoptosis, they are critical players in embryogenesis, and they are involved in the terminal differentiation of some tissue types. Alterations of both CBP and P300 have been implicated in tumorigenicity, and recent evidence suggest that they may act as tumor suppressor genes [47]. Germline mutations of CBP have been found in persons with Rubinstein-Taybi syndrome, who have an increased predisposition to cancer. CBP also is involved in translocations in various hematologic malignancies, including acute myelogenous leukemia [t(8;16)(p11;p13)]. Furthermore, loss of heterozygosity has been observed at the 22q13 locus (where P300 maps) in a majority of glioblastomas.

Chromosomal Translocations in Leukemia

The modular nature of transcription factors—including DNA binding domains, transactivation/transrepression domains, ligand binding domains, and protein interfaces—allows for a "mix-and-match" of effector regions not juxtaposed in normal cells, resulting in hybrid factors with aberrant binding or regulatory functions [44,48–50]. The classic and best studied examples of chromosomal translocations resulting in the formation of oncogenic transcription factors are seen in the human acute leukemias; some of the most common of these are described in the following sections (Fig. 6-13).

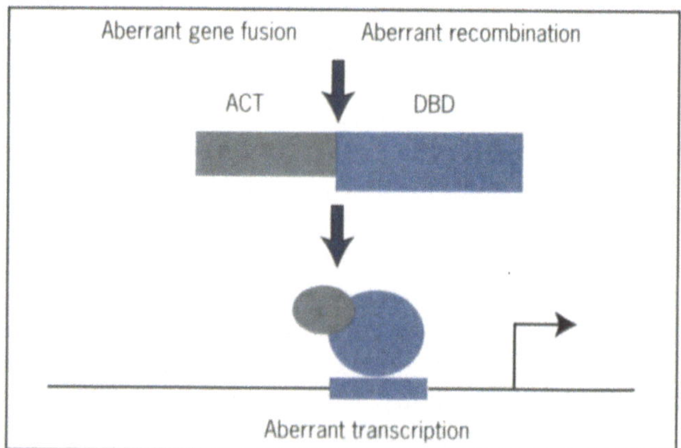

Figure 6-13. Many cancers are associated with the presence of novel fusion genes that have arisen from the aberrant recombination (translocation) between domains of two different transcription factors. These fusion genes are often responsible for the inappropriate activation or repression of genes involved in proliferation, cell cycle, and cell death.

PML-RARα

Acute promyelocytic leukemia (APL) is characterized by a translocation between chromosomes 15 and 17 that involves the (*PML*) and retinoic acid receptor (*RARα*) genes (Fig. 6-14) [51,52]. The translocation resulting in formation of the PML-RARα chimera is present in the vast majority of cases of APL, often as the only apparent chromosomal abnormality, and is believed to mediate leukemogenesis. Although the normal function of PML remains unclear, it is believed to act as a transcription factor. RARα is a member of the steroid hormone receptor family of transcription factors. Because RARα retains its DNA binding and ligand binding capacity within the context of the fusion protein, the PML/RARα fusion protein can interact with retinoid-responsive promoters in a ligand-dependent manner. Whether it is this gain of function of the fusion protein or the loss of function of the normal *PML* and *RARA* genes that leads to the malignant state is still under investigation. Nevertheless, the PML/RARα translocation provides a unique therapeutic opportunity, because it has been demonstrated that APLs that contain this chimeric protein are particularly sensitive to all-trans retinoic acid (ATRA). Although to date ATRA treatment in APL affords the only successful therapy directed at a fusion protein, it should be noted that chimeric proteins resulting from other chromosomal translocations do provide "tumor-specific" molecules that are promising targets for therapeutic intervention.

AML1 Chimeras

The most commonly altered transcription factor gene in human leukemia, *AML1*, [50,53,54] is a member of the CBP family of transcription factors and is normally expressed in hematopoietic tissues and during myeloid differentiation. Chromosomal translocations in several leukemias lead to the synthesis of AML1 fusion proteins, including AML1/ ETO [t(8;21)], AML-EVI-1 [t(3;21)], and TEL-AML1 [t(12;21)]. The best studied of these is AML-ETO, which is formed by one of the most common translocations in acute myelogenous leukemia in which the DNA binding domain of *AML1* is fused to most of the *ETO* gene. The resulting chimera can act as a dominant negative inhibitor of AML1 transactivation of its target genes. TEL/AML1 appears to act through a similar dominant-negative mechanism.

Hormone Receptors in Cancer

Hormone receptors are transcription factors that are activated upon binding of their respective ligands (discussed previously). They can be divided into receptors that are complexed with heat shock factors and unavailable for DNA binding in the absence of ligand (*eg*, receptors for glucocorticoid [GR], progesterone [PR], androgen [AR], and estrogen [ER]) and those that bind DNA in an inactive form in the absence of ligand (*eg*, receptors for thyroid hormone [TR], vitamin D [VDR], and retinoic acid). Mutations of hormone receptors are found in many types of cancer [55–57], although they are generally believed to be a marker of tumor progression or a therapeutic prognosticator rather than a transforming factor; however, this remains an area of controversy. For example, mutations in AR accompany the progression of prostate cancer to hormone independence. ER is elevated in some breast cancer patients; it is used as a clinical marker to predict response to antiestrogen therapy. Mutations in GR are associated with the development of glucocorticoid resistance in leukemia patients. Interestingly, a frameshift mutation in GR is associated with pituitary macroadenoma, where it may play a causative role in tumor formation. The avian homologue of TR, *erb*-a, is an oncogene, and mutated TR has been associated with neoplastic transformation of the liver in humans. RARα, as discussed previously, is a component of many chromosomal translocations found in a variety of leukemias, particularly APL.

TRANSCRIPTION: DRUG TARGET AND DRUG TARGETER

As the focal point of gene regulation and the target of mutations associated with the malignant state, tran-

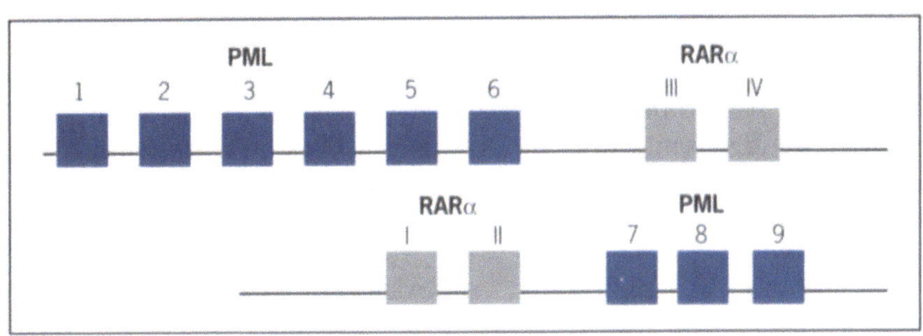

Figure 6-14. Acute promyelocytic leukemia is characterized by a translocation between chromosomes 15 and 17, generating a fusion protein containing regions from the PML and RARα genes.

scription represents an attractive target for therapeutic intervention. Moreover, the identification of cell-specific promoters and/or transcription factors that are aberrantly activated in tumors allows for the use of these promoters to target the synthesis of products toxic to cancer cells. Indeed, studies of drugs that target transcription [57–59] and of promoters that target gene products in a cell- or tumor-specific manner [60] are well underway.

TRANSCRIPTION AS A DRUG TARGET

Hormone Receptors

As described previously, hormone receptors are often altered in certain malignancies. The most successful transcription-directed therapy is aimed at the PML-RARα fusion protein associated with APL. Another hormone receptor that provides a chemotherapeutic target is the estrogen receptor (ER). The antiestrogen tamoxifen binds to ER and apparently causes a conformational change that precludes binding of estrogens, resulting in a receptor-ligand complex that is impaired in its transactivation function. This begins a cascade of changes in gene regulation, because many of the target genes of ER also encode transcription factors.

p53

Because *p53* is mutated in at least 50% of all cancers, it provides an inviting target for therapeutic intervention. Working on the hypothesis that loss of the wild-type *p53* results in the accumulation of mutations, dysregulated cell cycle progression, and inhibition of drug-induced apoptosis, several laboratories have been developing methods to introduce wild-type *p53* into human tumors. This approach is already in clinical trials, and preliminary results demonstrate synergistic effects between *p53* replacement and radiotherapy or chemotherapy.

Nuclear Factor-Y

Nuclear Factor-Y (NF-Y) is a trimeric transcriptional activator that regulates a number of genes involved in cell cycle and progression [61]. Part of its transactivation function results from its ability to recruit histone acetyltransferases to target promoters [29] Recently, we and others have shown that a novel marine natural product, ecteinascidin (ET-743), can inhibit the binding of NF-Y to its cognate element and inhibit activation of an NF-Y target gene [62,63]. ET-743 shows potent antitumor activity against a wide variety of malignancies and is currently in clinical trials.

NF-κB

NF-κB is a central mediator of the immune response as well as a critical component of apoptotic pathways. A number of drugs that alter the function of this transcription factor have been identified. In particular, the sesquiterpene lactone helenalin selectively alkylates the P65 subunit of NF-κB, rendering the protein inactive [64]. Another compound, capsaicin, downregulates the activity of NF-κB, in part by blocking the degradation of its inhibitory partner IκB [65]. Both capsaicin and helenalin have shown activity against a number of tumor types in vitro; more studies are needed to determine whether these antitranscription agents will prove clinically efficacious.

Histone Deacetylase

The oncoprotein PML-RARα, generated by chromosomal translocation in APL, has recently been shown to repress transcription by recruiting histone deacetylase. With this in mind, a number of groups have shown that HDAC inhibitors can overcome resistance to ATRA in APL cell lines and in an ATRA-resistant patient with APL, who achieved a complete remission following combination therapy with ATRA and the HDAC inhibitor sodium phenylbutyrate [66].

Targeted Gene Therapy

The identification of genes involved in neoplastic transformation and drug resistance has led to a significant effort to translate this molecular information into new therapeutic strategies. Advances in gene therapy, in which exogenous genes or antisense molecules can be introduced into cells to complement a mutated or deleted tumor suppressor or eliminate an oncogene, respectively, have made this approach feasible for some clinical applications. However, as with all chemotherapy, the primary goal of gene therapy as a treatment for neoplastic disease is the elimination of cancer cells while minimizing collateral toxicity to normal cells. Critical to the success of this strategy is the ability to selectively target gene expression to tumors. One approach to achieving this is to drive expression of exogenous genes using promoters that are preferentially activated in tumor cells. Currently, a number of cell-specific promoters are being used in gene transfer studies, each with unique properties and cell specificity (Table 6-1) [60].

For example, carcinoembryonic antigen (CEA) is an oncofetal antigen that is aberrantly expressed in colon and lung tumors. Investigators have shown that this expression is mediated by CEA promoter sequences (and presumably, altered expression of a transcription factor that interacts with these sequences) and have demonstrated that toxic genes linked to the CEA promoter are preferentially expressed in tumor cells that overexpress CEA. Similar observations have been made using promoters of other oncofetal proteins, including the alpha-fetoprotein promoter in hepatocellular carcinoma and nonseminomatous germ cell tumors of the testis; the testosterone-induced prostate-specific antigen promoter in prostate and prostatic tumors; and the oncogene *ERBB2* promoter in breast, pancreatic, gastric, and ovarian tumors and non–small cell lung cancer. Additional studies have employed promoters from genes that are activated in tumors during chemotherapy, radiation, or hyperthermia, including the multidrug resistance gene (*MDR1*), glucose-regulated protein (GRP78), and early growth

Table 6-1. Cell type–specific promoters for targeted gene expression

Promoter	Target cell/tissue
CD11a promoter	Leukocytes
CD11b promoter	Leukocytes
CD18 promoter	Leukocytes
β-Globin promoter/LCR	Erythroid cells
Immunoglobulin promoter	B lymphoma
Tie promoter	Endothelial cells
PEPCK promoter	Hepatocytes
Albumin promoter	Hepatocytes
ApoE enhancer	Hepatocytes
hAAT promoter	Hepatocytes
MMTV LTR	Mammary carcinoma
WAP promoter	Mammary carcinoma
β-casein	Mammary carcinoma
SPC promoter	Bronchiolar/alveolar epithelium
SPA, SPB	Bronchiolar/alveolar epithelium
MCK promoter	Undifferentiated myogenic cells
VLC1 promoter	Myoblasts
HIV LTR	Lymphocytes
Tat/Rev responsive elements	$CD4^+$ T cells
Tat-inducible element	$CD4^+$ T cells
CEA promoter	CEA-expressing malignancies
MUC-1 promoter	MUC-1–overexpressing malignancies
AFP promoter	Hepatocellular carcinoma
SLPI promoter	Carcinomas
Tyrosinase/TRP-1 promoters	Melanomas
c-*erb*B2 promoter	Breast, pancreatic, and gastric carcinomas
Myc-Max responsive element	Lung cancer
Egr-1 promoter	Irradiated tumors
Grp78 promoter	Anoxic, acidic tumor tissue
MDR1 promoter	Tumors treated with chemotherapy
HSP70 promoter	Tumors treated with hyperthermy

HIV—human immunodeficiency virus; LCR—locus control region; LTR—long terminal repeat; MMTV—mouse mammary tumor virus; PEPCK—phosphoenolpyruvate carboxylase; SPA/B/C— surfactant protein A/B/C.

(*Adapted from* Clary and Lyerly [60]; with permission.)

response gene (*EGR1*). Although this technology has not yet advanced to the stage where consistent cell-specific expression of exogenous genes can be achieved following systemic delivery of recombinant constructs, improvements in gene delivery systems that exploit the current knowledge of tumor-specific transcriptional regulatory elements and factors makes this a feasible goal.

CONCLUSION

Transcriptional regulation is remarkably complex. First, the highly ordered chromatin structure, which physically hinders the interaction between DNA and the transcriptional machinery, must be overcome via the regulation of histone-DNA interactions. This regulation is mediated by a variety of complexes that contain histone-modifying and chromatin-remodeling components. Next, the general transcription factors must assemble at specific promoters; the specificity and rate of assembly is regulated by the activity of transcriptional activators and repressors. Elongation and termination are additional levels at which transcriptional output can be controlled. Adding to this complexity, transcription of most genes is a dynamic process wherein the transcriptional machinery is continually responding to intracellular and extracellular signals. Given the extraordinary intricacy of this process, it is not surprising that alterations in transcriptional components can have profound effects on cell growth and death, leading to the malignant state. With this in mind, many researchers and pharmaceutical companies have begun to exploit our rapidly growing knowledge of transcriptional regulation and dysregulation in an effort to devise new transcription-based therapeutic regimens. These new approaches hold the promise of exquisite specificity with limited toxicity, and may hold the key to the prevention and treatment of many diseases, including cancer, in the years to come.

ACKNOWLEDGMENTS

Due to the broad nature of this chapter and space restrictions, the authors regret that the majority of literature cited are reviews rather than original research articles. We would like to thank members of the Scotto Laboratory for helpful discussions. The authors are supported by National Cancer Institute Grants P30-CA-08748 to Memorial Sloan-Kettering Cancer Center and RO1-CA-57307 to K. W. Scotto.

REFERENCES

1. Lewin B: *Genes V*. New York: Oxford University Press; 1994.
2. Raven PH, Johnson GB: *Biology*, edn 4. Boston: Wm.C. Brown Publishers; 1996:349–370.
3. Pugh F, Tjian R: Diverse transcriptional functions of the multisubunit eukaryotic TFIID complex. *J Biol Chem* 1992, 267:679–682.
4. Orphanides G, Lagrange T, Reinberg D: The general transcription factors of RNA polymerase II. *Genes Dev* 1996, 10:2657–2683.
5. Conaway RC, Conaway JW: General transcription factors for RNA polymerase II. *Prog Nucleic Acid Res Mol Biol* 1997, 56:327–346.
6. Hampsey M: Molecular genetics of the RNA polymerase II general transcriptional machinery. *Microbiol Mol Biol Rev* 1998, 62:465–503.
7. Aso T, Conaway JW, Conaway RC: The RNA polymerase II elongation complex. *FASEB J* 1995, 9:1419–1428.
8. Shilatifard A, Haque D, Conaway RC, Conaway JW: Structure and function of RNA polymerase II elongation factor ELL. Identification of two overlapping ELL functional domains that govern its interaction with polymerase and the ternary elongation complex. *J Biol Chem* 1997, 272:22355–22363.
9. Shore P, Sharrocks AD: The MADS-box family of transcription factors. *Eur J Biochem* 1995, 229:1–13.
10. Latchman DS: Transcription factors: an overview. *Int J Biochem Cell Biol* 1997, 29:1305–1312.
11. Kohn WD, Mant CT, Hodges RS: Alpha-helical protein assembly motifs. *J Biol Chem* 1997, 272:2583–2586.
12. Tan S, Richmond TJ: Eukaryotic transcription factors. *Curr Opin Struct Biol.* 1998, 8:41–48.
13. Treisman R: Regulation of transcription by MAP kinase cascades. *Curr Opin Cell Biol* 1996, 8:205–215.
14. Kaiser K, Meisterernst M: The human general co-factors. *Trends Biochem Sci* 1996, 21:342–345.
15. Darimont BD, Wagner RL, Apriletti JW, *et al.*: Structure and specificity of nuclear receptor-coactivator interactions. *Genes Dev* 1998, 12:3343–3356.
16. Torchia J, Glass C, Rosenfeld MG: Coactivators and co-repressors in the integration of transcriptional responses. *Curr Opin Cell Biol* 1998, 10:373–383.
17. Hampsey M, Reinberg D: Transcription: why are TAFs essential? *Curr Biol* 1997, 7:R44–R46.
18. Hahn S: The role of TAFs in RNA polymerase II transcription. *Cell* 1998, 95:579–582.
19. Struhl K, Moqtaderi Z: The TAFs in the HAT. *Cell* 1998, 94:1–4.
20. Lee TI, Young RA: Regulation of gene expression by TBP-associated proteins. *Genes Dev* 1998, 12:1398–1408.
21. Ogbourne S, Antalis TM: Transcriptional control and the role of silencers in transcriptional regulation in eukaryotes. *Biochem J* 1998, 331:1–14.
22. Boulikas T: Phosphorylation of transcription factors and control of the cell cycle. *Crit Rev Eukaryot Gene Expr* 1995, 5:1–77.
23. Hassig CA, Schreiber SL: Nuclear histone acetylases and deacetylases and transcriptional regulation: HATs off to HDACs. *Curr Opin Chem Biol* 1997, 1:300–308.

24. Wade PA, Wolffe AP: Histone acetyltransferases in control. *Curr Biol* 1997, 7:R82–R84.

25. Wu C: Chromatin remodeling and the control of gene expression. *J Biol Chem* 1997, 272:28171–28174.

26. Workman JL, Kingston RE: Alteration of nucleosome structure as a mechanism of transcriptional regulation. *Annu Rev Biochem* 1998, 67:545–579.

27. Allfrey VG: Structural modifications of histones and their possible role in the regulation of ribonucleic acid synthesis. *Proc Can Cancer Conf* 1966, 6:313–335.

28. Brownell JE, Zhou J, Ranalli T, *et al.*: Tetrahymena histone acetyltransferase A: a homolog to yeast Gcn5p linking histone acetylation to gene activation. *Cell* 1996, 84:843–851.

29. Jin S, Scotto KW: Transcriptional regulation of the MDR1 gene by histone acetyltransferase and deacetylase is mediated by NF-Y. *Mol Cell Biol* 1998, 18:4377–4384.

30. Armstrong JA, Bieker JJ, Emerson BM: A SWI/SNF-related chromatin remodeling complex, E-RC1, is required for tissue-specific transcriptional regulation by EKLF in vitro. *Cell* 1998, 95:93–104.

31. Klein CB, Costa M: DNA methylation and gene expression: introduction and overview. *Mutat Res* 1997, 386:103–105.

32. Siegfried Z, Cedar H: DNA methylation: a molecular lock. *Curr Biol* 1997, 7:R305–R307.

33. Razin A: CpG methylation, chromatin structure and gene silencing–a three-way connection. *EMBO J* 1998, 17:4905–4908.

34. Wolffe A: Packaging principle: how DNA methylation and histone acetylation control the transcriptional activity of chromatin. *J Exp Zool* 1998, 282:239–244.

35. Nan X, Ng HH, Johnson CA, *et al.*: Transcriptional repression by the methyl-CpG-binding protein MeCP2 involves a histone deacetylase complex. *Nature* 1998, 393:386–389.

36. Gonzalgo ML, Jones PA: Mutagenic and epigenetic effects of DNA methylation. *Mutat Res* 1997, 386:107–118.

37. Agarwal ML, Taylor WR, Chernov MV, *et al.*: The p53 network. *J Biol Chem* 1998, 273:1–4.

38. Mowat MR: p53 in tumor progression: life, death, and everything. *Adv Cancer Res* 1998, 74:25–48.

39. Taya Y: RB kinases and RB-binding proteins: new points of view. *Trends Biochem Sci* 1997, 22:14–17.

40. Sellers WR, Kaelin WG, Jr: Role of the retinoblastoma protein in the pathogenesis of human cancer. *J Clin Oncol* 1997, 15:3301–3312.

41. Dyson N: The regulation of E2F by pRB-family proteins. *Genes Dev* 1998, 12:2245–2262.

42. Bergmann L, Maurer U, Weidmann E: Wilms' tumor gene expression in acute myeloid leukemias. *Leuk Lymph* 1997, 25:435–443.

43. Menke AL, van der Eb AJ, Jochemsen AG: The Wilms' tumor 1 gene: oncogene or tumor suppressor gene? *Int Rev Cytol* 1998, 181:151–212.

44. Sanchez-Garcia I: Consequences of chromosomal abnormalities in tumor development. *Annu Rev Genet* 1997, 31:429–453.

45. Facchini LM, Penn LZ: The molecular role of Myc in growth and transformation: recent discoveries lead to new insights. *FASEB J* 1998, 12:633–651.

46. Luque I, Gelinas C: Rel/NF-kappa B and I kappa B factors in oncogenesis. *Semin Cancer Biol* 1997, 8:103–111.

47. Snowden AW, Perkins ND: Cell cycle regulation of the transcriptional coactivators p300 and CREB binding protein. *Biochem Pharmacol* 1998, 55:1947–1954.

48. Barr FG: Chromosomal translocations involving paired box transcription factors in human cancer. *Int J Biochem Cell Biol* 1997, 29:1449–1461.

49. Look AT: Oncogenic transcription factors in the human acute leukemias. *Science* 1997, 278:1059–1064.

50. Mitani K: Leukemogenesis by the chromosomal translocations. *Leukemia* 1997, 11(Suppl 3):294–296.

51. Grimwade D, Solomon E: Characterisation of the PML/RAR alpha rearrangement associated with t(15;17) acute promyelocytic leukaemia. *Curr Top Microbiol Immunol* 1997, 220:81–112.

52. Tenen DG, Hromas R, Licht JD, Zhang DE: Transcription factors, normal myeloid development, and leukemia. *Blood* 1997, 90:489–519.

53. Gelmetti V, Zhang J, Fanelli M, *et al.*: Aberrant recruitment of the nuclear receptor corepressor-histone deacetylase complex by the acute myeloid leukemia fusion partner ETO. *Mol Cell Biol* 1998, 18:7185–7191.

54. Wang J, Hoshino T, Redner RL, *et al.*: ETO, fusion partner in t(8;21) acute myeloid leukemia, represses transcription by interaction with the human N-CoR/mSin3/HDAC1 complex. *Proc Natl Acad Sci USA* 1998, 95:10860–10865.

55. Tenbaum S, Baniahmad A: Nuclear receptors: structure, function and involvement in disease. *Int J Biochem Cell Biol* 1997, 29:1325–1341.

56. Ing NHO, Bert W: The steroid hormone receptor superfamily: molecular mechanisms of action. In *Molecular Endocrinology: Basic Concepts and Clinical Correlations.* 1995:195–215.

57. Gewirtz AM, Sokol DL, Ratajczak MZ: Nucleic acid therapeutics: state of the art and future prospects. *Blood* 1998, 92:712–736.

58. Cavaliieri F: Drugs that target gene expression: an overview. *Crit Rev Eukaryot Gene Expr* 1996, 6:75–85.

59. Vasquez KM, Wilson JH: Triplex-directed modification of genes and gene activity. *Trends Biochem Sci* 1998, 23:4–9.

60. Clary BM, Lyerly HK: Transcriptional targeting for cancer gene therapy. *Surg Oncol Clin North Am* 1998, 7:565–574.

61. Maity SN, de Crombrugghe B: Role of the CCAAT-binding protein CBF/NF-Y in transcription. *Trends Biochem Sci* 1998, 23:174–178.

62. Mantovani R, LaValle E, Bonfani M, *et al.*: Effect of ecteinascidin (ET-743) on the interaction between transcription factors and DNA. *Proc NCI-EORTC* 1998, 10:139.

63. Jin S, Gorfajn B, Faircloth G, Scotto KW: Ecteinascidin 743, a transcription-targeted chemotherapeutic that inhibits MDR1 activation. *Proc Natl Acad Sci USA* 2000 [in press].

64. Ly GKA, Schmidt TJ, Pahl HL, Merfort I: The anti-inflammatory sesquiterpene lactone helenin inhibits the transcription factor NF-κB by directly targeting p65. *J Biol Chem* 1998, 273:33508–33516.

65. Singh SNK, Aggarwal BB: Capsaicin (8-methyl-N-vanillyl-6-nonenamide) is a potent inhibitor of nuclear transcription factor-kappa B activation by diverse agents. *J Immunol* 1996, 157:4412–4420.

66. Warrell R, He L-Z, Richon V, *et al.*: Therapeutic targeting of transcription in acute promyelocytic leukemia by use of an inhibitor of histone deacetylase. *J Natl Cancer Inst* 1998, 90:1621–1625.

CHAPTER

7

DNA Repair

Mark R. Kelley
Leonard C. Erickson

The knowledge of DNA repair and its relation to cancer is expanding at a breathtaking rate. This chapter explores DNA repair and focuses on two of the four main DNA repair pathways: the direct reversal of DNA damage typified by O-6-methylguanine DNA methyltransferase (MGMT, also known as alkylguanine transferase [AGT]) and DNA base excision repair (BER). These two pathways are of particular importance because they have direct implications for the development of experimental therapeutic techniques and gene therapy. The two other pathways, nucleotide excision repair (NER) and mismatch repair (MMR), also are discussed (Table 7-1).

CANCER THERAPEUTIC AGENTS AND DNA DAMAGE

Cancer therapeutic agents induce cytotoxic DNA damage by using a variety of mechanisms, many of which result in apoptosis [1]. The effects of some of these lesions are shown in Table 7-2. Overwhelming evidence has shown that the major mechanism of tumor cell resistance to nitrosoureas, such as the chloroethylnitrosoureas (CENUs), results from the DNA repair activity of MGMT. This DNA repair protein is thought to protect cells from the cytotoxic DNA interstrand cross-link produced by CENUs by removing chloroethyl adducts from the O-6 position of guanine before these adducts can rearrange to form a lethal cross-link. Although nitrosoureas are alkylating agents, the ability to form cross-links within a single base pair makes them different in their mode of action from more classic alkylating agents, which cross-link between adjacent base pairs. Alkylating agents, such as the clinically useful agents mafosfamide and cyclophosphamide, and the classic laboratory agent methyl methanesulfonate (MMS), generate electrophilic species that react with nucleophilic sites of DNA bases [1] and are subject to DNA BER [2]. These alkylating agents methylate the O-6 position of guanine and the N-3 position of adenine and guanine, as well as a number of other nucleophilic sites in DNA that are both toxic and mutagenic [1]. Thiotepa is another alkylator that forms aminoethyl adducts with adenine and guanine, resulting in depurination and ring-opened sites [3]. Similar to the O-6-alkylguanine lesion, alkylated adducts are repaired predominantly by the DNA BER pathway.

DNA damage caused by cisplatin, an alkylator-mimetic anticancer agent that generates cross-linked DNA species with a minority of monoalkylated products was initially thought to be repaired by the NER pathway, although cisplatin also has been shown to generate oxidative DNA damage that may be repaired by BER [1]. Furthermore, the production of cross-linking generally proceeds through an initial monoadduct that could be repaired via the BER pathway. Recent data demonstrate the involvement of MMR in cisplatin repair [4,5]. Bleomycin is a radiomimetic agent that generates free radicals capable of abstracting hydrogen from deoxyribose sugars in DNA, resulting in the formation of 3′-phosphoglycolates that block DNA synthesis [6] and are amenable to BER. It has been demonstrated that activated bleomycin reacts with the C-4′ position of the sugar residue, generating a 4′-oxidized apurinic/apyrimidinic (AP) site along with strand breaks [7]. Additionally, 4′-oxidized AP sites have been shown to be excellent substrates for AP endonuclease activity [7]. These results indicate that the BER pathway is involved in the repair of bleomycin-induced 4′-oxidized AP sites. Daunorubicin is an anthracycline that intercalates into DNA, altering topoisomerase II function and that also generates free radicals from the ring system to produce effects similar to those of bleomycin [8]. Radiation induces DNA dam-

Table 7-1. The four main DNA repair pathways in mammalian cells

Direct reversal repair (MGMT)
O-6MeGua
NER
XP, CS, TTD
Transcription-coupled repair
Base excision repair (BER)
Alkylated DNA, oxidative DNA damage
Mismatch/recombinational repair
HNPCC

CS—Cockayne's syndrome; HNPCC—hereditary nonpolyposis colon cancer; NER—nucleotide excision repair; TTD—trichothiodystropy; XP—xeroderma pigmentosum gene.

Table 7-2. Types of DNA lesions

Missing base
Altered base
Incorrect base
Bulge due to insertion or deletion
Linked pyrimidines
3′-Deoxyribose fragments
Cross-linkage of strands
Strand breaks

Table 7-3. Effects of various types of common DNA damage on mammalian cells

AP sites
Cytotoxic
Mutagenic
O-6-guanine
Cytotoxic
Mutagenic
8-oxoG
Promutagenic
SSB
Cytotoxic
Lacking 3′-OH and 5′-P for polymerase

8-oxoG—C-8 oxidation of guanine; AP—apurinic/apyrimidinic; SSB—sugar-phosphate backbone.

age through reactive oxygen intermediates that produce single- and double-strand breaks along with ring-opened species similar to those observed with bleomycin and endogenous oxidative DNA damage. This damage (at least the oxidative DNA adducts) can be repaired by the DNA BER pathway (Table 7-3) [9]. There are many more clinically relevant chemotherapeutic agents, the complete discussion of which is beyond the scope of this chapter.

DIRECT REVERSAL REPAIR

The most direct mechanisms for repairing DNA are those that simply reverse the damage. MGMT, which removes methyl groups from DNA, is an example of this class of repair mechanism. The MGMT protein irreversibly transfers the alkyl group from the O-6 position of guanine (O^6-MeGua), that is associated with both mutagenesis and carcinogenesis, to a cysteine residue within its own primary structure (conserved active site PCHRV) (Fig. 7-1). This is a stoichiometric reaction that leads to inactivation of the protein; also referred to as a suicide enzyme. If left unrepaired, O^6-MeGua adducts can mispair with thymine, causing a G:C-to-A:T transition, which is associated with both mutagenesis and carcinogenesis.

The mammalian MGMT, like its bacterial counterpart, ADA, has several unique features (Fig. 7-1). First, this protein acceptor molecule removes a single alkyl group from the O-6 position of guanine, covalently binds the alkyl group to a cysteine residue in the MGMT molecule, and subsequently is inactivated. This stoichiometric reaction allows for one repair event per MGMT molecule in the tumor cell. Second, there is no evidence for reactivation of the alkylated transferase molecule; therefore, new repair activity requires de novo protein synthesis. Finally, the *MGMT* gene appears to be inactivated or downregulated (methylation repair deficient [Mer^-]) in approximately 20% of all human tumor cell lines examined [10]. However, only occasionally are low levels of the transferase observed in human tumor specimens [11]. Collectively, these data suggest that strategies that deplete MGMT of the Mer^+ tumor cell, prior to therapy with CENU might provide effective chemotherapy against a tumor that would otherwise be resistant to these agents (Fig. 7-2) [10,11].

Streptozotocin (STZ) inactivation of MGMT has been observed in human peripheral blood mononuclear cells treated with STZ in vitro, or isolated from patients receiving STZ chemotherapy [11]. This inactivation is thought to occur when MGMT removes STZ-induced alkyl groups from the DNA; however, some inactivation may occur from direct interaction of MGMT with the drug. Evidence for the inactivation of MGMT by pretreatment of highly resistant Mer^+ human tumor cells with STZ recently has been reported [11]. Using a restriction enzyme-oligonucleotide assay, it has been demonstrated that STZ causes inactivation of MGMT, production of increased levels of interstrand cross-linking by 1,3-bis(2-chloroethyl)-1-nitrosourea (BCNU; Fig. 7-2), and several logs of synergistic cell kill [11]. The maximum effects of the two agents were observed when STZ was administered 1 hour prior to or simultaneously with the BCNU. Reversal of the STZ→BCNU schedule showed a marked decrease in the achievable cell kill [11].

Unfortunately, DNA methylating agents such as STZ are mutagenic and potentially carcinogenic, and may produce synergistic host toxicity. Because of these potential adverse effects, numerous laboratories have studied alternative methods for depleting resistant tumor cells of MGMT. It has previously been

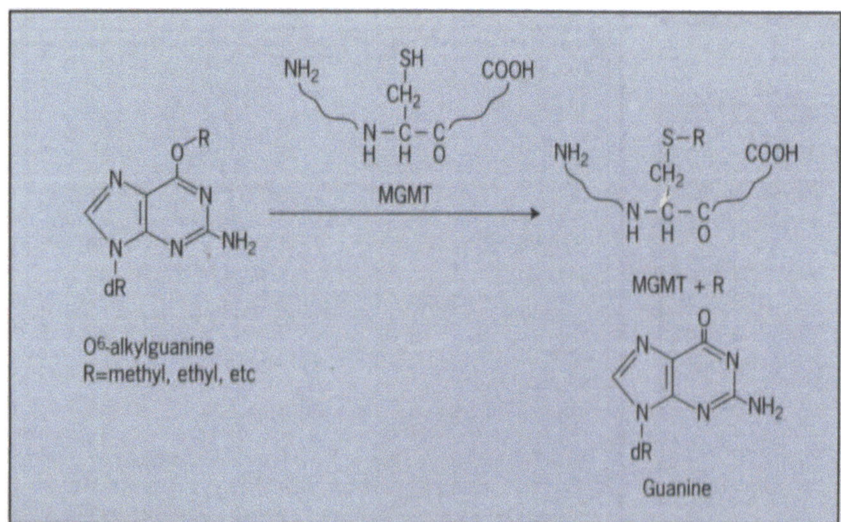

Figure 7-1. Mechanism of action of the O-6-methylguanine DNA methyltransferase (MGMT) with O-6-alkylguanine. The MGMT protein irreversibly transfers the alkyl group from the O-6 position of guanine to a cysteine residue within the conserved active site PCHRV of the MGMT protein. Only one alkyl group per protein molecule can be transferred through a stoichiometric reaction. There is no cleavage of the DNA, and the guanine is restored to its original unaltered state. If left unrepaired, O-6-methylguanine adducts can mispair with thymine, causing a G:C to A:T transition, which is associated with both mutagenesis and carcinogenesis.

reported that CENU agents themselves may react with MGMT to inactivate some of the cellular repair proteins [11]. Several groups have studied the potential of the free base O-6 methylguanine (O-6MG) to serve as a substrate for MGMT and subsequently deplete tumor cells of MGMT (Fig. 7-3). Karran [12] reported that O-6MG can deplete MGMT in human lymphoma cell lines and speculated that the depletion was accomplished by misincorporation of O-6MG into tRNA, which is subsequently repaired by MGMT. Other researchers who have been unable to demonstrate incorporation of the free base into any macromolecules have not confirmed this mechanism. However, the depletion of MGMT by the free base has been previously documented [11] in a series of studies showing that pretreatment of a variety of tumor

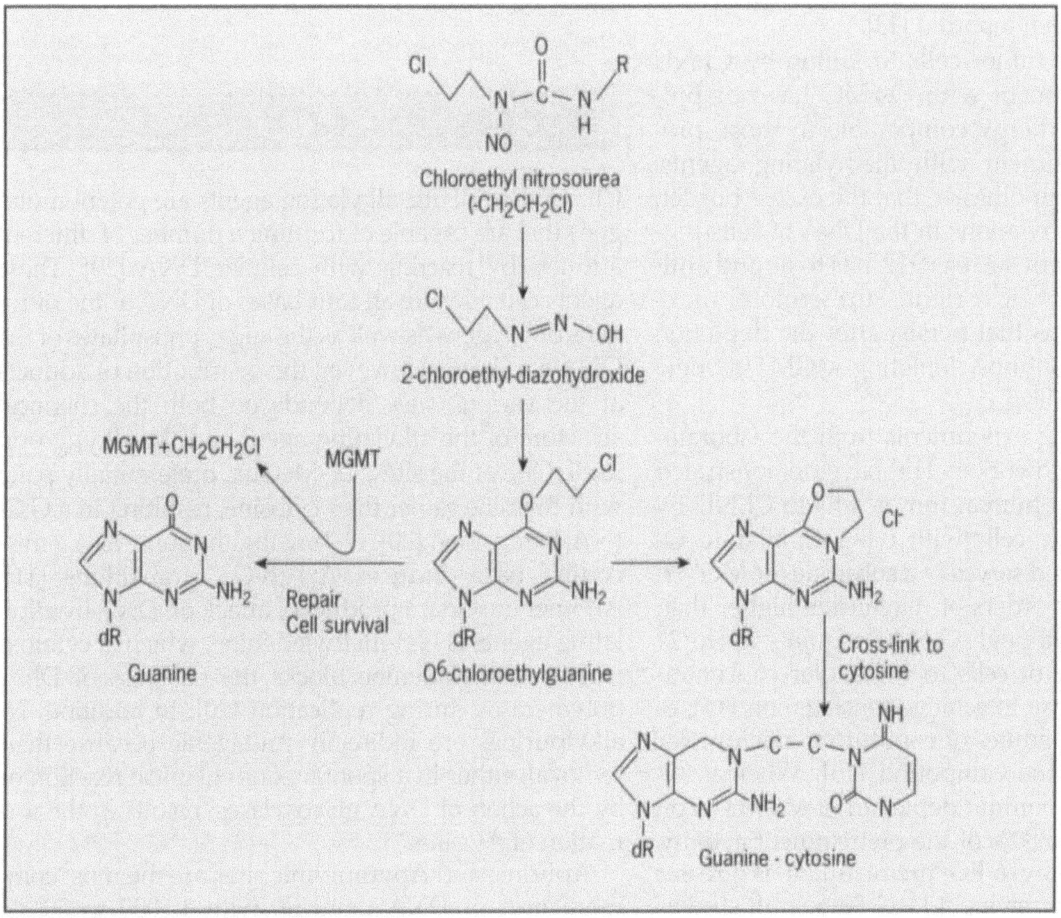

Figure 7-2. Chloroethyl nitrosourea mechanism of cell killing. Chloroethyl nitrosourea can alkylate the O-6 position of guanine and either be removed by MGMT, leading to cell survival, or rearranged, which causes an interstrand cross-link producing an ethyl bridge between N-1 of guanine and N-3 of cytosine in the opposite strand. This cross-linking produces cell cytotoxicity.

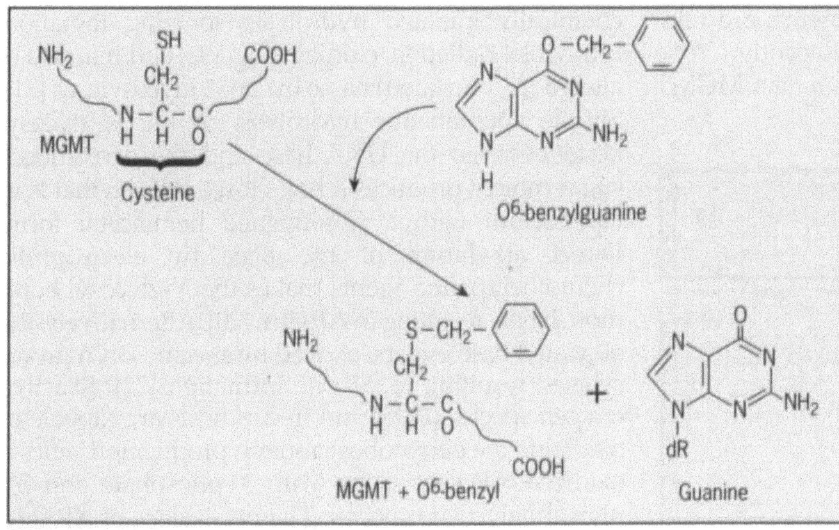

Figure 7-3. Mechanism of cellular depletion using O-6-benzylguanine. Pretreatment of cells with O-6-benzylguanine results in O-6-methylguanine DNA methyltransferase (MGMT) acting on the O-6-benzylguanine as it serves as a substrate for MGMT, but with an affinity orders of magnitude higher than that of O-6-methylguanine. This method allows for the sensitization of cells to chloroethyl nitrosourea by occupying most, if not all, of the MGMT molecules in a cell for a given time period. This is particularly advantageous in cases such as brain tumors, in which MGMT levels are elevated over those in the surrounding normal tissue.

cell lines with O-6MG partially depletes MGMT activity in those cells and leads to synergistic cell kills with a variety of CENUs and other chloroethylating agents. In similar studies, a series of Mer^+ human tumor cell lines could be sensitized to killing with CENU by pretreatment with O-6MG, but this sensitization was not observed in several Mer^- cell lines. In rats exposed to bolus doses of O-6MG, depletion of MGMT was observed in a variety of tissues [13]. Depletion of MGMT in human tumor xenografts by O-6MG also has been reported [13].

Sensitization of tumor cells to killing by CENU following pretreatment with O-6MG has not produced levels of synergy comparable to those produced by pretreatment with methylating agents, such as STZ. We hypothesize that the excess burden of unrepaired methylations in the DNA of cells pretreated with an agent such as STZ has toxic and antitumor effects in its own right. Furthermore, unrepaired methylations that persist after the depletion of MGMT may continue depleting MGMT as new molecules are synthesized.

Recently, exciting experiments from the laboratories of Dolan and coworkers [15] have demonstrated the sensitization of human tumor cells to CENU by pretreatment of the cells with 6-BG. Similar to O-6MG, this compound serves as a substrate for MGMT, but has an affinity orders of magnitude higher than that of O-6MG. Although O-6MG requires up to 24 hours of exposure of cells to millimolar concentrations of the free base to achieve sensitization [14], 6-BG requires only minutes of exposure to micromolar concentrations of the compound [15]. Whereas O-6MG–mediated maximum depletion of MGMT is on the order of 75% to 80% of the pretreatment activity, MGMT depletion by 6-BG pretreatment is greater than 95% of the pretreatment level. Xenograft studies using 6-BG and BCNU have demonstrated excellent synergistic activity.

Alkyltransferases from other species, including yeast and *Escherichia coli* (ADA) proteins, are relatively resistant to depletion by 6-BG. Recently, Crone and coworkers [16,17] reported mammalian MGMT mutants with increased resistance to 6-BG due to changes in the amino acid sequence around the critical active site located at cysteine 145 [16–18]. To date, little data are available regarding the relative resistance to 6-BG depletion of the wild-type MGMT, mutant MGMTs, or ADA proteins in primary bone marrow cells in vitro, although Reese and coworkers [19] recently demonstrated the utility of one MGMT mutant in human $CD34^+$ cells. (*see* section on gene therapy.)

Table 7-4. Causes of apurinic/apyrimidinic (AP) sites in cells
Spontaneous
Glycosylases
Ionizing radiation
Chemicals/antibiotics
Oxidative damage

DNA BASE EXCISION REPAIR

Chemotherapeutic alkylating agents are potent mutagens that are capable of forming a number of different adducts by reacting with cellular DNA [20]. These agents can alkylate all four bases of DNA at the nitrogens or oxygens as well as the sugar phosphates of the DNA backbone. However, the distribution of adducts at the various sites depends on both the chemical structure of the alkylating agent and the alkyl group itself. One of the sites, O^6-MeGua, preferentially pairs with thymine rather than cytosine, resulting in a G:C-to-A:T transition [20]. O-4-methylthymine, also a miscoding base, induces A:T-to-G:C transitions [11]. Another important product of attack on DNA by alkylating agents is N-3-methyladenine, which is cytotoxic. N-3-methyladenine blocks the progress of DNA polymerases during replication [20]. In addition, *N*-alkylpurines are indirectly mutagenic because their removal, either in a spontaneous chemical reaction or by the action of DNA glycosylases, results in the formation of AP sites.

Apurinic and Apyrimidinic sites are the most common form of DNA damage, with 10,000 to 20,000 apurinic and 500 apyrimidinic sites produced per cell each day under normal physiologic conditions (Table 7-4) [20]. AP sites are generated from spontaneous and chemically initiated hydrolysis, ionizing radiation, ultraviolet radiation, oxidizing agents, and removal of altered (*eg*, alkylated) bases by DNA glycosylases [21]. Simple spontaneous hydrolysis of the *N*-glycosyl bond between the DNA base and the deoxyribose sugar moiety produces a ring-closed AP site that is in equilibrium with a ring-opened hemiacetal form. Direct alkylation of the base by electrophilic chemotherapeutic agents makes the *N*-glycosyl bond more labile, resulting in AP sites [20]. Alternatively, the alkylated base may be excised by specific DNA glycosylases, resulting in AP site formation [22]. Reactive oxygen species (ROS) and free radicals are capable of oxidizing the deoxyribose moiety, producing 1′ and 4′ oxidized AP sites along with 3′-phosphate and 3′-phosphoglycolate species. The persistence of AP sites in DNA results in a block to DNA replication, cytotoxic mutations, and genetic instability [23].

Other damaged adducts or alterations of DNA that occur following alkylation involve the ring-opening of DNA bases that occurs following alkylation at the N-7 position of guanine. For example, *N,N′,N′′*-triethylenethiophospharamide (thiotepa) can be reduced to aziridine, which results in depurination and formation of aminoethyl adducts of guanine and adenine [3]. N-7-aminoethylguanosine becomes unstable and degrades by imidazole ring-opening and depurination. These ring-opened bases are repaired by members of the BER pathway, such as the yeast and human *OGG1* (8-oxoguanine glycosylase) genes [24–26].

Although many DNA-damaging agents may not directly produce AP sites in DNA, the manner in which they physically or chemically modify DNA may be the target for a class of DNA repair enzymes known as DNA glycosylases, whose action ultimately leads to the formation of AP sites in DNA (Fig. 7-4). DNA glycosylases remove a damaged base, creating an AP site in the DNA, which then is acted on by an AP endonuclease (APE/REF-1) [21,27]. Cytotoxic lesions such as N-3-methyladenine, N-7-methylgua-

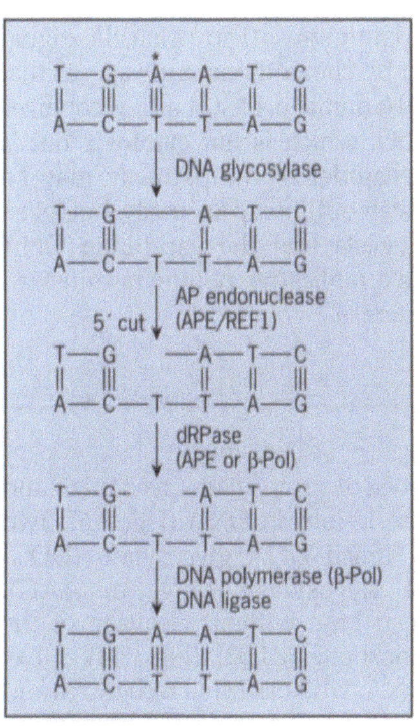

Figure 7-4. The DNA base excision repair (BER) pathway in mammalian cells. This pathway, arbitrarily designated "A," represents one of the two presumed pathways for repairing a single damaged base in DNA. Only four enzymes are needed to complete the repair of a damaged base, such as alkylated N-3-adenine, a lesion formed by alkylating agents that is cytotoxic to cells. A glycosylase removes the damaged base (*Asterisk*), leaving the sugar-phosphate backbone intact, and incision on the 5′ side of the baseless site occurs through a hydrolytic mechanism. The resulting termini are "polished" by a deoxyribosephosphate hydrolase (dRPase) which removes the 5′ phosphoribosyl. This step is followed by insertion of a new base by DNA polymeraseβ and ligation by DNA ligase I. AP/REF-1— apurinic/apyrimidinic; APE— apurinic/apyrimidinic endonuclease. β-pol—DNA polymeraseβ.

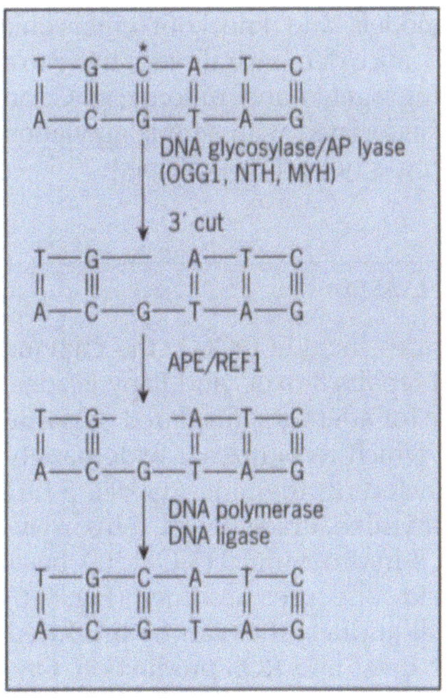

Figure 7-5. The DNA base excision repair (BER) pathway with combined glycosylase–apurinic/apyrimidinic (AP) lyase. The BER pathway "B" is similar to pathway "A" except that the first two steps are combined into a single enzyme called a glycosylase/AP lyase. These enzymes remove the damaged base (*Asterisk*) and cleave the DNA backbone at the 3′ side of the AP site through AP lyase activity, producing a 5′-phosphate and a 3′-phosphate. The 3′-phosphate must be acted on for BER to continue, and it appears this occurs through one of the numerous functions of the AP endonuclease (APE/REF-1). APE/REF-1 can act as a 3′-diesterase to remove this 3′-phosphate; this step is followed by correct repair of the gapped DNA [84,85]. The missing base can then be filled in with DNA polymeraseβ and ligated by DNA ligase I [21,27,28].

nine, and N-3-methylguanine are released by the *N*-methylpurine DNA glycosylase (MPG) enzyme [28]. AP sites produced by *N*-glycosylase action on damaged bases formed directly by agents such as bleomycin or by spontaneous hydrolysis are incised by AP endonucleases either 5′ to the AP site (class II AP endonuclease) (Fig. 7-4) or 3′ to the AP site (class I AP lyase) (Fig. 7-5) [21,27,29]. Repair is completed by loss of the abasic residue (5′-phosphoribosyl residue by deoxyribosephosphate hydrolase [dRPase]), followed by insertion of a new base by DNA beta-polymerase, and ligation. The rate-limiting protein in BER pathways may be cell-type– and lesion-type–specific, and only limited data are currently available with respect to which one or ones may be the rate-limiting step in this pathway. For example, previous data have shown that in some cells MPG is not the rate-limiting step in the BER pathway for the repair of alkylation DNA damage [29]. However, in vitro studies by Ramana and coworkers [30] have shown that APE/REF-1 is rate limiting in the repair of ROS-induced DNA strand breaks.

A second closely related pathway for removing and repairing a damaged base by BER involves a complex glycosylase associated with AP lyase activity [27,31] (Fig. 7-5). Removal of the damaged base and incision of the DNA backbone occurs via a single enzyme, in contrast to the previously described repair involving separate glycosylase (MPG) and APE enzymes. Examples of mammalian combined glycosylase/AP lyases include the human OGG1 and NTH1 (human homologue of the *E. coli* endonuclease III gene). The OGG1 glycosylase/AP lyase recognizes and initiates repair of ring-opened bases such as formamidopyrimidine-guanine (Fapy-Gua) and methylated formamidopyrimidine (N-7-methylformamidopyrimidine [7-methyl-Fapy-Gua]). These lesions are produced by alkylating agents such as thiotepa, by endogenous oxidative stress (Fapy-Gua, 8-oxoguanine [8-oxoG]), and by chemotherapeutic agents that create oxidative DNA damage. OGG1 also recognizes and removes 8-oxoG, which is not cytotoxic but is mutagenic. The remainder of the pathway may be similar to the pathway outlined previously, however, some evidence suggests that the gap-filling DNA polymerase may be a replicative polymerase instead of DNA beta-polymerase.

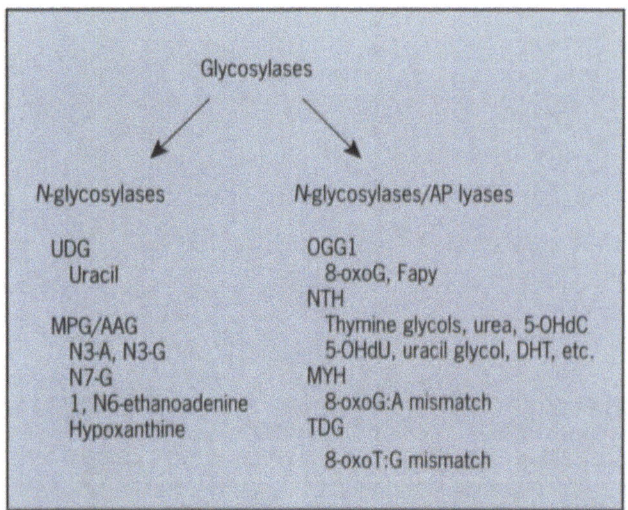

Figure 7-6. DNA glycosylases can be grouped into two classes: simple and those with associated apurinic/apyrimidinic (AP) lyase activity. Simple glycosylases remove the damaged base without cutting the DNA sugar-phosphate backbone. Complex glycosylases remove the damaged base but also cut the DNA at the 3′ side through an AP lyase activity. The former are predominantly involved in the removal of alkylated bases and uracil from DNA. The latter are responsible for the repair of oxidative DNA lesions (OGG1 and NTH), recognition and removal of 8-oxoG:A mismatches (MYH) or T:G mismatches (TDG). AAG—5-OHdC—5-hydroxycytosine; 5-OHdU—5-hydroxyuracil; 8-oxoG—C-8 oxidation of guanine; DHT—dihydrothymine; Fapy—formamdiopyrimidine; MPG—methylpurine glycosylase; UDG—uracil DNA glycosylase.

Simple Glycosylases

In humans, a number of glycosylases recognize and remove various base lesions in DNA (Fig. 7-6). Two main glycosylases, uracil DNA glycosylase (UDG) and methylpurine glycosylase (MPG, or AAG), remove the damaged base without cleavage of the sugar-phosphate backbone [31,32] (Fig. 7-4). UDG removes uracil in DNA, whereas MPG recognizes and removes N-3-adenines, N-3-guanine, N-7-guanine, 1, N-6-ethanoadenine, and hypoxanthine. The substrate specificity for MPG has recently been verified using animal knockout models and knockout embryonic stem cells [33]. MPG$^-$ mice demonstrate sensitivity to a number of alkylating agents and mitomycin C, an agent not normally associated with simple alkylation [33]. The latter finding is not yet unexplained.

Glycosylase/AP Lyases

Glycosylase/AP lyases include OGG1, the enzyme that recognizes and repairs 8-oxoG and Fapy lesions; MYH, a glycosylase for adenines mispaired opposite 8-oxoG; and NTH, which recognizes a wide variety of DNA adducts including thymine glycols, 5-OH and 6-OH dihydrothymine, uracil glycol, 5-hydroxycytosine (5-OHdC), 5-hydroxyuracil (5-OHdU), beta-ureidoisobutyric acid, and urea residues (Fig. 7-6) [34,35]. These are all adducts that can be produced following oxidative stress and ROS production. One other combined glycosylase/AP lyase that has been isolated from human cells is the thymine (T:G) mismatch DNA glycosylase (TDG) [36]. All of these enzymes remove the damaged base and cleave the DNA backbone at the 3′ side of the AP site through an AP lyase activity, producing a 5′-phosphate and 3′-phosphate. The 3′-phosphate must be acted on for BER to continue, and it appears that this occurs through one of the numerous functions of the AP endonuclease (APE/REF-1; discussed later). APE/REF-1 can act as a 3′-diesterase to remove this 3′-phosphate and allow subsequent repair of the gapped DNA [32].

DNA BETA-POLYMERASE AND DNA LIGASE I

Following removal of the damaged base and cutting of the sugar-phosphate backbone, a single base can be replaced by DNA beta-polymerase, followed by ligation of the 3′-OH and 5′-phosphate by DNA ligase I. DNA beta-polymerase also has been shown to have dRPase activity similar to that of APE/REF-1 (Figs. 7-4 and 7-5) [32]. Whether APE/REF-1 or DNA beta-polymerase performs this latter function in vivo is still unknown. Mouse knockout experiments of the DNA beta-polymerase gene show embryonic lethality at midgestation (day E10.5), about the time the central nervous system begins to develop more fully. DNA beta-polymerase is more highly expressed in the central nervous system than in other tissues, which may partially explain this stage of embryonic lethality. Fortunately, DNA beta-polymerase–deficient cell lines have been established by collecting cells before day E10.5. These cells are sensitive only to monofunctional alkylating agents [37]. DNA ligase I knockout mice are embryonic lethal at day E6.5 [32].

AP ENDONUCLEASES

APE/REF-1 is a multifunctional protein with roles in DNA BER, oxidative signaling, transcription factor regulation, cell cycle control, and apoptosis. The major cellular enzymes initiating repair of AP sites (class II AP endonucleases) have been identified and characterized in bacteria, yeast, *Drosophila*, and mammals [21,27]. These repair proteins hydrolyze the phosphodiester backbone immediately 5′ to an AP site, generating an abasic deoxyribose-5-phosphate that is released by a 5′- dRPase or 5′-exonuclease and is followed by DNA synthesis and ligation. These enzymes also have repair activity for 3′-terminal oxidative lesions [21,38]. By hydrolyzing 3′-blocking fragments from oxidized DNA, these enzymes can produce normal 3′-hydroxyl nucleotide termini, permitting DNA repair synthesis. As discussed previously, DNA BER (Fig. 7-4) requires the major human AP endonuclease APE/REF-1 for AP site recognition and cleavage 3′ to the AP site via a hydrolytic mechanism (Fig. 7-7). However, APE/REF-1 also is required in the other BER pathway, probably as a 3′-repair diesterase (Fig. 7-5) [21,27,29,39]. The predominant human class II AP endonuclease, APE/REF-1 [40], is a multifunctional protein that not only is responsible for repair of AP sites but also functions as a reduction-oxidation (redox) factor, maintaining transcription factors in an active reduced state (Fig. 7-7). The other type of "AP endonuclease" is an enzyme with combined glycosylase and AP lyase activity and may constitute the major pathway for the repair of oxidative DNA damage.

The APE/REF-1 protein also has been shown to stimulate the DNA binding activity of Fos-Jun dimers, NF-kappaB, Myb, AP1 proteins, Pax 5 members of the ATF/CREB family, and hypoxia-inducible factor (HIF1alpha) [41–43] (Fig. 7-8). Mutational analysis has revealed that cysteine residue 65 in the N-terminal region of AP endonuclease participates in maintaining the critical sulfhydryls in a functionally reduced state for certain transcription factors [44]. The proto-oncogenes *jun* and *fos* encode proteins that bind specific DNA sequences as a dimer complex, termed activator protein-1 (AP1), to regulate gene expression. Each AP1 binding factor (Fos, Jun) contains a cysteine

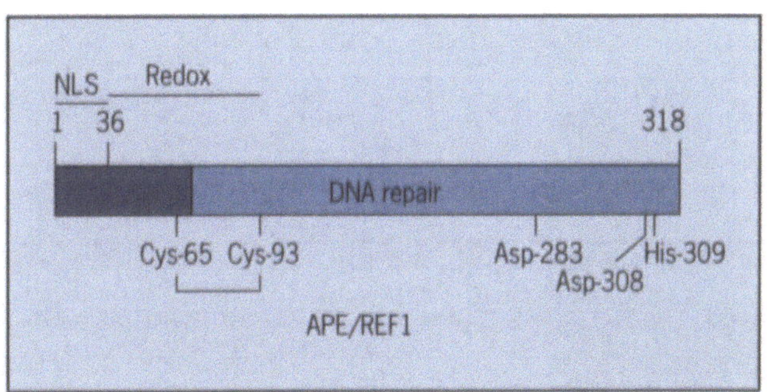

Figure 7-7. The human apurinic/apyrimidinic (AP) endonuclease (APE/REF-1) is a multifunctional DNA repair/redox enzyme. APE/REF-1 is a 318–amino acid protein with two domains; the amino end is involved in the reduction-oxidation of a wide variety of proteins. The cysteines at positions 65 and 93 are involved in this activity. The AP endonuclease repair domain is located near the carboxy-terminus, involving amino acids at 283, 308, and 309 in the active site. Mutations of cysteine 65 destroy all redox activity of APE/REF-1, whereas mutations of amino acids 283, 308, and 309 abolish AP endonuclease activity. The nuclear localization signal (NLS) is found in the first 36 amino acids of the protein. Truncation of APE/REF-1, leaving a protein that begins with amino acid 61, results in a protein having almost full AP endonuclease activity but no redox activity [49].

residue within the DNA binding motif that prevents DNA binding if oxidized and augments DNA binding if reduced. Therefore, the DNA binding activity of these proteins is sensitive to redox [45]. APE/REF-1, which is the major AP1 redox activity in HeLa cells, represents a novel redox component of the signal transduction processes that regulates eukaryotic gene expression [41] and identifies APE/REF-1 as a critical player in DNA repair and redox regulation. Recent developments also have intimately linked APE/REF-1 as a major controlling factor for P53 activity through a redox mechanism [46] and have established its interaction with P53 in vivo (Fig. 7-9) [47].

Recently, APE/REF-1 also has been shown to be inversely related to apoptosis levels in blood cells (Fig. 7-10) [48]. The HL-60 cell line (a myeloid leukemia cell line) can be induced to differentiate along the granulocytic or monocytic/macrophage lineage. Treatment of HL-60 cells with retinoic acid and dimethylsulfoxide (DMSO; granulocytic) or phorbol 12-myristate 13-acetate (PMA; monocytic) results in apoptosis and downregulation of APE/REF-1 expression at both the RNA and protein levels. Moreover, double-labeling experiments using APE/REF-1 immunohistochemistry and the TdT terminal transferase end-labeling assay for apoptosis demonstrated that individual cells

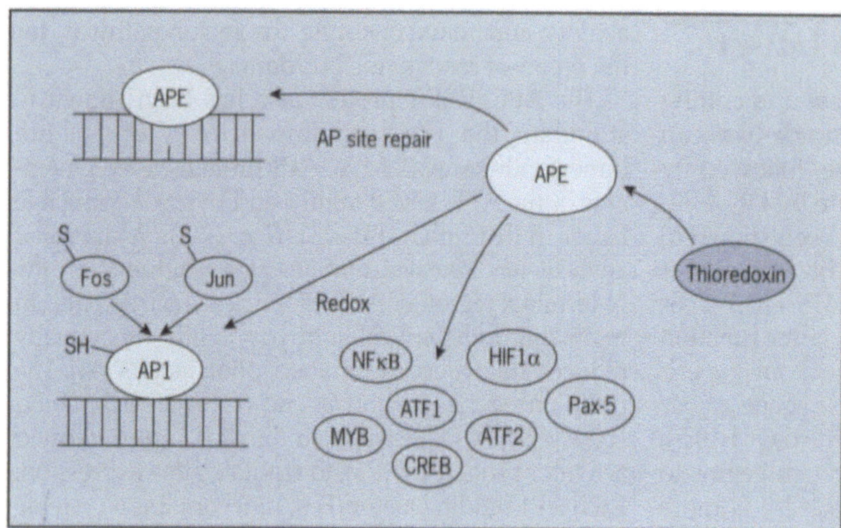

Figure 7-8. Multiple roles of apurinic/apyrimidinic (AP) endonuclease (APE/REF-1) in mammalian cells. APE/REF-1 functions as a DNA repair enzyme with AP endonuclease activity as well as diesterase and exonuclease activity. It also removes 3′ oxidative blocking lesions. APE/REF-1 redox function has been implicated in the reduction-oxidation of numerous proteins, most of which must be reduced to specifically bind to DNA. These include *Fos-Jun* dimers (AP1), as well as NF-κB and Myb proteins, members of the ATF/CREB family, and hypoxia-inducible factor (HIF1α) [67–71]. Recent developments also have indicated APE/REF-1 as a major controlling factor for P53 activity through a redox mechanism [74,75]. APE/REF-1 also has been shown to interact with thioredoxin following cellular stimulation with phorbol esters [78].

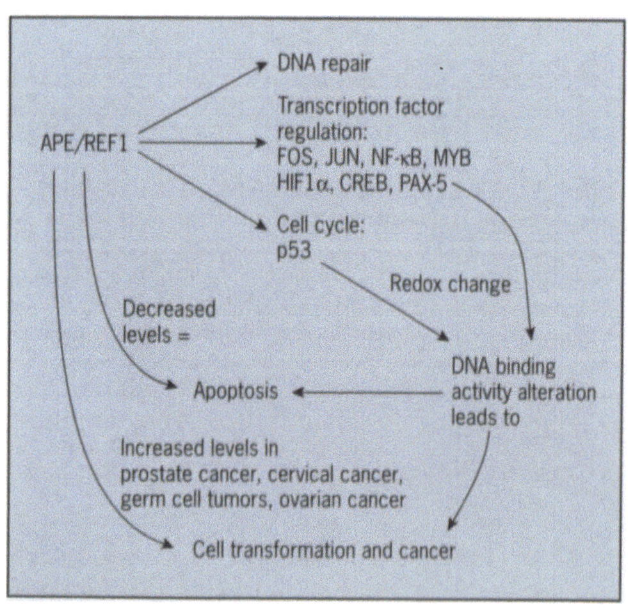

Figure 7-9. In addition to the role of apurinic/apyrimidinic (AP) endonuclease in DNA repair and redox regulation of proteins, APE/REF-1 has been implicated in apoptosis and has demonstrated altered levels in certain cancers. Recently, APE/REF-1 also has been shown to be inversely related to apoptosis levels in blood cells [48]; these studies established that downregulation of APE/REF-1 expression is associated with programmed cell death in cells of the myeloid lineage [48]. Elevated levels of APE/REF-1 also have been found in cervical and prostate cancer as well as germ cell tumors and have been shown to alter its cellular location from the nucleus to the cytoplasm in ovarian cancers [52].

undergoing apoptosis lose expression of APE/REF-1 regardless of their state of differentiation (Fig. 7-11) [48]. Blocking apoptosis by overexpression of the *BCL2* proto-oncogene in HL-60 cells or by a *BCR-abl* related mechanism in K562 cells and subsequent differentiation resulted in morphologic differentiation but no loss of APE/REF-1 expression [48]. These studies established that downregulation of APE/REF-1 expression is associated with programmed cell death in cells of the myeloid lineage.

Recent data have demonstrated that APE/REF-1 can be phosphorylated in vitro [49], possibly adding another level of post-translational regulation in the control of APE/REF-1 function (Fig. 7-12). Whether the phosphorylation affects only the repair activity and not the redox activity of APE/REF-1 is under close scrutiny; thus, evaluation of the impact of each of these functions on differentiation, growth, apoptosis, and sensitivity to therapeutic agents will be important. APE/REF-1 also has been shown to be part of a path-

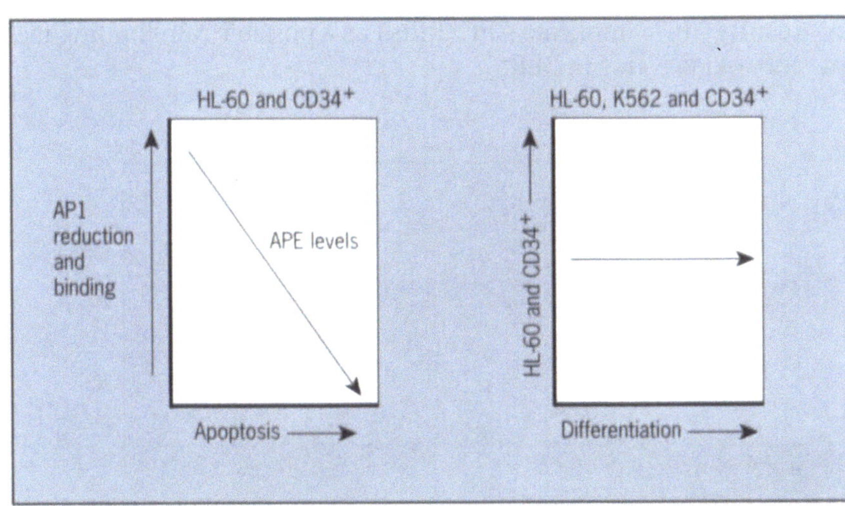

Figure 7-10. Apurinic/apyrimidinic (AP) endonuclease (APE/REF-1) is inversely related to apoptosis levels in a myeloid leukemia cell line. As the apoptosis level increases in HL-60 cells following stimulation to undergo apoptosis, the level of APE/REF-1 decreases. There is no change in the level of APE/REF-1 when the cells differentiate, but apoptosis is blocked [48]. These results also have been seen in human CD34$^+$ cells treated ex vivo (Williams & Kelley, unpublished observation).

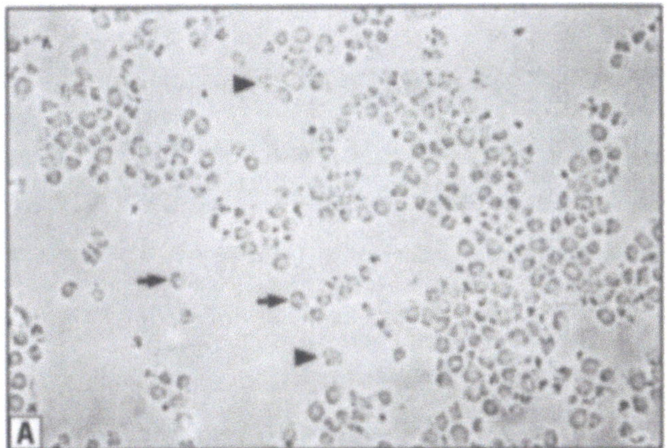

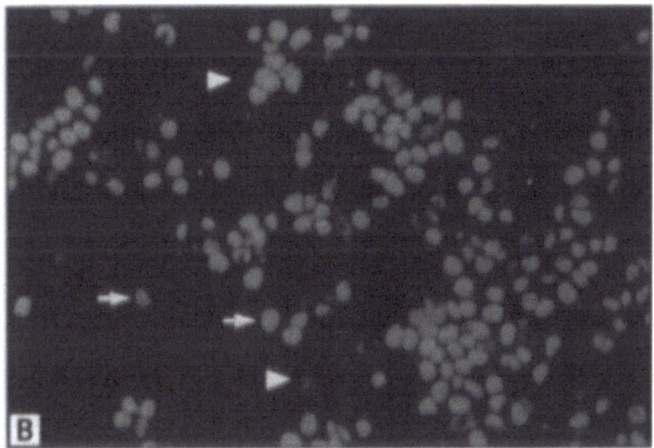

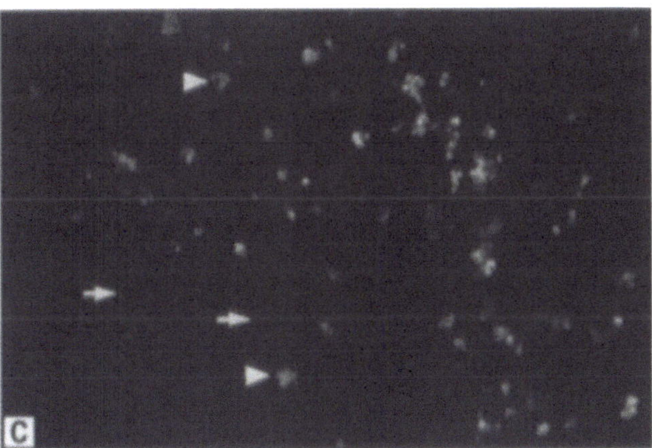

Figure 7-11. Inverse relation of apurinic/apyrimidinic (AP) endonuclease (APE/REF-1) and apoptosis in HL-60 cells. **A**, A 50:50 mixture of undifferentiated and differentiated HL-60 cells was cytospun onto slides. **B**, The sample was assayed for APE/REF-1 using polyclonal antibody to APE/REF-1 detected with rhodamine. **C**, The sample was also assayed for DNA fragmentation using TdT terminal transferase end-labeling (TUNEL) assay detected with fluorescein. Cells positive for APE/REF-1 (*arrows*) are negative for TUNEL (*arrowheads*). (*From* [48]; with permission.)

way that involves thioredoxin, which moves from the cytoplasm to the nucleus, interacting with APE/REF-1 [50]. Finally, elevated levels of APE/REF-1 have been found in cervical cancer, prostate cancer, and germ cell tumors (Fig. 7-13) [51,52]. APE/REF-1 appears to form a unique link between the DNA BER pathway, oxidative signaling, transcription factor regulation, cancer, apoptosis, and cell cycle control (Fig. 7-9).

Decreased APE/REF-1 Expression

Decreased APE/REF-1 expression results in increased sensitivity to chemotherapy and oxidative DNA damage. Studies using antisense APE/REF-1 in HeLa cells indicate that cells can be made hypersensitive to alkylating and oxidative agents by depleting the cell of APE/REF-1 (Table 7-5); similar findings have been obtained in rat glioma cells [53]. Mouse knockout experiments have shown that the loss of APE/REF-1 renders the mice embryonic lethal on days E5 to E9. In addition, no cell lines have been established that are completely deficient of APE/REF-1, indicating the importance of APE/REF-1 in cell viability and its dominant role in repair and redox. Furthermore, these findings implicate APE/REF-1 as a possible rate-limiting factor in BER.

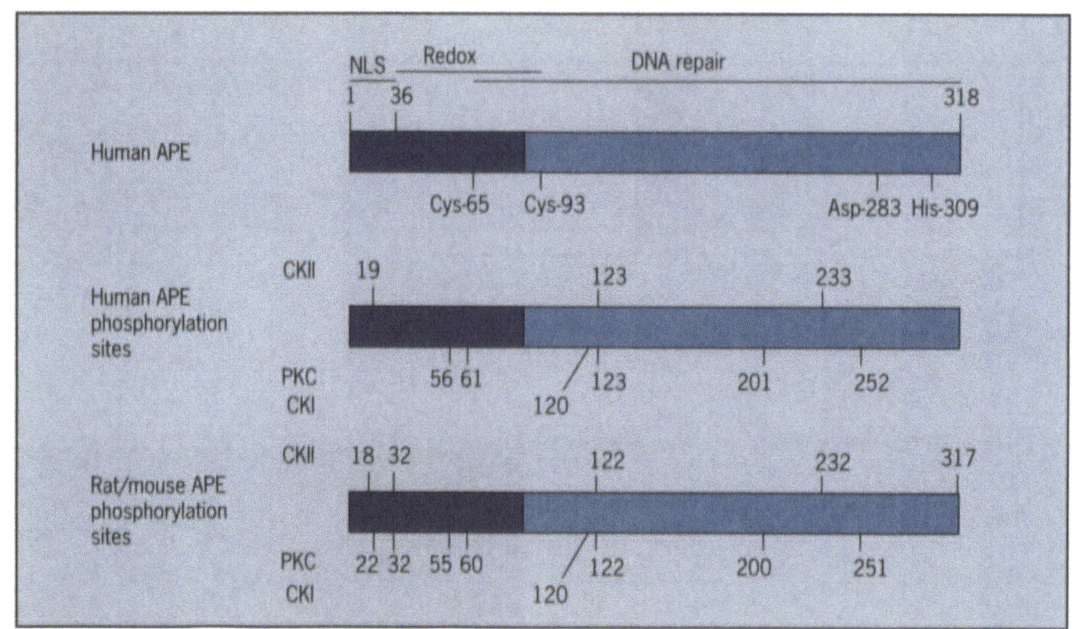

Figure 7-12. Phosphorylation sites of mammalian apurinic/apyrimidinic (AP) endonuclease (APE/REF-1). A number of theoretical phosphorylation sites have been identified in APE/REF-1 for casein kinase I (CKI), casein kinase II (CKII), or protein kinase C (PKC). Although in vitro all enzymes phosphorylated APE/REF-1, only CKII inhibited the AP endonuclease repair activity of APE/REF-1 [49]. This adds another dimension to the regulation of APE/REF-1 function in cells. These results must be confirmed in vivo, and the role of phosphorylation on redox function also needs to be determined. NLS—nuclear localization signal.

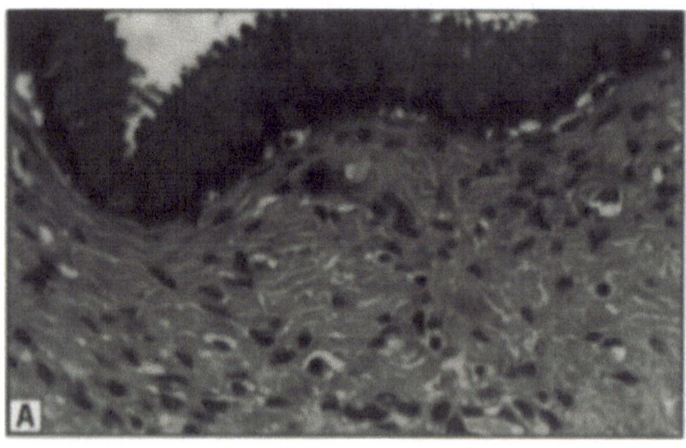

Figure 7-13. Altered levels of apurinic/apyrimidinic (AP) endonuclease (APE/REF-1) in human cervical cancer tissue samples. Normal tissue shows APE/REF-1 staining in nuclei at a much lower level than in the dysplastic tissue. Cells in the CIN1 tissue show increased levels of APE/REF-1 staining, both in intensity and number of cells. This increase is mainly in the nuclei, although some cells have increased APE/REF-1 levels in the cytoplasm as well. **A** and **E**, Hematoxylin and eosin staining of normal and CIN1 cervical tissue, respectively. **B**, Normal tissue with preimmune antibody. **C** and **D**, Normal tissue stained with APE/REF-1 antibody. *(continued)*

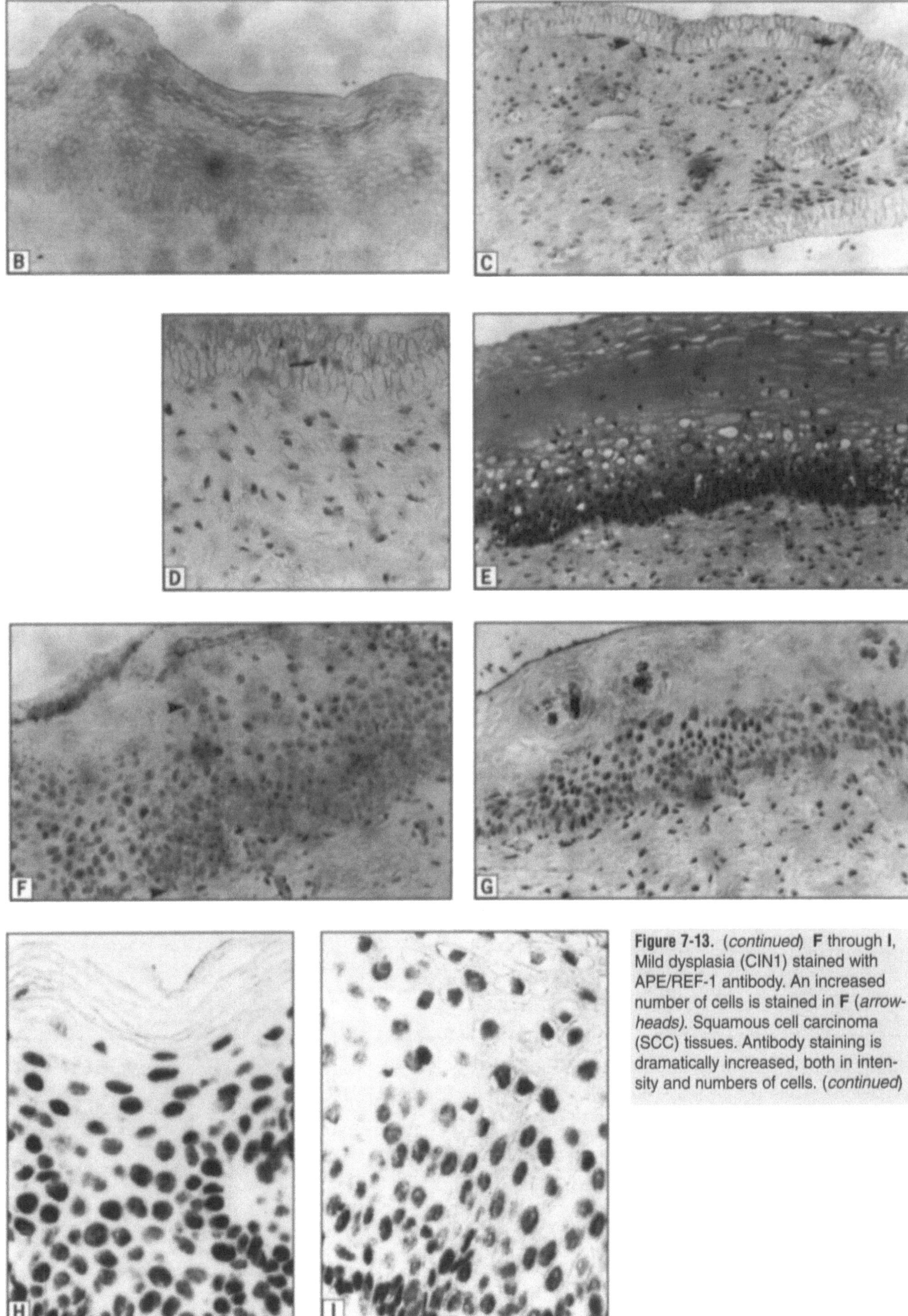

Figure 7-13. (*continued*) **F** through **I**, Mild dysplasia (CIN1) stained with APE/REF-1 antibody. An increased number of cells is stained in **F** (*arrowheads*). Squamous cell carcinoma (SCC) tissues. Antibody staining is dramatically increased, both in intensity and numbers of cells. (*continued*)

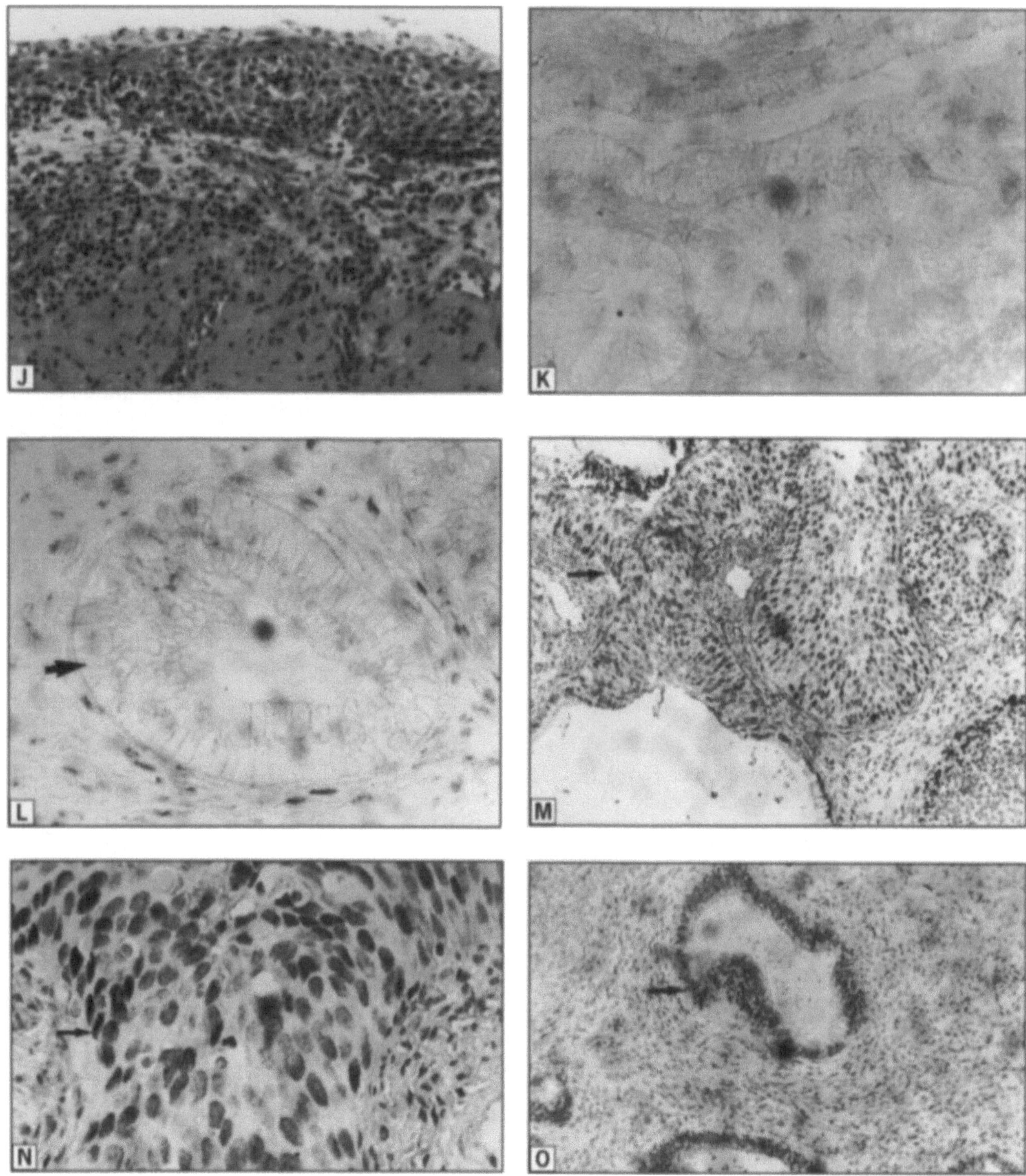

Figure 7-13. (*continued*) **J**, Hematoxylin and eosin staining of reactive epithelial change tissue. **K**, Preimmune control on normal cervix tissue. **L**, Normal cervix tissue with APE/REF-1 antibody. There is little staining of the endocervical gland (*arrow*). **M**, APE/REF-1 staining of SCC-G3. **N**, Magnified region corresponding to the region marked with an *arrow* in *D*. **O**, High level of APE/REF-1 staining of the endocervical glands in SCC tissues (*arrows*). These glands do not stain nearly as intensely in normal tissue (see *arrow* in **C**). (*From* [52]; with permission.)

Oxidative DNA Damage and Repair

Reactive oxygen species (ROS), such as superoxide radicals, hydrogen peroxide (H_2O_2), and hydroxyl radicals can be generated during aerobic metabolism of oxygen [54]. ROS have been implicated in the etiology of many human diseases and are significant contributors to mutagenesis, carcinogenesis, and tumor promotion [55]. Tumor promoters such as phorbol esters are known to indirectly induce certain types of DNA damage through their production of ROS (Fig. 7-14) [55]. ROS are critical to the toxicity resulting from treatment with ionizing radiation, antitumor drugs such as bleomycin, and agents such as adriamycin and VP-16 that form free-radical intermediates during enzymatic activation. Furthermore, almost half of the approved anticancer drugs used in the United States can form ROS (free radicals) [56].

One of the major products of DNA damage that results from ROS and chemotherapeutic agents is 8-oxoguanine, also referred to as 7,8-dihydro-8-oxodeoxyguanine, 8-hydroxyguanine, or 8-oxoG (Fig. 7-14). 8-oxoG is a premutagenic lesion that has been implicated in carcinogenesis via its G→C to T→A mediated transversions. Previous studies have found an increase in 8-oxoG levels in the liver of patients

Table 7-5. Apurinic/apyrimidinic (AP) endonuclease protection

Agent	Lesions	Sensitivity to AP endonuclease depletion
Monofunctional alkylating agents (MMS)	AP sites Base damage	Yes
Peroxides (H_2O_2)	AP sites Strand breaks	Yes
Ionizing radiation	AP sites Base damage Strand breaks	Yes
Redox cycling drugs (paraquat)	AP sites Strand breaks	Yes
Ultraviolet light	Pyrimidine dimers	No

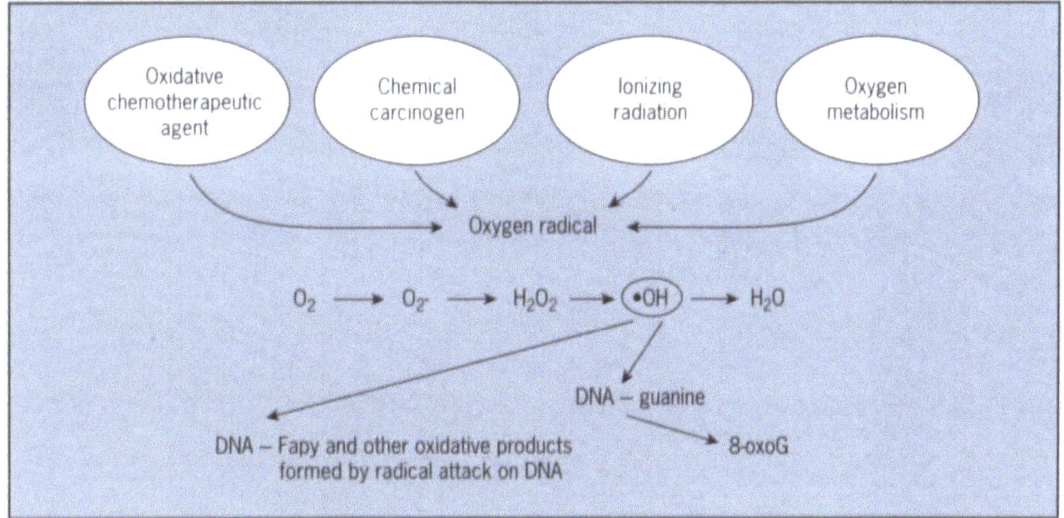

Figure 7-14. Numerous agents can produce oxygen free radicals in mammalian cells. The production of oxygen free radicals leads to the eventual production of hydrogen peroxide (H_2O_2) and, with iron present (through the Fenton reaction), the production of hydroxyl (OH) radicals that can damage DNA, leading to a variety of adducts. The most commonly measured of these adducts is 8-oxoguanine (8-oxoG) [91]. Fapy—formamdiopyrimidine.

with chronic hepatitis, leading to hepatocellular carcinoma (HCC), one of the most frequent human cancers worldwide [57]. G→C to T→A transversions occur frequently in the *P53* gene, leading to HCC [58]. Elevated levels of 8-oxoG have been found in Long-Evans cinnamon rats, an inbred strain that develops HCC, leading to the conclusion that oxygen radicals and oxidative DNA damage play a role in the carcinogenesis that occurs in these rats [59]. Oxidative stress is proposed to play a critical role in the pathogenesis of several neurologic disorders, including Parkinson's disease, Alzheimer's disease, and even aging. Furthermore, recent observations that both DNA adducts and oxidative base damage are increased in the brains of patients with Parkinson's disease and in spinal cord tissue of patients with amyotrophic lateral sclerosis support the idea that oxidative DNA damage may contribute to the observed loss of neurons in various neurologic disorders [60,61]. Therefore, understanding how oxidative DNA damage is repaired or not repaired is also critical to understanding the pathology of various neurologic disorders.

Numerous cancer chemotherapeutic agents are oxidative DNA damage promoters via their free-radical production. For example, MMC is a free-radical producer through a one-electron reduction to a semiquinone radical that, in the presence of oxygen, produces H_2O_2 and hydroxyl radicals, leading to DNA damage [62]. Another example is VP-16, one of the most active agents in the treatment of small cell lung cancer, testicular cancer, malignant lymphomas, and a variety of pediatric cancers. It has been suggested that VP-16 exerts its antitumor activity via hydroxyl radical production [62].

ROS damage chromosomal DNA, giving rise to strand breaks, AP sites, DNA-protein cross-links, and modified purine and pyrimidine bases. As mentioned previously, one of the major products of DNA damage resulting from ROS is 8-oxoG. The occurrence of this nucleotide is important in terms of mutagenesis as well as carcinogenesis, because it can pair with either cytosine or adenine and thereby cause G:C-to-T:A transversions [63]. Although the removal of 8-oxoG is important in preventing mutations, other ROS-damaged DNA that may be more important, particularly as it relates to cytotoxicity is the removal of guanine residues whose imidazole rings have been opened to form 2,6-diamino-4-hydroxy-5-*N*-methyl formamidopyrimidine (Fapy lesions) (Fig. 7-15). These lesions closely resemble those formed by ionizing radiation through the action of . OH and . H. The removal of Fapy lesions from damaged DNA has been shown to be mediated through the action of a Fapy-DNA glycosylase (human OGG1), which possesses both *N*-glycosylase and beta,delta-elimination activities, as discussed previously [26,64]. Therefore, the Fapy-DNA glycosylase OGG1 recognizes and initiates repair of 8-oxoG and Fapy lesions produced by oxidative DNA damage. Another means of correcting an 8-oxoG

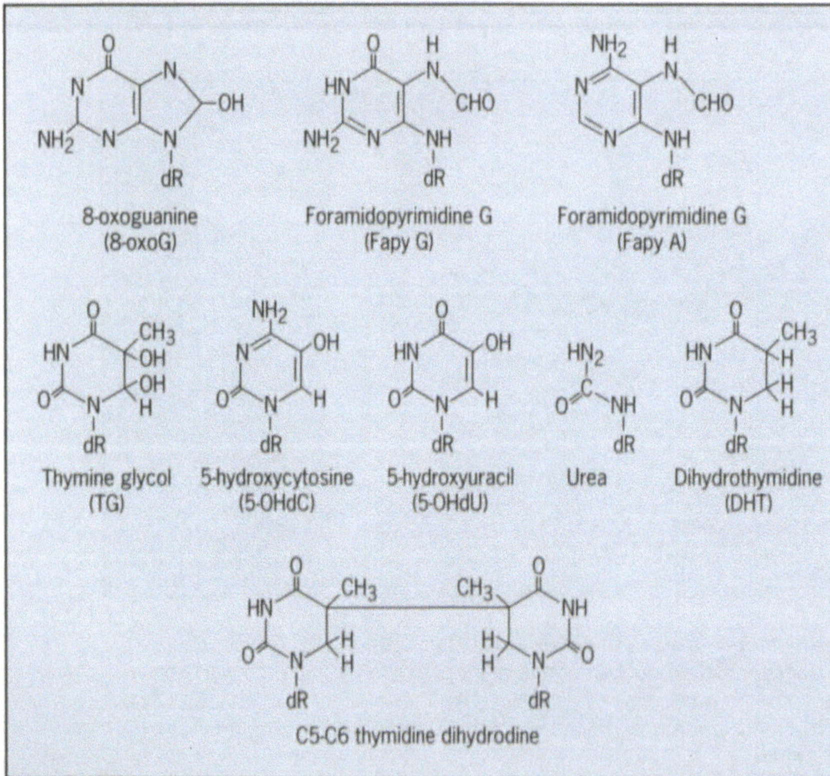

Figure 7-15. Oxidative DNA base modifications. Numerous DNA lesions formed following oxidative damage to DNA. Shown are some of the more significant modifications for cytotoxicity, mutagenicity, or makers of oxidative DNA damage (*eg*, 8-oxoguanine).

lesion is to excise the adenine residue that becomes misincorporated opposite 8-oxoG (Fig. 7-16). The human MYH DNA repair enzyme removes the adenine residues and subsequent removal of the 8-oxoG occurs via the OGG1 pathway [65] (Fig. 7-16).

Along with 8-oxoG being present in oxidatively damaged DNA, 8-oxo-deoxyguanosine (8-oxo-dGTP) is formed in the nucleotide pool during normal cellular metabolism and following oxidative stress [66]. The 8-oxo-dGTP nucleotide can be incorporated in DNA dur-

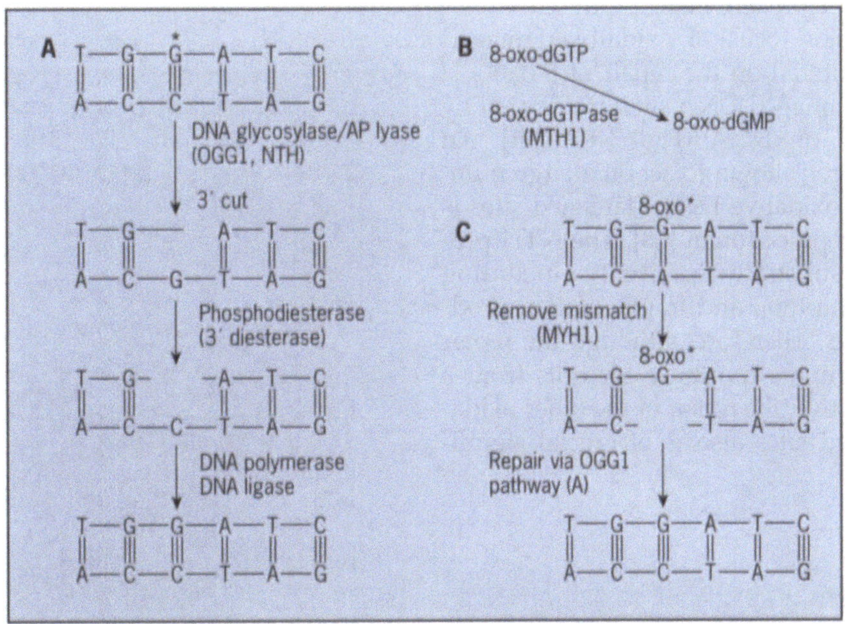

Figure 7-16. Pathways involved in the repair or removal of 8-oxoguanine (8-oxoG). **A**, In the first pathway, OGG1 removes 8-oxoG or formamdiopyrimidine (Fapy) lesions through a combined glycosylase–apurinic/apyrimidinic (AP) lyase activity, followed by the polishing of DNA ends with a phosphodiesterase, insertion of the normal base (guanine) by DNA polymeraseβ, and ligation with DNA ligase I. For other oxidative damaged bases, the NTH glycosylase/AP lyase enzyme performs the initial step. **B**, Another scheme involves MTH1, which prevents the incorporation of 8-oxoG into DNA or RNA by DNA or RNA polymerase, respectively. MTH1 converts 8-oxo-dGTP, formed in the nucleotide pool by oxidative stress, to 8-oxo-dGMP, which is not used by DNA or RNA polymerase [20,104,105]. **C**, Another way to correct 8-oxoG found in DNA involves the MYH1 enzyme, which recognizes the 8-oxoG:A mismatch that occurs following DNA replication and removes the A opposite the 8-oxoG, replacing it with the correct cytosine. The 8-oxoG altered base still remains in the DNA and must be removed by OGG1 (**A**) to prevent a continuous cycle.

Table 7-6. Oxidative repair genes

Human gene*	Cellular location	Oxidative DNA adducts recognized
OGG1 (mutM)	Nucleus	8-oxoG, FapyG, FapyA
MTH (mutT)	Cytoplasm	8-oxo-dGTPase
MYH (mutY)	Nucleus	8-oxoG:A mismatches
NTH (endonuclease III)	Nucleus	Thymine glycol, 5-OH DHT, 6-OH DHT, DHT, uracil glycol, 5-OHdC, 5-OHdU, β-ureidoisobutyric acid, urea, AP sites

**Escherichia coli homologue.*

5-OHdC—5-hydroxycytosine; 5-OHdU—5-hydroxyuracil; 8-oxoG—C-8 oxidation of guanine; AP—apurinic/apyrimidinic; DHT—dihydrothymine; FapyA— formamdiopyrimidine A; FapyG— formamdiopyrimidine G.

ing polymerization and can result in a mispairing unless repaired. MTH converts 8-oxo-dGTP in the nucleotide pool to the monophosphate and prevents the misincorporation of 8-oxo-dGTP into DNA (Fig. 7-16). Recently, it has been shown that MTH also recognizes 8-oxo-rGTP [67], which could become incorporated into RNA during gene transcription, leading to missense or nonsense proteins being produced.

Although a major focus of oxidative-damaged DNA has been centered on the repair of 8-oxoG, a number of other damaged DNA sites are created by free-radical attack on DNA (Fig. 7-15) [34]. An enzyme that has been shown to act on a large number of these other oxidative DNA–damaged sites is the human NTH repair protein [68]. The NTH protein has broad substrate specificity, including numerous ring saturation and fragmentation products of pyrimidines. Therefore, although the repair of 8-oxoG is of prime importance for cells from a mutagenic perspective, the repair of the other oxidative DNA damaged sites also is of crucial significance (Table 7-6).

MISMATCH REPAIR

Mismatches can occur in DNA due to incorrect incorporation by DNA polymerases, damage to the nucleotide precursors in the cellular nucleotide pool, or damage to DNA. The MYH MMR protein that removes 8-oxoG:A mismatches following oxidative DNA damage is technically an MMR enzyme, but it functions in a manner different than that of the MMR system (discussed later). In the MMR system, the MYH protein acts as a glycosylase/AP lyase, removing the single mismatched base. The MMR system has been extensively studied in bacteria (the MutHLS system); until a few years ago, the human or mammalian homologues to the bacterial system were unknown. However, a number of events enabled the cloning, initial characterization, and vigorous research into mammalian MMR. Broadly defined, mismatch repair is the recognition and correction of incorrectly paired nucleotides in DNA that results in a large fragment of DNA from the mismatched strand being excised and a new DNA strand being synthesized (Fig. 7-17).

Genetic instability of simple repeat (microsatellite) sequences in somatic and hereditary colorectal cancer led to the discovery that the mismatch DNA repair system was defective in hereditary nonpolyposis colon cancer (HNPCC). Currently, there are six homologues of the *E. coli mutS* gene, termed *MSH* genes in humans (Fig. 7-17) [69,70]. MSH2, MSH3, and MSH6 are found in the nucleus, MSH1 is located in the mitochondria, and MSH4 and MSH5 are part of the recombination system. The human MSH2 protein forms a complex with MSH6 and MSH3. When paired with MSH6, the heterodimer is termed MutSalpha and repairs base-to-base and insertion/deletion mismatches. MSH2 and MSH3 form a complex called MutSbeta, which binds to insertion/deletion mispairings. MSH2

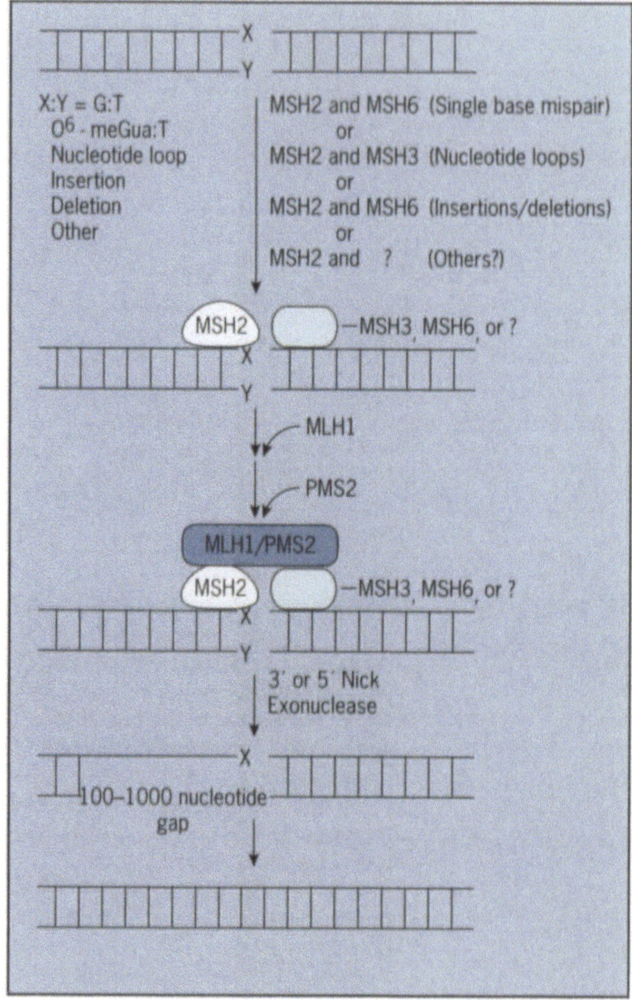

Figure 7-17. Mismatch repair pathway in mammalian cells. The initial step involves the binding of the MSH2 protein with MSH6 as a complex, in the case of single base mispairs such as G:T or O-6-methylguanine (O^6-MeGua):T, with MSH3 for nucleotide loops, insertions, or deletions, and with other proteins that have not yet been fully characterized [84,85]. Following the binding of MSH2 and MSH6 complex, for example, MLH1 and PMS2 bind to each other and the MSH2/MSH6 complex. The complex produces a 3′ or 5′ nick followed by exonuclease activity, resulting in a 100- to 1000-nucleotide gap in the strand with the incorrectly paired base. The gap is filled in, and the DNA is returned to its correct form. This repair system is used following an error in DNA replication in which a mismatch is produced. It is still unknown in mammalian cells how the system differentiates between the parental and daughter strands of DNA to repair the mismatched base.

can bind to mismatches by itself, but the binding is an order of magnitude lower than when interacting with MSH3 or MSH6 [69,71]. There are at least 16 genes that code for homologues of the *E. coli mutL* gene, termed *MLH* or *PMS* in humans [71].

The MMR system is deficient in HNPCC, with mutations in four of the players in the MMR pathway; MSH2, MSH6, MLH1, and PMS2 [69,72–75]. This discovery led to the mutator hypothesis, which proposes that cells deficient in MMR accumulate somatic mutations in proto-oncogenes and tumor suppressor genes [76]. In other words, defective MMR leads to defective proofing of DNA following replication, resulting in an accumulation of mutations, which is a prerequisite for tumorigenesis. Further analysis has shown that in the majority of cases of HNPCC, sporadic tumors with microsatellite instability are mutated in MLH1 or MSH2, and only a few mutations are seen in MSH3, MSH6, PMS1, and PMS2 [77,78]. PMS1 and PMS2 are members of the MLH1 family. Therefore, more than 60% of sporadic tumors with microsatellite instablity are not defective in the known MMR family members. Recent analysis demonstrates that more than 90% of HNPCC cases have mutations in either MSH2 or MLH1 [69]. The MMR system also appears to have overlapping activities with the NER system, particularly the transcription-coupled repair (TCR) process. This process is discussed in the following section.

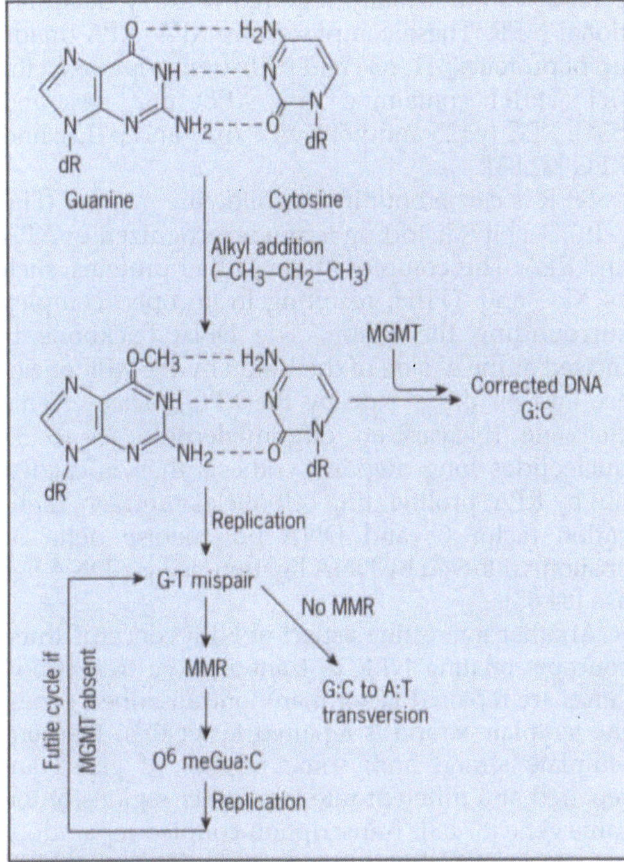

Figure 7-17. Mismatch repair pathway in mammalian cells. The initial step involves the binding of the MSH2 protein with MSH6 as a complex, in the case of single base mispairs such as G:T or O-6-methylguanine (O^6-MeGua):T, with MSH3 for nucleotide loops, insertions, or deletions, and with other proteins that have not yet been fully characterized [84,85]. Following the binding of MSH2 and MSH6 complex, for example, MLH1 and PMS2 bind to each other and the MSH2/MSH6 complex. The complex produces a 3′ or 5′ nick followed by exonuclease activity, resulting in a 100- to 1000-nucleotide gap in the strand with the incorrectly paired base. The gap is filled in, and the DNA is returned to its correct form. This repair system is used following an error in DNA replication in which a mismatch is produced. It is still unknown in mammalian cells how the system differentiates between the parental and daughter strands of DNA to repair the mismatched base.

Human cell lines with mutations in *MSH2*, *MSH6*, or *MLH1* are resistant to a number of alkylating agents. Furthermore, mutations in *MSH2* and *MLH1* are resistant to cisplatin [79]. Biochemical analysis demonstrated that the MSH2 protein can bind to DNA containing cisplatin and cis-ethylenediaminedichloroplatinum (II) but not to trans-diamminedichloroplatinum (II) or trans-diethylenetriamine-dichloroplatinum (II) DNA complexes [4,5]. MSH2 and MSH6 heterodimers also bind O^6-MeGua and O-4-methylthymine residues, whereas MSH2 binds thymine-thymine dimers [69]. These data imply a relation between MMR and NER repair. Finally, in cell lines, and more recently in mouse knockout models, it has been shown that cells deficient in MGMT and MMR are more resistant to alkylating agents than cells that are deficient in MGMT but have a competent MMR system [80]. This implies that cells that are MMR deficient cannot attempt to repair the mismatch that would occur following the replication of DNA with an O^6-MeGua lesion, allowing the cells to replicate (Fig. 7-18). However, the mutation rate would be elevated in these cells. Cells with a competent MMR system would attempt to repair the O-6-methylguanine-thymine lesion, but without MGMT present, they would become caught in a futile cycle, leading to chromosome alterations such as double-strand breaks, and cytotoxicity (Fig. 7-18).

Knockout mouse models for MSH2 have clearly shown the role of MMR in cancer susceptibility [81]. Homozygous MSH2-deficient mice are viable and fertile, but approximately 30% develop leukemia or lymphoma within the first 5 months of life and die of the disease by 1 year [82]. The majority of mice that live longer than 6 months also develop gastrointestinal and skin tumors [83]. Various cells from these homozygous MSH2 knockout mice demonstrate a lack of mispair binding and microsatellite instability [69].

NUCLEOTIDE EXCISION REPAIR

Nucleotide excision repair (NER) is a complex system that removes helix-distorting or bulky adducts from DNA, particularly UV-induced photoproducts acquired by cells on exposure to sunlight [84,85]. NER also plays a supporting or back-up role in the repair of O^6-MeGua and AP sites [22,84,86]. These lesions are removed from DNA in a 25- to 32-long nucleotide stretch by endonuclease cleavage on either side of the damaged region (Fig. 7-19) [22]. Recent biochemical reconstitution studies have elucidated the minimum number of elements of NER in mammalian cells. These include the following factors: XPA, XPC, XPG, XPF, RPA, and TFIIH [22,84,86]. XP stands for the disease xeroderma pigmentosum, of which there are seven complementation groups (XPA through XPG). However, in cell line studies, it appears that at least 14 proteins in six complexes are actually required to carry out functional NER. These complexes are XPA; RPA (made up of proteins p11, p34 and p70); transcription factor IIH (TFIIH; containing XPB, XPD, p62, p44, and p34); XPC (p125 and p58); XPF (p33 and p112); and XPG [22,84].

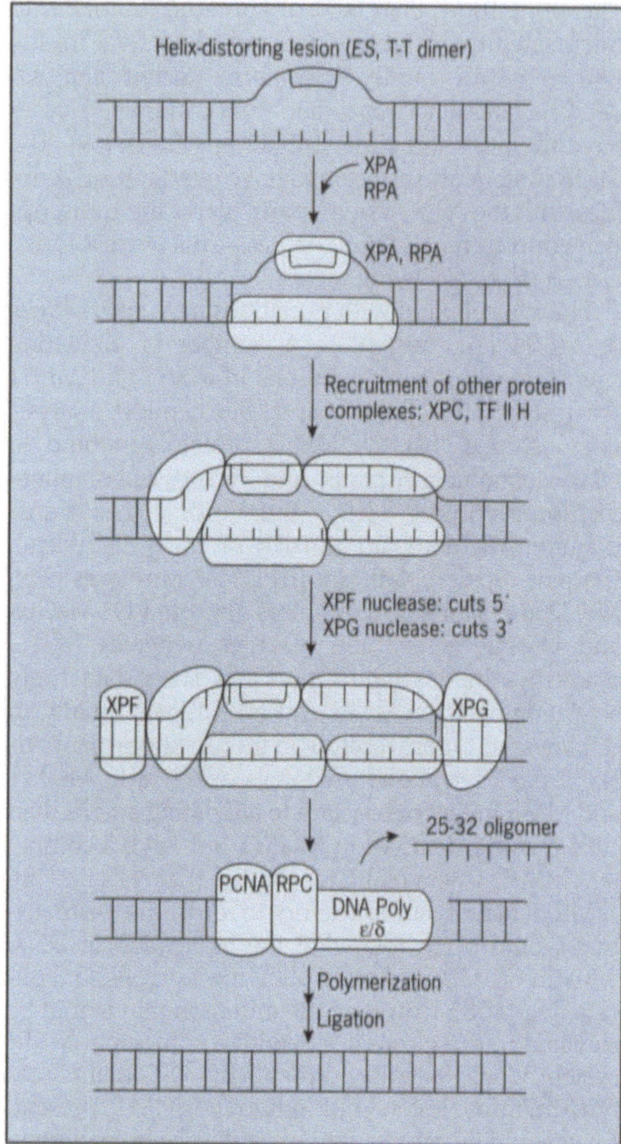

Figure 7-19. The nucleotide excision repair (NER) pathway in mammalian cells XPA and RPA (three-protein complex) recognize recognition of a helix-distorting lesion. This complex is recognized and attracts other proteins such as XPC (two-protein complex) and TFIIH (five-protein complex), resulting in an open structure surrounding the lesion. The DNA backbone is incised at the 5′ side of the lesion by the XPF nuclease (two-protein complex) and on the 3′ side by the XPG nuclease. This cleavage releases oligonucleotides 25 to 32 nucleotides in length. Repair synthesis is then carried out by RPA, proliferating cell nuclear antigen (PCNA), RPC, and DNA polymerase δ or ϵ, followed by DNA ligation using a DNA ligase [84,85].

NER is carried out in the following manner (Fig. 7-19). A helix-distorting lesion is recognized by XPA and RPA. This complex attracts other proteins, such as XPC and TFIIH, resulting in an open complex surrounding the lesion. The DNA backbone is incised at the 5′ side of the lesion by the XPF nuclease and on the 3′ side by the XPG nuclease. This cleavage releases an oligonucleotide 25 to 32 nucleotides long. Repair synthesis then is carried out by RPA, proliferating cell nuclear antigen, replication factor C, and DNA polymerase delta or epsilon, followed by DNA ligation using a DNA ligase [84,85].

Another interesting aspect of NER concerns three concepts relating NER to transcription: transcribed genes are repaired faster than nontranscribed genes; the template strand is repaired faster than the nontemplate strand and; some regions of genes are repaired at a different rate than other regions of the same gene [87,88]. Transcription-coupled repair does not require XPC, but does require five factors of NER and two additional factors: CSA and CSB. CSA and CSB are products of genes. Mutations in either of these two genes lead to Cockayne's syndrome, which has the phenotype of neuroskeletal abnormalities but does not have the predisposition to skin cancer induced by sunlight as does XP [85,89].

Xeroderma pigmentosum is a human disease that results in increased risk for sunlight-induced skin cancer and was initially shown to be due to a defect in UV-damaged DNA repair [89]. Further research demonstrated that the various complementation groups (XPA–XPG) of XP have defects in the NER pathway, and the cloning and characterization of these defects has led to the identification of the protein factors involved in NER (*eg*, XPA, complementation group A; XPC, complementation group C). As mentioned previously, patients with Cockayne's syndrome are also defective in NER, but their defect lies in the preferential repair of damage and not in global NER, producing a phenotype of progressive growth retardation, microcephaly, and leukodystrophy [89]. A third NER disease is trichothiodystrophy, which is distinguished by short stature, microcephaly, mental retardation, and sensitivity to sunlight [89]. Mutations in trichothiodystrophy have been found in XPD, part of the TFIIH transcription factor complex that functions as a helicase. XPD is involved in transcription and excision repair. Therefore, mutations in XPD can affect excision repair leading to XP or transcription leading to trichothiodystrophy [89]. All three of these diseases are autosomal recessive and rare.

GENE THERAPY AND DNA REPAIR

The use of multi-agent chemotherapy protocols has produced dramatic increases in the survival rates of patients with many cancers. In addition, dose intensification has been used increasingly in attempts to increase patient survival rates in both adult and pediatric cancers. DNA alkylating agents have been an important part of most dose-intensification protocols. Despite increased use of myeloid growth factor and stem cell support, myelosuppression continues to be a dose-limiting toxicity of many alkylating agents. This is particularly true in patients with relapsed disease who were treated with intensive chemotherapy during the induction and consolidation phases of initial therapies. An example of this is the severe bone marrow toxicity seen with the use of BCNU, which is commonly used to treat patients with brain tumors, lymphomas, and breast, lung, and gastrointestinal cancers [11,13]. The toxicity to bone marrow cells is most likely due to low levels of DNA repair activity that would otherwise help to protect cellular DNA from the damaging consequences of BCNU treatment [11,13]. One strategy to overcome this limited DNA repair capacity is to transduce bone marrow cells with specific genes that encode repair enzymes that act on the DNA lesions produced by BCNU or other alkylating agents. This recently has been accomplished with murine and human bone marrow cells by retroviral-mediated transduction of human *MGMT*, the protein product of which acts to repair BCNU-generated chloroethyl groups at the O-6 position of guanine [90,91].

The positive impact of increased-dose-intensity therapy on response rate and survival duration has been demonstrated in childhood Burkitt's lymphoma, metastatic breast cancer, neuroblastoma, testicular cancer, osteogenic sarcoma, Ewing's sarcoma [92], and most recently in childhood acute myelocytic leukemia [91]. However, despite the increasing use of growth factor support, myelosuppression is a major impediment to dose intensification in humans, and this is particularly true in patients with relapsed disease who were initially treated with intensive chemotherapy. One approach to circumvent the dose-limiting myeloid toxicities of chemotherapy agents has been the use of recombinant vectors to introduce and express various genes important in chemotherapy resistance in bone marrow–derived cells [91]. One area of research involves using DNA repair proteins in retroviral vectors as a mechanism to generate resistance to CENUs and other alkylating agents [90,91]. Retroviral-mediated gene transfer is an effective means of transduction of murine hematopoietic stem and progenitor cells [93]. This is important because the major limitation in gene transfer experiments has been inefficient transduction of reconstituting stem cells. However, studies with animal models have proved much more successful than initial studies with human progenitor cells [91,94,95]. Although therapeutic success has been slow in human gene therapy trials, the use of recombinant retroviral vectors has proven to be safe [96].

Along with DNA repair genes being transferred to bone marrow progenitor cells, a number of other genes have been or currently are being used to protect cells, particularly those of the bone marrow, from the damaging effects of chemotherapy [91,97]. These genes include those encoding protein products that can remove the drug from the cell (*eg*, multidrug resistance; P-glycoprotein), conjugate the drug to a cellular substrate rendering it inactive (glutathione-*S*-transferase [GST]), alter the drug's chemical structure by converting it to a less active form (aldehyde dehydrogenase), or act through other mechanisms such as superoxide dismutase and dihydrofolate reductase [91,97]. In all of these examples, the addition of these gene products via gene transfer results in significant drug resistance in hematopoietic progenitors both in vitro and in vivo.

The ability of MGMT to protect against CENU cytotoxicity, as discussed previously, led to one of the first uses of DNA repair genes in gene therapy . CENUs have been shown to be effective agents in the treatment of several human cancers, particularly brain tumors. Because the major determinant of CENU-induced cytotoxicity is the alkylation of guanine at the O-6 position followed by the formation of interstrand DNA cross-links by rearrangement to produce an ethyl bridge between N-1 of guanine and N-3 of cytosine in the opposite strand (Figs. 7-2 and 7-18) [11,13], the overexpression of MGMT affords protection against nitrosoureas. In most cases, the level of MGMT protein in mammalian cells correlates with CENU sensitivity [10,11,13]. The amount of MGMT protein expressed in human and murine bone marrow cells is considerably lower than that in other tissues and contributes to the inefficient repair of CENU-induced DNA damage in blood cells [90]. Therefore, the ability to increase the level of MGMT expression in bone marrow cells via retroviral-mediated gene transfer, is a good "proof of principle" starting point demonstrating the utility of DNA repair genes for gene therapy and cellular protection [91].

O-6-Methylguanine DNA Methyltransferase

Numerous laboratories have demonstrated that transduction of murine or human hematopoietic stem or progenitor cells via a retroviral vector encoding the human MGMT cDNA protects bone marrow cells from CENU-induced myelotoxicity [19,90,94,95,97]. In other studies, a model of CENU-induced fatal bone marrow suppression was developed and used to demonstrate that the reconstitution of murine bone marrow with hematopoietic stem cells expressing vector-derived human MGMT protected mice from BCNU-induced bone marrow hypoplasia and peripheral blood pancytopenia [90,94]. Bone marrow cells harvested from these mice were more resistant to BCNU in vitro and demonstrated a higher level of MGMT DNA repair activity compared with BCNU-treated mock-infected control mice [94]. Furthermore, a significant reduction in short-term CENU-related mortality in BCNU-treated mice transplanted with MGMT-expressing hematopoietic stem cells was found[94], and positive results on long-term survival, immunologic recovery, and drug-induced mortality were also demonstrated [95].

O-6 Benzylguanine Depletion of O-6-Methylguanine DNA Methyltransferase Coupled With O-6-Methylguanine DNA Methyltransferase Bone Marrow Protection

Many human tumors have demonstrated resistance to CENUs in vitro associated with persistent or increased expression of MGMT [13]. However, it has been shown that human MGMT can be depleted by a variety of compounds, including STZ and 6-BG (Fig. 7-3) [13]. These compounds act as substrates for the MGMT protein, which can remove only one alkyl group per molecule in a stoichiometric reaction. This allows for a "window of opportunity" in which one can follow the MGMT tumor depletion with a chemotherapeutic agent such as a CENU, before the tumor cell can replenish its MGMT protein level. This combination of tumor 6-BG depletion used in conjunction with bone marrow protection is currently under investigation. Furthermore, recent studies have shown that site-directed mutants of the MGMT protein can be created that are resistant to 6-BG while still being active on O^6-MeGua [18]. One of these MGMT mutant clones has been used in human $CD34^+$ cells [19]. These 6-BG resistant mutants will be of great use for bone marrow transduction in patients undergoing 6-BG treatment to sensitize tumors to nitrosoureas.

Base Excision Repair Gene Therapy

Because alkylating chemotherapeutic agents generate many types of DNA adducts in addition to O^6-MeGua and some of these adducts are cytotoxic (*eg*, N-3-adenine) or mutagenic, we have begun a series of experiments using the members of the BER pathway (*eg*, MPG, APE/REF-1, beta-polymerase, DNA ligase I) to protect cells from the cytotoxic and mutagenic effects of alkylating agents (Fig. 7-20). We also have begun to characterize the members of the BER pathway that can protect against oxidative DNA-damaging agents (*eg*, OGG1, NTH, MTH, MYH) [98], given that many chemotherapeutic agents have multiple actions in damaging DNA and that a number of cancer chemotherapeutic agents are oxidative DNA damage promoters via their free-radical production. For example, as discussed in the BER section, MMC is a free-radical producer that, in the presence of oxygen, produces H_2O_2 and hydroxyl radicals, leading to oxidative DNA damage [62],and the formation of oxygen free radicals is highly correlated with MMC-induced tumor cell killing. Other examples of such agents are cisplatin and VP-16, both of which exert a portion of their antitumor activity via hydroxyl radical production [62].

In addition to the use of human DNA repair genes, nonmammalian DNA repair genes have been used successfully for protection of cells against DNA-damaging agents (Fig. 7-20). For example, we and others [3] have shown that the *E. coli Fpg* gene can be used in expression systems in mammalian cells to protect against the chemotherapeutic alkylating agent thiotepa. Overexpression of *Fpg* protects cells from the cytotoxic effects of the replication-blocking lesions (the ring-opened guanines). This result recently has been confirmed using mouse 3T3 cells, and these cells were shown to be protected using the human *OGG1* gene as well [99]. Recently, the T4 DNA ligase gene has been shown to modulate bleomycin-induced DNA damage, decreasing chromosome irregularities and allowing increased cell survival in Chinese hamster ovary cells [100]. Along these same lines, the yeast AP endonuclease APN1 has been shown to protect mammalian cells against MMS, menadione (a redox cycling drug), and H_2O_2 (an oxidative DNA-damaging agent) when overexpressed. The *E. coli* homologue of *Apn1*, endonuclease IV, has been shown to have much higher affinity for 4′-oxidized AP sites in DNA that can be created by bleomycin [7,101]. Overexpression of *Apn1* in mammalian cells has been shown to protect against H_2O_2 and MMS [102]. These findings have been tested further, using the yeast *Apn1* gene overexpressed in mouse 3T3 and human HeLa cells and it was found that the yeast APN1 protein does protect against the cytotoxic effects of bleomycin. Current research in this area involves following up these findings and testing the protective ability of APN1 against various chemotherapeutic drugs, such as bleomycin, alkylating agents, redox cycling drugs, and ionizing radiation in primary bone marrow cells and transgenic mouse models. The use of DNA repair genes, both mammalian and nonmammalian, in retroviral-mediated gene therapy has the potential to protect against a large number of clinically relevant chemotherapeutic agents.

DNA Repair Fusion Proteins

Because alkylating agents are known to generate many different types of DNA modifications, we hypothesized that added protection to nontarget tissues could be achieved by linking various DNA repair proteins together in a fusion protein construct expressed in a single retrovirus. In principle, a variety of DNA repair enzymes can be fused to form proteins that recognize a broad spectrum of DNA lesions. As a model of this general approach, human APE/REF-1 was linked to MGMT, thereby providing not only for the repair of O-6 modifications of guanine but also for an activity directed toward baseless sites and modified 3′ termini in DNA (Fig. 7-20) [103]. All of these lesions are a consequence of chloroethyl-nitrosourea (CNU)–generated DNA damage. In vitro analysis of repair function and protection studies in cell lines using this construct have shown that both the MGMT and APE/REF-1 domains are fully functional in a fused format and can protect cells from BCNU and simple alkylating agents such as MMS [103]. The data generated provide evidence that combined domains of DNA BER enzymes can be used to generate multi-active, highly efficient DNA repair proteins for gene therapy.

CONCLUSIONS

With the rapid and recent cloning of a number of DNA repair genes in humans and the linking of DNA

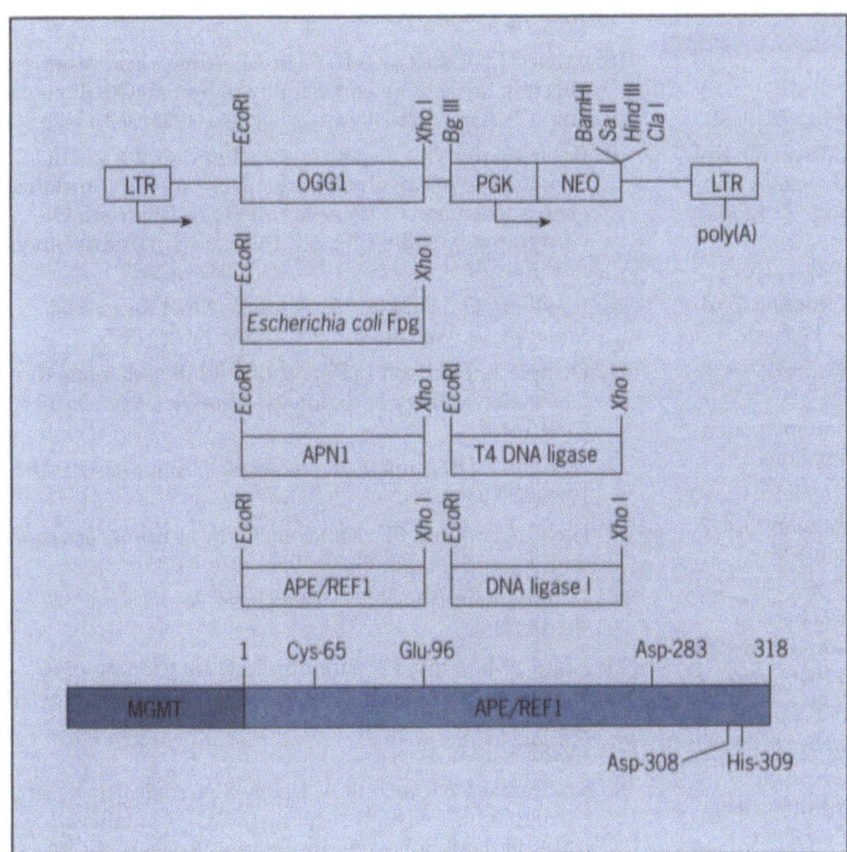

Figure 7-20. Retroviral DNA repair constructs used in the protection of cells from chemotherapy by gene therapy. A number of DNA repair proteins, when overexpressed in mammalian cells, have been shown to protect cells against various laboratory and chemotherapeutic agents as well as from ionizing radiation. Genes that have been used and are currently being considered for gene therapy include mammalian DNA repair genes as well as those from *Escherichia coli* (*Fpg*), bacteriophage (T4 DNA ligase), and yeast (*APN1*). As additional DNA base excision repair (BER) genes are cloned and characterized, they will be incorporated into this analysis. Of particular interest is the area of oxidative DNA damage and repair, because almost half of anticancer chemotherapeutic agents currently approved for use in the United States can form reactive oxygen species and cause oxidative DNA damage [56,104]. This type of DNA damage has been implicated in aging, Alzheimer's disease, Parkinson's disease, and amyotrophic lateral sclerosis (ALS) [60,61,105].

repair genes (such as those involved in MMR) to human cancers, such as HNPCC, interest in this field has increased rapidly and demonstrates the increased need for basic research into the regulation and role that the various DNA repair genes and their associated pathways play in preventing mutations and carcinogenesis. The renewed interest in the area of DNA repair will enable these findings to be assimilated rapidly into translational paradigms, allowing these findings to be used in clinical settings for cell protection, such as with gene therapy of bone marrow cells, or in modulating the expression of these genes to sensitize cells to chemotherapy and radiation therapy. With this increased interest in the relation between DNA repair genes and cancer, the near future should be filled with many exciting and useful findings.

ACKNOWLEDGMENTS

Drs. Kelley and Erickson are supported by National Institutes of Health (NIH)/National Cancer Institute (NCI) Program Project Grant PO1-CA75426. Dr. Kelley also is supported by NIH grants RR09884 and ES07815. Dr. Erickson also is supported by NIH grant CA45628.

REFERENCES

1. Lawley PD, Phillips DH: DNA adducts from chemotherapeutic agents. *Mutat Res* 1996, 355:13–40.
2. Barzilay G, Walker LJ, Rothwell DG, Hickson ID: Role of the HAP1 protein in repair of oxidative DNA damage and regulation of transcription factors. *Br J Cancer* 1996, 74:S145–S150.
3. Gill RD, Cussac C, Souhami RL, Laval F: Increased resistance to N,N',Ndouble'-triethylenethiophosphoramide (thiotepa) in cells expressing the *Escherichia coli* formamidopyrimidine-DNA glycosylase. *Cancer Res* 1996, 56:3721–3724.
4. Gradia S, Acharya S, Fishel R: The human mismatch recognition complex hMSH2-hMSH6 functions as a novel molecular switch. *Cell* 1997, 91:995–1005.
5. Fishel R, Ewel A, Lescoe MK: Purified human MSH2 protein binds to DNA containing mismatched nucleotides. *Cancer Res* 1994, 54:5539–5542.
6. Povirk LF: DNA damage and mutagenesis by radiomimetic DNA-cleaving agents: bleomycin, neocarzinostatin and other enediynes. *Mutat Res* 1996, 355:71–89.
7. Haring M, Rudiger H, Demple B, *et al.*: Recognition of oxidized abasic sites by repair endonucleases. *Nucleic Acids Res* 1995, 22:2010–2015.
8. Olson RD, Mushlin PS: Doxorubicin cardiotoxicity: analysis of prevailing hypotheses. *FASEB J* 1990, 4:3076–3086.
9. Price A: The repair of ionizing radiation-induced damage to DNA [review]. *Semin Cancer Biol* 1993, 4:61–71.
10. Pieper RO: Understanding and manipulating O6-methylguanine-DNA methyltransferase expression. *Pharmacol Ther* 1997, 74:285–297.
11. Erickson LC: The role of O-6 methylguanine DNA methyltransferase (MGMT) in drug resistance and strategies for its inhibition. *Semin Cancer Biol* 1991, 2:257–265.
12. Karran P: Possible depletion of a DNA repair enzyme in human lymphoma cells by subversive repair. *Proc Natl Acad Sci USA* 1985, 82:5285–5289.
13. Pegg AE: Mammalian O6-alkylguanine-DNA alkyltransferase: regulation and importance in response to alkylating carcinogenic and therapeutic agents. *Cancer Res* 1990, 50:6119–6129.
14. Dolan ME, Young GS, Pegg AE: Effect of O6-alkylguanine pretreatment on the sensitivity of human colon tumor cells to the cytotoxic effects of chloroethylating agents. *Cancer Res* 1986, 46:4500–4504.
15. Dolan ME, Moschel RC, Pegg AE: Depletion of mammalian O6-alkylguanine-DNA alkyltransferase activity by O6-benzylguanine provides a means to evaluate the role of this protein in protection against carcinogenic and therapeutic alkylating agents. *Proc Natl Acad Sci USA* 1990, 87:5368–5372.
16. Crone TM, Pegg AE: A single amino acid change in human O6-alkylguanine-DNA alkyltransferase decreasing sensitivity to inactivation by O6-benzylguanine. *Cancer Res* 1993, 53:4750–4753.
17. Crone TM, Goodtzova K, Edara S, Pegg AE: Mutations in human O6-alkylguanine-DNA alkyltransferase imparting resistance to O6-benzylguanine. *Cancer Res* 1994, 54:6221–6227.
18. Crone TM, Goodtzova K, Pegg AE: Amino acid residues affecting the activity and stability of human O6-alkylguanine-DNA alkyltransferase. *Mutat Res* 1996, 363:15–25.
19. Reese JS, Koc ON, Lee KM, *et al.*: Retroviral transduction of a mutant methylguanine DNA methyltransferase gene into human CD34 cells confers resistance to O6-benzylguanine plus 1,3-bis(2-chloroethyl)-1-nitrosourea. *Proc Natl Acad Sci USA* 1996, 93:14088–14093.
20. Friedberg EC, Walker GC, Siede W: *DNA Repair and Mutagenesis*. Washington, DC: ASM Press; 1995.
21. Demple B, Harrison L: Repair of oxidative damage to DNA: enzymology and biology. *Annu Rev Biochem* 1994, 63:915–948.
22. Wood RD: DNA repair in eukaryotes. *Annu Rev Biochem* 1996, 65:135–167.
23. Loeb LA, Preston BD: Mutagenesis by apurinic/apyrimidinic sites. *Annu Rev Genet* 1986, 20:201–230.
24. Cunningham RP: DNA glycosylases. *Mutat Res* 1997, 383:189–196.
25. Arai K, Morishita K, Shinmura K, *et al.*: Cloning of a human homolog of the yeast Ogg1 gene that is involved in the repair of oxidative DNA damage. *Oncogene* 1997, 14:2857–2861.
26. Sandigursky M, Yacoub A, Kelley MR, *et al.*: The yeast 8-oxoguanine DNA glycosylase (OGG1) contains a DNA deoxyribophosphodiesterase (dRpase) activity. *Nucleic Acids Res* 1997, 25:4557–4561.

27. Doetsch P, Cunningham R: The enzymology of apurinic/apyrimidinic endonucleases. *Mutat Res* 1990, 23:173–201.
28. Mitra S, Kaina B: Regulation of repair of alkylation damage in mammalian genomes [review]. *Prog Nucleic Acid Res Mol Biol* 1993, 44:109–142.
29. Mitra S, Hazra TK, Roy R, *et al.*: Complexities of DNA base excision repair in mammalian cells. *Mol Cells* 1997, 7:305–312.
30. Ramana CV, Boldogh I, Izumi T, Mitra S: Activation of apurinic/apyrimidinic endonuclease in human cells by reactive oxygen species and its correlation with their adaptive response to genotoxicity of free radicals. *Proc Nat Acad Sci USA* 1998, 95:5061–5066.
31. Krokan HE, Standal R, Slupphaug G: DNA glycosylases in the base excision repair of DNA. *Biochem J* 1997, 325:1–16.
32. Wilson DM III, Thompson LH: Life without DNA repair. *Proc Natl Acad Sci USA* 1997, 94:12754–12757 .
33. Engelward BP, Dreslin A, Christensen J, *et al.*: Repair-deficient 3-methyladenine DNA glycosylase homozygous mutant mouse cells have increased sensitivity to alkylation-induced chromosome damage and cell killing. *EMBO J* 1996, 15:945–952.
34. Wallace SS: DNA damages processed by base excision repair: biological consequences. *Int J Radiat Biol* 1994, 66:579–589.
35. Wallace SS: Recognition and processing of oxidative DNA lesions. *Biochem Cell Biol* 1997, 75:477–478.
36. Neddermann P, Gallinari P, Lettieri T, *et al.*: Cloning and expression of human G/T mismatch-specific thymine-DNA glycosylase. *J Biol Chem* 1996, 271:12767–12774.
37. Sobol RW, Horton JK, Kuhn R, *et al.*: Requirement of mammalian DNA polymerase beta in base-excision repair. *Nature* 1996, 379:183–186.
38. Ramotar D: The apurinic-apyrimidinic endonuclease IV family of DNA repair enzymes. *Biochem Cell Biol* 1997, 75:327–336.
39. Suh D, Wilson DM, Povirk LF: 3'-Phosphodiesterase activity of human apurinic/apyrimidinic endonuclease at DNA double-strand break ends. *Nucl Acids Res* 1997, 25:2495–2500.
40. Demple B, Herman T, Chen DS: Cloning and expression of APE, the cDNA encoding the major human apurinic endonuclease: definition of a family of DNA repair enzymes. *Proc Natl Acad Sci USA* 1991, 88:11450–11454.
41. Xanthoudakis S, Curran T: Identification and characterization of Ref-1, a nuclear protein that facilitates AP-1 DNA-binding activity. *EMBO J* 1992, 11:653–665.
42. Yao KS, Xanthoudakis S, Curran T, *et al.*: Activation of AP-1 and of a nuclear redox factor, Ref-1, in the response of HT29 colon cancer cells to hypoxia. *Mol Cell Biol* 1994, 14:5997–6003.
43. Huang LE, Arany Z, Livingston DM, *et al.*: Activation of hypoxia-inducible transcription factor depends primarily upon redox-sensitive stabilization of its alpha subunit. *J Biol Chem* 1996, 271:32253–32259.
44. Walker LJ, Robson CN, Black E, *et al.*: Identification of residues in the human DNA repair enzyme HAP1 (Ref-1) that are essential for redox regulation of Jun DNA binding. *Mol Cell Biol* 1993, 13:5370–5376.
45. Okuno H, Akahori A, Sato H, *et al.*: Escape from redox regulation enhances the transforming activity of Fos. *Oncogene* 1993, 8:695–701.
46. Jayaraman L, Murthy KGK, Zhu C, *et al.*: Identification of redox/repair protein Ref-1 as a potent activator of p53. *Genes Dev* 1997, 11:558–570.
47. Melra LB, Cheo DL, Hammer RE, *et al.*: Genetic interaction between HAP1/REF-1 and p53 [letter]. *Nat Genet* 1997, 17:145.
48. Robertson KA, Hill DP, Xu Y, *et al.*: Downregulation of AP endonuclease expression is associated with the induction of apoptosis in differentiating myeloid leukemia cells. *Cell Growth Differ* 1997, 8:443–449.
49. Yacoub A, Kelley MR, Deutsch WA: The DNA repair activity of human redox/repair protein APE/REF-1 is inactivated by phosphorylation. *Cancer Res* 1997, 57:5457–5459.
50. Hirota K, Matsui M, Yodoi J: AP-1 transcriptional activity is regulated by a direct association between thioredoxin and Ref-1. *Proc Natl Acad Sci USA* 1997, 94:3633–3638.
51. Kelley MR, Xu Y, Tritt R, Robertson KA: The multifunctional DNA base excision repair and redox protein, AP endonuclease (APE/REF-1), and its role in germ cell tumors. In *Germ Cell Tumors,* vol 4. Edited by Jones I, Harnden P, Joffe JK. London: John Libbey & Co.; 1998: 81–86.
52. Xu Y, Moore DH, Broshears J, *et al.*: The apurinic/apyrimidinic endonuclease (APE/REF-1) DNA repair enzyme is elevated in premalignant and malignant cervical cancer. *Anticancer Res* 1997, 17:3713–3719.
53. Ono Y, Furuta T, Ohmoto T, *et al.*: Stable expression in rat glioma cells of sense and antisense nucleic acids to a human multifunctional DNA repair enzyme, APEX nuclease, *Mutat Res* 1994, 315:55–63.
54. Jaruga P, Dizdaroglu M: Repair of products of oxidative DNA base damage in human cells. *Nucleic Acids Res* 1996, 24:1389–1394.
55. Frenkel K: Carcinogen-mediated oxidant formation and oxidative DNA damage. *Pharmacol Ther* 1992, 53:127–166.
56. Southorn PA: Free radicals in medicine. II. Involvement in human disease. *Mayo Clin Proc* 1988, 63:390–408.
57. Shimoda R, Nagashima M, Sakamoto M, *et al.*: Increased formation of oxidative DNA damage, 8-hydroxydeoxyguanosine, in human livers with chronic hepatitis. *Cancer Res* 1994, 54:3171–3172.
58. Oda T, Tsuda H, Scarpa A, Sakamoto M: p53 gene mutation spectrum in hepatocellular carcinoma. *Cancer Res* 1992, 52:6358–6364.
59. Yamamoto F, Kasai H, Togashi Y, *et al.*: Elevated level of 8-hydroxydeoxyguanosine in DNA of liver, kidneys and brain of Long-Evans cinnamon rats. *Jpn J Cancer Res* 1993, 84:508–511.

60. Alam ZI, Daniel SE, Lees AJ, *et al.*: A generalised increase in protein carbonyls in the brain in Parkinson's but not incidental Lewy body disease. *J Neurochem* 1997, 69:1326–1329.
61. Levay G, Ye Q, Bodell WJ: Formation of DNA adducts and oxidative base damage by copper mediated oxidation of dopamine and 6-hydroxydopamine. *Exp Neurol* 1997, 146:570–574.
62. Clarke AA, Philpott NJ, Gordon-Smith EC, Rutherford TR: The sensitivity of Fanconi anaemia group C cells to apoptosis induced by mitomycin C is due to oxygen radical generation, not DNA crosslinking. *Br J Haematol* 1997, 96:240–247.
63. Tajiri T, Maki H, Sekiguchi M: Functional cooperation of MutT, MutM and MutY proteins in preventing mutations caused by spontaneous oxidation of guanine nucleotide in *Escherichia coli*. *Mutat Res* 1995, 336:257–267.
64. Shinmura K, Kasai H, Sasaki A, *et al.*: 8-Hydroxyguanine (7,8-dihydro-8-oxoguanine) DNA glycosylase and AP lyase activities of hOGG1 protein and their substrate specificity. *Mutat Res DNA Repair* 1997, 385:75–82.
65. Slupska MM, Baikalov C, Luther WM, *et al.*: Cloning and sequencing a human homolog (hMYH) of the *Escherichia coli* mutY gene whose function is required for the repair of oxidative DNA damage. *J Bacteriol* 1996, 178:3885–3892.
66. Sakumi K, Furuichi M, Tsuzuki T, *et al.*: Cloning and expression of cDNA for a human enzyme that hydrolyzes 8-oxo-dGTP, a mutagenic substrate for DNA synthesis. *J Biol Chem* 1993, 268:23524–23530.
67. Taddei F, Hayakawa H, Bouton M, *et al.*: Counteraction by MutT protein of transcriptional errors caused by oxidative damage. *Science* 1997, 278:128–130.
68. Aspinwall R, Rothwell DG, Roldan-Arjona T, *et al.*: Cloning and characterization of a functional human homolog of *Escherichia coli* endonuclease III. *Proc Natl Acad Sci USA* 1997, 94:109–114.
69. Fishel R, Wilson T: MutS homologs in mammalian cells. *Curr Opin Genet Dev* 1997, 7:105–113.
70. Fishel R, Lescoe MK, Rao MRS, *et al.*: The human mutator gene homolog MSH2 and its association with hereditary nonpolyposis colon cancer. *Cell* 1993, 75:1027–1038.
71. Peltomaki P: DNA mismatch repair gene mutations in human cancer. *Environ Health Perspect* 1997, 105:775–780.
72. Fishel R, Kolodner RD: Identification of mismatch repair genes and their role in the development of cancer. *Curr Opin Genet Dev* 1995, 5:382–395.
73. Kolodner RD: Mismatch repair: mechanisms and relationship to cancer susceptibility. *Trends Biochem Sci* 1995, 20:397–401.
74. Prolla TA, Pang Q, Alani E, *et al.*: MLH1, PMS1, and MSH2 interactions during the initiation of DNA mismatch repair in yeast. *Science* 1994, 265:1091–1093.
75. Kolodner RD, Hall NR, Lipford J, *et al.*: Human mismatch repair genes and their association with hereditary non-polyposis colon cancer. *Cold Spring Harb Symp Quant Biol* 1994, 59:331–338.
76. Vogelstein B, Kinzler KW: The multistep nature of cancer [review]. *Trends Genet* 1993, 9:138–141.
77. Nicolaides NC, Papadopoulos N, Liu B, *et al.*: Mutations of two PMS homologues in hereditary nonpolyposis colon cancer. *Nature* 1994, 371:75–80.
78. Papadopoulos N, Nicolaides N, Wei Y, *et al.*: Mutation of a mutL homolog in hereditary colon cancer. *Science* 1994, 263:1625–1629.
79. Aebi S, Kurdi-Haidar B, Gordon R, *et al.*: Loss of DNA mismatch repair in acquired resistance to cisplatin. *Cancer Res* 1996, 56:3087–3090.
80. Kawate H, Sakumi K, Tsuzuki T, *et al.*: Separation of killing and tumorigenic effects of an alkylating agent in mice defective in two of the DNA repair genes. *Proc Nat Acad Sci USA* 1998, 95:5116–5120.
81. de Wind N, Dekker M, Berns A, *et al.*: Inactivation of the mouse Msh2 gene results in mismatch repair deficiency, methylation tolerance, hyperrecombination, and predisposition to cancer. *Cell* 1995, 82:321–330.
82. Reitmair AH, Schmits R, Ewel A, *et al.*: MSH2 deficient mice are viable and susceptible to lymphoid tumours. *Nat Genet* 1995, 11:64–70.
83. Reitmair AH, Redston M, Cai JC, *et al.*: Spontaneous intestinal carcinomas and skin neoplasms in Msh2-deficient mice. *Cancer Res* 1996, 56:3842–3849.
84. Lindahl T, Karran P, Wood RD: DNA excision repair pathways. *Curr Opin Genet Dev* 1997, 7:158–169.
85. Chaney SG, Sancar A: DNA repair: enzymatic mechanisms and relevance to drug response. *J Natl Cancer Inst* 1996, 88:1346–1360.
86. Wood RD: Nucleotide excision repair in mammalian cells. *J Biol Chem* 1997, 272:23465–23468.
87. Hanawalt PC: Transcription-coupled repair and human disease. *Science* 1994, 266:1957–1958.
88. Hanawalt PC, Donahue BA, Sweder KS: Repair and transcription. Collision or collusion? *Curr Biol* 1994, 4:518–521.
89. Woods GC: DNA repair disorders. *Arch Dis Child* 1998, 78:178–184.
90. Moritz T, Mackay W, Glassner BJ, *et al.*: Retrovirus-mediated expression of a DNA repair protein in bone marrow protects hematopoietic cells from nitrosourea-induced toxicity in vitro and in vivo. *Cancer Res* 1995, 55:2608–2614.
91. Moritz T, Williams DA: *Transfer of Drug Resistance Genes to Hematopoietic Precursors. Encyclopedia of Cancer,* vol 3. New York: Academic Press; 1997:1765–1776.
92. Antman K, Ayash L, Elias A III, *et al.*: High-dose cyclophosphamide, thiotepa, and carboplatin with autologous marrow support in women with measurable advanced breast cancer responding to standard-dose therapy: analysis by age. *J Natl Cancer Institute Monogr* 1994, 16:91–94.
93. Williams DA, Lemischka IR, Nathan DG, Mulligan RC: Introduction of new genetic material into pluripotent haematopoietic stem cells of the mouse. *Nature* 1984, 310:476–480.

94. Maze R, Carney JP, Kelley MR, *et al.*: Increasing DNA repair methyltransferase levels via bone marrow stem cell transduction rescues mice from the toxic effects of 1,3-bis(2-chloroethyl)-1-nitrosourea, a chemotherapeutic alkylating agent. *Proc Natl Acad Sci USA* 1996, 93:206–210.

95. Maze R, Kapur R, Kelley MR, *et al.*: Reversal of 1,3-bis(2-chloroethyl)-1-nitrosourea-induced severe immunodeficiency by transduction of murine long-lived hemopoietic progenitor cells using O6-methylguanine DNA methyltransferase complementary DNA. *J Immunol* 1997, 158:1006–1013.

96. Cornetta K, Tricot G, Broun ER, *et al.*: Retroviral-mediated gene transfer of bone marrow cells during autologous bone marrow transplantation for acute leukemia. *Hum Gene Ther* 1992, 3:305–318.

97. Koc ON, Allay JA, Lee K, *et al.*: Transfer of drug resistance genes into hematopoietic progenitors to improve chemotherapy tolerance *Semin Oncol* 1996, 23:46–65.

98. Kelley Hansen WK, *et al.*: Use of DNA base excision repair (BER) genes in gene therapy; translational applications. 30th Annual Meeting of the Environmental Mutagen Society; Washington, D.C., 1999.

99. Xu Y, Hansen WK, Clapp W, *et al.*: Retroviral mediated protection against chemotherapeutic agents using the DNA base excision repair genes fpg and OGG1. American Association of Cancer Research 89th Annual Meeting; New Orleans, 1998.

100. Ortiz T, Flores MJ, Pinero J, *et al.*: T4 DNA ligase reduces chromosome damage and enhances cell survival in CHO cells treated with bleomycin. *Cytogenet Cell Genet* 1997, 78:197–201.

101. Takeuchi M, Lillis R, Demple B, Takeshita M: Interactions of *Escherichia coli* endonuclease IV and exonuclease III with abasic sites in DNA. *J Biol Chem* 1994, 269:21907–21914.

102. Tomicic M, Eschbach E, Kaina B: Expression of yeast but not human apurinic/apyrimidinic endonuclease renders Chinese hamster cells more resistant to DNA damaging agents. *Mutat Res* 1997, 383:155–165.

103. Hansen WK, Deutsch WA, Yacoub A, *et al.*: Creation of a fully-functional human chimeric DNA repair protein: combining O6-methylguanine DNA methyltransferase (MGMT) and AP endonuclease (APE/REF-1) DNA repair proteins. *J Biol Chem* 1998, 273:756–762.

104. Sinha BK: Free radicals in anticancer drug pharmacology. *Chem Biol Interact* 1989, 69:293–317.

105. Alam ZI, Jenner A, Daniel SE, *et al.*: Oxidative DNA damage in the parkinsonian brain: an apparent selective increase in 8-hydroxyguanine levels in substantia nigra. *J Neurochem* 1997, 69:1196–1203.

CHAPTER

8

Carcinogenesis

James Norris
Deanne King

THE MULTISTEP PROCESS OF CARCINOGENESIS

Carcinogenesis describes the process that transforms a normal cell into a malignant cell. Knudsen studied the inheritance of retinoblastoma and theorized that carcinogenesis is a multistep process [1]. He proposed the idea that two mutations are necessary for the development of retinoblastoma. Some individuals have an inherited predisposition to retinoblastoma, resulting in bilateral presentation at an early age. In this multifocal form, only one exogenous mutation is required, because the first mutation is inherited (Fig. 8-1*A*). In the sporadic form, the disease is unifocal and characterized by later onset (Fig. 8-1*B*). In this case, "two hits" must occur in the same cell—a much rarer event.

Table 8-1 provides definitions of terms relevant to carcinogenesis. The process of carcinogenesis can be divided into three stages: initiation, promotion, and progression (Fig. 8-2). Each stage of carcinogenesis has unique properties (Table 8-2). The initial insult of the initiator is genotoxic, causing a mutation in the DNA, often by formation of an adduct. The mutation becomes irreversible once cell division occurs and often remains in a latent phase until the cell is stimulated to divide. This proliferative stimulus, provided by the promoter, leads to epigenetic changes that induce proliferation and are often reversible; however, some effects may be irreversible, such as mutations caused by free radicals formed during metabolic stress. A promoter alone or a promoter preceding an initiator does not result in cancer. Following initiation, a tumor may then progress. Progression is a state of genomic instability represented by karyotypic changes, multiple mutations, and greater malignant potential. This instability results in a more aggressive phenotype characterized by increased tumor size, invasiveness, metastasis, anaplasia, increased growth rate, drug resistance, and escape from immune surveillance. A complete carcinogen exhibits all three properties. Fearon and Vogelstein [2] have proposed a model for colorectal cancer that involves multiple steps of progression in addition to initiation and promotion (Fig. 8-3). Carcinogens are likely to influence all three stages. In this model of colorectal cancer, many gene mutations are commonly acquired during the course of tumor development.

CARCINOGENS

Promoters often interact with a signal transduction pathway. This interaction may lead to uncontrolled proliferation of the initiated cell. Several promoters have a defined target (Table 8-3), whereas for other promoters the mechanism of action remains to be elu-

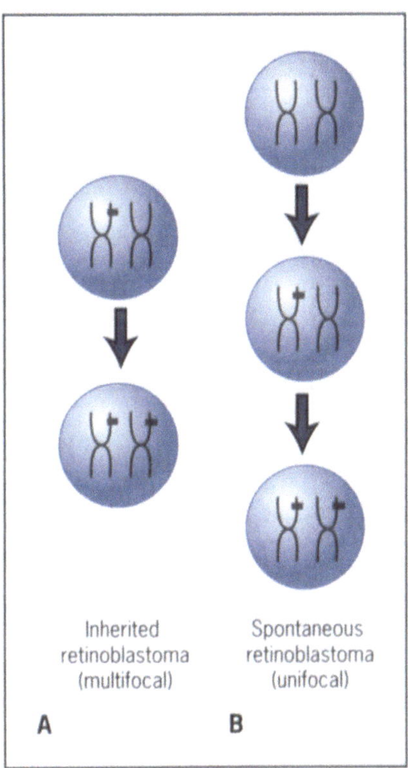

Figure 8-1. **A**, In the multifocal form of retinoblastoma, only one mutation is needed, because the first mutation is inherited. **B**, In unifocal cases of retinoblastoma, two spontaneous hits must occur in the same cell.

Table 8-1. Definitions relevant to carcinogenesis

Term	Definition
Initiators	Electrophiles that interact with nucleophiles in the cell (*ie*, DNA, RNA, and protein). The most deleterious interaction is with DNA leading to mutation, often by adduct formation.
Promoters	Substances that mediate their effect through epigenetic changes, often interacting with elements of signal transduction pathways, altering regulation and leading to clonal expansion of initiated cells. Promoters are not carcinogenic or mutagenic, can be reversed by withdrawal, must be given after an initiator, and require prolonged exposure to cause tumor formation.
Progression	State in tumor development where genomic instability exists, as evidenced by the occurrence of many mutations, and the cells develop a more aggressive and malignant phenotype.
Genotoxic	Carcinogens that interact chemically with DNA (*eg*, cause adduct formation).
Genetic change	Alteration in DNA sequence (*ie*, point mutation, deletion, insertion, gain or loss of entire chromosome).
Epigenetic change	Any change in phenotype not resulting from an alteration of DNA sequence (*ie*, DNA methylation, changes in transcriptional or translational regulation).

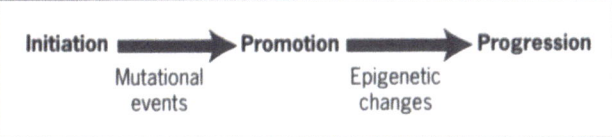

Figure 8-2. Carcinogenesis as a multistep process.

cidated. Chemicals are established as carcinogens in a variety of ways. The clinical association with special subsets of the population, along with geographic and demographic distributions of various forms of cancer, provide epidemiologic evidence. Numerous carcinogens have been discovered by a clinical association with the development of malignancy. Chemicals can also be identified as possible carcinogens by using laboratory tests, including cell, tissue, and organ culture as well as by using animal studies. Because many carcinogens are mutagens, the Ames test can be used to identify potential carcinogens by their ability to revert point mutants to the normal phenotype in *Salmonella typhimurium*. To identify procarcinogens, the assay can be modified and performed in the presence of a fraction of liver microsomal enzymes that may convert many procarcinogens into the active form. Mouse skin studies helped prove the validity of the multistep model of tumorigenesis. Different chemicals were applied to the skin at different intervals, and those that produced an irreversible change that led to neoplasia upon addition of a known promoter were defined as initiators. Similarly, chemicals that would induce a tumor upon repeated administration after an initial dose of a known initiator were defined as promoters. A chemical that is associated with an appearance of a novel cancer or that results in a change in the rate or frequency of tumor formation on exposure, renders a chemical suspect as a carcinogen. These criteria apply to both animal studies and human observations.

Biotransformation

Often, compounds are converted to an active carcinogen in the body through a process of biotransformation. Most procarcinogens are metabolized to carcino-

Table 8-2. Comparison of the stages of carcinogenesis

Initiation	Promotion	Progression
Irreversible	Reversible	Irreversible
Additive	Nonadditive	Additive
Genetic mutations	Nongenetic	Chromosomal aberrations
Dose dependent		
No measurable threshold	Minimal threshold	
No maximum response	Maximum response	

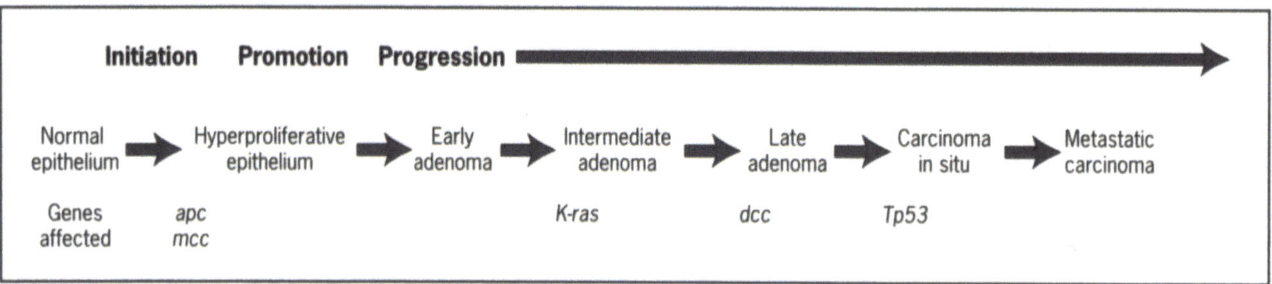

Figure 8-3. Progression of colon cancer.

Table 8-3. Promoters and their mechanism of action

Promoter	Active site
Phorbol esters	Protein kinase C
Steroid hormones and agonists	Androgen and estrogen receptors
Tetrachlorodibenzo-p-dioxin	Aryl hydrocarbon receptor

genic compounds by enzymes in the smooth endoplasmic reticulum and are referred to as microsomal. Many of these enzymes use cytochrome p450 and are mixed-function oxidases that perform both oxidations and reductions. These phase I reactions convert molecules to more polar substances and sometimes create a more carcinogenic compound. Phase II reactions conjugate the chemical to a substrate such as glutathione, sulfuric acid, or amino acids (Fig. 8-4). Individual rates of metabolism, which are a result of genetic, hormonal, environmental, and gender- and age-related influences, play a role in different susceptibilities to different procarcinogens.

Aflatoxin, a fungal carcinogen often found in grains, requires activation through a pathway that has a 2,3-epoxide intermediate that reacts with DNA, forming an adduct (Fig. 8-5). In a similar manner, polycyclic amines require metabolic activation to the reactive epoxide form by the microsomal enzyme aryl hydrocarbon hydroxylase.

Genotoxic Versus Epigenetic Carcinogens

Carcinogens can be classified as genotoxic (directly interacting with DNA) or as epigenetic (altering the phenotype of the cell without a change in the DNA sequence; Table 8-4). Genotoxic compounds may act directly or may require activation by biotransformation. Compounds that act epigenetically often stimulate cell division and hence are commonly promoters. Epigenetic changes are heritable but are not due to a change in DNA sequence. Rather, they are changes in gene transcription due to alteration in DNA methylation, transcriptional activation, translational control, and posttranslational modification. These changes are reversible, yet they can be inherited by genomic imprinting.

A variety of DNA structural changes are caused by carcinogens (Table 8-5) [3]. Electrophilic attack of the carcinogen commonly leads to formation of numerous types of adducts, depending on the specific carcinogen. Irradiation leads to breaks in both single- and double-stranded DNA that may lead to mutations after incorrect DNA repair.

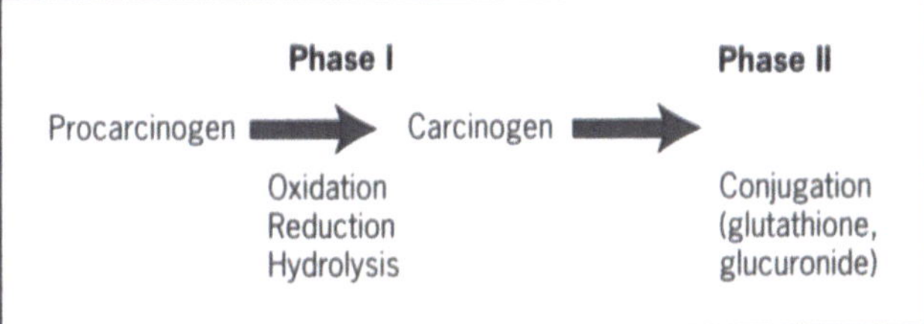

Figure 8-4. Compounds can be converted to an active carcinogen in the body through the two-phase process of biotransformation.

Major Cellular Targets of Carcinogens

There are a number of cellular targets for carcinogens (Table 8-6). Proto-oncogenes are normal cellular genes, many of which are involved in signal transduction, that become inappropriately activated to oncogenes via mutation. Tumor suppressor genes normally serve as checkpoints during the cell cycle. Apoptosis-regulating genes normally allow for death of damaged cells and maintenance of the balance between proliferation and senescence. DNA repair enzymes decrease the number of spontaneous and induced mutations. Most of these mutations lead to either a mutator state or to a state of uncontrolled growth, leading to genomic instability coupled with proliferation, followed by the onset of cancer.

The activation of proto-oncogenes to oncogenes can occur through a variety of genetic mechanisms (Table 8-7) [4]. The activation of oncogenes is frequently a dominant effect; *ie*, only one allele must be mutated to produce an altered phenotype. Tumor suppressor genes and DNA repair enzymes usually require a double hit: either two somatic mutations or one inherited mutation and one hit from a carcinogen,

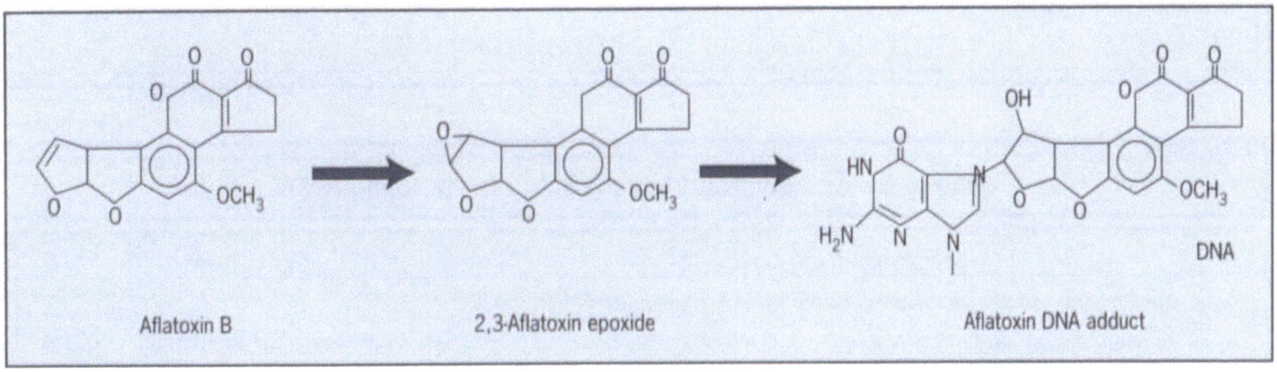

Figure 8-5. Aflatoxin B, a fungal carcinogen often found in grains, requires activation through a pathway that has a 2,3-epoxide intermediate that reacts with DNA, forming an adduct.

Table 8-4. Classification of carcinogens

Genotoxic
Direct electrophile that interacts with DNA
Procarcinogen compound that requires metabolic activation to interact with DNA
Epigenetic
Hormones that interact with receptors in the cell, often functioning as a promoter
Solid-state: mechanism unknown, possibly induces proliferation

as exemplified in Knudsen's model of retinoblastoma, although dominant negative mutations, such as p53, can modify activity in the presence of a normal allele.

CLASSIFICATION

The International Agency for Research on Cancer (IARC) classification system for the carcinogenicity of various compounds is based on medical and occupational exposure in humans, animal studies, and reactivity to DNA (Table 8-8). The evidence of carcinogenicity is weighted more heavily in humans than in animal studies.

Table 8-5. Interaction of carcinogens with DNA

Carcinogen	Structural change
Aromatic amines	C-8 and N-2 guanine adducts
	N-6 adenine adducts
Polycyclic hydrocarbons	N-2 guanine adducts
	N-2 adenine adducts
Methylating agents	O-6 guanine adducts
	O-2, O-4 thymine adducts
	Depurination
Aflatoxin B1	N-7 guanine adducts
Ultraviolet radiation	Thymine dimers
	Single- and double-stranded breaks
	Cross-linking of DNA and protein
Ionizing radiation	Single- and double-stranded breaks
	Cross-linking of DNA and protein

Table 8-6. Cellular targets of carcinogens

Gene	Result
Proto-oncogenes	Increased or unregulated proliferation or differentiation
Tumor suppressor genes	Loss of regulatory control over the cell cycle
Apoptosis-regulating genes	Loss of ability to undergo apoptosis
DNA repair enzymes	Increased mutation rates

Table 8-7. Genetic alterations leading to carcinogenesis

Genetic alteration	Causative agents
Gene amplification (*eg*, double minutes, homologously staining regions)	
Point mutations (*eg*, transitions, transversions, insertions, deletions)	Thymine dimer and adduct formation
Chromosomal rearrangements (*eg*, deletions, inversions, translocations)	Double- and single-stranded DNA breaks
Insertional mutagenesis (*eg*, proviral insertion, transposition)	Viruses and transposons

Environmental Carcinogens

Exposure to a number of chemicals in the environment can cause cancer (Table 8-9). In 1894, textile factory workers were found to have an increased incidence of bladder cancer (Fig. 8-6). Aromatic amines in the dyes used in these factories were determined to be the cause. Since that time, exposure to a number of aromatic amines has been associated with an increase in bladder cancer rates (Table 8-10). Sir Percival Potts noted in 1775 that scrotal skin cancer rates were high in chimney sweeps. He attributed these rates to soot and coal tar. Research performed 150 years later on mice and rabbits confirmed that the tar is carcinogenic on repeated exposure and is associated with a long latency period. Benzopyrenes were identified as the carcinogenic chemical component.

Cigarettes are associated with a number of cancers (Table 8-11). Most lung cancers are attributable to cigarette smoking, including adenocarcinoma, large cell carcinoma, and oat cell carcinoma (Fig. 8-7). Additionally, lung cancer rates dramatically increase in those who both smoke and are exposed to asbestos. Similarly, alcohol synergizes with the carcinogens in cigarette smoke in the formation of oral, esophageal, and laryngeal tumors. Several carcinogens have been identified in cigarette smoke, including benzopyrenes, dibenzanthracene, and nitrosamines, but the possibility exists that more remain to be discovered. Also contained in cigarette smoke are several promoting substances such as phenolic compounds and terpenes [5]. Asbestos can produce an inflammatory response in the lung, and exposure to asbestos can produce lung adenocarcinoma and mesothelioma. Mesotheliomas are almost invariably associated with asbestos exposure (Fig. 8-8). Angiosarcoma of the liver is associated with vinyl chloride exposure and thorium oxide, a radiologic dye (Fig. 8-9). The liver is a fairly common target of

Table 8-8. Classification of carcinogens devised by the International Agency for Research on Cancer

Group	Description
1	Sufficient evidence exists to show carcinogenicity
2a	Evidence suggests probably carcinogenic
2b	Evidence suggests possibly carcinogenic
3	Nonclassifiable as to carcinogenicity
4	Evidence suggests unlikely to be carcinogenic

Table 8-9. Environmental carcinogens

Carcinogen	Associated cancer
Organic chemicals	
Aromatic amines	
4-Aminobiphenyl	Bladder carcinoma
Aniline (benzidine)	Bladder carcinoma
2-Naphthylamine	Bladder carcinoma
Polycyclic hydrocarbons	
Benzopyrene	Lung carcinoma
Dimethylbenzanthracene	Lung carcinoma
Methylcholantrene	Lung carcinoma
Other organics	
Benzene	Leukemia
Carbon tetrachloride	Lung cancer, leukemias, lymphomas
Ethylene dibromide	Squamous cell carcinoma
Vinyl chloride	Angiosarcoma of the liver
Others	
Asbestos	Mesotheliomas (pleura and peritoneum)

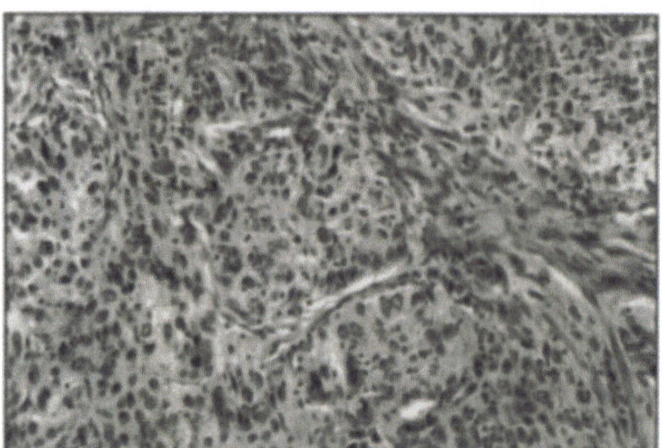

Figure 8-6. Transitional cell carcinoma of the urinary bladder.

Table 8-10. Carcinogens causing bladder carcinoma

4-Aminobiphenyl
Benzidine (aniline)
Chlornaphazine
Cyclophosphamide
Phenacetin-containing analgesic
2-Napthylamine

Table 8-11. Cancers associated with cigarette smoking

Lung
Adenocarcinoma
Small cell (oat cell) carcinoma
Squamous cell carcinoma
Large cell carcinoma
Esophagus
Larynx
Oral cavity
Bladder
Kidney
Pancreas

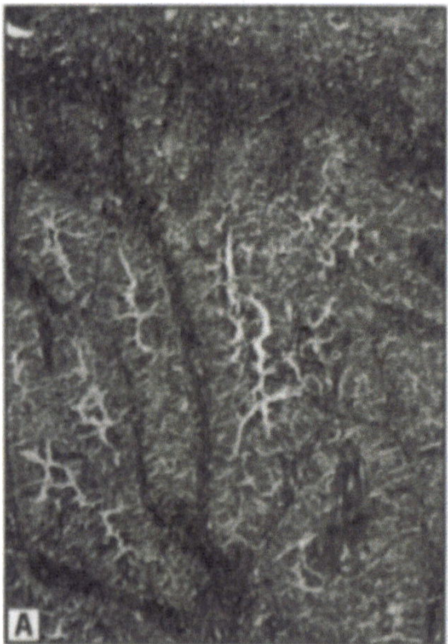

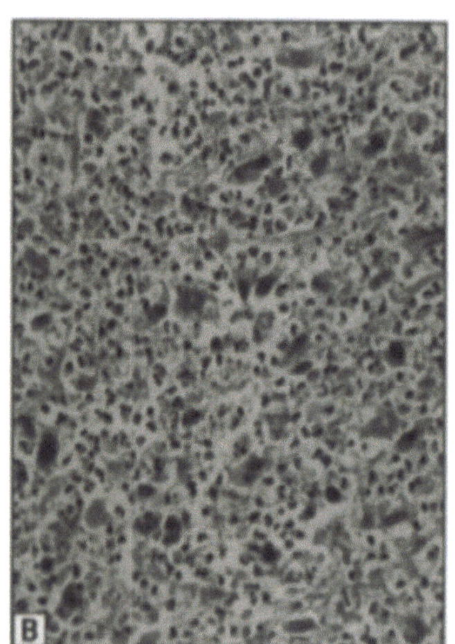

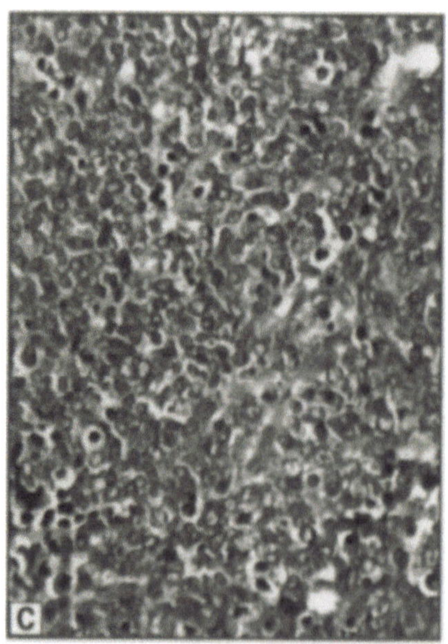

Figure 8-7. Lung cancers associated with cigarette smoking. **A**, Adenocarcinoma, which is comprised of columnar cells of increased size and nuclear atypia, forming glandular structures. **B**, Large cell carcinoma comprised of large anaplastic cells. **C**, Oat cell carcinoma, with cells characteristic of a small cell anaplastic carcinoma.

procarcinogens because it is the site of the majority of biotransformation reactions.

Hormonal Carcinogens

Steroid hormones diffuse into the cell and bind intracellular receptors that then translocate to the nucleus to alter gene transcription. This function enables steroid hormones to act as promoters. Many cancers are associated with hormones (Table 8-12). Estrogens exert a proliferative response in many tissues, including the endometrium, whereas progesterone induces differentiation, promotes the oxidation of estradiol to the less potent estrone, and decreases the amount of estrogen receptor [6]. Unopposed estrogen, or an increase in estrogen without a concomitant increase in progesterone, leads to an increased risk for endometrial cancers as evidenced by an association between endometrial cancer and exogenous estrogen exposure, obesity (adipocytes synthesize estrogen), estrogen-secreting tumors, estrogen replacement therapy, and a long reproductive span. Estrogens are metabolized to reactive quinones by cytochrome p450 reductases. The semiquinone intermediate in this redox cycling is a free radical that can damage protein or DNA (Fig. 8-10). Diethylstilbestrol (DES), a synthetic estrogen previously used to prevent miscarriages, can pass transplacentally to the fetus.

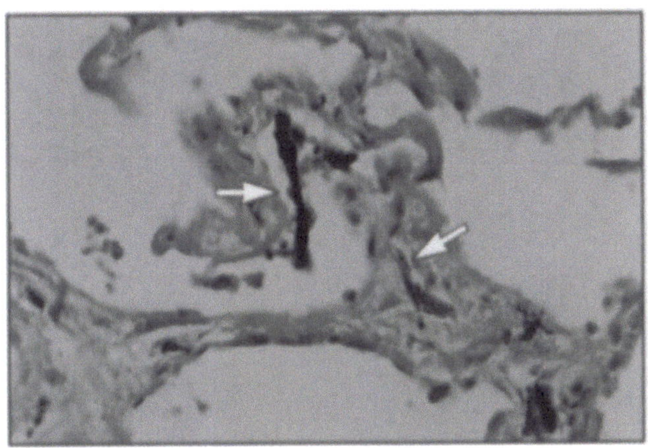

Figure 8-8. Mesothelioma caused by asbestos. The asbestos fibers can be seen as fibers in the lung tissue (*arrows*).

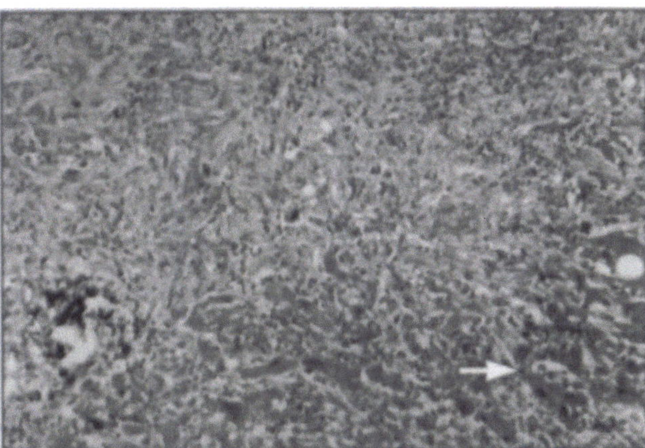

Figure 8-9. Angiosarcoma of the liver after thorium oxide exposure. An area of thorium oxide deposition is indicated (*arrow*), and some liver sinusoids can be seen in the lower right corner.

Table 8-12. Sex hormones associated with cancer

Hormones	Associated cancer
Diethylstilbestrol	Clear cell adenocarcinoma of the vagina in female offspring
	Breast cancer
Estrogen	Endometrial adenocarcinoma
	Breast carcinomas
	Fibrocystic disease of the breast (benign)
	Liver
	Kidney
Tamoxifen	Endometrial hyperplasia
Combined oral contraceptives	Hepatocellular carcinoma
	Cervical cancer (in conjunction with human papillomavirus)

Female offspring of women who took DES show a marked increase in the incidence of clear cell adenocarcinoma of the vagina.

Pharmacologic Carcinogens

Many chemotherapeutic agents are alkylating agents that damage the DNA of dividing cells, and affect both tumor cells and cells in the immune system. Patients treated with these drugs have a higher incidence of leukemias and lymphomas, presumably due to DNA damage to bystander cells during chemotherapy (Table 8-13). Cancers commonly associated with the use of antineoplastic drugs include large cell lymphoma, small noncleaved cell lymphoma, and small cleaved cell lymphoma (Fig. 8-11).

Dietary Carcinogens

Many compounds consumed in a normal diet are associated with various forms of cancer (Table 8-14). Diets high in smoked meats, salted fish, pickled foods, nitrates, and nitrites are correlated with increases in gastric cancer. Many nitrates and nitrites consumed in the diet are converted to nitrosamines and nitrosamines in the gastrointestinal tract. Aflatoxin B1 is a toxin excreted by *Aspergillus flavus* and is sometimes found in grains and peanuts stored

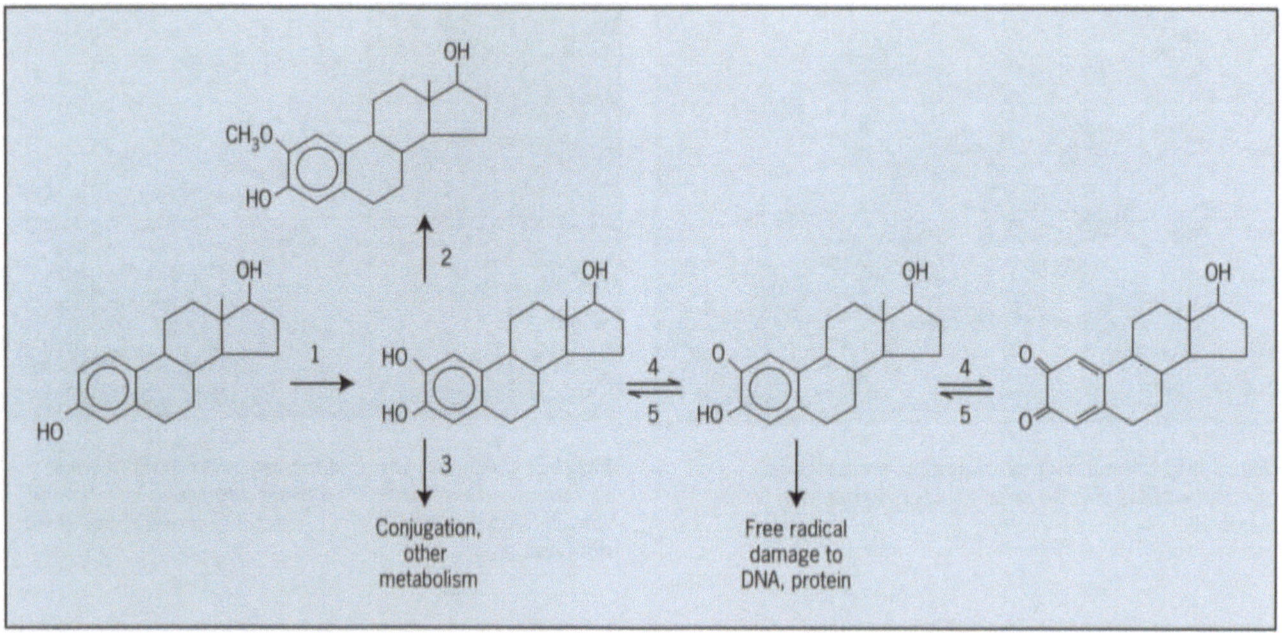

Figure 8-10. Quinine forms of estrogens. The semiquinone intermediate in this redox cycling is a free radical that can cause damage to protein or DNA.

Table 8-13. Pharmacologic carcinogens

Carcinogen	Associated cancer
Antineoplastics	
Chlornaphazine	Bladder
Busulfan	Leukemia
Chlorambucil	Leukemia
Cyclophosphamide	Leukemia
Melphalan	Leukemia
Immunosuppressants	
Azathioprine	Lymphoma
Cyclosporine	Lymphoma

in damp areas. Aflatoxin B1 has been implicated in the development of hepatocellular carcinoma (Fig. 8-12), particularly in China and Africa in conjunction with hepatitis B exposure, which results in acute liver damage and reparative proliferation.

METAL CARCINOGENS

Numerous metals have been implicated in a variety of cancers (Table 8-15). Respiratory carcinomas occur more frequently in miners of a number of ores (Table 8-16); the inhalation of ore dust is thought to be responsible. Nickel is a cause of nasal carcinoma.

RADIATION AND CARCINOGENESIS

Radiation can induce DNA damage leading to carcinogenesis (Table 8-17). Natural ultraviolet (UV) radiation, particularly the higher frequency UVB component, can cause skin cancers. The excitation by UV irradiation causes damage via two mechanisms: the formation of thymine dimers and the creation of

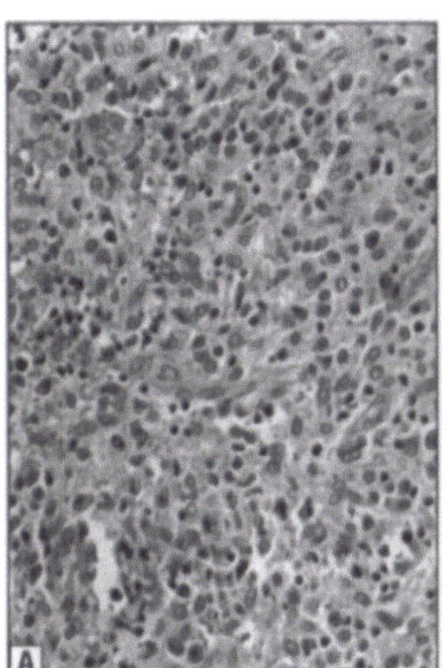

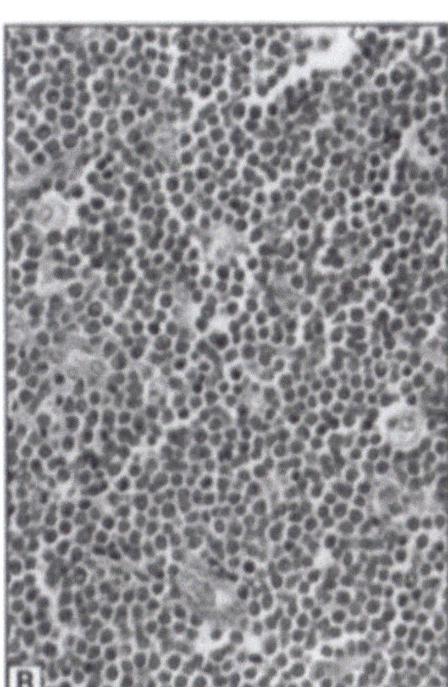

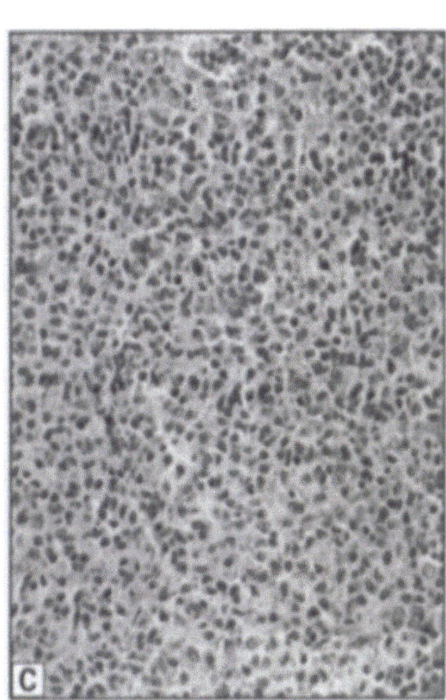

Figure 8-11. Some common postchemotherapy lymphomas include large cell lymphoma (*A*), small noncleaved cell lymphoma (*B*), and small cleaved cell lymphoma (*C*).

Table 8-14. Dietary carcinogens

Carcinogen	Associated cancer
Aflatoxin B1	Hepatocellular carcinoma
Nitrosamides	Gastric
Nitrosomethyl urea	Brain and kidney
Nitrosamines	Gastric
Dimethylnitrosamine	Gastric
Diethylnitrosamine	Gastric

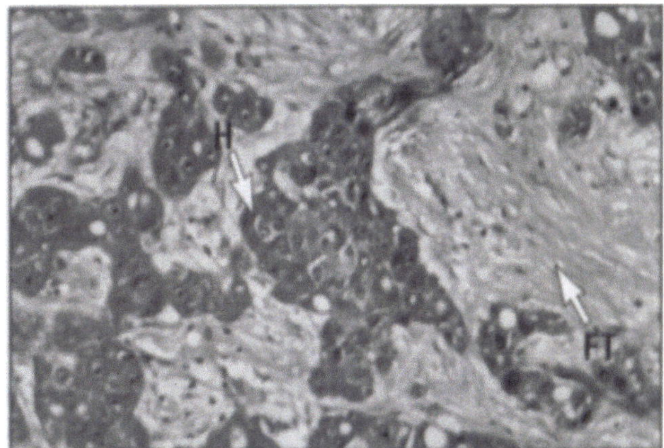

Figure 8-12. In hepatocellular carcinoma, sheets of atypical cells resembling hepatocytes (H) with nuclear abnormalities are nestled in fibrous tissue (FT).

breaks in the DNA (Fig. 8-13). Thymine dimers are the most common result of UV irradiation (Fig. 8-14). The adjacent thymines are excited, forming a cyclobutane ring that leads to distortion of the bases and of base pairing. These defects normally are corrected by nucleotide excision repair; however, incorrect repair or replication of unrepaired thymine dimers can lead to mutations.

Table 8-15. Metal carcinogens

Carcinogen	Associated cancer
Arsenic	Skin, lung, and liver carcinoma
Beryllium	Respiratory tract carcinoma
Cadmium	Prostate and kidney carcinoma
Chromium	Respiratory tract carcinoma
Nickel	Respiratory tract carcinoma
Uranium	Lung carcinoma

Table 8-16. Metals associated with respiratory tract carcinomas

Metal	Associated cancer
Arsenic	Lung
Chromium	Lung, nasal cavity, sinus, larynx
Nickel	Nasal sinus, lung
Uranium	Lung

Table 8-17. Physical carcinogens

Carcinogen	Associated cancer
Radiation	Melanoma, basal, and squamous cell
Ultraviolet light	Carcinomas of the skin
Ionizing radiation	Leukemia, lung cancer, bone cancer, skin cancer, thyroid cancer

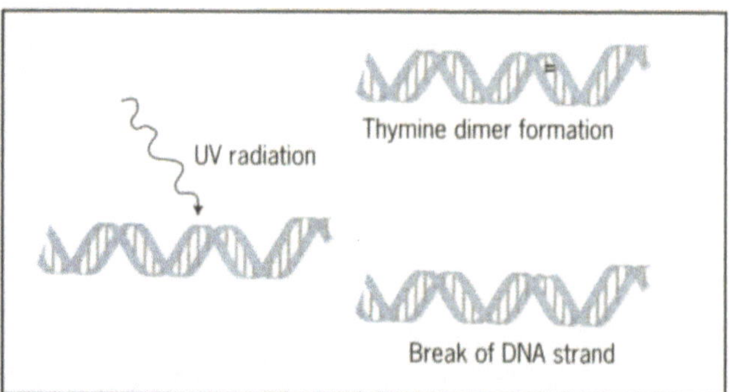

Figure 8-13. Ultraviolet (UV) radiation–induced DNA damage. UV irradiation most commonly leads to the formation of thymine dimers (*A*), but may also produce breaks in the DNA (*B*).

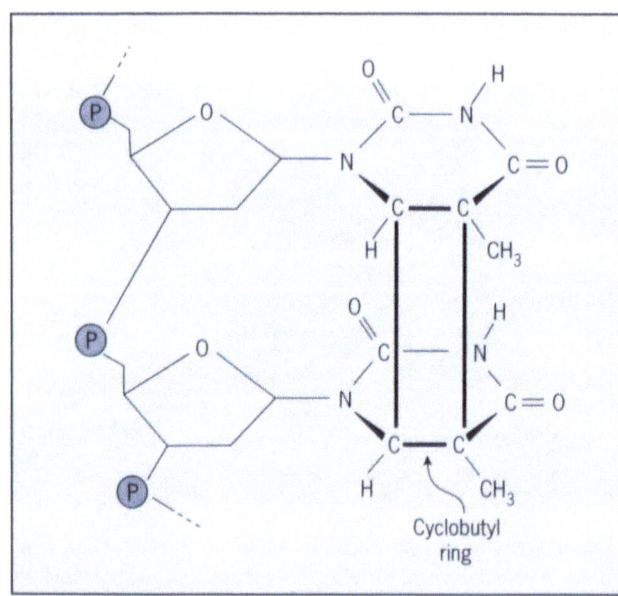

Figure 8-14. Thymine dimers.

DNA Damage and Repair Defects Associated With Carcinogenesis

DNA repair defects predispose certain individuals to cancer (Table 8-18). Because UV radiation damages the DNA, defects in DNA repair pathways predispose to cancers after exposure to radiant energy. Xeroderma pigmentosum is the best characterized DNA repair defect. Affected individuals are unable to repair the thymine dimers formed by UV irradiation. As a result, patients have a higher incidence of skin cancer. Ataxia telangiectasia, Fanconi's anemia, and Bloom's syndrome result from other defects in DNA repair and are associated with a higher frequency of mutations and increased cancer rates.

Ultraviolet Radiation–Associated Carcinogenesis

Many premalignant and malignant conditions are associated with UV radiation (Table 8-19). Exposure to UV radiation increases the occurrence of actinic (solar) keratosis (Fig. 8-15*A*), a dysplastic lesion consisting of hyperkeratosis macroscopically, and atypia and hyperplasia of the lower epidermis microscopically. Squamous and basal cell carcinomas of the epidermis are associated with UV exposure (Fig. 8-15*B*). Dysplastic nevi have a high malignant potential in individuals with an autosomal dominant form of the trait and a low risk in individuals without this form of the trait. Malignant melanoma is most commonly due to UV irradiation and is more fatal than either squamous or basal cell carcinoma because of its high metastatic potential.

Ionizing Radiation

DNA damage can also result from ionizing radiation and occurs via two pathways. The direct pathway involves the direct interaction of the radiation with the DNA (Fig. 8-16*A*) and is more dominant when the radiation consists of higher-energy particles such as neutrons or "α"particles (nuclei of helium atoms consisting of two protons and two neutrons). Water is often the target of radiation during the indirect process, resulting in the formation of the reactive hydroxyl free radical (OH•) that then reacts with DNA (Fig. 8-16*B*). This process is more significant

Table 8-18. DNA repair defects that predispose to cancer

Xeroderma pigmentosum
Ataxia telangiectasia
Fanconi's anemia
Bloom's syndrome

Table 8-19. Premalignant and malignant conditions associated with ultraviolet radiation

Condition	Associated cancer
Actinic (solar) keratosis	Squamous cell carcinoma
	Basal cell carcinoma
Dysplastic nevi	Melanoma

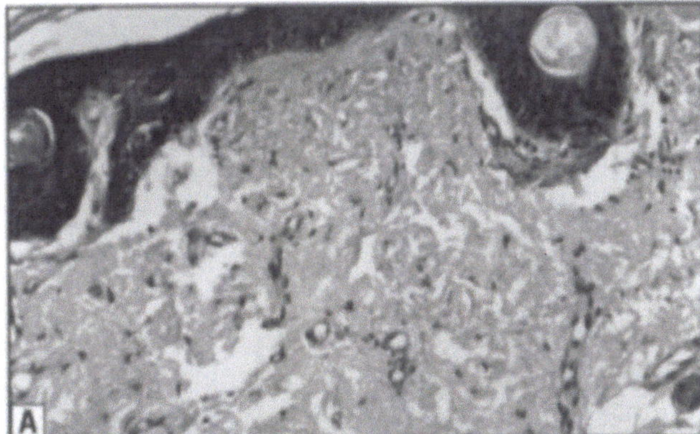

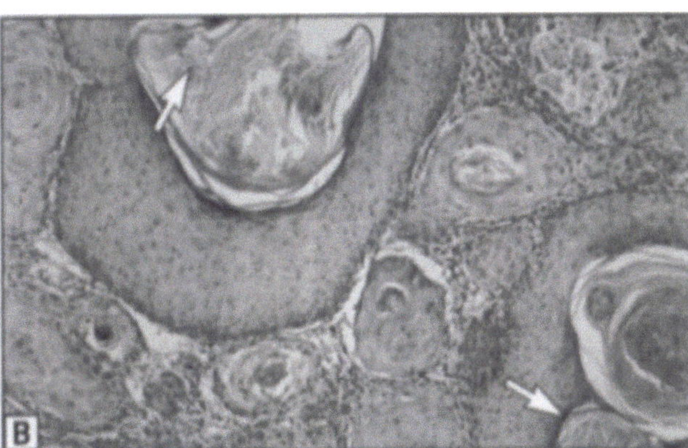

Figure 8-15. A, Actinic keratosis shows irregular accumulation of keratin and collagen degeneration in the superficial dermis. **B**, Squamous cell carcinoma displays keratin accumulations (*arrows*) and epithelial cells with enlarged and atypical nuclei.

than the direct action observed with x-ray irradiation. Both pathways lead to single-strand breaks, base damage, sugar damage, and least frequently, double-strand breaks.

Incorrect repair of two separate double-stranded DNA breaks can lead to a number of chromosomal alterations. If the two breaks occur on the same chromosome, the segment between the breaks may be lost if the repair process joins the incorrect ends of the breaks (Fig. 8-17*A*). The small circular DNA that results will be lost during cell division. If the ends of the two intermediates are relegated to the opposite cleavage site, an inversion can occur (Fig. 8-17*B*). If the breaks are on two separate chromosomes but are in close proximity, improper repair can lead to a translocation.

There is much anecdotal evidence of ionizing radiation–induced cancers (Table 8-20). In cases in which a specific population has been exposed to ionizing radiation, there have been increases in the frequency of certain cancers. Radiation therapy can induce cancer such as adenomas.

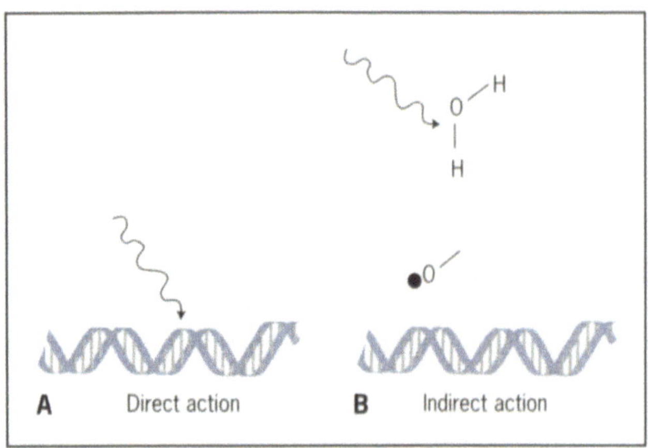

Figure 8-16. DNA damage resulting from ionizing radiation. **A**, The direct pathway involves direct interaction of radiation with the DNA. **B**, Water is often the target of radiation in the indirect process, resulting in the formation of the reactive hydroxyl free radical (OH•) that then reacts with DNA.

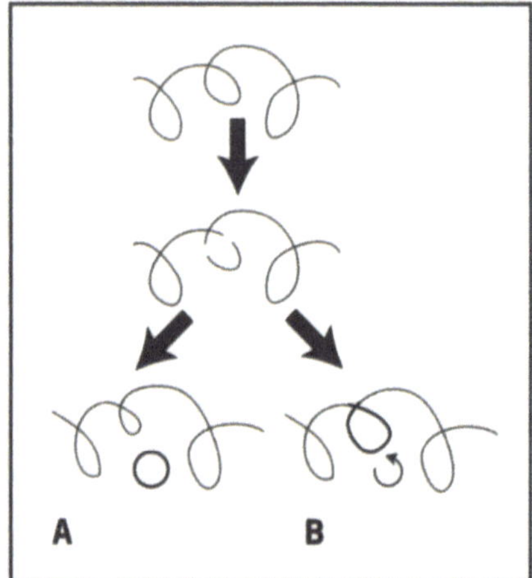

Figure 8-17. Repair of double-stranded DNA breaks. Incorrect repair of two separate double-stranded DNA breaks on the same chromosome can result in a deletion when the segment between the breaks is lost (*A*) or inversion if the ends of the two intermediates are re-ligated to the opposite cleavage site (*B*).

Table 8-20. Anecdotal evidence for ionizing radiation–induced cancers

Cancer	Population affected
Skin cancers	Early radiologists working with x-ray machines
Leukemia	Survivors of atomic bombs in Hiroshima and Nagasaki
Lung cancer	Miners of uranium and radium ore
Bone tumors	Radium dial painters (ingested radium was deposited into growing bones, leading to irradiation of surrounding bone)
Leukemia	Ankylosing spondylitis patients treated with radiotherapy in Britain from 1935 to 1944
Thyroid tumors	Patients treated with radiotherapy for enlarged thymus

REFERENCES

1. Knudsen AG Jr: Mutation and cancer: statistical study of retinoblastoma. *Proc Natl Acad Sci USA* 1971, 68:820–823.
2. Fearon ER, Vogelstein B: A genetic model for colorectal tumorigenesis. *Cell* 1990, 61:759–767.
3. Pitot HC: The molecular biology of carcinogenesis. *Cancer* 1993, 72(Suppl 3):962–970.
4. Couch DB: Carcinogenesis: basic principles. *Drug Chem Toxicol* 1996, 19:133–148.
5. Weisburger JH, Horn CL: The causes of cancer. In *Textbook of Clinical Oncology*. Edited by Holleb AI, Fink DJ, Murphy GP. Atlanta: American Cancer Society, Inc; 1991:80–98.
6. Key TJ, Beral V: Sex hormones and cancer. *International Agency for Research on Cancer Scientific Publications* 1992, 116:255–269.

CHAPTER

9

Pharmacology of Anticancer Drugs

Dwayne Dexter

It is estimated that 1.2 million new cases of cancer will be diagnosed in the United States in 2000. Although treatment advances encompassing several disciplines, including surgery, radiation treatment, and medical oncology, have reduced the mortality rate from cancer by 16% between 1950 and 1995 (excluding lung and bronchus cancer), 560,000 people per year still succumb to this disease in the United States [1]. Surgery is the best treatment for well-localized and accessible solid tumors and is often curative for many tumor types if they are detected early. However, chemotherapy remains the only alternative for tumors that have metastasized or are inaccessible to surgery or radiation. The role of chemotherapy in the success of cancer treatment regimens provides hope that further drug discoveries will have a continuing substantial impact on this disease. A thorough understanding of how current anticancer agents function in the context of tumor and cellular physiology will contribute to further rational drug discovery and improve existing regimens. This chapter reviews chemotherapeutic approaches to cancer treatment with an emphasis on drug class and mechanisms of action. The reader is referred to several excellent monographs, and the references therein, for a more detailed discussion on the pharmacology of these agents [2–7].

The historical success of chemotherapeutic approaches to cancer treatment can be traced over the last half of the 20th century. Since the first directed efforts in the mid-1940s to develop anticancer compounds using mustard gas agents, the U.S. Food and Drug Administration has approved more than 70 drugs for use as anticancer agents (Fig. 9-1). Currently, many tumor types are treated with multimodality therapy that usually includes a combination of chemotherapy and surgery or radiation therapy. Adjuvant therapy (surgery and/or radiation therapy, followed by chemotherapy) has increased survival rates of patients with several solid tumors such as is found in breast cancer. Neoadjuvant therapy (chemotherapy followed by surgery and/or radiation therapy) also is being employed as a first-line treatment for several solid tumor types. The rationale behind this approach is to not only shrink or reduce the primary tumor burden before local control by surgery or radiation therapy but also to initiate treatment of potential metastases before local control is completed. Many effective anticancer drugs and clinical protocols have dramatically increased the 5-year survival rates of patients with several cancer types (Table 9-1). Unfortunately, for many solid, slow-growing tumors, treatment advances have failed to significantly increase survival rates.

In general, tumor responsiveness is directly related to the proliferative rate, or doubling time, of the tumor. Table 9-2 compares the doubling times of some tumor types with anticancer drug responses. This comparison suggests that cancers with a high proliferative rate are more susceptible to the cytotoxicity of anticancer drugs than those with slower proliferative rates. Furthermore, the clinical effectiveness of chemotherapy is often limited by tumor heterogeneity. As shown in Figure 9-2, tumors are clonal popula-

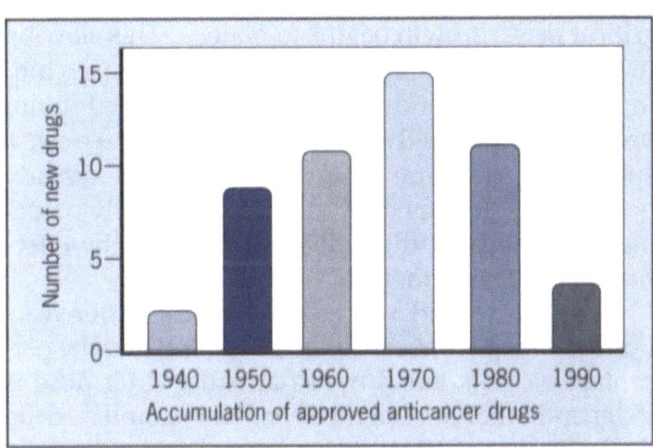

Figure 9-1. Rate of accumulation of approved anticancer drugs.

Table 9-1. Five-year survival rates in 1955 and 1994 by type of cancer, %

Tumor	1955	1994
Breast	60	87
Prostate	43	95
Testis	57	96
Hodgkin's lymphoma	30	83
Childhood cancers (0–14 years of age)	20	75
Liver	1	6
Pancreas	1	4
Lung and bronchus	6	15
Esophagus	4	13
Stomach	12	19

Table 9-2. Relation between tumor doubling time and response to chemotherapy

Tumor	Doubling time, *d*	Curable by chemotherapy
Burkitt's lymphoma	1	Yes
Choriocarcinoma	2	Yes
Acute lymphocytic leukemia	3–4	Yes
Hodgkin's lymphoma	3–4	Yes
Colon cancer	80	No
Non–small cell lung cancer	90	No
Breast cancer	100	Sometimes

From *Pratt* et al. *[7]; with permission.*

tions of cells that typically arise from a single transformed cell. These clonal populations, however, are genetically unstable and can acquire different genetic mutations. These mutations result in a heterogeneous population of cells that has different biologic properties, including proliferation rates and sensitivities to anticancer drugs. Thus, for treatment regimens to effectively destroy tumors, they must not only kill highly proliferative drug-sensitive cells but must also be able to combat the most recalcitrant of tumor cells—slowly proliferating or nonproliferating cells with decreased drug susceptibility.

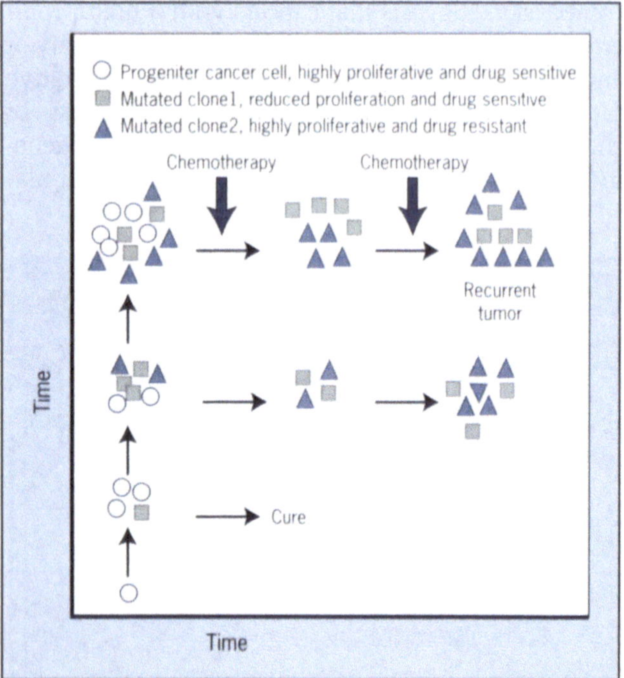

Figure 9-2. Effectiveness of chemotherapy is limited by tumor heterogeneity.

To understand the basic mechanisms of tumor regression, one must appreciate not only the kinetics of cell death but also the kinetics of tumor growth. Skipper and coworkers [8], at the Southern Research Institute, initially modeled tumor growth after classical experiments. Skipper's laws were based on experiments in which all tumor cells were proliferating. Although these laws still apply to the fundamental effects of chemotherapy on tumor growth, they are complicated by the fact that in actual tumors, a proportion of cells is nonproliferating.

Skipper's first law states that the doubling time of tumor cells remains constant regardless of tumor size. Simply put, the doubling time of a tumor with 50 cells is the same as one with 500,000 cells. Tumors, however, contain proliferating as well as nonproliferating cell fractions. Tumor growth consisting of these two populations is more appropriately modeled after a Gompertzian growth pattern (Fig. 9-3). Initially, cell growth follows an exponential growth cycle in which cell number or tumor volume doubles every unit of time. As the tumor reaches a certain critical mass, growth begins to plateau. This slowing in growth is the result of a number of factors, including a decreased ratio of dividing cells to total tumor volume (*ie*, reduced growth fraction). Moreover, a substantial decrease in growth rate has already occurred by the time that a tumor is clinically palpable. This fact will ultimately impinge on the effectiveness of chemotherapy.

Skipper's second law states that first-order reaction kinetics govern cell killing, meaning that the percentage of cells killed by a particular drug dose is independent of the cell number. For example, a drug

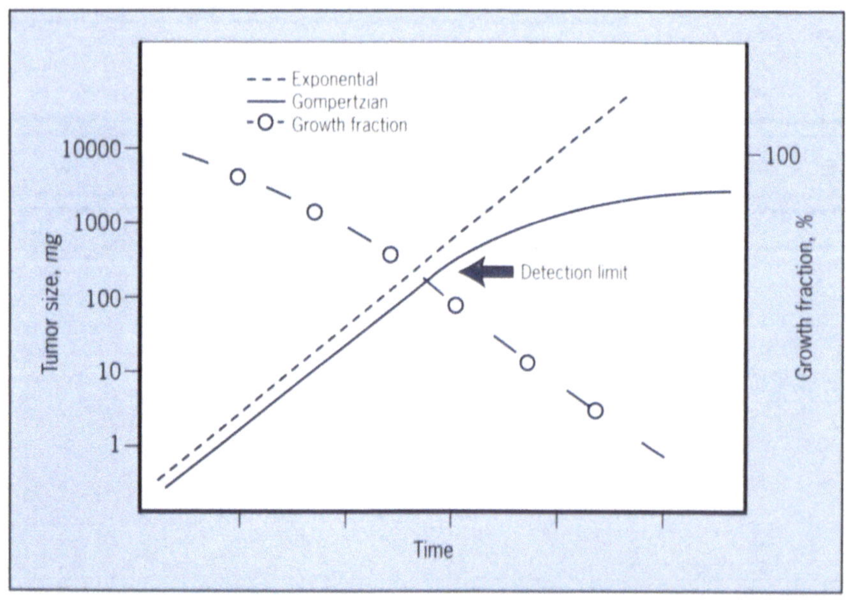

Figure 9-3. Exponential versus Gompertzian growth.

concentration that will reduce a cell population of 100 cells by 50% will also reduce a cell population of 1,000,000 cells by 50%. Figure 9-4 illustrates the difficulty of eliminating a tumor completely by chemotherapy. Dramatic increases in drug dose to obtain large cell kill (99.999%, 5 logs) achieves only a modest delay in tumor regrowth. It is evident from Table 9-2 and Figures 9-3 and 9-4 that early detection and treatment provide the greatest opportunity for maximum cell killing by chemotherapy. Two important principles are established by the first-order reaction kinetics of chemotherapy; the maximum tolerated dose (MTD) of drug should be used to achieve the greatest tumor cell kill possible, and multiple single-dose treatments may be more effective than single treatments given in increasing doses.

Clearly, proliferation rate correlates well with anticancer drug susceptibility. It is not surprising that most anticancer drugs interact with important cellular targets involved in the cell cycle. The increased proliferation rate and biochemistry of tumor cells make them more sensitive to many anticancer drugs during different phases of the cell cycle than their normal counterparts. Indeed, most current anticancer compounds are most active against highly proliferating cell populations. Consequently, many normal, rapidly dividing cells and tissues are also susceptible to these agents. The destruction of these types of normal cells, including normal bone marrow cells, epithelial cells of the gastrointestinal tract, and cells of the oral mucosa, often dictates the major dose-limiting toxicity for many treatment regimens.

A diagram of the cell cycle is shown in Figure 9-5 with anticancer drugs indicated at the phase of the cell cycle in which they are most effective. The differences in phase dependency of the various compounds can be exploited when developing combination therapies and drug schedules. In general, combination therapies of phase-specific drugs are most effective against rapidly dividing tumors, whereas combination therapies that include phase-nonspecific drugs are most active against large tumors or tumors with low growth fractions. Examples of both types of treatment strategies are shown in Table 9-3.

Cellular resistance mechanisms also reduce chemotherapy effectiveness. Resistance can be the result of intrinsic mechanisms—those genetically inherited and present before drug exposure—or it can be acquired as a result of drug exposure. Regardless of the type of resistance, decreased sensitivity of tumors to single-agent therapies or combination therapies (*ie*, multiple drug resistance [MDR]) is one of the leading causes of cancer treatment failure and patient death.

Early anticancer drug development relied mainly on empirical screening methods, and more sophisticated techniques are being employed to identify new anticancer agents. Improved drug discovery programs, coupled with increasing knowledge of cancer biology and a basic understanding of the pharmacokinetics and functions of successful drugs, may lead to improved cancer treatments. However, the promise of these newly directed approaches remains unfulfilled. Almost all of the current anticancer agents routinely employed in treatment regimens were discovered through empirical methods. Furthermore, although discreet differences in proliferating tumor cells and nonmalignant cells have been identified, the differences between proliferating and nonproliferating tumor cells are likely to yield targets for future drug intervention.

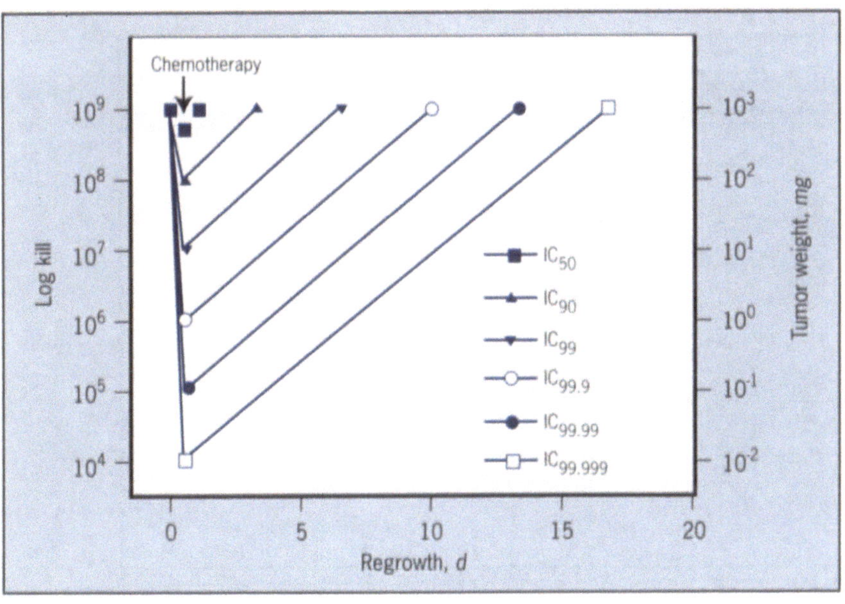

Figure 9-4. Chemotherapy treatment of a hypothetical tumor with different log kill concentrations of drug. Increasing concentrations provide only modest delay in tumor regrowth. IC—inhibitory concentration.

ALKYLATING AGENTS

The first directed development of an anticancer agent was based on mustard gas war research in the mid-1940s. These compounds were known to be alkylating agents (Table 9-4)—highly reactive electrophiles that can covalently interact with a number of nucleophilic groups, including amino, carboxyl, phosphate, and sulfhydryl groups. Physiologically, the major cytotoxic effect of most alkylating agents is the formation of a covalent bond with the nucleophilic groups in DNA. This interaction causes numerous alterations in DNA structure, in particular, interstrand and intrastrand cross-links, resulting in a disruption of normal cellular DNA replication processes that ultimately leads to cell death.

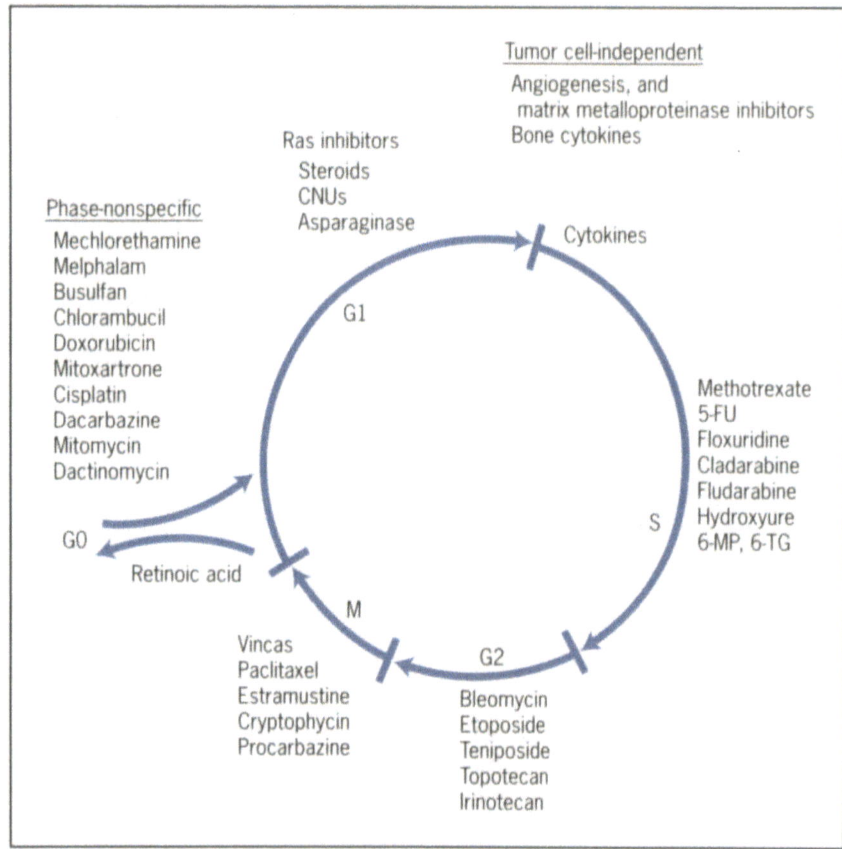

Figure 9-5. Cell cycle and phase specificity of anticancer drugs. During G1, there is normal cellular growth and accumulation of DNA synthesis metabolites. In S-phase, DNA synthesis (chromosomal duplication) takes place. G2 is the premitotic phase, during which validation of chromosomal duplication takes place. M-phase indicates mitosis. 5-FU—5-fluorouracil; 6-MP—6-mercaptopurine; 6-TG—6-thioguanine; CNUs—nitrosoureas.

Table 9-3. Combination therapy protocols

Drug	Day	Class	Cell cycle dependence
MOPP treatment regimen (repeat every 28 days)			
Mechlorethamine	1, 8	Alkylating	Nonphase
Vincristine	1, 8	Antimitotic	Phase
Procarbazine	1–14	Alkylating	Nonphase
Prednisone	1–14	Hormone	Nonphase
CA adjuvant treatment regimen (repeat every 21 days)			
Cyclophosphamide	1	Alkylating	Nonphase
Doxorubicin	1	Antibiotic	Nonphase

Nitrogen Mustards: Mechlorethamine, Chlorambucil, and Melphalan

Considerable evidence suggests that the major mechanism of action of the nitrogen mustards is the alkylation of the N-7 position of guanine in DNA (Fig. 9-6). Minor adduct formation has also been shown at the N-1 and O-6 positions of guanine, the N-1, N-3, and N-7 positions of adenine, the N-3 position of cytosine, and the O-4 position of thymidine. Of particular interest is the nonrandom nature of nitrogen mustard DNA damage and repair. Experimental evidence suggests that these agents may have gene-specific targets that are also targets for enhanced repair.

Cyclophosphamide (CPA) was developed as a nitrogen mustard prodrug and is the most frequently used member of this class of compounds. The rationale for this prodrug was based on the observation that many tumors have a high level of phosphoramidases, which could potentially activate prodrugs like CPA. Interestingly, although CPA was selected for further clinical development, its mechanism of toxicity was not associated with prodrug activation by tumor phosphoramidases. Subsequent studies showed that CPA metabolites, activated by liver enzymes, were the main cytotoxic agents. Ifosfamide, an isoform of CPA, also has been approved for use in treating several human tumors. Like CPA, it is activated by the liver; however, because of slightly different reaction kinetics, several of its major metabolites have been shown to cause increased neurotoxicity and greater incidence of hemorrhagic cystitis.

Dose-limiting urotoxicity of CPA and ifosfamide can be reduced by co-administration of sodium 2-mercaptoethane sulfonate (mesna). The protective role of this compound is highlighted in Figure 9-7 and is similar to the role of cellular reduced glutathione.

Platinum Complexes

Serendipity and astute observations led Rosenberg and coworkers [9] to identify the anticancer potential of platinum complexes. Their observation that electrolysis products from a platinum electrode inhibited *Escherichia coli* cell division led them to explore the antitumor activity of platinum complexed with chloride and ammonia groups. Among the initial compounds analyzed, cisplatin (*cis*-diaminedichloroplatinum[II]) was identified as having the best activity.

Cisplatin is a square, planar complex coordinated by a central platinum atom. Like other alkylating

Table 9-4. Alkylating agents

Drug	Major indications
Mechlorethamine	Hodgkin's lymphoma, NHL, CML, CLL, lymphosarcoma
Chlorambucil	CLL, malignant lymphoma
Melphalan	Multiple myeloma, ovarian cancer, breast cancer
Cyclophosphamide	Hodgkin's lymphoma, NHL, myeloma, neuroblastoma, ovarian cancer, breast cancer, SCLC, cutaneous T-cell lymphoma
Ifosamide	Testicular cancer
Cisplatin	Testicular cancer, ovarian cancer, transitional bladder cancer
Carboplatin	Ovarian cancer, SCLC, testicular cancer
Carmustine (BCNU)	Brain cancer, multiple myeloma, Hodgkin's lymphoma, NHL
Lomustine (CCNU)	Brain, Hodgkin's, lung, colon
Semustine (Me-CCNU)	Similar to CCNU, in particular gastrointestinal cancers
Streptozotocin	Metastatic islet cell carcinoma of the pancreas, malignant carcinoid cancer
Altretamine	Recurrent ovarian cancer
Mitomycin C	Anal cancer, stomach cancer, pancreatic cancer, superficial bladder cancer
Busulfan	CML, myeloablative therapy
Dacarbazine	Melanoma, Hodgkin's lymphoma, sarcoma
Procarbazine	Advanced stage Hodgkin's lymphoma, NHL, melanoma, bronchogenic cancer, medulloblastoma, multiple myeloma

CLL—chronic lymphocytic leukemia; CML—chronic myelogenous leukemia; GI—gastrointestinal; NHL—non-Hodgkin's lymphoma; SCLC—small cell lung cancer.

agents, cisplatin interacts with DNA, forming mainly dGpG diaminoplatinum adducts resulting in intrastrand cross-links (Fig. 9-8). Minor adducts of dApG and dGpXdG also have been detected. Because of cisplatin's severe dose-limiting toxicity (nausea, nephrotoxicity, ototoxicity, and peripheral neurotoxicity), less toxic compounds were developed. Of these, carboplatin has found clinical utility and appears to have the same mechanism of action as cisplatin.

NITROSOUREAS

All of the nitrosoureas (CNUs) alkylate DNA at the O-6 position of guanine. CNUs chloroethylate DNA, resulting in GC strand cross-linking. In addition, CNUs alkylate DNA in a sequence-specific manner, preferentially targeting contiguous regions of guanines. This sequence selectivity contributes to CNUs potent cytotoxicity but also to its mutagenic and carcinogenic potential. Early enthusiasm for the use of CNUs as anticancer agents was dampened by their severe dose-limiting toxicity, including myelosuppression, pulmonary fibrosis, and a significant incidence of secondary leukemias after long-term exposure. Unlike the chloroethyl nitrosoureas, streptozotocin is an antibiotic that has a methylnitrosurea moiety bound to a glucose molecule. Its mode of action is very similar to that of the CNUs.

AZIRIDINES

This group of diverse compounds includes synthetic drugs and natural antibiotics. The mechanism of

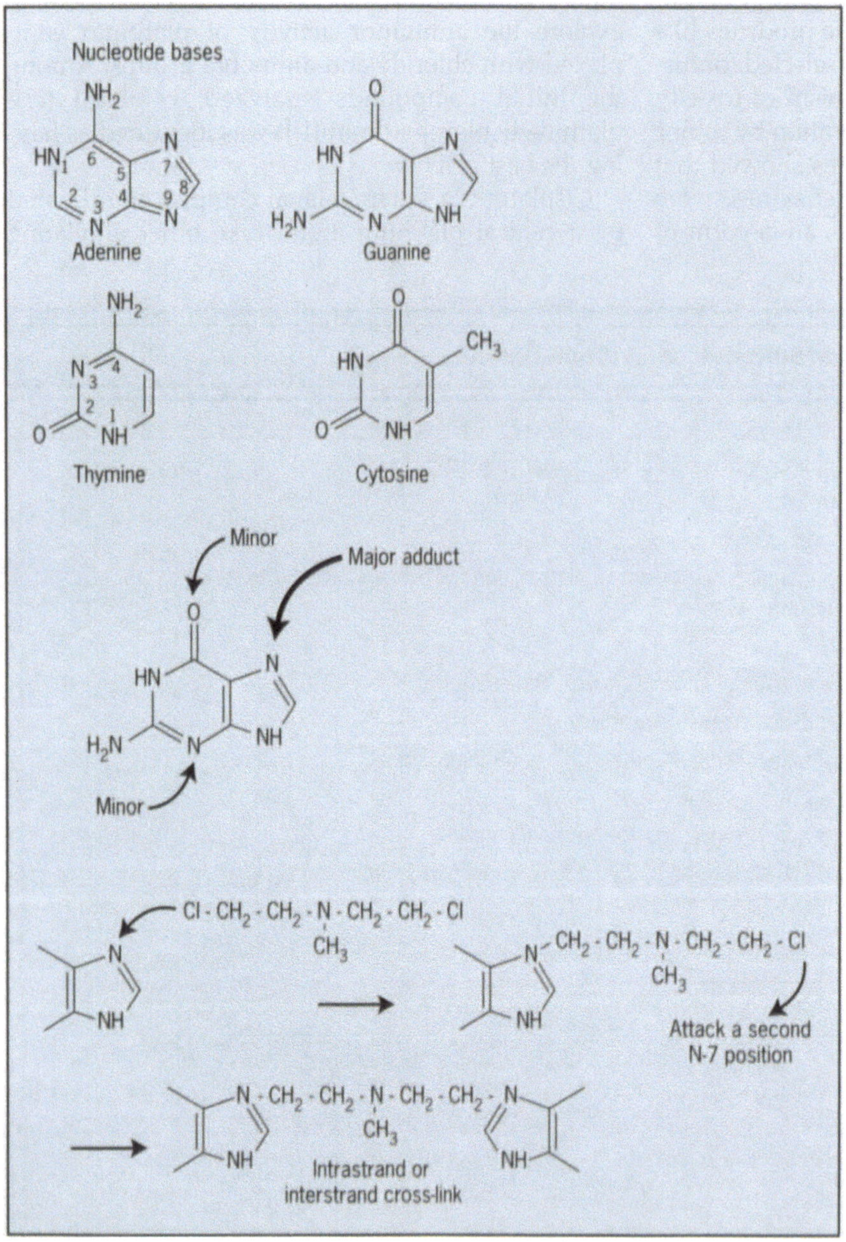

Figure 9-6. Alkylation of guanine by mechlorethamine.

action of aziridines is not well understood, but these drugs appear to be polyfunctional alkylating agents that can alkylate DNA on the N,O positions of several bases and attack the phosphate backbone of DNA.

Altretamine (hexamethylmelamine) functions predominantly as a mono-alkylator but appears to have some bifunctional alkylation activity. The parent drug does not have cytotoxic activity, but liver metabolites, namely demethylated species, are the major cytotoxic compounds. Altretamine has limited toxicity; its major dose-limiting toxicities are nausea and vomiting. Because myelosuppression is rarely dose limiting, altretamine, in combination with stem cell support protocols, has resurfaced as an agent used in high-dose chemotherapy regimens.

Mitomycin C is an antitumor antibiotic that has bifunctional alkylating capabilities. It initiates intrastrand cross-links between 5′ CG residues and also generates superoxide and hydroxyl radicals promoted by Cu^2 ions. Mitomycin C appears to be activated by an acidic environment.

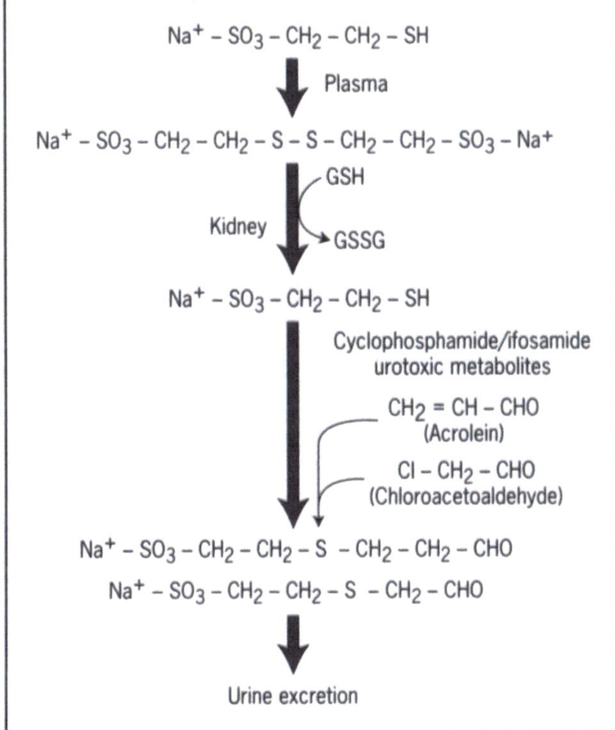

Figure 9-7. Supportive care with sodium 2-mercaptoethane sulfonate (mesna). GSH—glutathione; GSSH—glutathione disulfide.

Alkane Sulfonates

Busulfan is a bifunctional alkylating agent that alkylates the N-7 position of guanine. Evidence also suggests that it can promote DNA-protein cross-links, in particular, DNA-histone cross-links. Busulfan's major activity is a selective effect on cells with a myeloid lineage. Although busulfan was widely used to treat chronic myelogenous and granulocytic leukemias, it has been replaced with less toxic therapies. Recently, it has found new use in combination therapies used for bone marrow ablation followed by marrow transplantation.

N-Methyl Compounds

Methyl compounds are unique alkylating agents because they contain at least one *N*-methyl group in their structure. These compounds require host activation to mediate cytotoxicity. Furthermore, their uniqueness as alkylating agents is demonstrated by their lack of cross-resistance to other alkylating agents.

Antitumor Antibiotics

Antitumor antibiotics (Table 9-5) encompass a wide spectrum of structures and modes of action. The

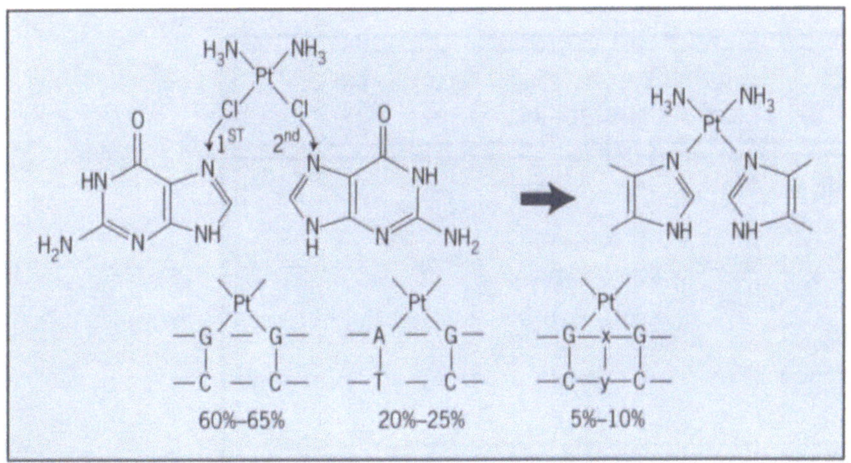

Figure 9-8. Cisplatin adducts.

majority of these compounds were isolated from various *Streptomyces* species. Chemical modifications of parent compounds and semisynthetic or synthetic analogues have been developed in an effort to improve clinical activity.

Doxorubicin, Daunorubicin, and Derivatives

Doxorubicin is one of the most widely used and effective anticancer compounds available today. Although several different modes of action have been ascribed to this group of compounds, their main cytotoxic effects appear to be related to their ability to intercalate into DNA and RNA (Table 9-6). Intercalation inhibits a number of DNA and RNA metabolic processes, in particular proper topoisomerase II activity (Fig. 9-9). Ultimately, accumulated single- and double- stranded DNA breaks result in cell death. Mitoxantrone is a member of this group that is interesting, less for its activity, but more for its manner of discovery. It was a developed as synthetic ballpoint pen ink, but its structure was recognized as having similarity to doxorubicin and other anthracyclines. This compound was found to have potent antitumor activity in the National Cancer Institute antitumor drug screen and was found also to have a mechanism of action similar to that of doxorubicin. Moreover, mitoxantrone appears to be as efficacious as doxorubicin in some treatment regimens but appears to lack the dose-limiting cardiotoxicity.

Dactinomycin

Although not widely used, dactinomycin (actinomycin D) was the first antitumor antibiotic successfully employed to treat cancer patients. It intercalates into DNA at GC base pairs, disrupting RNA polymerase activity and reducing protein synthesis. This activity has made actinomycin D a very useful reagent for cell biologists, in addition to its clinical role in the treatment of cancer.

Table 9-5. Antitumor antibiotics

Drug	Major indications
Doxorubicin	Breast cancer, ALL, AML, Hodgkin's lymphoma, NHL, germ cell cancer, SCLC, Wilms' tumor, ovarian cancer, bladder cancer, thyroid cancer, neuroblastoma, sarcoma
Daunomycin	ALL, AML
Idarubicin	ALL, AML, breast cancer
Epirubicin	Breast cancer, endometrial cancer, SCLC
Mitoxantrone	ALL, AML, NHL, breast cancer, bladder cancer
Dactinomycin	Pediatric solid tumors, Wilms' tumor, Ewing's sarcoma, osteogenic and soft tissue sarcoma, germ cell cancer
Plicamycin	Germ cell cancer, malignant hypercalcemia
Bleomycin	NHL, Hodgkin's germ cell cancer, squamous cell carcinoma

ALL—acute lymphocytic leukemia; AML—acute myelogenous leukemia; NHL—non-Hodgkin's lymphoma; SCLC—small cell lung cancer.

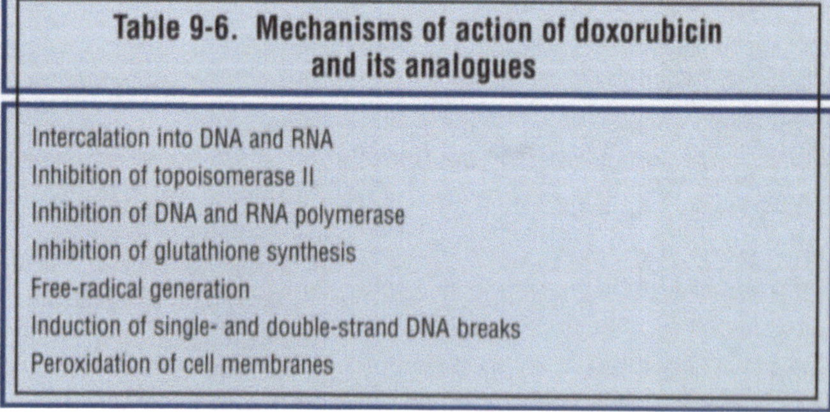

Table 9-6. Mechanisms of action of doxorubicin and its analogues

Intercalation into DNA and RNA
Inhibition of topoisomerase II
Inhibition of DNA and RNA polymerase
Inhibition of glutathione synthesis
Free-radical generation
Induction of single- and double-strand DNA breaks
Peroxidation of cell membranes

Bleomycin

This antibiotic is unique in that it requires a metal ion (Fe or Cu) to be effective. Bleomycin complexed with Fe^{++} will intercalate into DNA preferentially between GT and GC base pairs. Oxidation of Fe^{++} to Fe^{+++} results in localized oxygen free-radical formation, causing DNA strand breaks.

ANTIMITOTIC AGENTS

Antimitotic agents (Table 9-7) are commonly divided into two classes based on their action: topoisomerase inhibitors and microtubule poisons.

Topoisomerase Inhibitors

Podophyllotoxin, isolated from a plant extract, is a potent microtubule poison; however, its antitumor effectiveness is limited by its severe toxicity. Analogue synthesis led to the isolation of two glycosidic derivatives: etoposide and teniposide. Both analogues have potent antitumor activity; however, their mode of action does not involve microtubules. Subsequent work showed that the major cytotoxic effect of topoisomerase inhibitors was the result of DNA strand breaks. These lesions are the result of inhibition of topoisomerase II activity and the stabilization of topoisomerase II–DNA cleaveable complexes in a mechanism similar to that of doxorubicin (Fig. 9-9).

In addition to topoisomerase II inhibitors, topoisomerase I inhibitors have been recently introduced into the clinic. These inhibitors are analogues of camptothecin, a plant alkaloid that was identified in the 1960s as having antitumor properties. Camptothecin, however, had several drawbacks as an anticancer agent, including severe cytotoxicity (myelosuppression) and limited solubility. Analogue synthesis and screening determined that topotecan and irinotecan (CPT-11) were very potent, soluble analogues of camptothecin. All of these compounds introduce DNA strand breaks during DNA synthesis by stabilizing topoisomerase I–DNA cleaveable complexes.

Antimicrotubule Agents

The microtubule network is one of the major cytoskeletal structures of the cell. Microtubules serve multiple functions throughout the cell cycle; however, it is their pivotal role in chromosomal positioning and separation during mitosis that make them an attractive anticancer target. The first successful anticancer agents that targeted the microtubule network, the vinca alkaloids, were derived from the plant *Catharanthus roseus*. Clinically active compounds that make up this group include vincristine, vinblastine, and vinorelbine. The mechanism of action of the vinca alkaloids is thought to be mediated by their ability to depolymerize microtubules (Fig. 9-10*A*).

Paclitaxel is a natural product derived from the yew tree that was identified as an anticancer agent in the National Cancer Institute anticancer drug screening program. Paclitaxel has shown great promise as a single agent as well as in a number of combination therapy regimens. Paclitaxel, and its more water soluble analogue docetaxel, appear to mediate their activity by stabilizing or causing increased polymerization of microtubules.

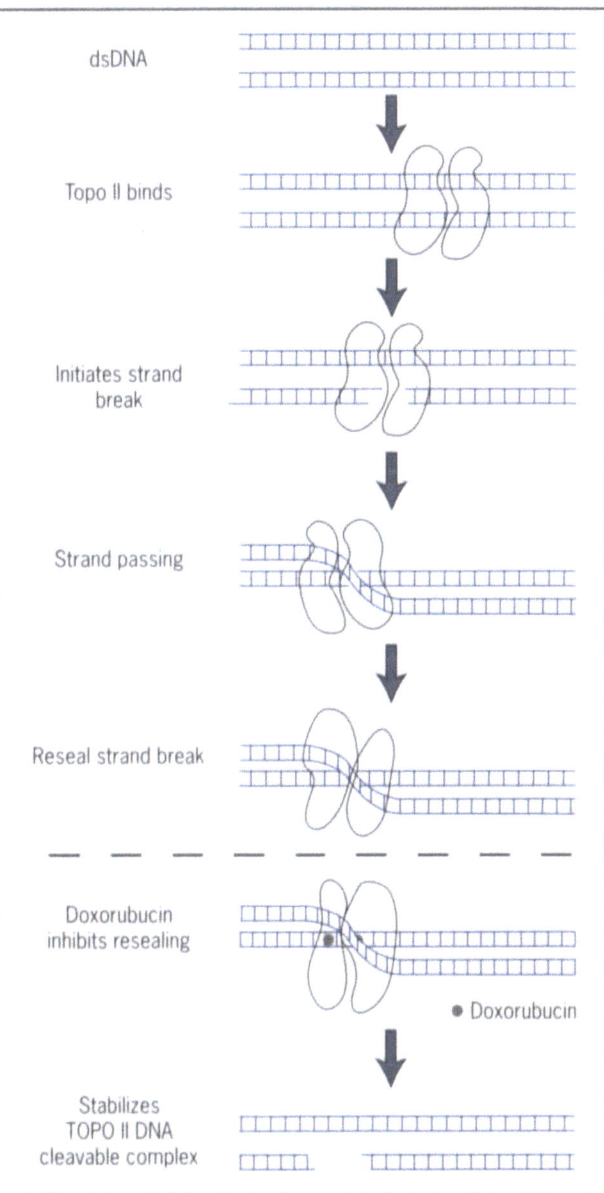

Figure 9-9. Inhibition of topoisomerase II by doxorubicin.

Estramustine was developed as a nor-nitrogen mustard analogue of estradiol to target steroid-responsive tumors such as prostate cancer. As with cyclophosphamide and podophyllotoxin analogues, the mechanism of action of estramustine was not that which was predicted by the developmental rationale. Estramustine, a potent anticancer agent, was shown to mediate its activity through microtubule alterations, not as a directed alkylating agent, and like the vinca alkaloids, it appears to be a depolymerizing agent. Interestingly, estramustine appears to preferentially accumulate in tumors with a high concentration of estramustine-binding protein, such as prostate and breast adenocarcinoma. This association may provide increased treatment efficacy for these tumors.

Cryptophycins were identified through a blind anticancer drug screening process and were found to exhibit very potent cytotoxic activity. Subsequent work showed that the mechanism of action was through inhibition of microtubule function. Importantly, cryptophycin has been shown to be 10- to 100-fold more potent than other microtubule inhibitors and circumvents cross-resistance mechanisms that limit the activity of other microtubule inhibitors [10].

Recently, Jordan and Wilson [11] have brought the classical cytotoxic mechanism of action of the antimicrotubule drugs into doubt through a series of studies. Briefly, they have shown that the concentration of these compounds that results in polymerization or depolymerization of the microtubule is well in excess of the concentration of drug shown to be cytotoxic. They have shown that these compounds, at doses that have profound effects on cell growth, do not promote polymerization or depolymerization of microtubules. Instead, these drugs alter the dynamic assembly and disassembly of microtubules during mitosis, which is critical for the microtubules to properly function (Fig. 9-10*B*).

ANTIMETABOLITES

The antimetabolites (Table 9-8) are a diverse group of compounds that ultimately mediate their action by a similar mechanism; disruption of DNA and RNA synthesis. Many antimetabolites resemble naturally occurring substrates of normal metabolic processes and usually require metabolic activation before entering their targeted metabolic pathway (Fig. 9-11).

5-Fluorouracil (5-FU) is the prototype of rational drug design. Based on the observation that uracil is preferentially captured by tumors, it was postulated that the addition of a fluoride group onto uracil might inhibit uracil-dependent enzymatic processes. 5-FU inhibits thymidylate synthetase. Floxuridine is a

Table 9-7. Antimitotic agents

Drug	Major indications
Topoisomerase II inhibitors	
Etoposide	Testicular cancer, SCLC, AML, ALL, Hodgkin's lymphoma, NHL
Teniposide	Pediatric ALL
Topoisomerase I inhibitors	
Topotecan	Ovarian cancer
Irinotecan (CPT-11)	Colorectal cancer
Microtubule poisons	
Vinblastine	Hodgkin's lymphoma, NHL, testicular cancer, breast cancer, bladder cancer, lung cancer, choriocarcinoma
Vincristine	ALL, Hodgkin's lymphoma, NHL, Wilms' tumor, Ewing's sarcoma, CLL, CML-blast, breast cancer, SCLC
Vinorelbine	NSCLC, breast cancer, prostate cancer, ovarian cancer, Hodgkin's lymphoma
Paclitaxel	Breast cancer, ovarian cancer, lung cancer, prostate cancer
Docetaxel	Breast cancer, head and neck cancer, lung cancer
Estramustine	Prostate cancer
Cryptophycin	Phase I trials

ALL—acute lymphocytic leukemia; AML—acute myelogenous leukemia; CLL—chronic lymphocytic leukemia; CML—chronic myelogenous leukemia; NHL—non-Hodgkin's lymphoma; NSCLC—non-small cell lung cancer; SCLC—small cell lung cancer.

metabolic precursor of 5-FU and functions in a similar manner. 6-Mercaptopurine (6-MP) and 6-thioguanine (6-TG) are purine analogues that inhibit normal purine biosynthesis and, following phosphorylation by hypoxanthine phosphoribosyltransferase, are incorporated into DNA, thus preventing DNA synthesis. Cytarabine (ARA-C) is a phosphorylated pyrimidine analogue that reduces the pool of deoxycytidine, which inhibits DNA and RNA synthesis. Methotrexate is a folate antagonist that competitively inhibits dihydrofolate reductase. Inhibition of dihydrofolate reductase results in a loss of folate and folate cofactors as well as precursors of purine and pyrimidine synthesis. Hydroxyurea inhibits the catalytic

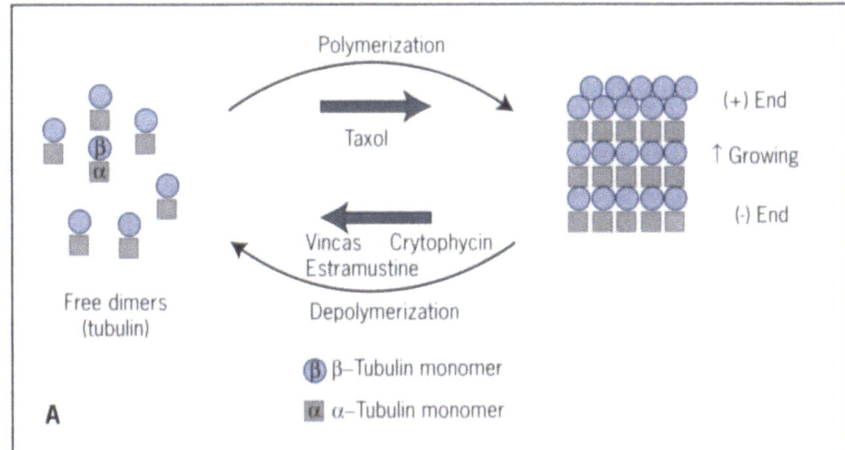

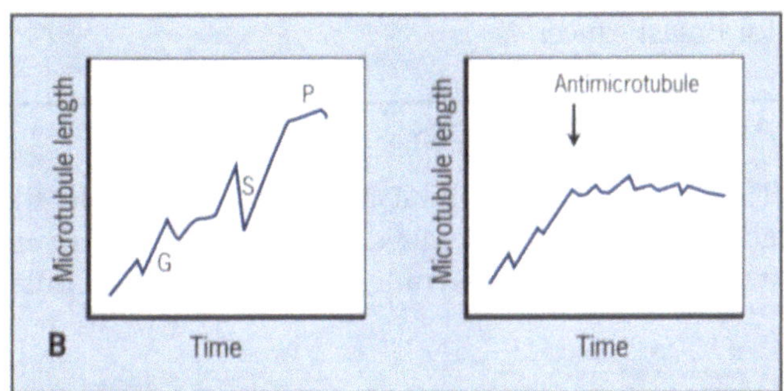

Figure 9-10. Alteration in microtubule equilibrium kinetics by antimicrotubule drugs. **A**, High concentrations. **B**, Low concentrations. On the left is a graphic representation of normal microtubule dynamics. G—growth; P—plateau; S—shortening. In the right panel, the addition of antimicrotubule agents suppresses microtubule dynamics.

Table 9-8. Antimetabolites

Drug	Major indications
5-Fluorouracil (5-FU)	Breast cancer, colon cancer, liver cancer, ovarian cancer, stomach cancer, pancreatic cancer, head and neck cancer
Floxuridine	Breast cancer, colon cancer, liver cancer, ovarian cancer, stomach cancer, pancreatic cancer, head and neck cancer
6-Mercaptopurine (6-MP)	Lymphocytic and myelogenous leukemia
6-Thioguanine (6-TG)	Lymphocytic and myelogenous leukemia
Cytarabine (ARA-C)	AML, ALL, CLL, meningeal cancer, leukemia
Methotrexate	Osteogenic sarcoma, ALL, lymphomas
Hydroxyurea	Melanoma, head and neck cancer, refractory CML, ovarian cancer
Cladribine	Hairy cell leukemia
Fludarabine	B-cell CLL

ALL—acute lymphocytic leukemia; AML—acute myelogenous leukemia; CLL—chronic lymphocytic leukemia; CML—chronic myelogenous leukemia.

activity of the M2 component of ribonucleotide reductase. This inhibition reduces the pool of deoxyribonucleotides, which in turn inhibits DNA synthesis. Cladribine (Leustatin; Ortho Biotech, Raritan, NJ) is a synthetic purine analogue that prevents proper DNA repair, leading to single-strand DNA breaks. Fludarabine is also a synthetic purine analogue that inhibits several DNA enzymatic processes, such as those that involve DNA polymerase alpha, ribonucleotide reductase, and DNA primase.

HORMONES AND ENZYMATIC THERAPIES

Hormonally sensitive tumors such as those of the breast and prostate are the major targets of most hormone-based therapies (Table 9-9). Hormones are extensively used in supportive care in cancer chemotherapy regimens; however, this survey reviews hormone use in the context of curative intent, which can include the use of agonists, antagonists, and surgical and chemical ablation.

ADRENOCORTICOIDS

Several glucocorticoid receptor agonists are available for use in cancer treatment regimens. Prednisone is one of the most frequently used agonists; it is part of the MOPP (mechlorethamine, vincristine, procarbazine, and prednisone) treatment for Hodgkin's lymphoma. Glucocorticoid receptor agonists ultimately interfere with the AP1 induction of growth responsive genes. This interference downregulates genes that drive cellular proliferation, ultimately causing cells to senesce or apoptose.

ESTROGEN AGONISTS AND ANTAGONISTS

Activation of estrogen receptors (ER) causes a number of cellular changes, leading to increased cellular proliferation (Fig. 9-12). Although ER agonists have found success in the treatment of breast and prostate cancer, they are often used as second- or third-line treatment strategies. It is the use of ER antagonists that has received the most attention. Anti-estrogens such as tamoxifen have been very successful in the clinic as single agents or in combination therapy for treating ER-positive breast cancer. Tamoxifen has had a substantial impact on overall disease-free survival for breast cancer patients in a number of clinical trials and is considered routine care for early-stage ER-positive breast cancer. Tamoxifen also is being considered as a chemopreventive agent for women at high risk for breast cancer.

AROMATASE INHIBITORS

These compounds inhibit aromatase activity in the adrenal gland and reduce the pool of precursors available for steroid synthesis. These chemical abla-

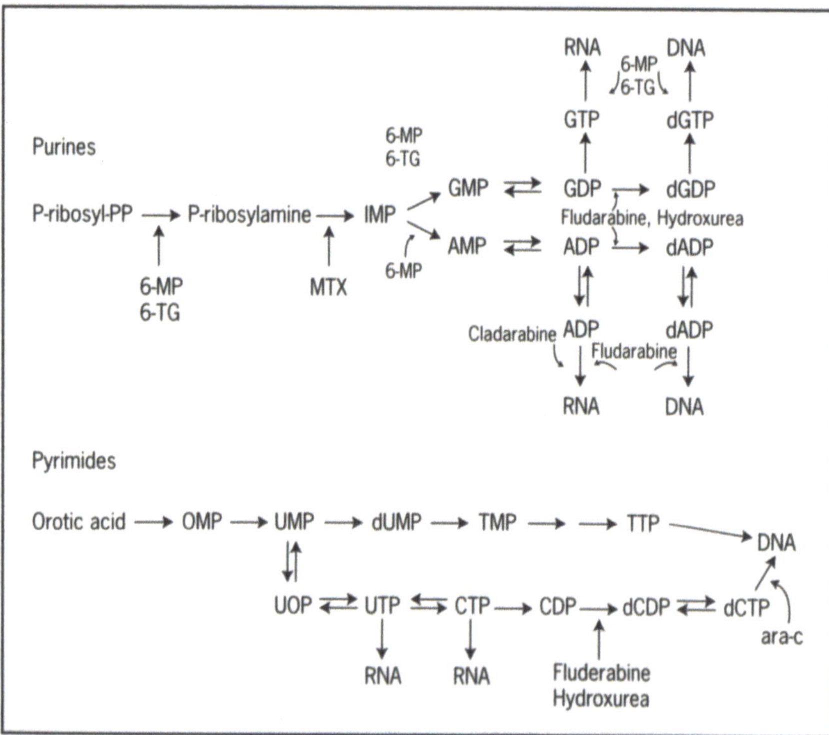

Figure 9-11. Antimetabolite mechanism of action. 5-FU—5-fluorouracil; 6-MP—6-mercaptopurine; 6-TG—6-thioguanine; A—adenosine; C—cytosine; DP—diphosphate; G—guanosine; I—inosine; MP—monophosphate; MTX—methotrexate; O—oratate; TP—triphosphate.

tion agents have found clinical use as third-line treatment options in breast cancer.

Androgen Agonists and Antagonists

These compounds are used to curb the growth of androgen-responsive prostate cancer. The nonsteroidal antagonist of androgen receptors, flutamide, blocks proliferative signals through the androgen receptor pathway. In addition, it negatively regulates the production of androgen products, thus reducing endogenous levels of androgen.

Enzymatic Agents

L-Asparaginase from *E. coli* has shown dramatic activity against acute lymphocytic leukemia (Fig. 9-13). *L*-Asparaginase converts asparagine to aspartic acid and ammonia. Tumors that lack the capability to synthesize endogenous asparagine are especially sensitive to this agent. Asparagine depletion results in diminished protein synthesis that ultimately impairs DNA and RNA synthesis.

Biologic Response Modifiers

The use of biologic response modifiers (*ie*, biotherapy) is an emerging treatment option for certain types of cancers. These modifiers are usually natural biologic substances whose normal role in cellular physiology is co-opted to alter tumor growth directly or to modify and enhance host immune responses against tumor antigens. Hematopoietic growth factors are the most commonly used biologic response modifiers in cancer therapy. They are important agents in supportive care because they decrease the incidence and severity of hematopoietic toxicities caused by cytotoxic drugs. Cytokines are currently the only biologic response modifiers used clinically to directly treat tumors. Cytokines are soluble protein factors that can act in a

Table 9-9. Hormones and enzymes

Drug	Major indications
Prednisone	Hodgkin's lymphoma, ALL, CLL, breast cancer
Tamoxifen	Postmenopausal and estrogen receptor (positive) breast cancer, chemopreventive (?)
Flutamide	Prostate
L-asparaginase	ALL, AML

ALL—acute lymphocytic leukemia; AML—acute myelogenous leukemia; CLL—chronic lymphocytic leukemia.

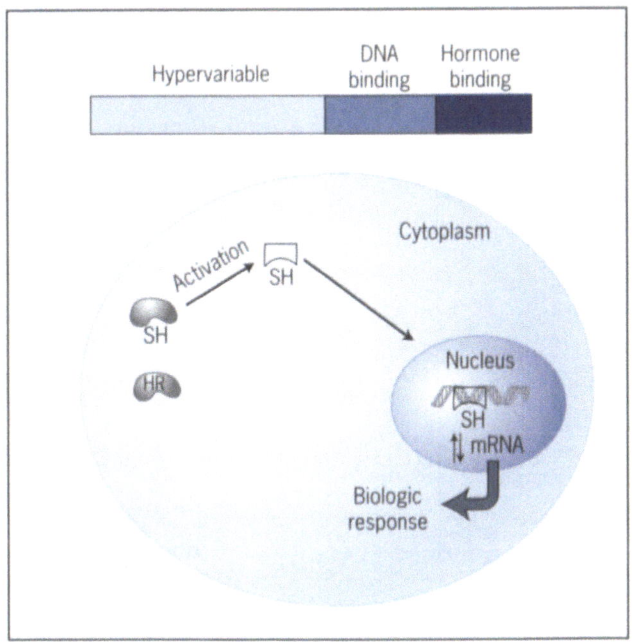

Figure 9-12. General structure and function of steroid receptors. SH—steroid hormone; HR—hormone receptor.

paracrine or autocrine manner to modify cell growth. Cytokines can directly target and inhibit the growth regulatory machinery of a tumor, or they can enhance the host immune response against the tumor. Interferons and interleukins are two of the most widely used biologic response modifiers. Although the exact mechanism of action of these cytokines is not understood, both function through membrane receptors to initiate a complex series of biochemical events that modulate tumor growth.

Monoclonal antibodies (mAb) also are used to directly target tumor antigens (Fig. 9-14). Because early studies indicated that passive immunomodulation of tumor growth by mAbs was not very effective, immunoconjugates were developed. These molecules conjugate mAbs with cytotoxic agents, targeting the cytotoxin to the tumor via tumor antigen-mAb interactions. Cytotoxic conjugates include radioisotopes, anticancer drugs, and toxins.

NOVEL APPROACHES TO CANCER CHEMOTHERAPY

As our understanding of tumor and cellular physiology increases, the number of possible targets for intervention also increases. High-throughput drug-discovery programs are also increasing the number of potential anticancer compounds. Highlighted in the following sections are four types of compounds that are the result of years of work in understanding the mechanisms of tumor growth (Table 9-10).

Differentiation Agents

Three observations have sparked interest in the use of retinoids as anticancer drugs: cytotoxic drug treatment induces, infrequently, differentiation of cancer cells, rendering these cells nonmalignant; deficiency in vitamin A (retinol) is associated with an increase in cancer; and animals deficient in vitamin A have increased hyperplasia that can be reversed by dietary supplementation with retinol.

The exact mechanism by which retinoic acid drugs cause differentiation is not clear; however, the retinoid acid receptors RAR and RXR transactivate and deactivate a number of genes (Fig. 9-15). These genes control a number of cellular processes, including apoptosis and terminal differentiation programs. The use of retinoic acid has found success in the clinic in the treatment of acute promyelocytic leukemia.

Angiogenesis Inhibitors

Most of the compounds reviewed in this survey directly target cancer cells. One of the more interesting and novel approaches to cancer chemotherapy

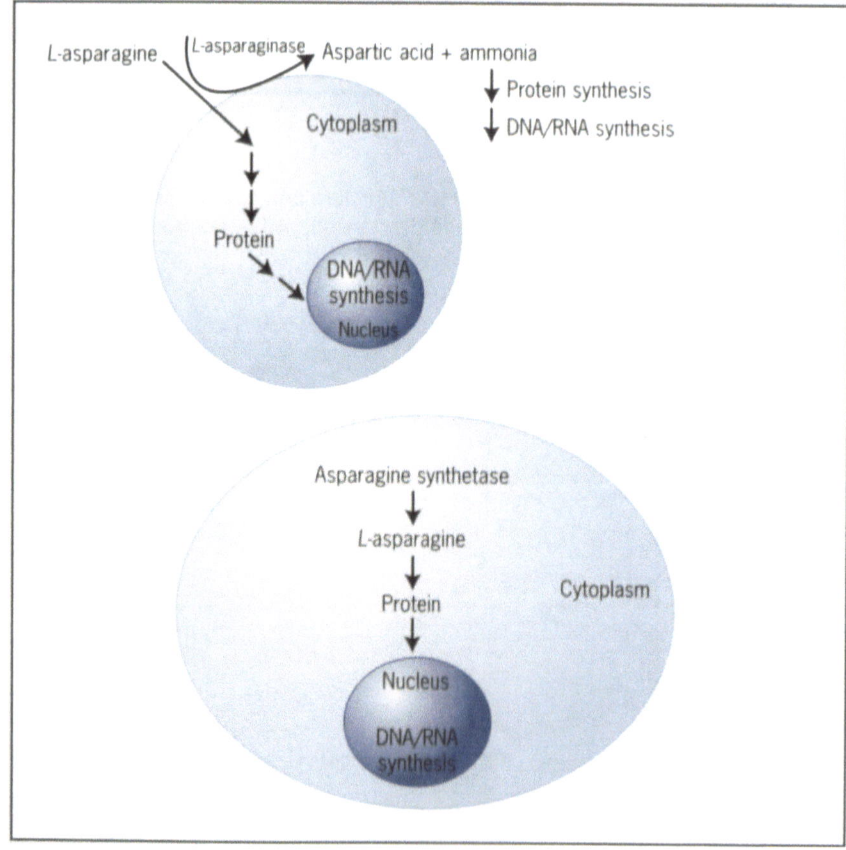

Figure 9-13. L-asparaginase activity on a sensitive cell (*A*) and a resistant cell (*B*).

is the development of anti-angiogenesis drugs. Angiogenesis refers to the processes involved in new blood vessel formation. Whereas angiogenesis has important physiologic roles in many areas, such as wound healing, there is ample evidence to suggest that it also plays a critical role in the continued growth and expansion of solid tumors. The pioneering work of Judah Folkman, Donald Ingber, and coworkers [12,13] provided proof that angiogenesis inhibition can be an effective anticancer treatment. Angiogenesis inhibitors include bacterial and fungal antibiotics, natural biologics (IFN-α2a), and synthetic compounds. The general mechanism of action of these compounds is the inhibition of proliferation of capillary endothelial cells, which ultimately reduces blood supply (and thus nutrients, oxygen, and waste removal) to the tumor. Initial phase I studies have shown minimal toxicity associated with these compounds.

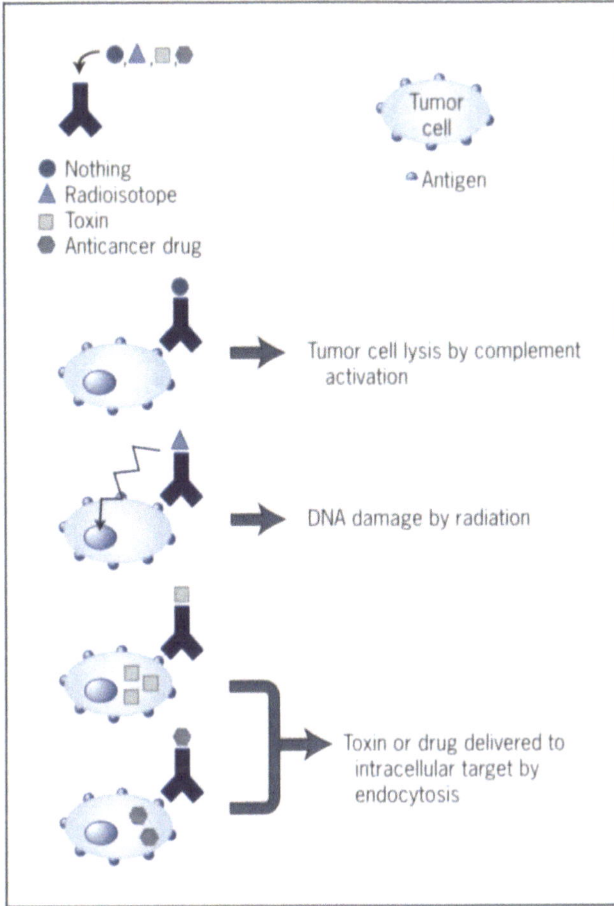

Figure 9-14. Monoclonal antibody cytotoxicity.

Table 9-10. Novel anticancer agents
Differentiation agents
All-*trans* retinol
All-*trans* retinoic acid
13-*cis* retinoic acid
9-*cis* retinoic acid
Angiogenesis/metalloproteinase inhibitors
TNP-470
Batimastat
Marimastat
AG3340
FTase inhibitors
L-744, 749
R115777
SCH 66336

Matrix Metalloproteinase Inhibitors

In addition to appropriate blood supply, the physical space required for tumor growth necessitates a reorganization of local tissue structure (*ie*, tissue remodeling). This remodeling not only provides the physical space for tumor growth but also plays a key role in angiogenesis and metastasis. Key components in tissue remodeling are the matrix metalloproteinases (MMPs). Several families of MMPs have been identified and have been shown to be overexpressed by tumors. Furthermore, endogenous MMP inhibitors have been identified. Thus, there is a rationale for developing MMP inhibitors that, like angiogenesis inhibitors, target tumors indirectly. Several MMP inhibitors are currently in phase I clinical trials (Table 9-10) [14]. Of particular interest is the dual action of some of these inhibitors. Not only do they prevent localized tissue remodeling around the tumor, but they also have been shown to be potent angiogenesis inhibitors.

Signal Transduction

The expansive increase in knowledge of the molecular and biochemical events responsible for cellular proliferation, and their roles in tumorigenesis have significantly increased the potential anticancer drug target repertoire. Autocrine, paracrine, and endocrine factors that mediate their effects through cellular receptors drive cell growth. These cellular receptors transduce their signal directly to the nucleus (*eg*, estrogen receptor) or initiate a signaling cascade that activates a complex array of downstream effectors. In either case, it is usually a defect in one or more of these pathways that initiates and sustains tumor growth. Significantly, it is the interconnection of these pathways and the concentration of the effector molecules that establish cell growth parameters. Obvious targets include growth factor receptors and their downstream effector molecules. Numerous downstream effectors present themselves as potential anticancer drug targets, including tyrosine kinases, protein kinase C, cyclin-dependent kinases, phosphatases, phospholipases, and activators of programmed cell death. One of the most significant and relevant targets is p21 Ras.

The three human *RAS* genes (*H-ras*, *N-ras*, and *K-ras*) encode low-molecular-weight G proteins of 21 kD termed p21. Mutations in *RAS* have been found in 30% to 50% of all human solid tumors, 50% of colon tumors, and 90% of pancreatic tumors. In both normal and transformed cells, p21 RAS undergoes a series of post-translational modifications that result in its anchoring to the plasma membrane (Fig. 9-16). This membrane localization is an absolute requirement for its signal-transducing functions to occur. The first modification attaches a farnesyl moiety to the

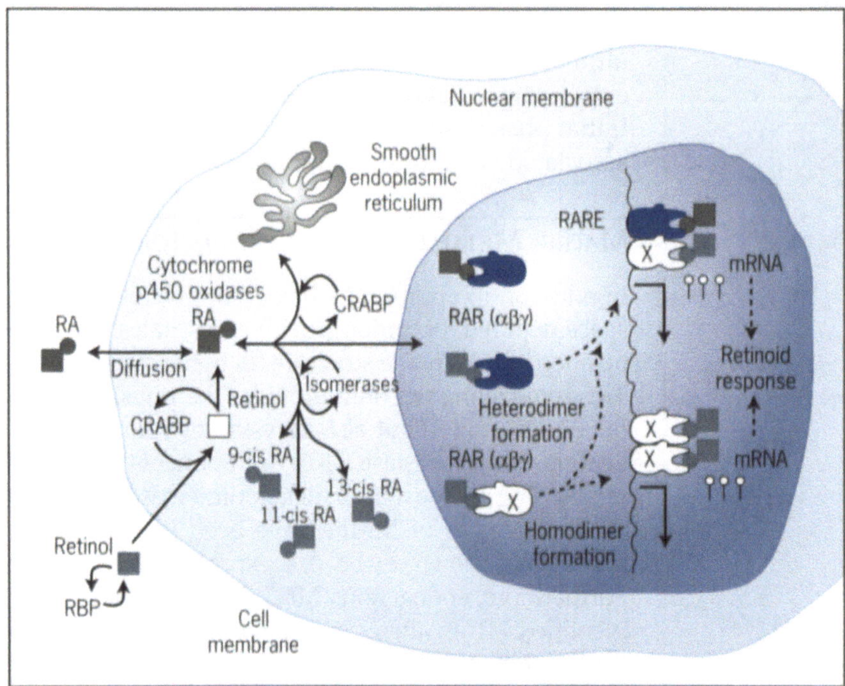

Figure 9-15. Metabolism of all-*trans* retinoic acid (RA). CRABP—cellular retinoic acid binding proteins; CRBP—cellular retinol binding proteins; RAR—retinoic acid receptor; RARE—retinoic acid response element; RBP—retinol binding protein; RXR—retinoid "X" receptor. (*From* Warrell *et al.* [15]; with permission.)

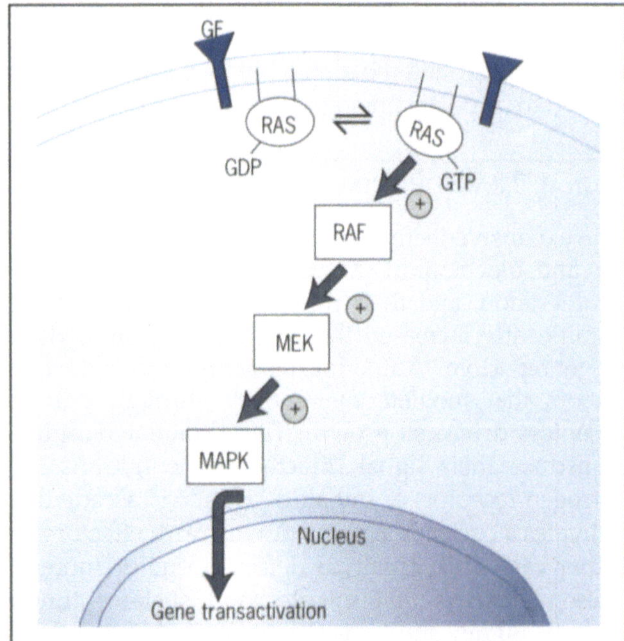

Figure 9-16. *RAS* activation by growth factor receptors requires membrane localization.

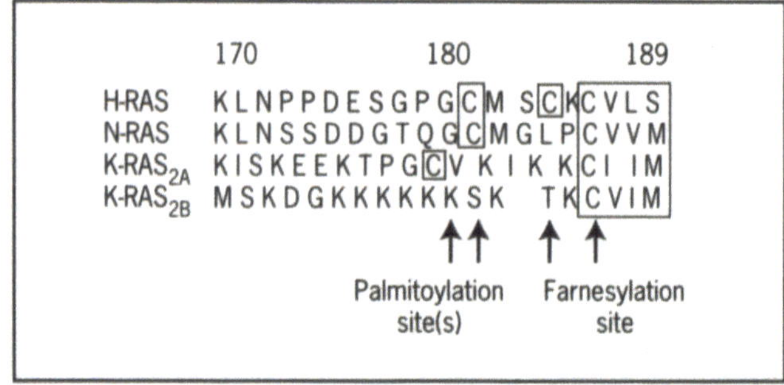

Figure 9-17. C-termini of human p21 proteins (the CAAX motif).

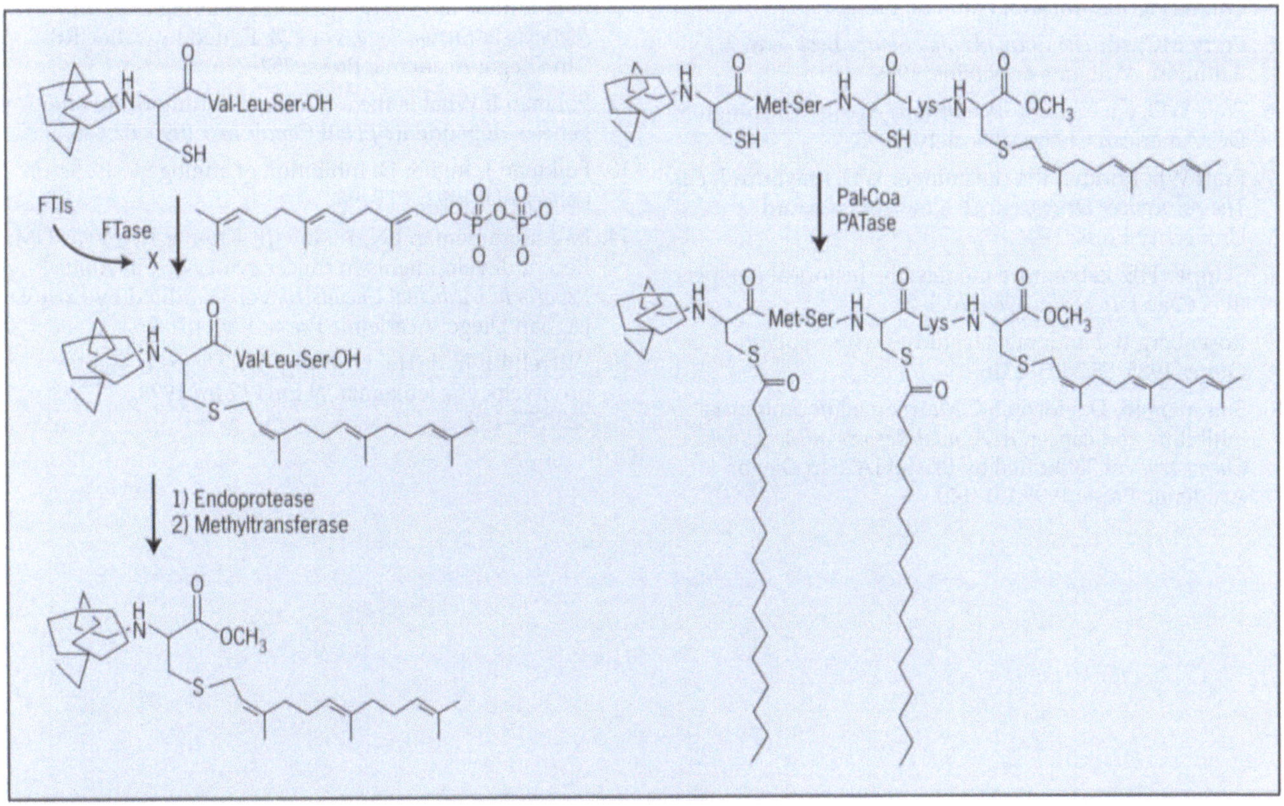

Figure 9-18. Posttranslational processing of H-*ras* p21. FTase—Farnesyl transferase; FTI—farnesyl transferase inhibitor; Pal-CoA—Palmitoyl-CoA; PATase—Palmitoyl acyltransferase.

cysteine that is four amino acid residues away from the C-terminus of the protein, referred to as the CAAX motif; this modification is required for subsequent processing steps (Figs. 9-17 and 9-18). Most drug development attention has focused on the first step catalyzed by farnesyl protein transferase, which has been isolated, cloned, and used in screening assays to identify farnesyl protein transferase inhibitors. Current approaches involve the development and refinement of CAAX peptidomimetics, as well as the isolation of natural product inhibitors.

Ultimately, the enormous amount of time and effort spent on understanding the underlying causes of cancer will yield more directed therapies. Clearly, cancer is a disease of the genome, with mutations in important growth regulatory genes driving tumorigenesis. Clinical strategies that target these alterations—gene therapy and chemoprevention—may reverse or prevent genetic defects that ultimately result in cancer. However, new technologies need to be developed to take advantage of gene therapy, such as better expression vectors and delivery vehicles. A greater understanding of the mutagenic and carcinogenic processes coupled with pharmacogenetics will also aid in the development of chemopreventive strategies. With declining cancer mortality rates (except those related to smoking), it is clear that we have begun to make progress in the battle against cancer, and advances in chemotherapy will continue to be part of the arsenal against this disease.

ACKNOWLEDGMENT

This chapter is dedicated to those cancer patients whose courage and foresight have saved countless lives and increased the use of the phrase "cancer survivor."

REFERENCES

1. Ries LAG, Kosary CL, Hankey BF, *et al*, eds: *SEER Cancer Statistics Review, 1973-1995.* Bethesda: National Cancer Institute; 1998.
2. Grochow LB, Ames MM, eds: *A Clinician's Guide to Chemotherapy: Pharmacokinetics and Pharmacodynamics.* Baltimore: Williams & Wilkins; 1998.
3. Fischer DS, Knobf MT, Durivage HJ, eds: *The Cancer Chemotherapy Handbook,* edn 5. St. Louis: Mosby-Year Book; 1997.

4. Teicher BA, ed: *Cancer Therapeutics: Experimental and Clinical Agents.* Totowa: Humana Press; 1997.
5. Perry MC, ed: *The Chemotherapy Source Book,* edn 2. Baltimore: Williams & Wilkins; 1996.
6. Foye WO, ed: *Cancer Chemotherapy Agents.* Washington, DC: American Chemical Society; 1995.
7. Pratt WB, Rudden RW, Ensminger WD, Mayburn J, eds: *The Anticancer Drugs,* edn 2. New York: Oxford University Press; 1994.
8. Skipper HE: Laboratory models: the historical perspective. *Cancer Treat Res* 1986, 70:3–7.
9. Rosenberg B: Fundamental studies with cisplatin. *Cancer* 1985, 55:2303–2316.
10. Summers JB, Davidson SK: Matrix metalloproteinase inhibitors and cancer. In *Annual Reports in Medicinal Chemistry,* vol 33. Edited by Bristol JA. San Diego: Academic Press; 1998:131–140.
11 Jordan MA, Wilson L: Use of drugs to study role of microtubule assembly dynamics in living cells. In *Methods in Enzymology,* vol 298. Edited by Vallee RB. San Diego: Academic Press; 252–276.
12. Fokman J: What is the evidence that tumors are angiogenesis-dependent? *J Natl Cancer Inst* 1990, 82:4–6.
13. Folkman J, Ingber D: Inhibition of angiogenesis. *Semin Cancer Biol* 1992, 3:89–96.
14. Balasubramanian BN, Kadow JF, Kramer RA, Vyas DM: Recent developments in cancer cytotoxics. In *Annual Reports in Medicinal Chemistry,* vol 33. Edited by Bristol JA. San Diego: Academic Press; 1998:151–162.
15. Warrell RP Jr, deThé H, Wang Z-Y, Degos L. Acute promyelocytic leukemia. *N Engl J Med* 1993, 329:177–189.

CHAPTER

10

Drug Resistance

Kenneth D. Tew

The expression or development of a drug-resistant phenotype is one of the major contributing factors in the failure of cancer chemotherapy. At the onset of treatment, most human cancers are composed of many millions of actively dividing tumor cells. Although clonal in origin, heterogeneity is a common trait even within a single tumor mass. Standard anticancer drugs are chemicals that exert a toxic effect on the tumor cell population, producing a biologic stress response. Thus, drug treatment creates the optimal environment for the selection of "fit" cells that are able to survive the insult. This chapter outlines numerous factors that contribute to a drug-resistant phenotype. Because of the diversity of drug targets, a wide array of cellular adaptations are apparent. In some instances, the changes are overlapping or redundant, perhaps reflecting the important survival advantage of multiple cellular protective processes.

GENERAL CONSIDERATIONS

Because many of the drugs used in cancer chemotherapy are toxic, a complex array of adaptive responses can create a resistant phenotype. Some of these responses occur at the whole-organism level, whereas others take place at the cellular level. Natural selection of protective traits has led to redundancies in many of the mechanisms that protect the cell.

Drug resistance and ultimate cell survival depend on both the rate and extent of drug-induced damage. Various arbitrary threshold values may determine which type of cellular drug resistance mechanism is most effective. It is also possible for a cell to invoke more than one type of damage-control system, sometimes in a sequential or temporal fashion (Fig. 10-1).

Table 10-1 provides an overview of the major classes of anticancer agents and those drug resistance mechanisms that have been characterized. Although resistance mechanisms are often applicable to specific drug classes, there are indications of generality in some instances (*eg*, disabled apoptosis). In many cases, homology between fungal genes and newly discovered human genes has permitted functional identification. Table 10-2 provides a partial listing of genes reported to have a role in mediating drug resistance in yeast. Other genes involved in the stress response have been described, and many of these also share homology and functional similarity to human counterparts. There are many parallels evident in the selection of, or resistance in, yeast and mammals.

Most tumors contain heterogeneous cell populations. The expression of drug resistance can have an equally varied phenotype (Fig. 10-2). Some drugs are ineffective in the initial treatment regimen, frequently because the tumor cells have genetic properties that circumvent the drug's cytotoxicity, providing natural resistance. Frequently, early drug treatment can achieve several logarithms of cell kill. A few cells may exist within the heterogeneous population that have intrinsic resistance properties to subsequent drug treatment. Repopulation with these clonal variants will then occur. This is an example of intrinsic resistance within the population, selected through Darwinian principles. The acquired resistance phenotype can occur following repeated exposure to a particular drug. At least two factors can contribute to the development of resistance. First, chronic drug exposure can cause some surviving cells to induce the expression of protective "stress response" genes. Because increased expression of these genes is maintained in this population, the cells will have an acquired resistant phenotype. Second, some anticancer drugs have mutagenic properties and may cause mutations in key cellular "target" genes. Repopulation of the tumor can occur with these adapted cells, conferring an acquired resistant phenotype.

Even with novel detection techniques, solid tumors are generally discovered only when they are 1 mm or more in volume (1 million cells). Chemotherapy is frequently begun when the primary tumor consists of 10^6 to 10^9 cells. Commonly, the initial tumor response results in disease remission. Regrowth leads to relapse, which is generally followed by a second round of chemotherapy. A second remission may be achieved, and in some cases, a cure may be obtained. More commonly, however, chemoresistant clones of cells take over and subsequent chemotherapeutic treatments prove ineffective. Failure of the initial chemotherapy to eradicate or slow the growth of the tumor indicates a natural resistant phenotype (Fig. 10-3).

The majority of preclinical studies of drug resistance have made use of drug resistant model cell lines that may be obtained by using several approaches. Often, a heterogeneous tumor cell population is treated with incrementally increasing concentrations of the selected drug, with or without pretreatment with a mutagen to enhance the likelihood of selecting mutant resistant cells. Growth and subculture take place over several weeks, during which intermediate resistance may be obtained. An arbitrary level of resistance is reached, and individual cells are removed and cloned. Growth of these clones is followed by drug testing and other characterization procedures, and the extent of resistance is measured by a standard in vitro cell-growth assay. Although some model cell lines can achieve very high levels of resistance (>10,000-fold), it is not unusual to achieve 5- to 10-fold resistance to the selecting agent (Fig. 10-4).

Figure 10-5 illustrates various pathways by which drug resistance to anticancer agents can be expressed [1]. Numerous drugs and xenobiotics can cause induction of gene expression through transcription activation. It is generally accepted that agents can be categorized into monofunctional and bifunctional inducers [2]. The latter type of inducer frequently requires binding to the aryl hydrocarbon (Ah) receptor or some intermediate metabolic process. Eventually, drug effects are manifest at some regulatory element level within the gene, resulting in transcription activation (Fig. 10-6).

Chronic sublethal exposure to drugs results in the induction and overexpression of gene products that protect the cell. There are advantages and disadvantages to inducing overexpression of an individual gene product versus a pleiotropic response in which a broader range of gene products is over-

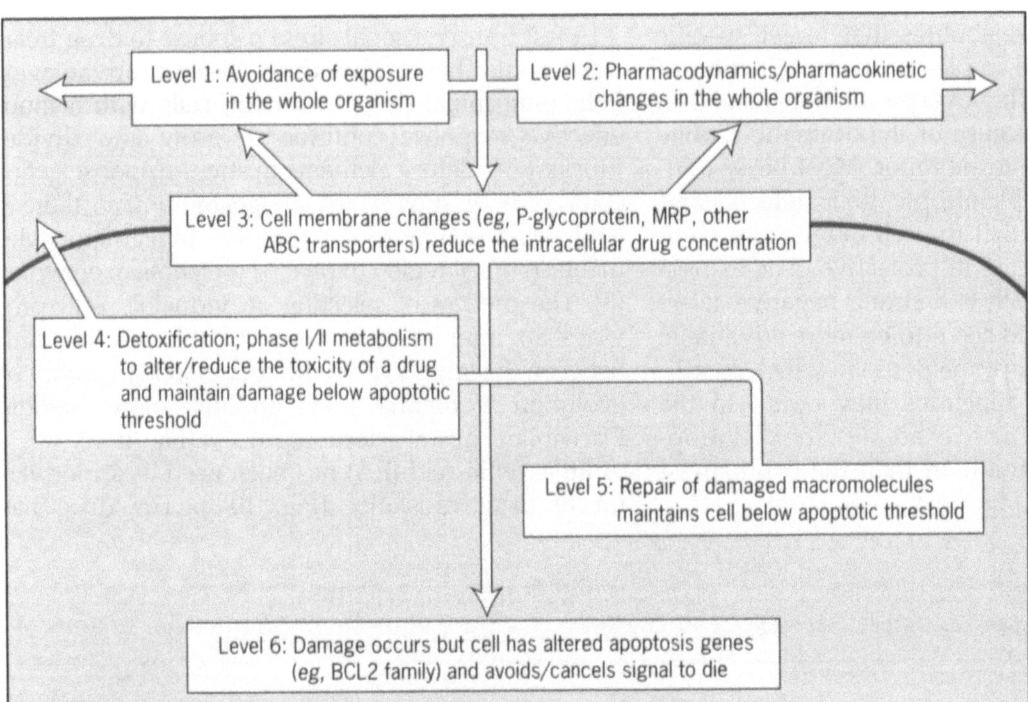

Figure 10-1. Factors influencing acquired resistance to drugs and xenobiotics.

Table 10-1. Drug resistance mechanisms for specific anticancer drugs

	Mechanism										
Drug Type	GSH/GST	Other altered phase I/II	MRP	MDR1 gene	Mer+ phenotype	Enhanced DNA repair	Topoisomerase I/II§§	Altered microtubules	Overexpressed or mutant target enzymes	Altered receptors	Altered expression of apoptosis genes
Nitrogen mustard	†	‡				†					†
Nitrosoureas	†				†	†					†
Platinums	†		†			†					†
Bleomycin	†	†				†					†
Anthracyclines	†		†	†		†	†		¶		†
Epipodophyllotoxins			†	†			†		¶		†
Antimitotics		§	†	†				†			†
Camptothecins						†	†		¶		†
Antifolates		†		*					†		†
Other antimetabolites		†		†					†		†
Retinoids		§	†							†	†
Steroids				†						†	†
Biological response modifiers										†	†

**P glycoprotein or other "drug transporters."*

†Mechanism identified for this drug type.

‡Cyclophosphamide resistance has been linked to different phase II enzymes.

§Some examples of these drugs are substrates for cytochrome P450.

§§Underexpression of topoisomerases.

¶Includes BCL2, Bax, NFκb, n-ras, MDM2, and so on.

MRP—multidrug-resistance protein; GSH—glutathione; GST—glutathione-S-transferase.

expressed. For antimetabolites that target specific enzymes, there are examples of overproduction of the target enzyme. This overproduction results in cellular protection because of the dramatic change in the ratio of target to inhibitor. Most other anticancer drugs have pleiotropic toxic effects, and there are indications that the cell mobilizes a similarly pleiotropic increase in protective gene expression. Because cell death is a strong negative selection force, there would seem to be more advantage in mounting a pleiotropic response in which coordination of protective functions may occur. In the majority of drug resistance examples, the pleiotropic response is more common than the overexpression of a specific gene product.

A fast transcriptional stress response to drug treatment could have significant selective advantages. Following initial drug treatment, cells with a more effective response continue to grow and divide. Efficient regulatory elements in stress-response genes could provide such an advantage. In humans, there is evidence of polymorphic expression of regulatory elements in the 5′ region of phase I metabolism enzymes [3]. The process of selecting an inducible trait provides an interesting example of the possible link between the largely discredited Lamarckian theory of evolution of organic traits and the more credible Darwinian natural selection process (Fig. 10-7).

Ethacrynic acid (EA) has been used as a modulator of drug resistance (Fig. 10-8). The drug has

Table 10-2. Drug resistance genes from the yeast protein database

Gene synonym	Protein	Cellular location	Comments
PDR1	Transcription factor	Nucleus	Has Zn-Cys binuclear cluster domain. PDR-dominant mutations give resistance to cycloheximide and oligomycin.
PDR3	Transcription factor	Nucleus	Related to PDR 1. Can be mutated to confer multidrug resistance. Has fos/jun DNA-binding homology domain.
PDR5	ABC transporter	Integral Plasma Membrane	Overexpression leads to cycloheximide, sulfomethyluron, and other drug resistance; properties similar to mammalian P-glycoproteins.
PDR6	Regulatory protein	?	Regulates proteins involved in membrane permeability.
PNT1	?	Membrane?	Has potential transmembrane domain. Overproduction causes resistance to pentamidine
ROD1	?	Particulate organelles	Overproduction linked with Ca:/Zn' and O-dinitrobenzene resistance.
STE6	ABC transporter	Integral plasma membrane	12 transmembrane domains. Homologous to P glycoprotein. Transports "mating factors."
YAP1	Transcription factor	Nucleus	Member of jun family; can bind API sites. Involved in oxidative stress response.
YBR 180W	Membrane transport facilitator	Integral membrane	12 predicted transmembrane domains.
YGR 138C	Putative drug transporter	Integral membrane	Similar to other fungal methotrexate resistance proteins.
YHR 048W	Membrane transport facilitator	Integral membrane	Similar to other fungal cycloheximide resistance proteins. Has ATP/GTP-binding site motif.
YNR 070W	?	Integral membrane?	
YOL 158C	Major facilitator superfamily	Integral membrane?	Homology with other resistance proteins.

ABC—ATP-binding cassette.

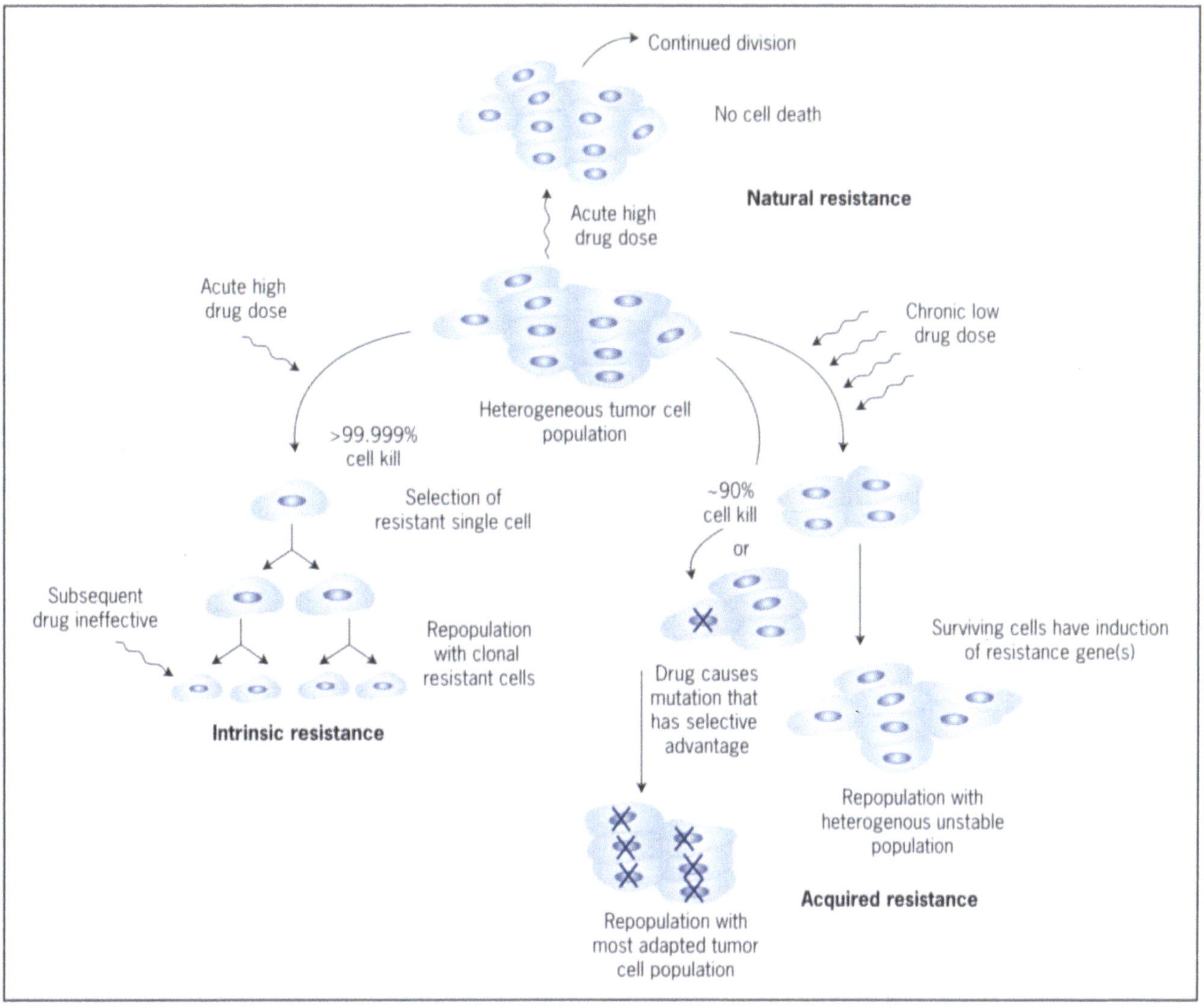

Continued division
No cell death
Natural resistance
Acute high drug dose
Acute high drug dose
Chronic low drug dose
Heterogeneous tumor cell population
>99.999% cell kill
Selection of resistant single cell
Subsequent drug ineffective
Repopulation with clonal resistant cells
Intrinsic resistance
~90% cell kill
or
Drug causes mutation that has selective advantage
Surviving cells have induction of resistance gene(s)
Repopulation with heterogenous unstable population
Acquired resistance
Repopulation with most adapted tumor cell population

Figure 10-2. Types of drug resistance.

Tumor cell burden
10^{12}
10^9
10^6
10^3
Treatment initiation
No treatment
1 cm
1mm
Average detectable mass
Remission
Regrowth
More chemotherapy
Chemo-resistant tumor
Failure
"Cure"
"Cure"
20
40
Time

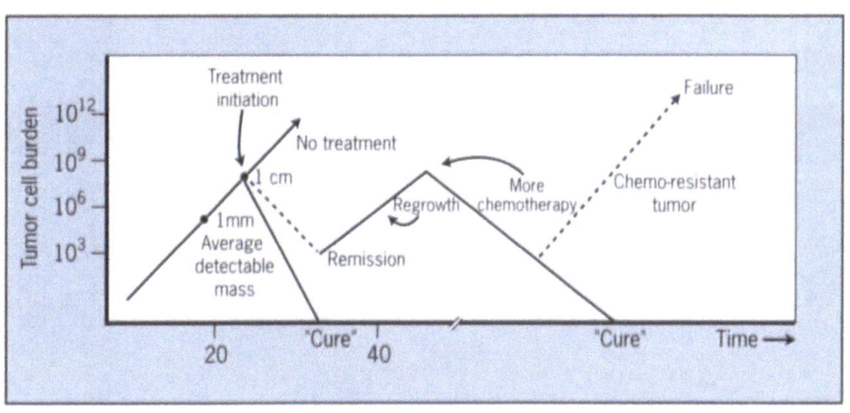

Figure 10-3. Detection and chemotherapeutic treatment of human cancer.

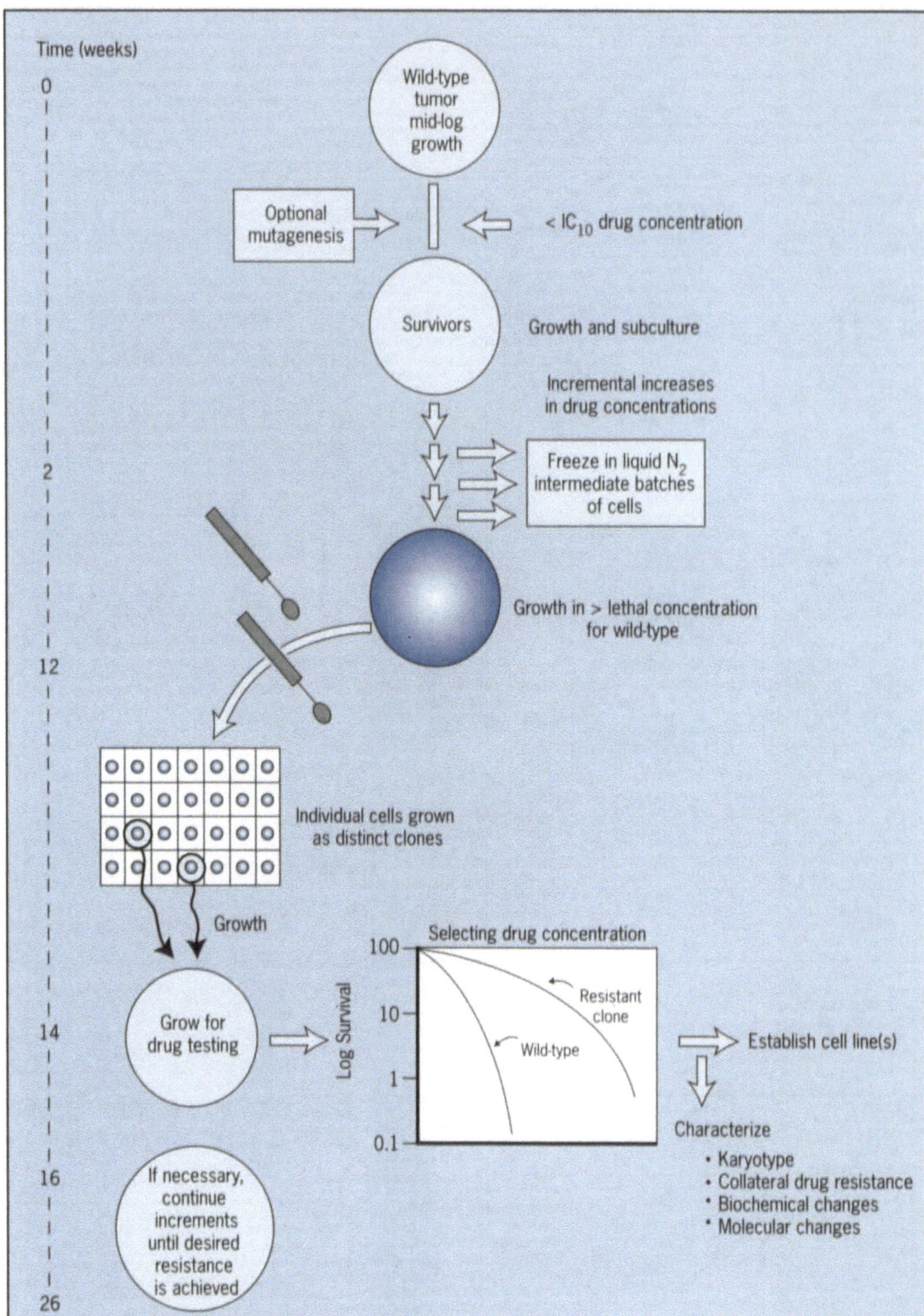

Figure 10-4. Strategy for the selection of drug-resistant cell lines.

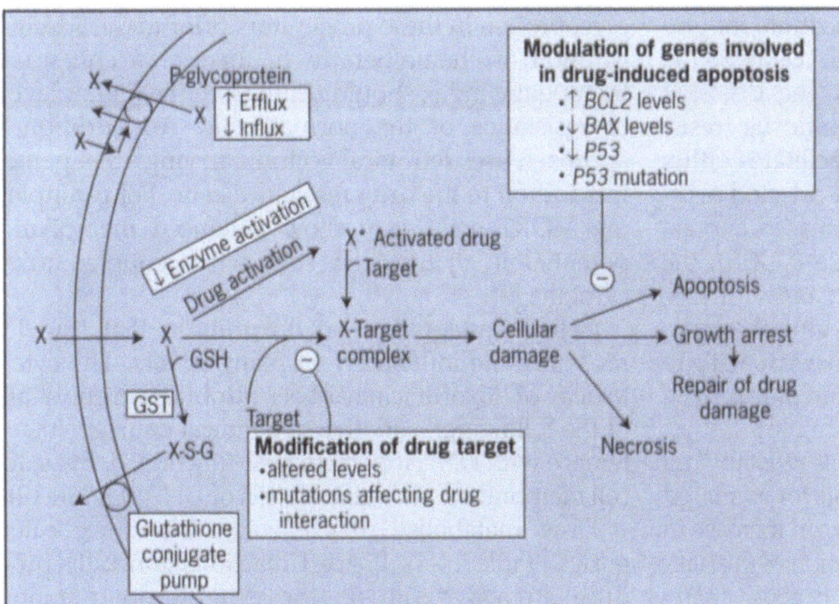

Figure 10-5. Various pathways by which mechanisms of resistance to anticancer agents can be expressed. *Asterisk* indicates active center. GSH—glutathione; GST—glutathione-S-transferase. (*Adapted from* Laing and Tew [1]; with permission.)

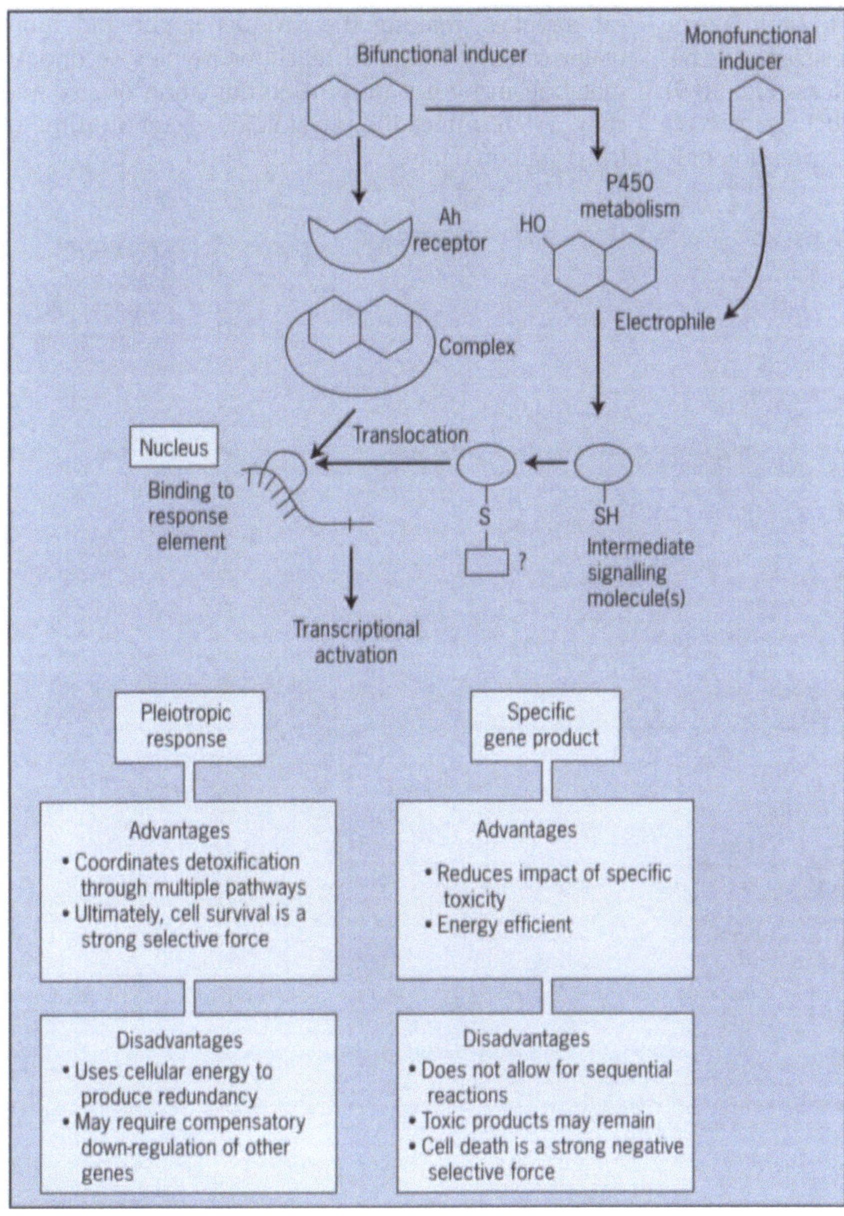

Figure 10-6. Gene induction and comparison of a specific versus pleiotropic response to drug exposure.

Michael addition chemistry and is a substrate for glutathione-S-transferases (GSTs), which catalyze its conjugation with glutathione (GSH). The EA-GSH conjugate is a substrate for the multidrug resistance–related protein (MRP), which facilitates efflux of the conjugate from the cell. In an EA-selected resistant cell line, there is a coordinate increased expression of γ-glutamyl cysteine synthetase (γGCS), the rate-limiting enzyme in de novo GSH biosynthesis; GSTπ, the enzyme that catalyzes the glutathionylation reaction; and MRP [4]. The cellular capacity to coordinate the metabolism and excretion of this drug results in a fivefold resistance to the drug [5].

Table 10-3 shows that in many drug-resistant cell lines, more than one mechanism accounts for increased levels of the gene product. For example, an increase in transcription can result from a prolongation of the half-life of both transcript and protein [6]. Because many housekeeping genes are unaffected, a selective effect seems to be limited to protective gene products.

Early clinical trials have attempted to capitalize on the principle of introducing drug resistance genes into hematopoietic stem cell progenitors (Fig. 10-9). Retroviral vectors carrying the *MDR1* gene have been used in an attempt to cause overexpression of P-glycoprotein in these progenitors prior to the administration of chemotherapy. In theory, an enhanced therapeutic index should result from the higher level of resistance of the normal cells. An additional approach uses retroviral vectors carrying other genes in addition to the drug resistance gene. For example, the *MDR1* gene may show enhanced therapeutic potential in cytotoxic T cells when coupled to a cytokine [7].

Cellular adaptations to doxorubicin that lead to resistance are influenced by many factors. The cytotoxicity of doxorubicin has been attributed to one or all of the following: oxidative free radical damage, interference with DNA topoisomerase function, damage to cell membranes, and intercalation of DNA (Fig. 10-10).

Drug metabolism reactions fall into three categories (Table 10-4). Phase I reactions generally produce an active site on the drug through minor changes in chemical structure. Phase II reactions frequently result from the attachment of bulkier chemical moieties, making the product larger and more water soluble. Phase III reactions involve secondary metabolism by gut flora. A combination of size and charge determines the physiologic excretion route of the drug conjugate.

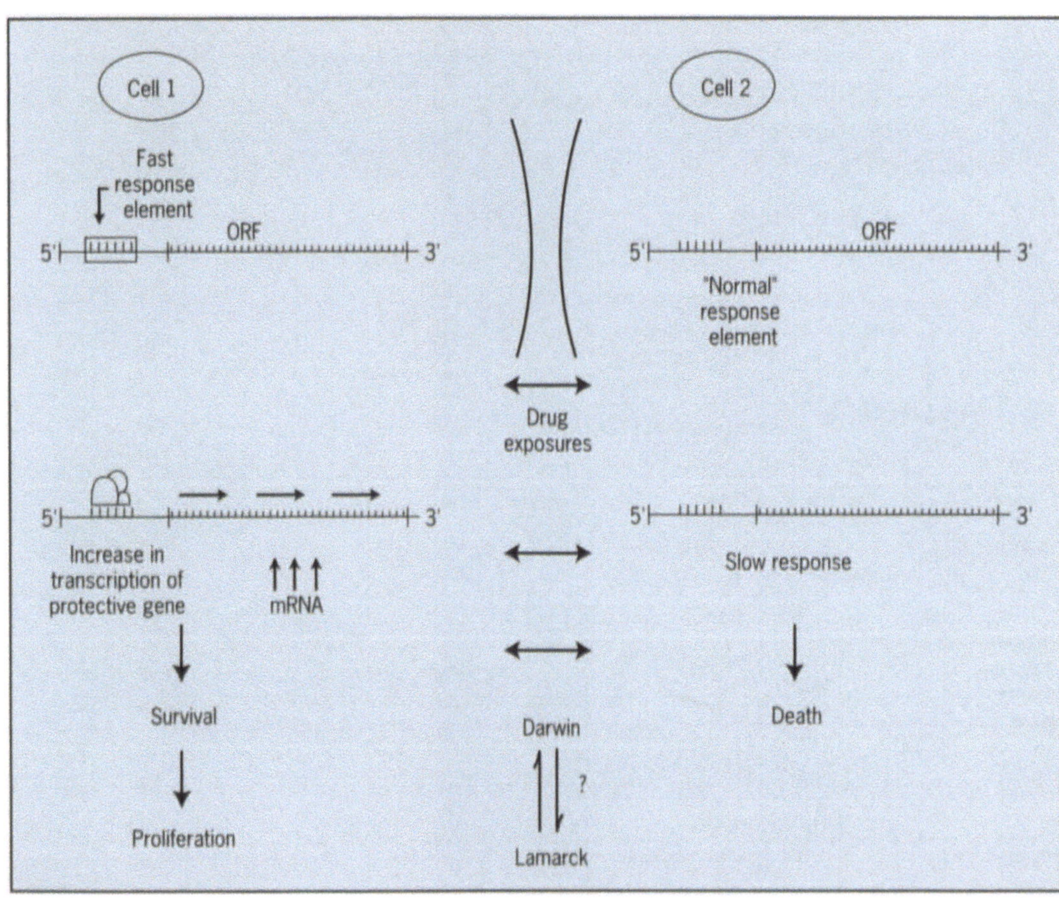

Figure 10-7. Selection of regulatory elements as a resistance mechanism.

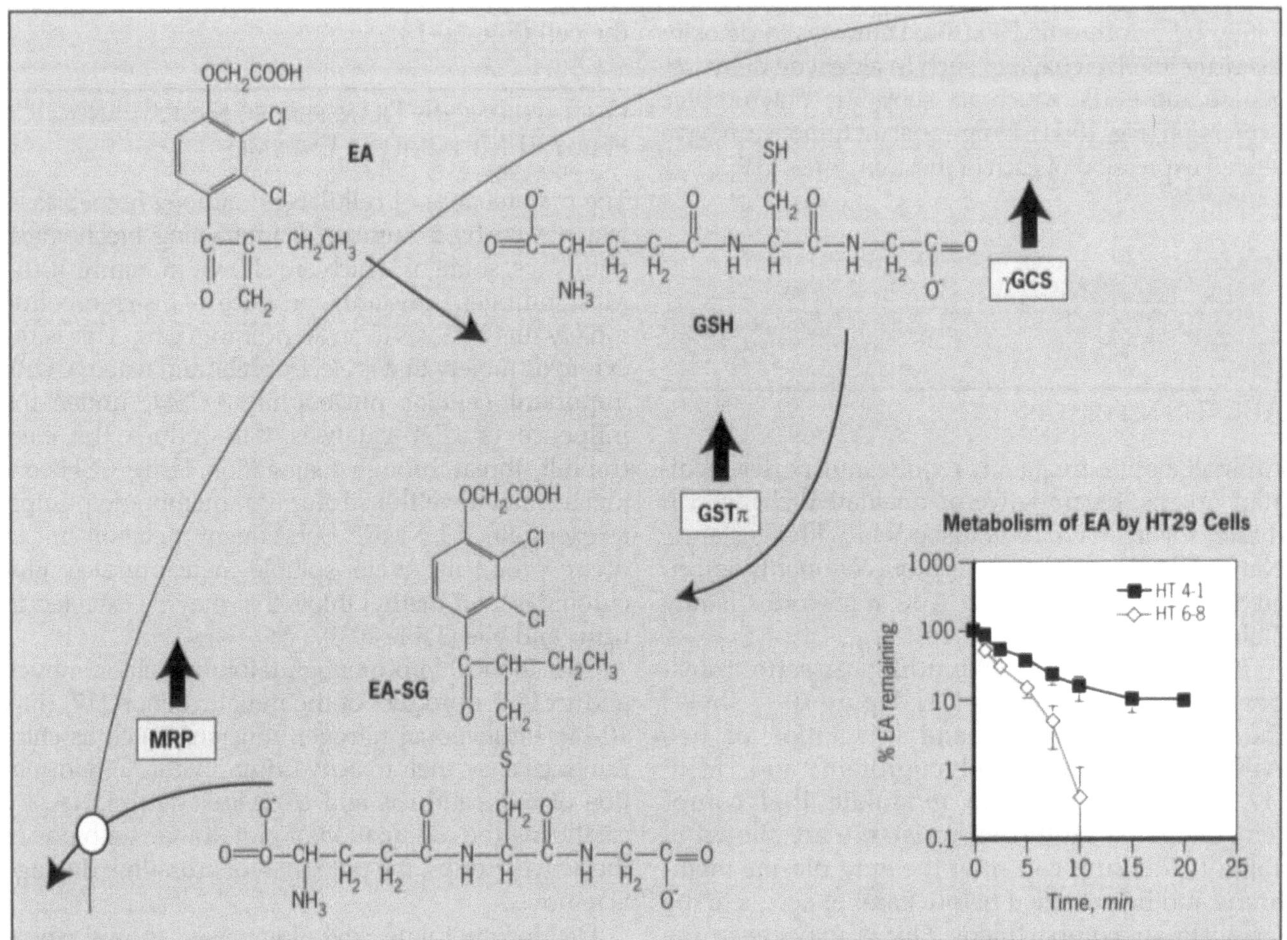

Figure 10-8. Coordinate gene regulation resistance to ethacrynic acid (EA). The cellular capacity to coordinate the metabolism and excretion of this drug (*inset*) results in a fivefold resistance to the drug (*Bars* indicate ± SEM). HT6-8 are resistant cells. γGCS— γ-glutamyl cysteine synthetase; GSH—glutathione; GST—glutathione-S-transferase; MRP—multidrug resistance–related protein; EA-SG—glutathione conjugate of EA.

Table 10-3. Transcripts overexpressed in EA-resistant HT-68 cell line

Gene product	Increase in mRNA	Transcript half-life, h (increase over WT)
Glutathione S-transferase π	Threefold	8.4 (twofold)
γ-Glutamylcysteine synthetase	Threefold	14.5 (twofold)
Multidrug resistance–related protein	Threefold	ND
Dihydrodiol dehydrogenase	20-fold	13.8 (sixfold)
NAD(P)H quinone oxidoreductase	Two to threefold	ND
SSP 3521 (putative transcription factor)	Two to threefold	ND
Glyoxalase-1	No change	ND
Glyceraldehyde-3-phosphate dehydrogenase	No change	11.7 (0.6-fold)
β-Actin	No change	7.9 (0.7-fold)
β-Tubulin	No change	8.7 (0.7-fold)

EA—ethacrynic acid; ND—not determined.

Cyclophosphamide is a prodrug that requires activation by cytochrome P4502B6. Pathways to detoxify the drug involve enzymes such as aldehyde dehydrogenase and GSTs, which are subject to polymorphic expression (Fig. 10-11). Drug-resistant tumors can have altered expression of each of these enzymes [8,9].

MECHANISMS OF DRUG RESISTANCE

ABC TRANSPORTERS

Antimetabolites frequently require transporter-mediated uptake. Quantitative or qualitative changes in these proteins have been associated with resistance. Natural product resistance is more commonly associated with members of the ABC transporter family (Table 10-5) [10].

Table 10-6 lists ATP-binding cassette transporters in human disease [11]. Figure 10-12 shows the predicted structure and orientation of two ABC transporters: P-glycoprotein and MRP [12,13]. Agents used to modulate P-glycoprotein–mediated multidrug resistance are shown in Table 10-7. Drugs can enter the lipid plasma membrane and be extruded before gaining access to the intracellular compartment. Drugs may reach the intracellular compartment, be returned to the lipid bilayer, and then be effluxed. Efflux is directly from the cytoplasm via P-glycoprotein to outside the cell (Fig. 10-13).

GLUTATHIONE-S-TRANSFERASE SYSTEM AND PHASE II METABOLISM ENZYMES

The maintenance of cellular glutathione homeostasis is achieved by a number of interacting biochemical pathways, some of which are shown in Figure 10-14. Most nitrogen mustards produce a bis-chloroethyl moiety that cyclizes to an aziridinium ring. This is the cytotoxic moiety that is electrophilic and reactive with important cellular nucleophiles. GSH, under the influence of GST catalysis, can reduce the electrophilic threat through conjugation. Drug–GSH conjugates may be effluxed through membrane pumps, as exemplified by MRP. Subsequent metabolism can occur, producing water-soluble mercapturates, glucuronides, and methyl thiols that may be excreted in urine and bile (Table 10-8).

The monochloro-monoglutathionyl chlorambucil adduct is the product of the initial reaction [17] (Fig. 10-14). Bifunctional nitrogen mustards such as chlorambucil exert their toxicity primarily through formation of monoadducts and cross-links with DNA. By catalyzing the conjugation of glutathione with one of the active groups, the potential for cross-link damage is removed.

Dichloromethane dehalogenase shows some homology with the human θ-class GST family. This enzyme is believed to be the early progenitor of the

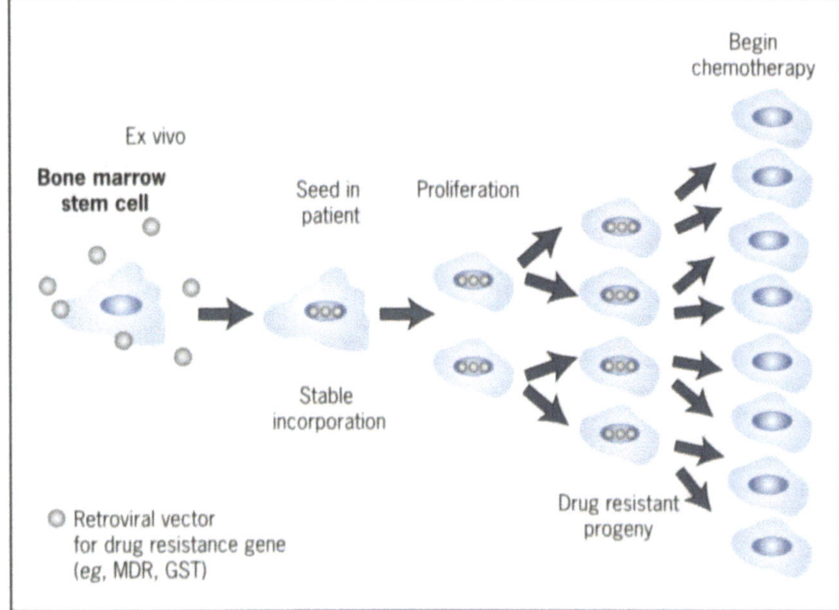

Figure 10-9. Gene therapy exploiting drug-resistance genes. MDR—multidrug resistance.

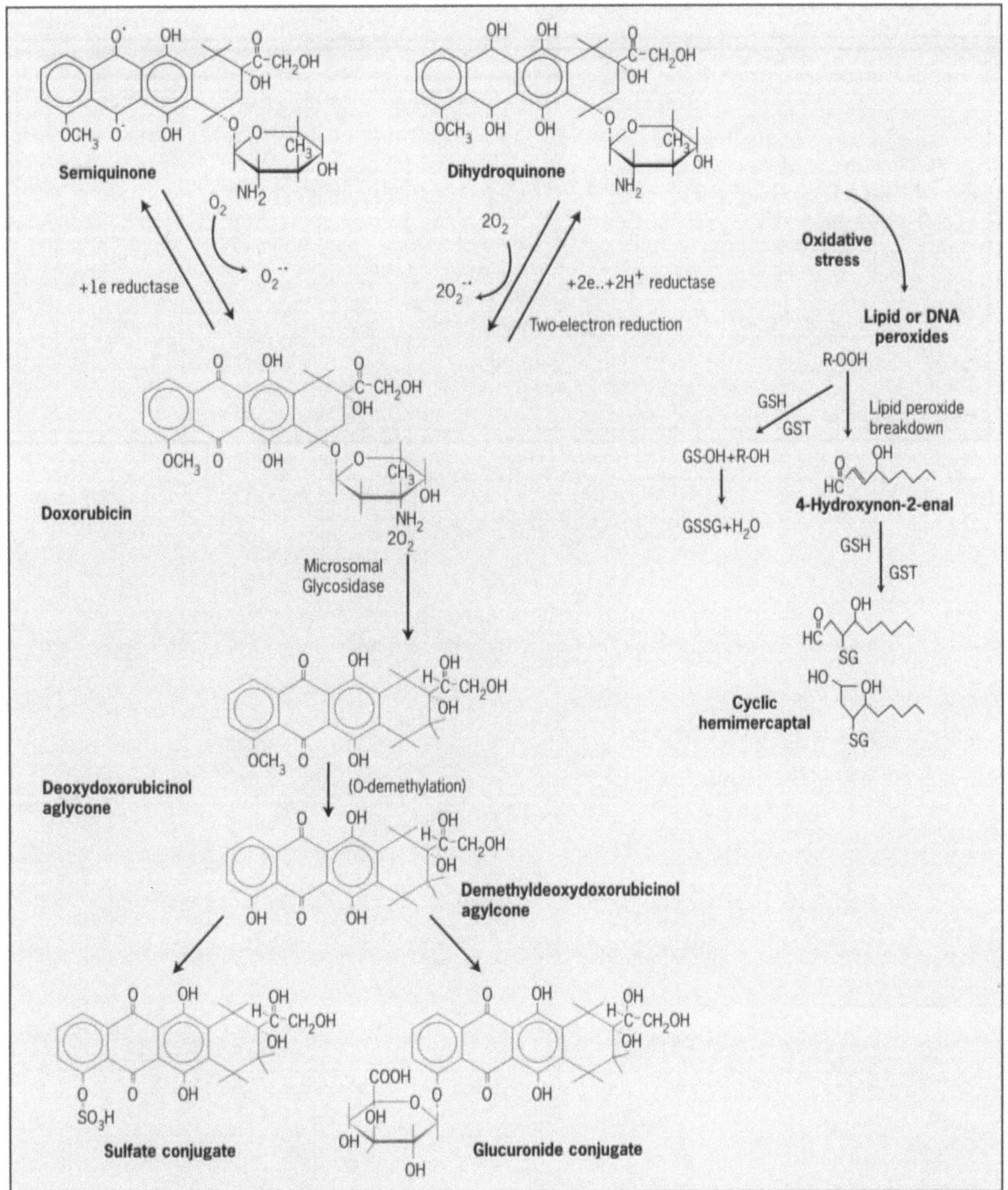

Figure 10-10. Doxorubicin as an example of multiple mechanism–mediated resistance. The metabolic pathway shows how each of these mechanisms may be affected and where cellular adaptations can lead to resistance; for example, direct DNA damage repair and topoisomerase II mediated damage; detoxification enzymes for oxidative stress; and other phase II metabolism. GSH—glutathione; GST—glutathione-S-transferase.

Table 10-4. Drug metabolism reactions

	Example reactions	
	Phase I	Phase II
Phase I: Small changes in drug structure, often producing a reactive functional group	Oxidation	Glutathionylation
Phase II: Conjugation reactions, usually influencing drug solubility	Reduction	Glucuronidation
Phase III: Secondary metabolism by gut flora	Hydrolysis	Sulfation
	Hydration	Acetylation
	Isomerization	Methylation
	(frequently cytochrome p450)	

Excretion routes for drugs		
Drug MW	Charge	Excretion route
300–500	+/-	Urine and/or bile
> 50	Uncharged or -ve	Bile
Phase II metabolite	-ve	Bile

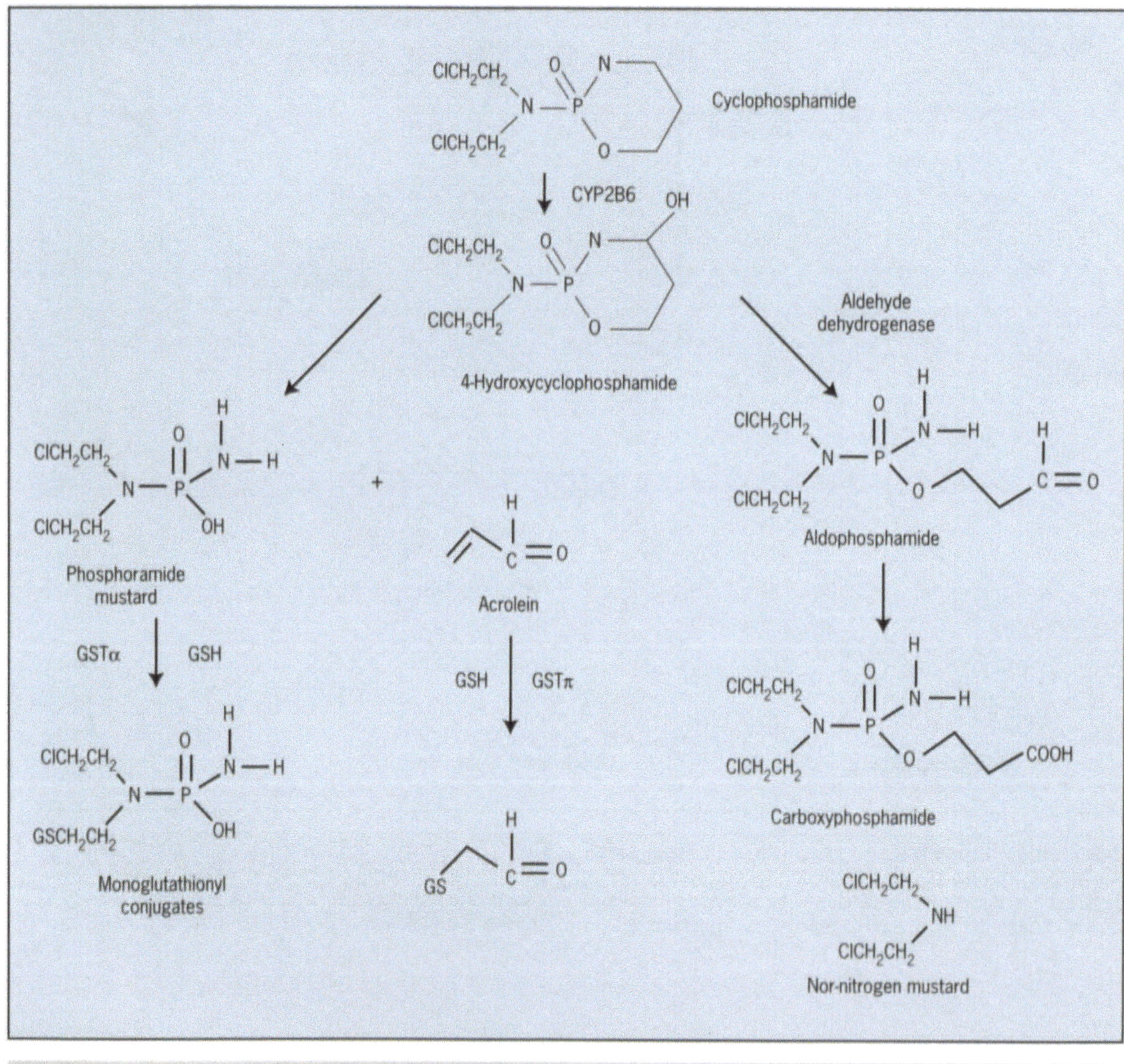

Figure 10-11. Cyclophosphamide activation and detoxification.

Table 10-5. Drugs affected by transporter resistance mechanisms

Antimetabolites	Natural products
Methotrexate	Anthracyclines
Cytosine arabinoside	Daunorubicin
6-Thioguanine	Doxorubicin
	Vinca alkaloids
	Vincristine
	Vinblastine
	Epidophyllotoxins
	Etoposide
	Teniposide
	Actinomycins
	Actinomycin D
	Taxanes
	Taxol
	Taxotere

Table 10-6. ATP-binding cassette transporters in human disease

Transporter name	Associated disease
ABC1	Tangier disease type 1
ABCR	Stargardt macular dystrophy
ABC7	X-linked sideroblastic anemia
MDR1	Anticancer drug resistance
MRP1	Anticancer drug resistance
MRP2	Dubin-Johnson syndrome
CFTR	Cystic fibrosis
SUR1	Familial persistent hyperinsulinemic hypoglycemia of infancy
ALDP	Adrenoleukodystrophy

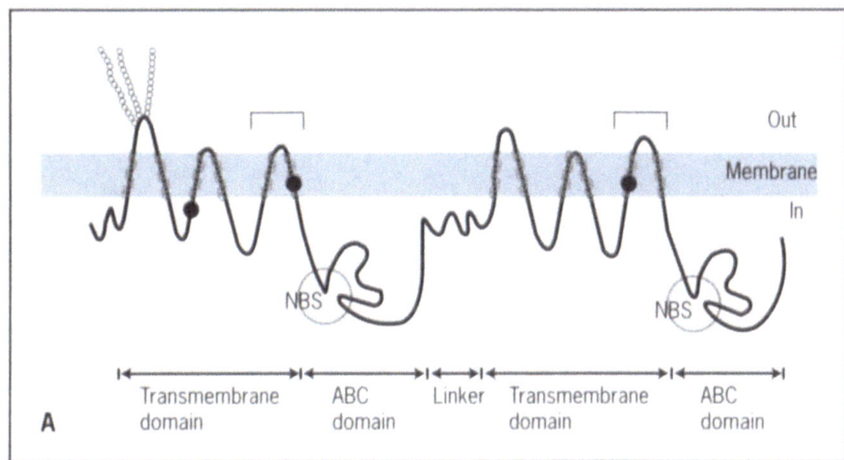

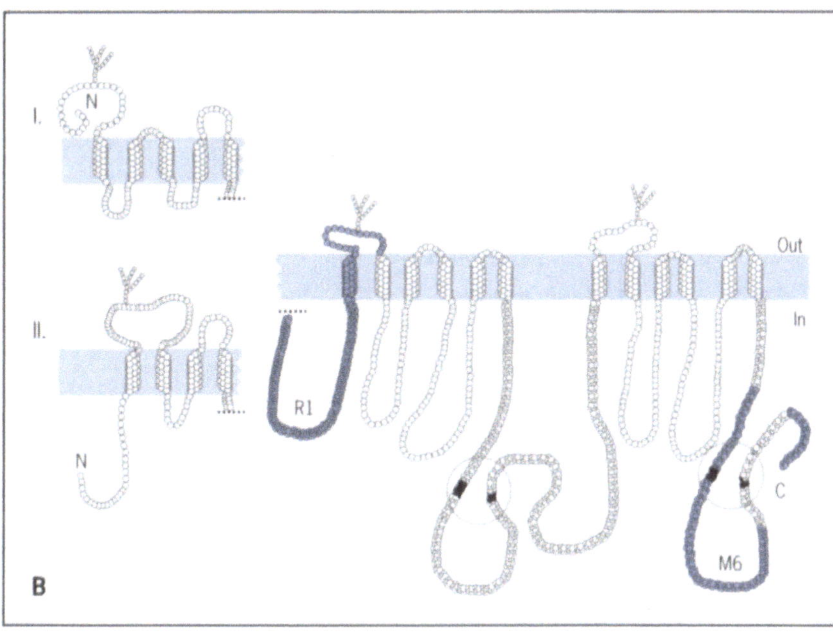

Figure 10-12. Predicted structure and orientation of two ABC transporters. **A,** The P-glycoprotein. *Chains* indicate the predicted N-linked glycosylation sites; *dots* indicate positions of the amino acid residues subject to mutations that alter the substrate specificity of P-glycoprotein. **B,** Human multidrug resistance–related protein (MRP). The numbers indicate alternative possibilities for the arrangement of transmembrane helices in the *N*-terminal membrane-bound domain. *Solid lines* indicate *N*-linked glycosylation sites; a possible extra glycosylation site is indicated by the *dotted line* [12,13]. NBS—nucleotide binding sites.

remaining GST family members [18]. Although many of the drugs listed in Table 10-9 can be conjugated to GSH, not all are substrates for GSTs. Initial treatments with a cancer drug at sublethal doses cause a stress response in the tumor cell. Subsequent rounds of treatment are blocked by the enhanced protective machinery. In principle, modulation uses a reasonable nontoxic drug in combination with the anticancer drug, and the modulator counteracts the cellular defense mechanism [14] (Fig. 10-15). A phase I

Table 10-7. Examples of modulators of the MDR phenotype

Agent class	Example
Calcium channel blockers	Verapamil; Dihydropyridines
Calmodulin inhibitors	Phenothiazines
Coronary vasodilators	Dipyridamole
Indole alkaloids	Reserpine
Quinolines	Quinine, Chloroquine
Acridines	Quinacrine
Benzylisoquinoline alkaloids	Cepharanthines
Lyosomotropic agents	Chloroquine, Monensin
Isoprenoids	Methylbenzyl-decaprenylamine
Steroids	Progesterone
Estrogen antagonists	Tamoxifen
Antibiotics	Cephalosporin
Anthracycline analogues	*N*-acetyl daunorubicin
Protein kinase inhibitors	Staurosporine
Immunosuppressive drugs	Cyclosporins
Diuretics	Amiloride analogues
Detergents	Triton X- I 00
Peptides	Various

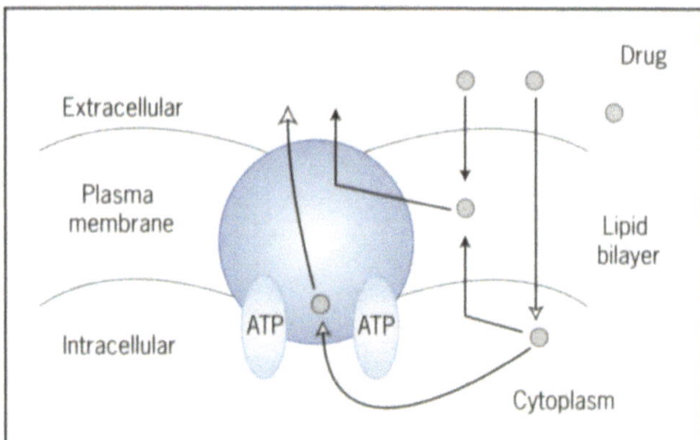

Figure 10-13. Possible drug efflux routes via membrane ABC transporters.

Table 10-8. Examples of drugs subject to GSH-based metabolism

Nitrogen mustards	Free radical damage
Chlorambucil	Anthracyclines
Melphalan	Radiation
Cyclophosphamide (phosphorarmide mustard/acrolein)	Ultraviolet light
Other alkylating agents	Peroxidative damage
Busulfan	Hydroxyalkenals
Thio-TEPA	Base propenals
Platinum drugs	DNA hydroperoxides
Nitrosoureas	Modulators
BCNU	Ethacrynic acid
CCNU	Ter 199
	Prodrugs
	Ter 286

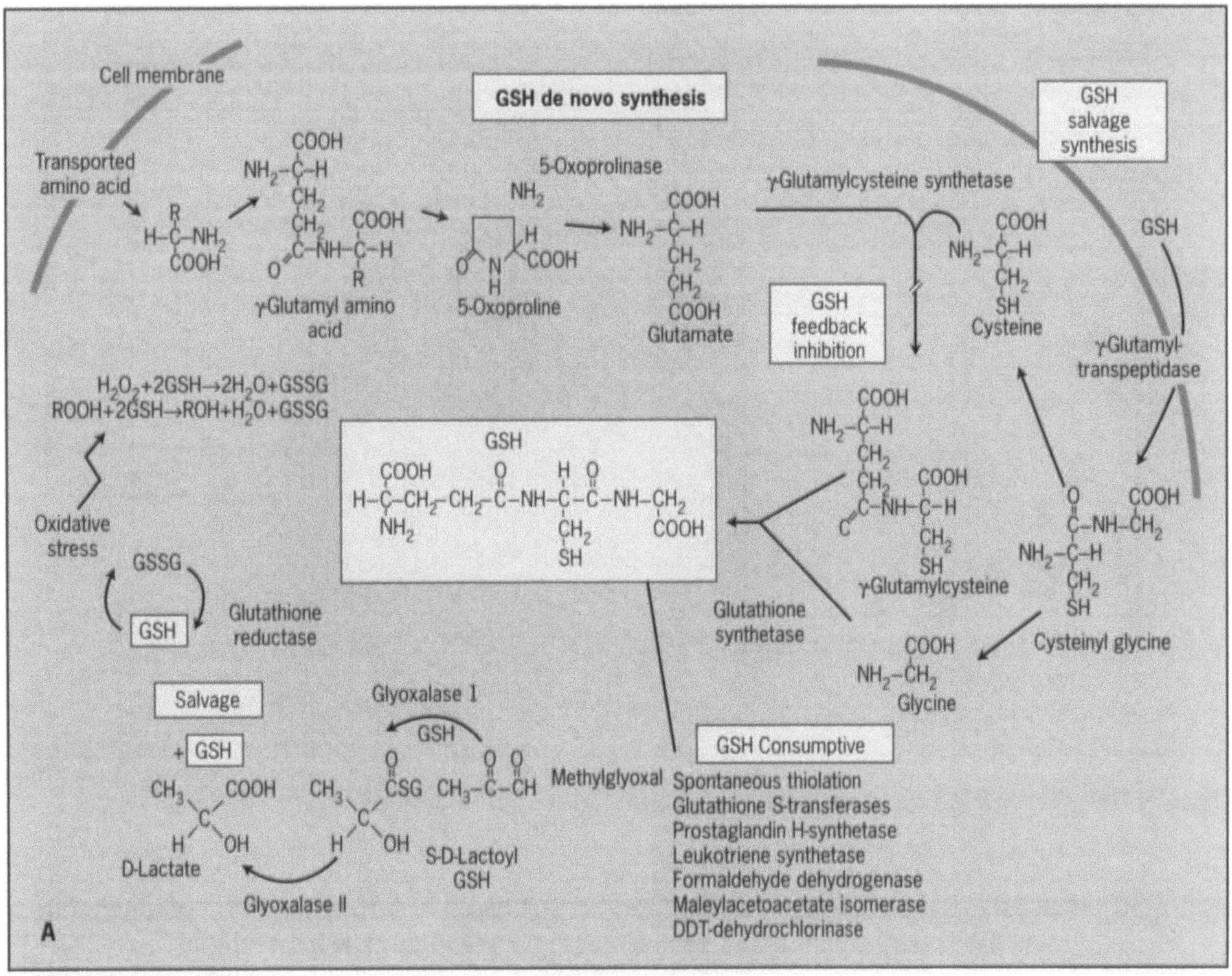

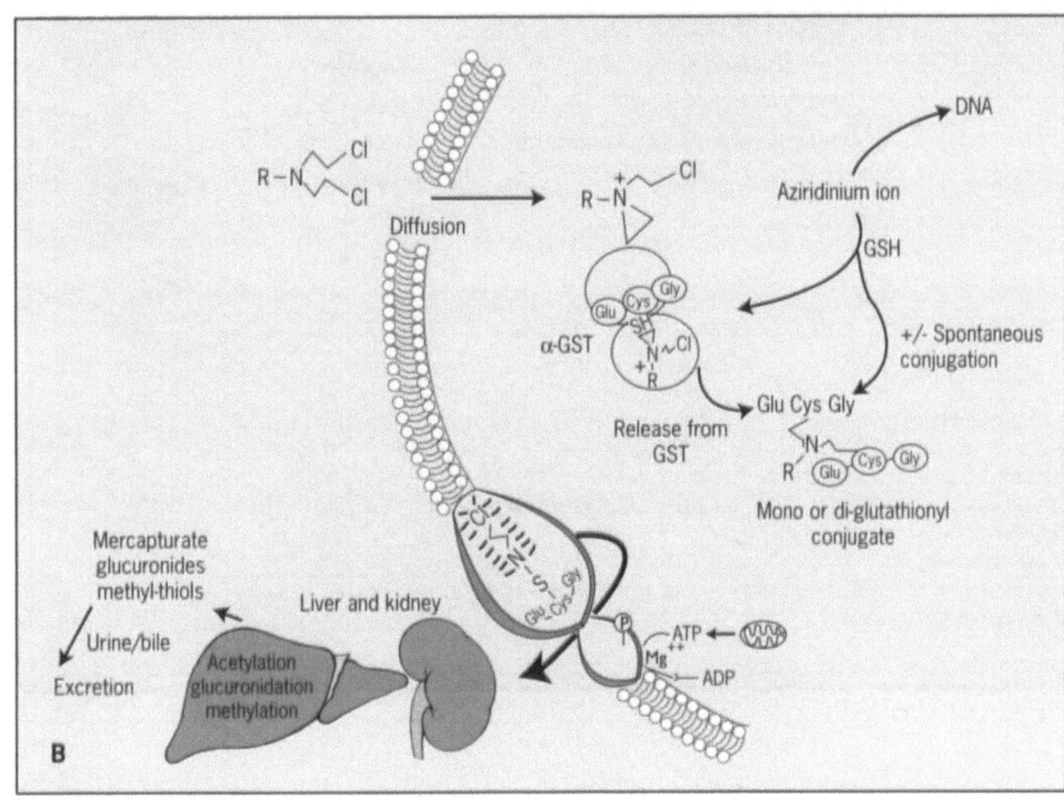

Figure 10-14. Glutathione S-transferase (GST)–catalyzed conjugation of glutathione (GSH) with chlorambucil. **A,** GSH de novo synthesis. **B,** Metabolic fate of alkylating species. Both the rate and extent of conjugate formation is increased in the presence of GST-α. This GST isozyme has the most efficient catalytic constant for the reaction [17]. (*continued*)

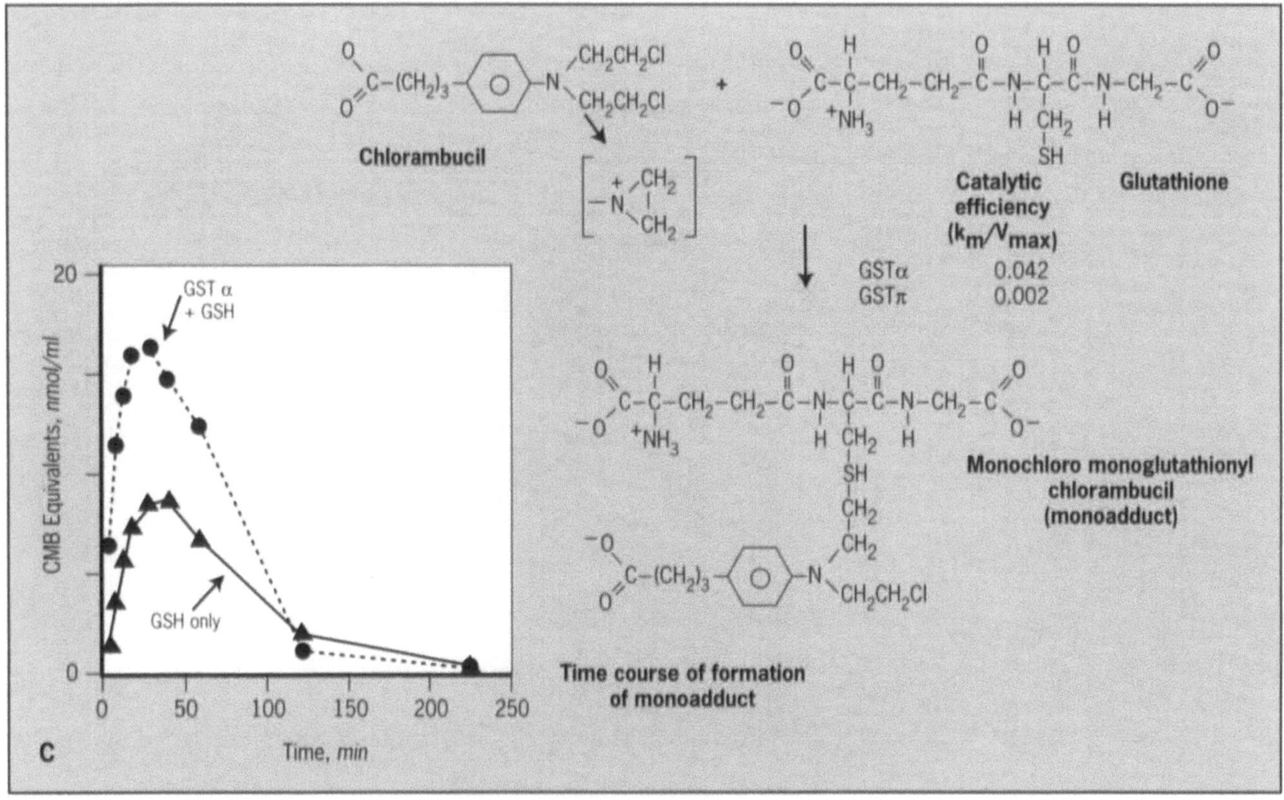

Figure 10-14. (*continued*) **C,** Time course of formation of monoadduct. GSH—glutathione.

Table 10-9. Anticancer drugs as substrates for glutathione S-transferases*

Convincing substrate/kinetic data exist	No definitive proof of catalysis exists	Indirect evidence exists†
Chlorambucil‡	Antimetabolites	Bleomycin
Melphalan‡	Antimicrotubule drugs¶	Hepsulfam
Nitrogen mustard‡	Topoisomerase I and II inhibitors	Mitomycin C
Phosphoramide mustard§,¶		Adriamycin
Acrolein¶		Cisplatin
Carmustine**		Carboplatin
Hydroxyalkenals††		
Ethacrynic acid		
Steroids‡‡		

**The catalyzed reaction is assumed to involve conjugation with glutathione (GSH) through thioether bond formation.*
†Indirect evidence can include low levels of resistance conveyed by transfection.
‡The aziridinium intermediate of the nitrogen mustards is the main GST substrate.
§The antimicrotubule drug estramustine is an inhibitor of GST, but there is no direct evidence that it iS 2 substrate.
¶Metabolites of cyclophosphamide.
***GST catalyzes a denitrosation of carmustine.*
††Most electrophilic anticancer drugs produce lipid peroxidation, degradation of which produces a variety of hydroxyalkenals.
‡‡GST can act as transporter ligands for some steroids.

clinical trial was carried out using EA as a modulator of the alkylating drug thiotepa [19]. The principle was that EA would influence the GSH-GST defense mechanism used to detoxify thiotepa. The appropriateness of the modulator was assessed by using peripheral mononuclear cells as a surrogate tissue. A decrease in GST activity was found following EA administration. The relevance of the approach was supported by data from patients with chronic lymphocytic leukemia. These patients initially respond to chlorambucil-containing drug regimens but frequently relapse after numerous cycles of therapy (Fig. 10-16). Analysis of lymphocytes from drug-resistant patients showed an elevation of GST activity [20], providing stimulus for the commencement of a phase II clinical trial.

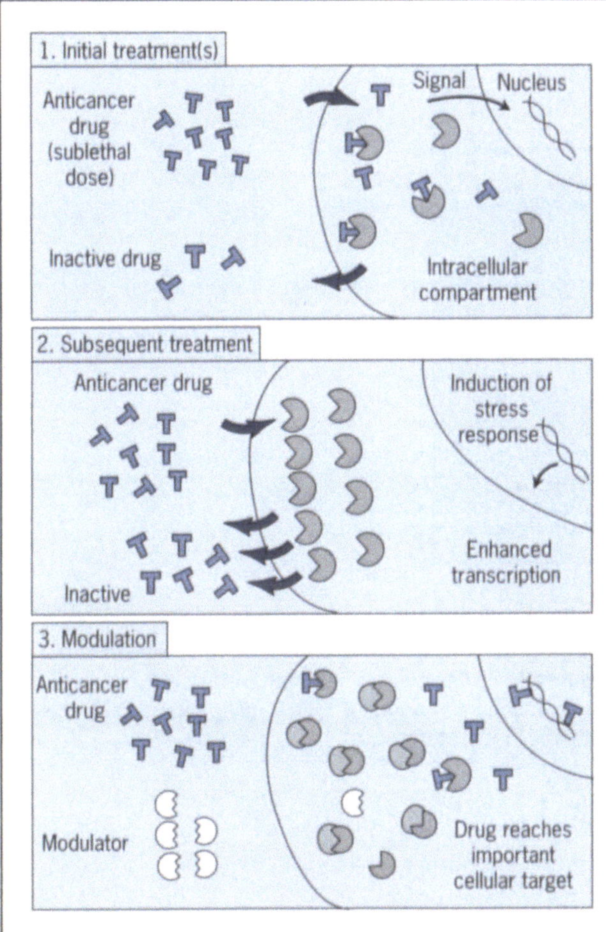

Figure 10-15. Principles of modulation of drug resistance. This model shows how cellular adaptations to initial drug treatment may result in increased drug target. Modulation confers the capacity to alter this target with a different second drug.

Ter 199 (Fig. 10-17; Table 10-7) is a second-generation drug resistance modulator [15]. The GST-mediated activation of a prodrug, Ter 286, is shown in Figure 10-18 [16]. Ter 286 was designed as a prodrug that can be activated by GSTπ. Because many tumors have elevated expression of GSTπ, the underlying premise behind drug design was that some enhancement in therapeutic index may be achieved in a tumor that activates more drug than does the corresponding normal tissue. Mechanistically, active chloroethylating moieties are released by proton abstraction at the tyrosine active site of GSTπ, and these moieties have antitumor properties [16].

Many tumor cells can activate DNA damage repair pathways [21] and express resistance (Table 10-10). Two of the most common pathways are direct base excision and nucleotide excision repair. Although enhanced repair can account for drug resistance, the majority of the drugs listed have also been associated with other resistance mechanisms discussed elsewhere in this chapter.

Complexity and redundancy are hallmarks of genes that control DNA integrity. Many of the genes listed in Table 10-11 are defective in a variety of human genetic diseases. Not all are involved in the damage repair pathways that are linked with drug resistance.

Recognition, excision, and repair of a typical intrastrand cross-link is shown in Figure 10-19. This mechanism is also effective in protecting against other drugs that cause intrastrand cross-links, providing a broader range of drug resistance.

DNA Repair Mer Phenotype

Alkylation of guanine by methylating, ethylating, or chloroethylating agents is shown in Figure 10-20. The base excision scheme complements a similar type of repair carried out by O^6-alkylguanine transferase, or the so-called "Mer" phenotype. The Mer phenotype has been most extensively characterized in nitrosourea-resistant cells. Early animal testing at the National Cancer Institute predicted nitrosoureas would be an extremely active class of drugs in mouse tumor models. Mouse tumors were later found to be deficient in O^6-alkylguanine transferase, a factor that contributes to their chemosensitivity. Unfortunately, a large number of human tumors have significant levels of this enzyme, making the nitrosoureas less therapeutically effective. Chapter 7 provides more details regarding DNA repair.

Both preclinical and clinical studies are underway using modulators of O^6-alkylguanine transferase. The end result is that the initial methyl guanine is removed

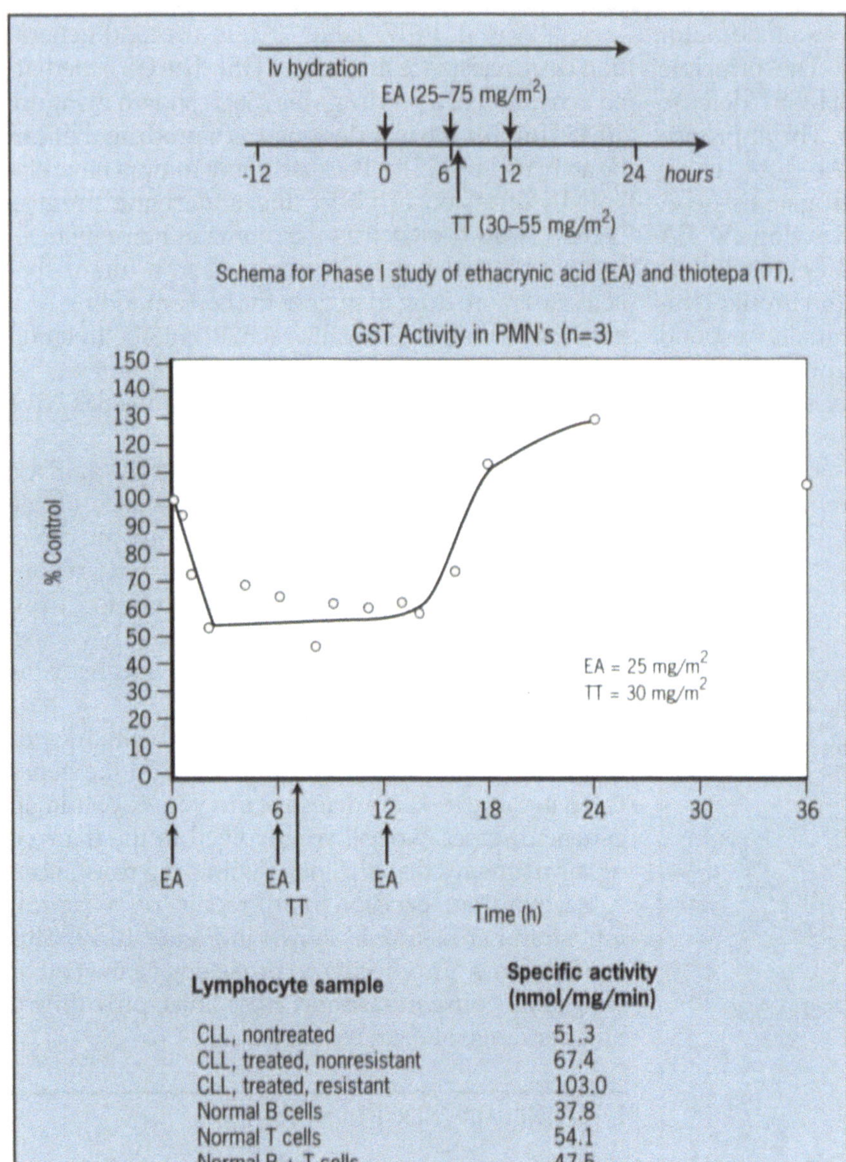

Lymphocyte sample	Specific activity (nmol/mg/min)
CLL, nontreated	51.3
CLL, treated, nonresistant	67.4
CLL, treated, resistant	103.0
Normal B cells	37.8
Normal T cells	54.1
Normal B + T cells	47.5

Figure 10-16. Clinical modulation protocol using ethacrynic acid (EA). **A**, Drug schedule. **B**, Effects of EA on GST activity in peripheral mononuclear cells. **C**, GST activity in lymphocytes of patients (normal or CLL). TT—thiotepa.

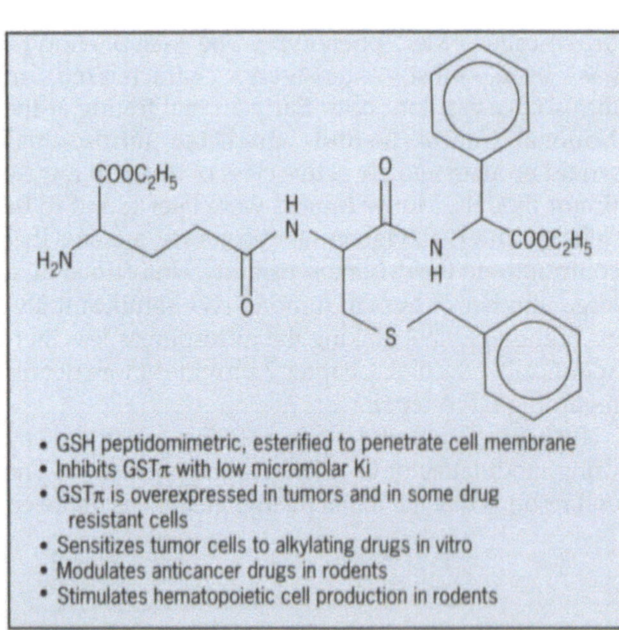

- GSH peptidomimetric, esterified to penetrate cell membrane
- Inhibits GSTπ with low micromolar Ki
- GSTπ is overexpressed in tumors and in some drug resistant cells
- Sensitizes tumor cells to alkylating drugs in vitro
- Modulates anticancer drugs in rodents
- Stimulates hematopoietic cell production in rodents

Figure 10-17. Structure of Ter 199, a second-generation drug-resistance modulator. GSH—glutathione; GST—glutathione-S-transferase.

by the enzyme, resulting in suicide inactivation. This then permits a cross-link to form from the carmustine treatment. This cross-link is the cytotoxic event that eventually gains therapeutic advantage [22] (Fig. 10-21).

TOPOISOMERASES

Drugs affected by topoisomerase-mediated resistance mechanisms are listed in Table 10-12, and topoisomerase I interactions with DNA are shown in Figure 10-22.

Topoisomerase I becomes covalently linked to the 3′ DNA terminus, whereas the 5′ DNA terminus has a hydroxyl moiety. DNA breakage and relaxation results as a consequence of the formation of the cleaveable complex. Drugs such as camptothecin trap the cleaveable complex and cause direct protein DNA adducts. Additional DNA damage results from the

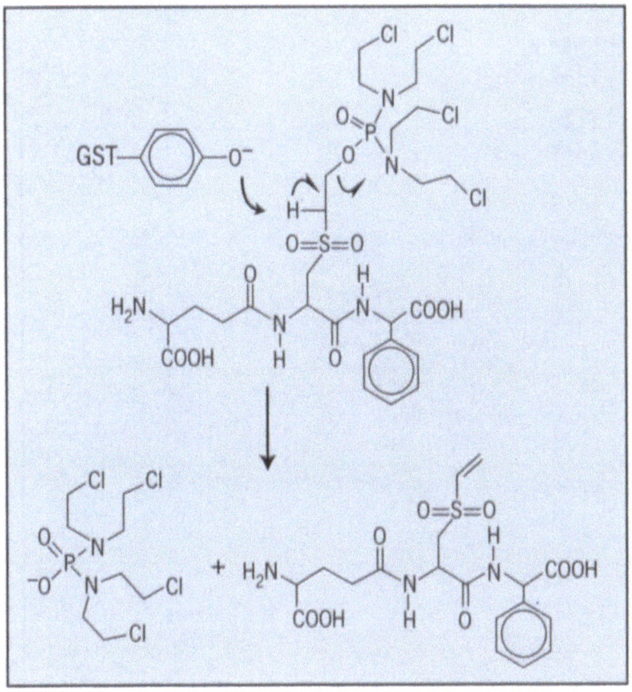

Figure 10-18. Activation of Ter 286, a glutathione-S-transferase (GST)-activated alkylating agent prodrug.

Table 10-10. Anticancer drugs and DNA repair pathways

Drug class	Main cytotoxic lesion	Main repair pathway involved in resistance
Cisplatinum	Monoadducts and inter/intrastrand crossings	Nucleotide excision repair
Nitrogen mustards Chlorambucil, melphalan	Interstrand crosslinks	Nucleotide excision repair
Procarbazine, dacarbazine	Monofunctional alkylations	Base excision repair or suicide thiol exchange (Mer phenotype)
Nitrosoureas	Interstrand crosslink ≠ methylation monoadducts	Nucleotide excision repair or suicide thiol exchange (Mer phenotype)
Carmustine		
Streptozotocin		
Bleomycin	Apurinic sites/strand breaks (maybe double strand breaks)	Base excision repair (site specific recombination)
Free radicals from anthracyclines (quinones)	Base hydroperoxides	Base excision repair
Topoisomerase I poisons	Protein–DNA "adduct" ≠ DNA strand breaks	Base excision repair
Topoisomerase II poisons	Protein–DNA adduct ≠ DNA strand breaks	Base excision repair

Table 10-11. Human genes involved in DNA repair and metabolism

Gene	Function
0^6AGT (MGMT)	0^6-methyl guanine methyltransferase
LIG	DNA ligase
APE (REF-1, HAP1)	AP endonuclease and redox regulator of transcription activation by AFT/CREB, AP-1,and NF-κB
UNGI	Uracil DNA glycosylase
TDG	G/T mismatch-specific glycosylase to repair the 5-methyl-dC deamination product
AAG (ANPG, MPG)	3-methyl-adenine DNA glycosylase active in base excision repair
XPAC	NER damage recognition factor, Zn^{2+}-finger DNA binding protein that interacts with RPA
ERCC1	Complexes with ERCC4; homolog of yeast Rad IO
ERCC2	NER 5′-3′ helicase, defective in XPD and TTD
ERCC3	NER 3′-5′ helicase, defective in XPD and TTD
ERCC4	NER 5′ endonuclease
ERCC5	NER 3′ endonuclease
ERCC6	Defective in Cocayne's syndrome, a chromatin remodeling activator homolog of SWI/SNF with ATP-dependent helicase activity
CSA	Defective in Cocayne's syndrome, a WD-repeat protein that interacts with CSB protein and TFIIH of RNA pol II
XPCC	NER-genome overall repair, protein product interacts with pHHR23A and B
HHR23A	Single-strand DNA binding protein with ubiquitin-like N-terminus
HHR23B	Single-strand DNA binding protein with ubiquitin-like N-terminus
PCNA	Auxiliary factor for DNA pol δ required for NER
RPA1, 2, and 3	Three-subunit single-strand binding protein required for NER
hMSH2	Mismatch binding protein defective in Lynch's syndrome
GTBP	Heterodimeric partner of hMSH2 protein
hMLH1	Mismatch correction factor
hPMS1	*MutL* homolog
hPMS2	*MutL* homolog required for proper chromsomal synapsis in meiosis
MSH3 (Duc-1 MRP1)	Homolog of yeast *Msh3*
PMSR1-5	Gene family of *hPMS2* homologs
HRAD51	*Esherichia coli* RecA homolog, searches for homology between two DNA double-strands and promotes strand transfer
XRCCI	Single-strand DNA break repair required for DNA ligase III activity
XRCC2	Double-strand break repair
XRCC3	Single-strand DNA break rejoining and replication repair
XRCC5	DNA-end binding protein, Ku86, required for double-strand break repair and recombination
Ku70	Heterodimer partner of Ku86
XRCC7	DNA-PK_{cs} and PI-3 kinase required for double-strand break repair and recombination
FACC	Mutated in Fanconi's anemia, a disorder associated with defective repair of DNA crosslinks
RECQL	Rec Q DNA helicase homolog
BLM	Mutated in Bloom's syndrome, a genetic hyper-recombination disorder coupled with apparent DNA repair proficiency, BLM protein is a DNA helicase
TOP3	DNA topoisomerase III, putative suppressor of mitotic recombination, yeast TOP3, and SGS1 proteins physically interact
WRN	Defective in Werner's syndrome, a premature aging disorder, the protein product is a DNA helicase
ATM	PI-3 kinase involved in signal transduction, meiotic recombination, and cell cycle control
TP53	Facilitator of NER via interactions with TFIIH of RNA pol II, C-terminus of p53 protein mediates DNA renaturation and strand transfer

Adapted from Carothers [21].

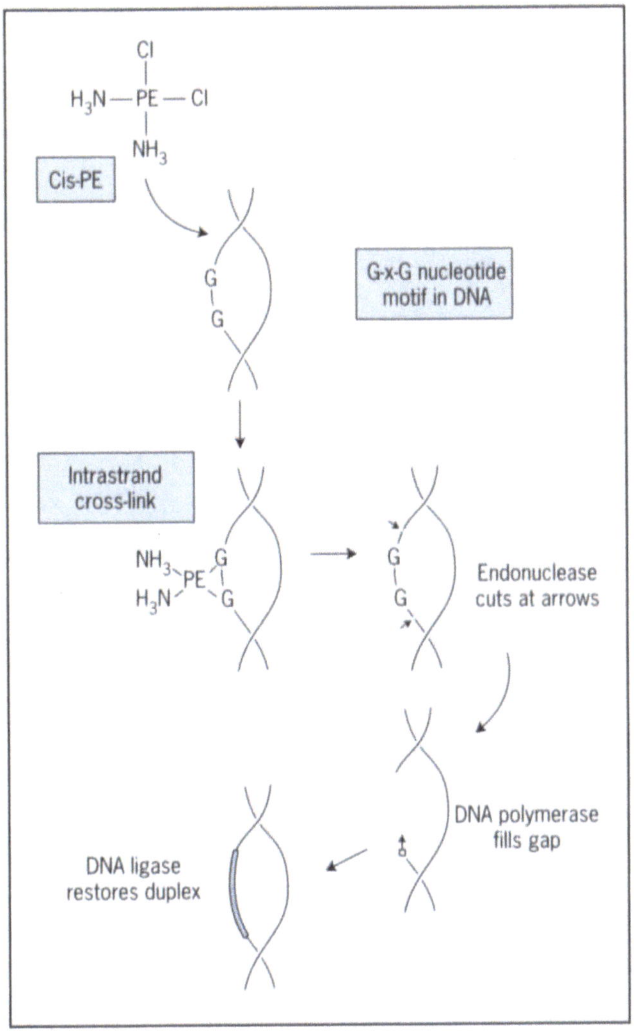

Cl
$H_3N—PE—Cl$
NH_3
Cis-PE
G
G
G-x-G nucleotide motif in DNA
Intrastrand cross-link
NH_3 PE G
H_3N G
G
G
Endonuclease cuts at arrows
DNA polymerase fills gap
DNA ligase restores duplex

Figure 10-19. Nucleotide excision repair following intrastrand cross-link formation by cisplatin.

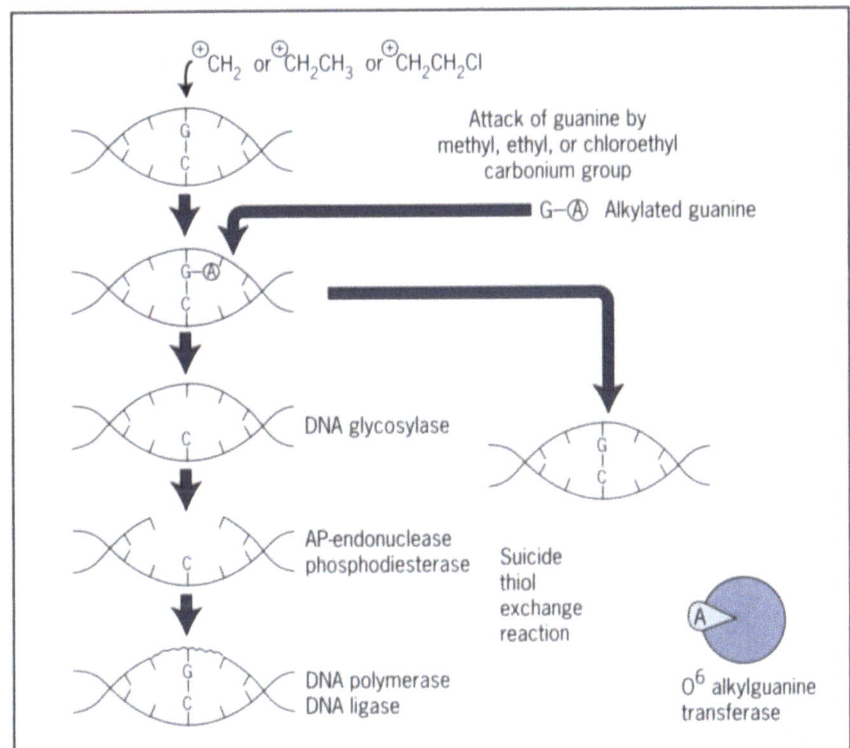

Figure 10-20. Steps in DNA base excision repair.

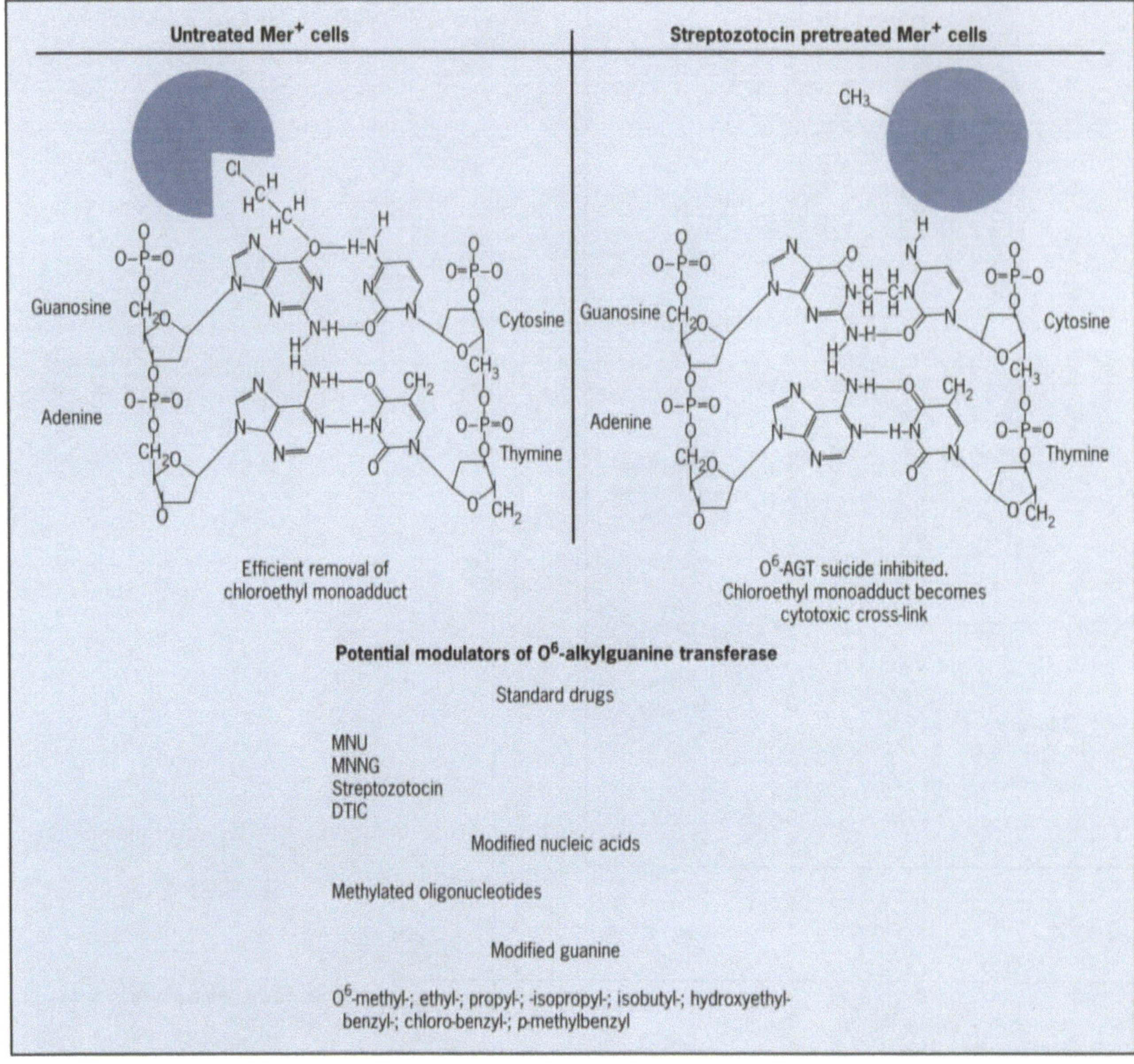

Figure 10-21. Modulation of the "Mer" phenotype. **Left**, Untreated Mer$^+$ cells. **Right**, Streptozotocin-pretreated Mer $^+$ cells.

Table10-12. Drugs affected by topoisomerase-mediated resistance mechanisms

	Topoisomerase I		
	Camptothecin	Topotecan	
	9-Aminocamptothecin	Irinotecan	
	Topoisomerase II		
Doxorubicin	Daunomycin	Etoposide	mAMSA
Daunorubicin	Mitoxantrone	Teniposide	

artifactual presence of the enzyme-DNA complex within the nucleic acid structure. In addition to DNA damage repair, other resistance mechanisms may involve downregulation of topoisomerase I or expression of mutant topoisomerase I with lowered affinity for the drug [23].

Although similar to topoisomerase I, the polarity of the enzyme DNA attachment is reversed for topoisomerase II. Resistance to topoisomerase II poisons has been shown to be a function of the following factors [23,24]: quantitative decreases in topoisomerase II expression, production of splice variants of topoisomerase II with different activities, increase in phosphorylation of topoisomerase II, and specific point mutations leading to the conversion of arginine residues at positions 449, 486, or 493 to glutamine (Fig. 10-23).

Antimitotic Drug Resistance

Drugs with reported antimitotic activity are listed in Table 10-13. The cellular morphology associated with resistance to antimitotic drugs [26-28] is shown in Figure 10-24. Microtubules associated with the centromeres of chromosomes are particularly sensitive to antimitotic drugs. The *arrowheads* in the inset of Figure 10-24 show the connection between spindle microtubules and chromosome centromeres. Antimitotic drug-resistant cells frequently maintain viable connections between the spindle and the chromosome, which in some cases can be shortened. Drug-sensitive cells may lose the integrity of this connection [27,28].

The adaptations listed in Table 10-14 have been reported in different antimitotic drug-resistant cell lines. Not all of these adaptations have been found in all cells studied.

Antifolate Resistance

Methotrexate is a primary example of the classic antifolate drug where resistance has been associated with each of the adaptations shown in Table 10-15 to achieve resistance [29]. The specific adaptation is generally contingent on the selection conditions. For example, incremental increases in concentrations of

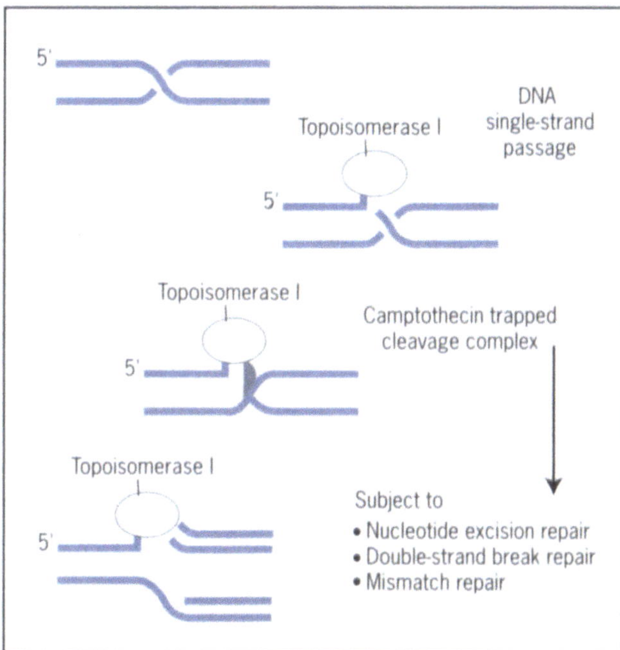

Figure 10-22. Topoisomerase I interactions with DNA.

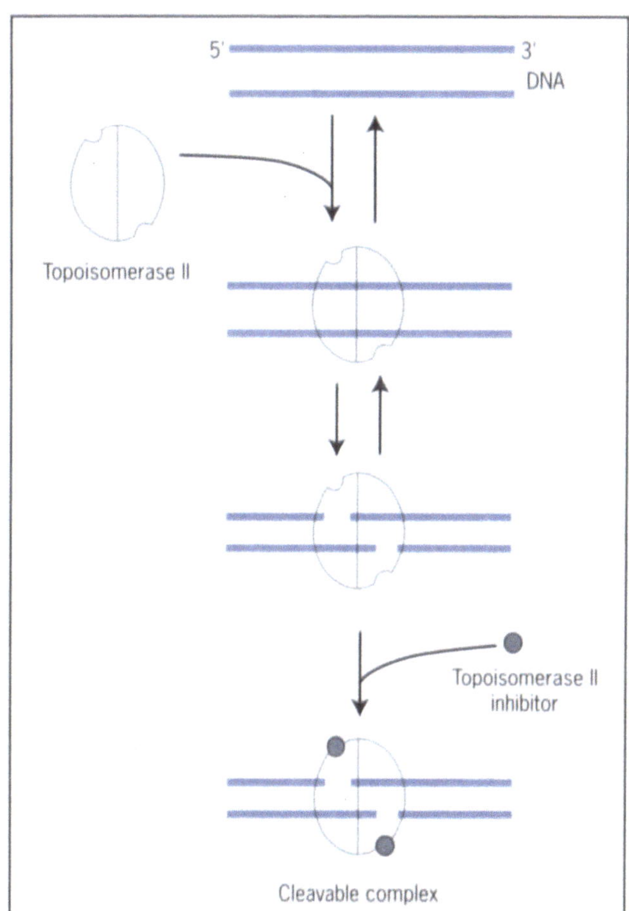

Figure 10-23. Topoisomerase II inhibitors trapping the enzyme–drug–DNA- cleavable complex formation.

drugs reaching high doses frequently yield dihydrofolate reductase overexpression. Shorter, repetitive treatments frequently produce polyglutamylation mutants. Single-step selections (low concentrations) generally produce transport mutants. At least one clinical correlation shown in resistant human leukemia cells has shown a loss of folypolyglutamate synthetase (FPGS) activity in the resistant cells.

Amplification of genes has been correlated with resistance to a diverse range of anticancer drugs and other toxins. Resistance to antimetabolites such as those listed in Table 10-16 results in a high frequency of gene duplication for target enzymes [30]. Many of these adaptations have been covered in detail in Chapter 1.

Altered Apoptotic Threshold

A partial listing of gene families that have been linked to induction and inhibition of apoptosis, and by

Table 10-13. Drugs with reported antimicrotubule activities

Benzimidazole carbamate(s)	Griseofulvin
Chalcones	Isopropyl-*N*-phenylcarbamate
Chlorpromazine	Maytansine
Coichicine/colcemid (colchicum alkaloids)	Nocodazole
Combretastatin	Podophyllotoxin derivatives
Cyclohexyl isocyanate and 2,4-dichlorobenzyl thiocyanate	Rhizoxin
Diethylstilbestrol	Rifampicin
Dihydropyridopyrazine(s)	Rotenone
Diphenylpyridazine derivatives	Steganacin
Dolastatin(s)/phomopsin A	Tubulozole
Ergot derivatives (ergocryptine/bromocryptine)	Taxol
Estramustine	Vincristine/vinblastine (vinca alkaloids)

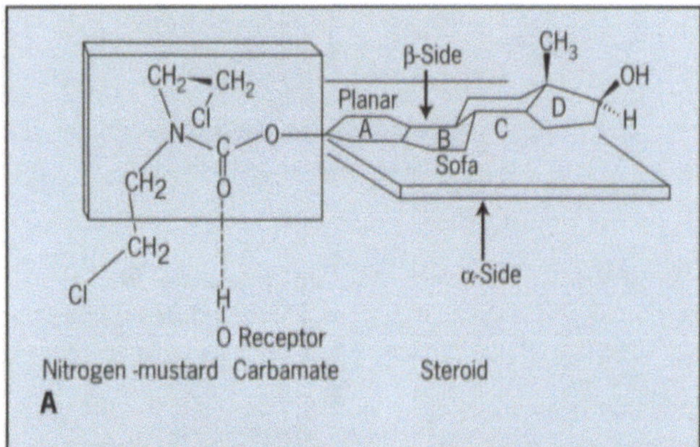

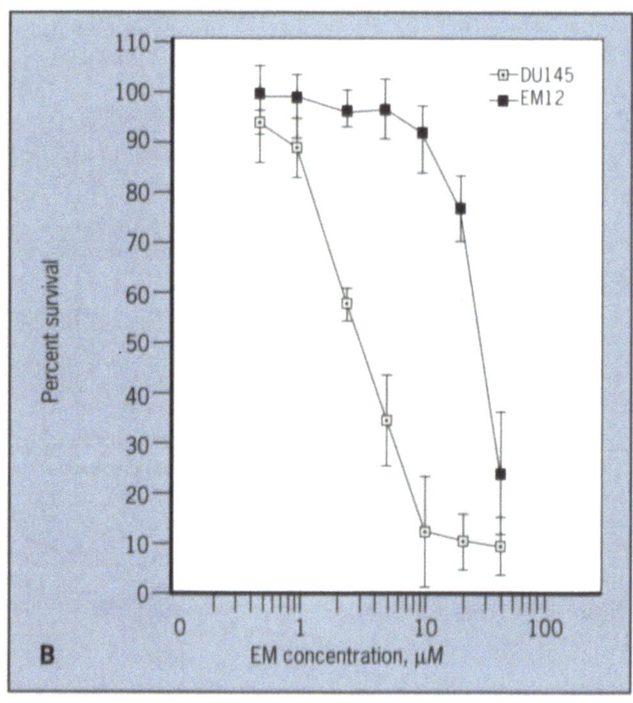

Figure 10-24. Cellular morphology associated with resistance to antimitotic drugs. **A,** The structure of estramustine is shown with potential intermolecular interactions illustrating how the drug binds to microtubule proteins. **B,** Sequential stepwise selection of an estramustine-resistant prostate carcinoma cell line resulting in approximately 5-fold resistance. *Bars* indicate ± SD. (*continued*)

extrapolation, drug resistance, is provided in Table 10-17 [31].

The ratio between proapoptotic and antiapoptotic proteins determines the potential for the cell to avoid entering programmed cell death. The overexpression of antiapoptotic proteins can thus lead to a drug-resistant phenotype [32]. Although examples of such overexpression have been found in several drug-resistant cell lines to date, in theory, such a resistance mechanism could apply to all drug types (Fig. 10-25).

Receptor Changes

Table 10-18 shows types of resistance in which receptor changes may affect drug activity. Retinoids and retinoic acid receptors [33] in cancer are shown in Figure 10-26.

A summary of some other characterized resistance mechanisms not covered in other parts of this chapter is shown in Table 10-19.

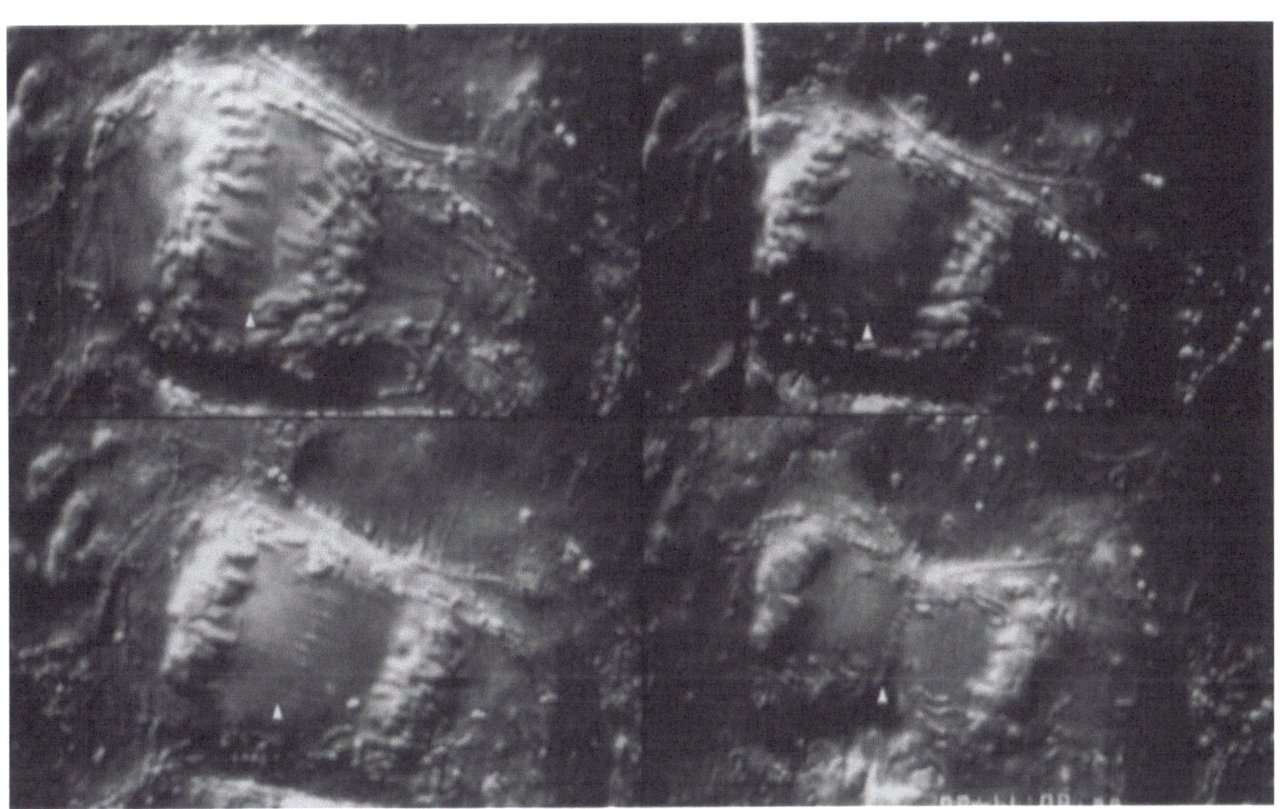

Figure 10-24. (*continued*) **C,** Various stages of mitosis. The video-enhanced differential interference contrast optics show the traverse of the cell from early anaphase (spindle fibers illustrated by *arrowhead, top left*) through late anaphase (interzonal microtubule bundles indicated by *arrowhead, bottom left*), to telophase (stem bodies indicated by *arrowhead, top right*), and cytokinesis, *bottom right* (midbody indicated by *arrowhead*). The *bar* represents 10 μm. (*Adapted from* Sheridan *et al.* [26]; with permission.)

Table 10-14. Cytoskeletal changes associated with resistance to antimitotic drugs
Quantitative and qualitative changes in α or β-tubulin isotypes
Mutation in β-tubulin isotypes affecting drug binding sites
Altered microtubule associated protein expression
Morphologic changes including smaller cell size and mitotic spindles
Altered expression of drug transporters

Table 10-15. Reported resistance mechanisms to classic antifolates
Alterations in transport
Increased expression of antimetabolite target enzyme
Mutated target enzyme with lower affinity for drug
Altered polyglutamation of the antifolate
Reduced folpolyglutamate synthetase
Increased γ-hydrolase activity

Table 10-16. Examples of DNA sequence amplification in antimetabolite-resistance cell lines

Gene amplified	Drug
Dihydrofolate reductase	Methotrexate
Adenosine deaminase	Deoxycoformycin
Adenylate deaminase	Coformycin
Ribonucleotide reductase	Hydroxyurea
Multienzyme CAD complex	Phosphonacetyl-L-apartate
Thymidylate synthetase	Fluorodeoxyuridine
UMP synthetase	Pyrazofurine
IMP-5'-dehydrogenase	Mycophenolic acid

Table 10-17. Gene families involved in drug resistance and apoptosis

Gene	Expression	Effect of increased levels on drug resistance and cell proliferation
bcl-2	Increases, then inhibits apoptosis	Increase
bax	Interferes with *bcl-2* and enhances apoptosis	Decrease
p53 tumor suppressor gene	Loss of gene function blocks apoptosis	Increase
myc oncogene	In the absence of growth factors, stimulates apoptosis	Decrease
E IA adenovirus oncogene	Equivalent to *bax*	Decrease
EIB adenovirus oncogene	Equivalent to *bcl-2*	Increase
mdm-2		?
ASKI (MAPKKK)	Increases, then induces apoptosis	Decrease
mutated n-*ras*	Point mutations activate gene product and decrease apoptosis	Increase

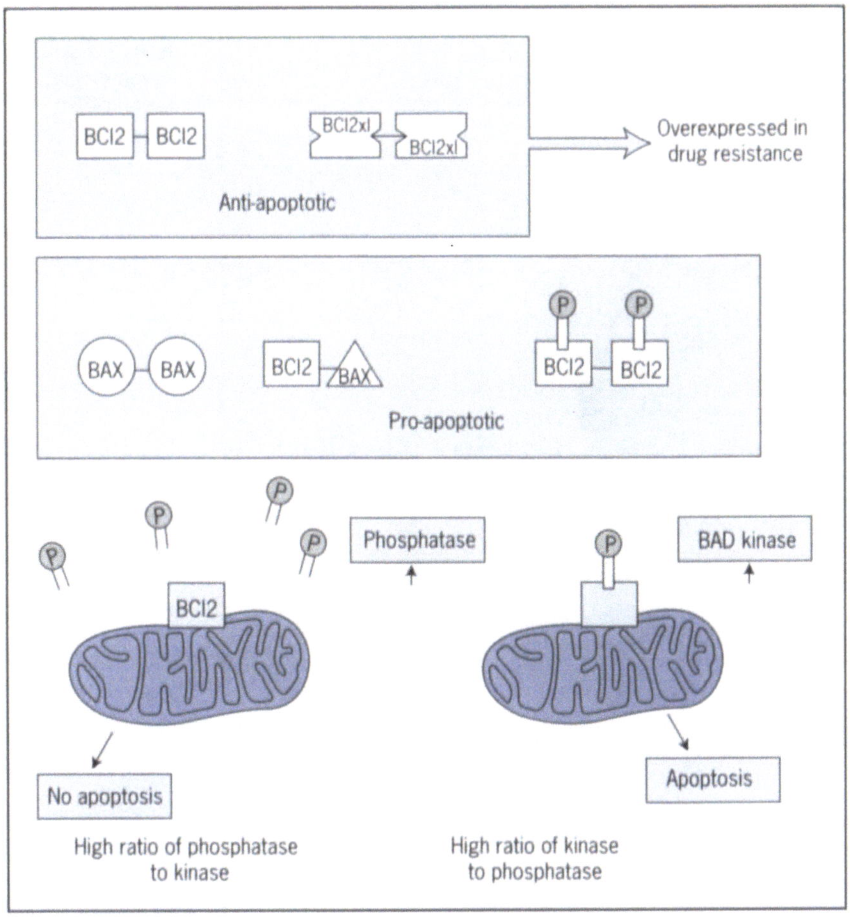

Figure 10-25. The expanding family of BCL-2 proteins.

Table 10-18. Resistance in which receptor changes may affect drug activity

Absence of expression of relevant receptor
Quantitative downregulation of receptor expression
Mutations in receptor and drug-binding domains
Alternative splicing of receptor transcripts
Homo- or heterodimerization
  stoichiometry of receptor subunits
Drug classes affected
  Estrogens
  Antiestrogens
  Androgens
  Retinoids
  Glucocorticoids

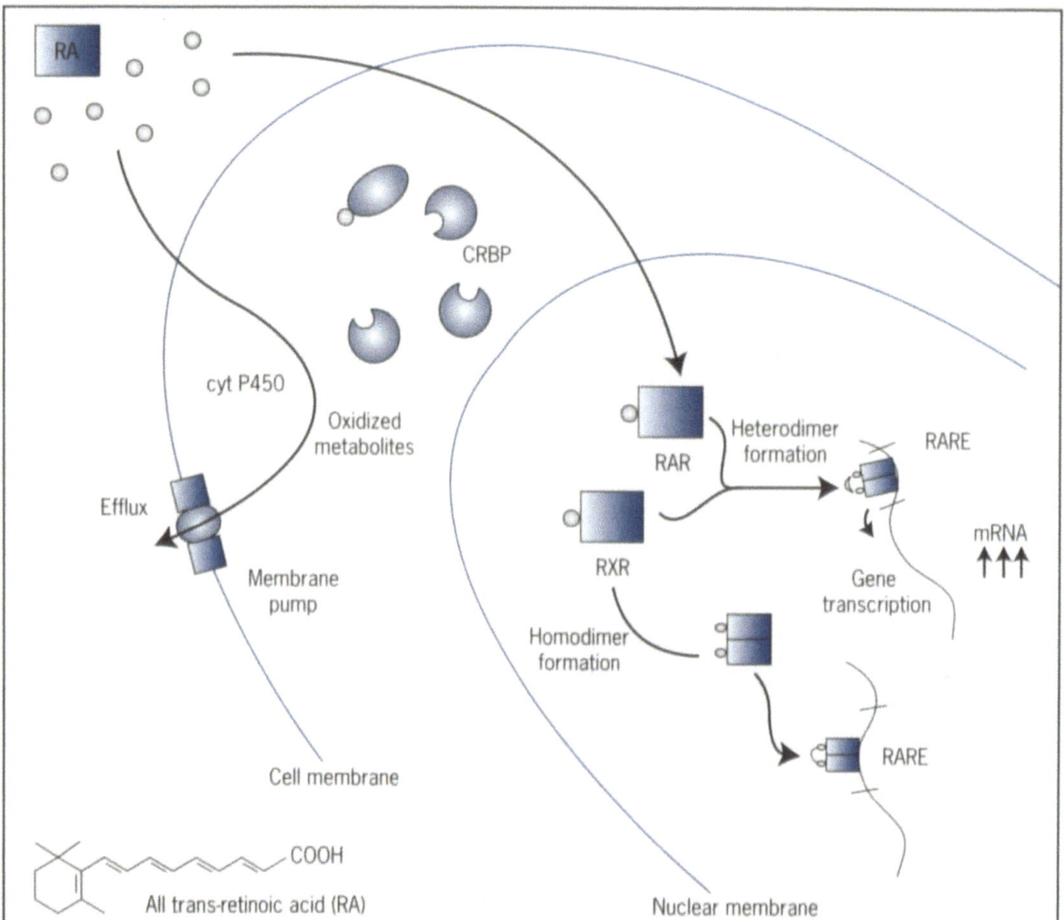

Figure 10-26. Retinoids and retinoic acid receptors in cancer.

Table 10-19. Other drug resistance mechanisms

Drug	Resistance correlate
Mytomycin C	Reduced levels of NADPH-quinone oxidoreductase (DT-diaphorase) [34]
Bleomycin	Increased bleomycin hydrolase [35]
Cisplatin (other alkylating agents)	Increased metallothionein [36]
"Antisense drugs"	Increased nucleases
Peptidomimetic agents	Increased proleolytic enzymes
Antibody conjugated drugs	Enhanced host recognition of antigen

REFERENCES

1. Laing N, Tew KD: Drug resistance to chemotherapy: mechanisms. In *Encyclopedia of Cancer*. Edited by Bertino JR. Academic Press; 1996:560–570.
2. Prestera T, Holtzclaw WD, Zhang Y, Talalay P: Chemical and molecular regulation of enzymes that detoxify carcinogens. *Proc Natl Acad Sci USA* 1993, 90:2965–2969.
3. Kato S: Cytochrome P450IIE1: genetic polymorphism, racial variation and lung cancer risk. *Cancer Res* 1992, 52:6712–6715.
4. Ciaccio PJ, Shen H, Kruh GD, Tew KD: Effects of ethacrynic acid exposure on conjugation and MRP mediated efflux in human colon tumor cells. *Biochem Biophys Res Commun* 1996, 222:111–115.
5. Kuzmich S, Vanderveer LA, Walsh ES, *et al.*: Increased levels of glutathione S-transferase pi-transcript as a mechanism of resistance to ethacrynic acid. *Biochem J* 1992, 281:219–224.

6. Shen H, Ranganathan S, Kuzmich S, Tew KD: Influence of ethacrynic acid on glutathione S-transferase π transcript and protein half-lives in human colon cancer cells. *Biochem Pharmacol* 1995, 50:1233–1238.

7. Moritz T, Williams DA: Transfer of drug resistance genes to hematopoietic precursors. In *Encyclopedia of Cancer*. Edited by Bertino JR. Academic Press; 1996:1765–1776.

8. Bunting KD, Townsend AJ: Protection by transfected rat or human class 3 aldehyde dehydrogenase against the cytotoxic effects of oxazaphosphorine alkylating agents in hamster V79 cell lines: demonstration of aldophosphamide metabolism by the cytosolic class 3 isozyme. *J Biol Chem* 1996, 271:11891–11896.

9. Tew KD: Glutathione associated enzymes in anticancer drug resistance: perspectives in cancer research. *Cancer Res* 1994, 54:4313–4320.

10. Roninson IB: Multidrug resistance. In *Encyclopedia of Cancer*. Edited by Bertino JR. Academic Press; 1996:1095–1107.

11. Kartner N, Ling V: Multidrug resistance in cancer. *Sci Am* 1989, 260:44–51.

12. Chen CJ, Chin JE, Ueda K, *et al.*: Internal duplication and homology with bacterial transport proteins in the MDR1 (P-glycoprotein) gene from multidrug-resistant human cells. *Cell* 1986, 47:381–389.

13. Cole SPC, Bhardwaj G, Gerlach JH, *et al.*: Overexpression of a transporter gene in a multidrug-resistant human lung cancer cell line. *Science* 1992, 258:1650–1654.

14. Tew KD, Houghton JA, Houghton PJ: *Preclinical and Clinical Modulation of Anticancer Drugs*. Boca Raton: CRC Press; 1993:125–196.

15. Flatgaard JE, Bauer KE, Kauvar LM: Isozyme specificity of novel glutathione S-transferase inhibitors. *Cancer Chemother Pharmacol* 1993, 33:63–70.

16. Lyttle MH, Satyam A, Hocker MD, *et al.*: Glutathione-S-transferase activates novel alkylating agents. *J Med Chem* 1994, 37:1501–1507.

17. Ciaccio PJ, Tew KD, LaCreta FP: Enzymatic conjugation of chlorambucil with glutathione is catalyzed by human glutathione S-transferases and inhibition by ethacrynic acid. *Biochem Pharmacol* 1991, 42:1504–1507.

18. Taylor J, Pemble S, Harris J, *et al.*: Evolution of GST genes. In *Structure and Function of Glutathione Transferases*. Edited by Tew KD, Pickett CB, Mantle TJ, *et al.*: Boca Raton: CRC Press; 1993:63–174.

19. O'Dwyer PJ, LaCreta F, Nash S, *et al.*: Phase I study of thio-TEPA in combination with the glutathione transferase inhibitor ethacrynic acid. *Cancer Res* 1991, 51:6059–6065.

20. Schisselbauer J, Silber R, Papadopoulous E, *et al.*: Characterization of lymphocyte glutathione S-transferase isozymes in chronic lymphocytic leukemia (CLL). *Cancer Res* 1990, 50:3569–3573.

21. Carothers AM: DNA damage, mutation, and repair. In *Encyclopedia of Cancer*. Edited by Bertino JR. Academic Press; 1996:484–500.

22. Zlotogorski C, Erickson LC: Pretreatment of human colon tumor cells with DNA methylating agents inhibits their ability to repair chloroethyl monoadducts. *Carcinogenesis (Lond)* 1984, 5:83–87.

23. D'Arpa P, Liu LF: Drug resistance: inhibitors of topoisomerases. In *Encyclopedia of Cancer*. Edited by Bertino JR. Academic Press; 1996:600–609.

24. Pommier Y: DNA topoisomerase II inhibitors. In *Cancer Therapeutics: Experimental and Clinical Agents*. Edited by Teicher B. Totowa, NJ: Humana Press; 1997:153–174.

25. Speicher LA, Sheridan VR, Godwin A, Tew KD: Resistance to the antimitotic drug estramustine is distinct from the multidrug resistant phenotype. *Br J Cancer* 1991, 64:267–273.

26. Sheridan VR, Speicher LA, Tew KD: The effects of estramustine on mitotic progression in DU 145 human prostatic carcinoma cells. *Eur J Cell Biol* 1991, 54:268–276.

27. Ranganathan S, Dexter DW, Benetatos CA: Increase of β_{III} and β_{Iva} tubulin isotypes in human prostate carcinoma cells as a result of estramustine resistance. *Cancer Res* 1996, 56:2584–2589.

28. Laing N, Dahloff B, Hartley-Asp B, *et al.*: The interaction of estramustine with tubulin isotypes. *Biochemistry* 1997, 36:871–878.

29. Melera PW: Drug resistance: inhibitors of folate metabolism. In *Encyclopedia of Cancer*. Edited by Bertino JR. Academic Press; 1996:587–599.

30. Hamlin JL: Drug resistance: DNA sequence amplification. In *Encyclopedia of Cancer*. Edited by Bertino JR. Academic Press: 1996, pp 571–586.

31. Hickman JA: Apoptosis induced by anticancer drugs. *Cancer Metastasis Rev* 1992, 11:121–139.

32. Lowe SW, Bodis S, McClatchey A, *et al.*: p53 Status and the efficacy of cancer chemotherapy in vivo. *Science* 1994, 266:807–810.

33. deThé H, Degos L: Retinoids/retinoic acid receptors in cancer. In *Encyclopedia of Cancer*. Edited by Bertino JR. Academic Press; 1996:1561–1570.

34. Rauth AM, Goldberg Z, Misra V: DT-diaphorase: possible roles in cancer chemotherapy and carcinogenesis. *Oncol Res* 1997, 9:339–349.

35. Sebti SM, Jani JP, Mistry JS, *et al.*: Metabolic inactivation: a mechanism of human tumor resistance to bleomycin. *Cancer Res* 1991, 51:227–232.

36. Kondo Y, Woo ES, Michalska AE, *et al.*: Metallothionein null cells have increased sensitivity to anticancer drugs. *Cancer Res* 1995, 55:2021–2023.

CHAPTER

11

Apoptosis and Cancer

Fruma Yehiely
Louis P. Deiss

Apoptosis, or Programmed Cell Death, is the activation of an inherent cellular suicide program that results in cell death [1]. There are two hallmarks in the death process. First, is a set of distinct morphologic changes such as membrane blebbing, cell shrinkage, and chromosomal condensation followed by chromosomal fragmentation. Second, is the rapid phagocytosis of the corpses of the dead cells, resulting in a limited local immune response. Recently it has been demonstrated that apoptosis plays a crucial role in cardiac damage and a variety of human diseases such as acute liver failure, Alzheimer's disease, and cancer [2]. The realization that apoptosis constitutes a major mechanism of tumor suppression has dramatically advanced tumor biology by leading to a number of novel approaches for preventing, diagnosing, and treating cancer. The guiding principles for understanding and manipulating the apoptotic response have emerged from studies of both lower eukaryotes and mammalian model systems [3]. These principles, as well as strategies designed to harness the apoptotic response, are described in this chapter.

CAENORHABDITIS ELEGANS CELL DEATH MACHINERY

The general principles of apoptosis were identified in the seminal work of Horvitz and coworkers [3–7], studying the 131 cell death events in the course of development of the nematode *Caenorhabditis elegans*. An elegant combination of genetic and biochemical approaches was used to define a limited number of genes that are essential for the killing process [3]. Evolutionary conservation of the cell death process between *C. elegans* and mammals facilitated the identification and analysis of the mammalian counterparts.

Genetic analysis of *C. elegans* Death (CED) mutants has revealed that the core of the cell killing activity resides in three genes; *ced-3*, *ced-4*, and *ced-9*. Whereas CED-3 and CED-4 are required for cell death, CED-9 inhibits the killing process [4–6]. Loss of CED-9 results in inappropriate cell killing only if CED-3 and CED-4 are intact [6]. In transgenic worms, overexpression of CED-3 or CED-4 results in cell death; the CED-4 induced killing requires CED-3, whereas CED-3 induced killing is independent of CED-4. Moreover, CED-4 is required for the inhibition of CED-3 induced killing by CED-9 [7,8]. These data suggest that functionally, the CED-9 protein is an antagonist to CED-4, which acts between CED-3 and CED-9 or parallel to CED-3, and the CED-3 protein is a downstream mediator [7,8]. Biochemical studies have validated this proposal and demonstrated that CED-3, CED-4, and CED-9 form a trimeric complex and that CED-4 is the bridging molecule [8,9].

CED-3 is a cysteine protease that cleaves at aspartic acid residues and is synthesized as an inactive proprotein [5]. Whereas CED-4/CED-4 interactions are inhibited by CED-9, the removal of CED-9, possibly by EGL-1, allows the assembly of two CED-4/CED-3 units by virtue of CED-4/CED-4 interactions [10–12]. The crowding of CED-3 driven by CED-4 interaction leads to CED-3 activation as shown in Figure 11-1 [10]. Such activation requires two proteolytic (presumably autocatalytic) events; cleavage of the amino terminal inhibitory pro-domain and an internal cleavage that generates a small and a large subunit. The active CED-3 protease is composed of two heterodimers, each comprised of a small and a large subunit.

Thus, the *C. elegans* system has provided the notion that proteolytic activation of a protease is a critical event in cell killing. This activation is mediated by molecular crowding driven by protein-protein interactions, and the entire killing process appears to be regulated by interactions between CED-3, CED-4, and CED-9.

MAMMALIAN CELL DEATH MEDIATORS

The *ced-3*, *ced-4* and *ced-9* genes have mammalian counterparts that play crucial roles in regulating cell killing. Not surprisingly, a single *C. elegans* gene is represented by a family of related mammalian genes, resulting in multiple functions and multiple levels of complex regulation. It is clear that these genes play a role in tumor formation and progression, and in order to manipulate cell death for the treatment of human cancer it is essential to understand their mode of action. Following, is a description of the families of mammalian CED-3, CED-4, and CED-9 homologs, their functions, and their relevance to cancer.

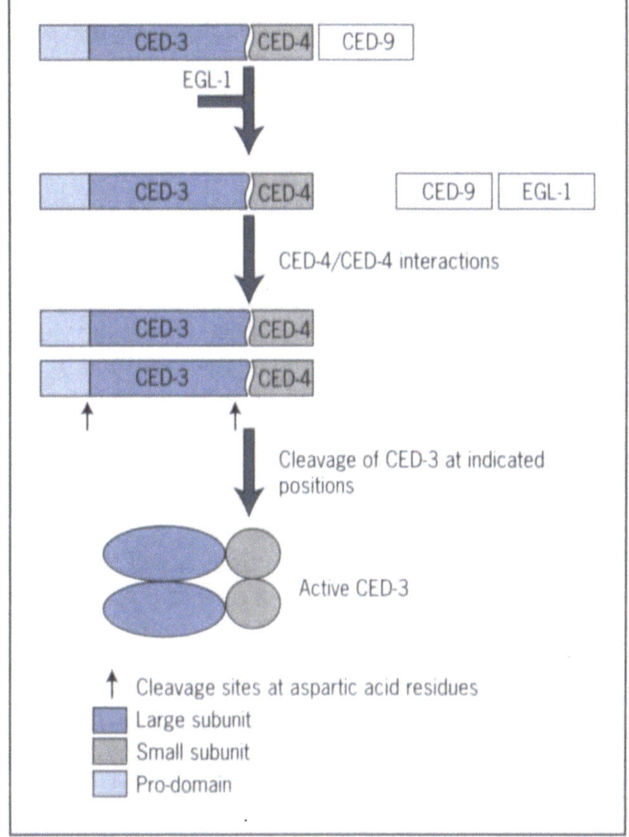

Figure 11-1. CED-3 activation model. CED-3, CED-4, and CED-9 assemble into an inactive trimeric complex in which CED-4 is the bridging molecule. An apoptotic trigger such as EGL-1 dissociates the trimer by binding to CED-9. The removal of CED-9 leads to oligomerization of CED-3/ CED-4 dimers due to CED-4 self-aggregation. Crowding of CED-3 leads to its proteolytic activation by two cleavage events: removal of the amino terminal inhibitory pro-domain and internal cleavage that generates a large and a small unit. Two dimers composed of both large and small units comprise the active CED-3.

CED-3 LIKE FAMILY

The cysteine protease Interleukin-1β converting enzyme (ICE, also called caspase-1), which cleaves Interleukin-1β, was the first identified mammalian homolog of CED-3. The finding that overexpression of ICE induces killing in mammalian fibroblasts validated the functional linkage between the nematode and mammalian genes [5]. Many mammalian CED-3 homologs have been described, all of which are cysteine proteases with aspartase activity (caspases) that undergo cleavage of the inhibitory domain and one or more additional cleavages (all adjacent to an aspartic acid residue) to generate the mature active caspase consisting of heterodimers of large and small subunits [8]. Whereas caspase-3, -6 and -7 contain short pro-domains that may serve only as protease inhibitors, caspase-1,-2,-4,-5,-8,-9, and -10 contain long pro-domains that are involved in protein–protein interactions. The structural features of the procaspases are summarized in Figure 11-2 [13].

In mammals there are two major routes of caspase activation. The first route, similar to the activation of CED-3, involves the molecular crowding of a pro-caspase. The second route involves direct proteolytic activation by other caspases or proteases, such as granzyme B. The crowding can be mediated by ligand–activated receptor clustering or by intermolecular dimerization as will be described for caspase-9. Granzyme B, which is produced by cytotoxic lymphocytes along with perforin, is inserted into target cells through a pore in the membrane that is generated by perforin.

Of all the receptors that mediate the activation of caspase-8, FAS (also called CD95 or APO1) was the first described in detail. Binding of FAS ligand induces trimerization of the receptor and binding of the FAS–associated protein with death domain (FADD) adaptor through the death domain (DD) found on both FAS and FADD. The recruited FADD binds to caspase-8 through the death effector domains (DEDs) present on each of the proteins. Binding leads to the activation of caspase-8 [14]. Two models have been proposed to explain the activation. In the first model, the two DEDs of caspase-8 interact in an intramolecular fashion, resulting in the folding of caspase-8 into an inactive state. The conformation induced by FADD binding to the trimerized FAS receptor exposes the DED on FADD, which in turn effectively binds to one of the two DED modules of caspase-8. This binding induces a structural change that leads to autocatalytic processing and activation of caspase-8. The second model of activation is based on crowding of caspase-8 at the trimerized FAS receptor that might promote transactivation of caspase-8 by a very low inherent activity of the proprotein. Similarly, ligand activated tumor necrosis factor Receptor-1 (TNFR1, also called p55 or CD120a) activates caspase-8 through the binding of the TNFR1 adaptor (TRADD) to FADD [15]. In vitro studies demonstrated that activated caspase-8 proteolytically activates all other caspases. In cells, caspase-8 activation leads to the activation of downstream effector caspases in a cascade fashion, resulting in cell death (Fig. 11-3). Thus, in the caspase cascade, activation of caspase-8 is a critical control point [8,13,14,16].

The role of caspases in cell killing has been demonstrated using a variety of genetic, biochemical, and pharmacologic approaches. Genetic studies indicate a critical role for CED-3 in developmentally regulated cell killing in *C. elegans* [5]. Similarly, analyses of null mice indicate a similar critical role for caspase-3 and -9 in developmentally regulated apoptosis (especially of neuronal cells) and in experimentally induced cell death [17–19]. In most cell lines, ectopic overexpression of long pro-domain containing caspases induces death. Both in vivo and in vitro, inhibitors of caspases (peptides, viral gene products, and dominant–negative caspases) inhibit cell killing induced by a variety of triggers [8,13]. Taken together, these data emphasize the important role of caspases in apoptosis. Although the mechanism by which caspases exert killing is not yet clear, it probably involves proteolytic cleavage of structural proteins and enzymes by the effector caspases and interference with mitochondrial functions, all of which ultimately lead to cell destruction, as shown at the bottom of Figure 11-3.

CED-4 LIKE FAMILY

The first mammalian homolog of CED-4, apoptosis protease activating factor-1 (APAF1), was identified by the elegant biochemical work of Wang and coworkers [20]. APAF1 interacts with caspase-9 and with cytochrome *c*, which is released into the cytosol during apoptosis. Similar to CED-4, APAF1 is sandwiched between its partners; assembly of the complex leads to the activation of caspase-9, which in turn activates caspase-3 [20]. A model for APAF1 mediated activation of caspase-9 proposes that binding of cytochrome *c* to APAF1 induces aggregation of APAF1 and the binding of caspase-9 through the caspase recruitment domain (CARD). Caspase-9 activation is possibly exerted by the transproteolytic cleavage of pro-caspase-9 that is promoted by its crowding. In addition, binding of ATP induces a conformational change that is required for caspase-9 processing and release from the complex. Thus, the mammalian APAF1 functionally resembles the *C. elegans* CED-4 in that it serves as a molecular scaffold to assemble and activate a caspase following an apoptotic stimulus. Whereas in *C. elegans* the apoptotic trigger might be the displacement of CED-9 from the CED-4/CED-3 complex by EGL-1, in mammals the inducer might be cytochrome *c* or a member of the EGL-like family that contains only BCL-2 homology domain 3 (BH3; Fig. 11-1 and 11-4). Because APAF1 binds to BCL-X_L, it is tempting to speculate that in mammals a complex

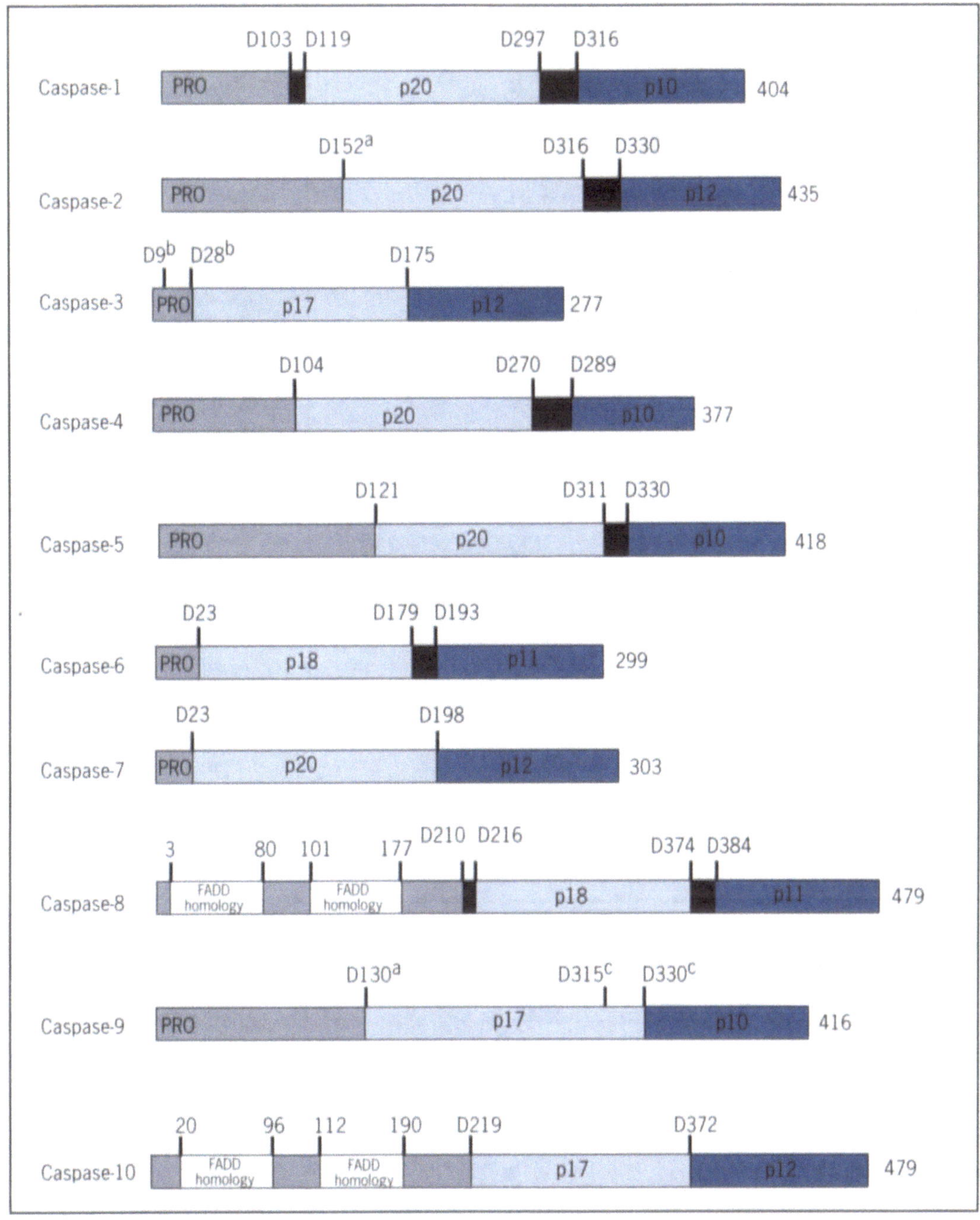

Figure 11-2. Structural features of the mammalian CED-3 family. The structural features of pro-caspases (cysteine proteases that cleave at aspartic acid) are indicated. PRO—amino terminal inhibitory pro-domain; D—aspartic acid residues (at the indicated positions) that are the sites of cleavage of the proenzymes; FAS-associated protein with death domain (FADD): the domains of caspase-8 and caspase-10 that are homologous to the death effector domain of FADD/MORT1. The large subunit (≈ 20 kD) and the small subunit (≈ 10 kD) are sometimes separated by a linker peptide (*black box*); a—exact cleavage site is not known; b—the cleavage site of caspase-3 may be at Asp-9 or Asp-28; c—caspase-9 is cleaved preferentially at Asp-330 by caspase-3 and at Asp-315 by granzyme B. (*Adapted from* Cohen [13]; with permission.)

comprised of $BCL\text{-}X_L$ (CED-9 like), APAF1 (CED-4 like), and caspase-9 (CED-3 like) might be activated by EGL-like proteins [21].

In APAF1 ablated mice, there is a significant reduction or delay in developmentally regulated cell death events, especially in the central nervous system

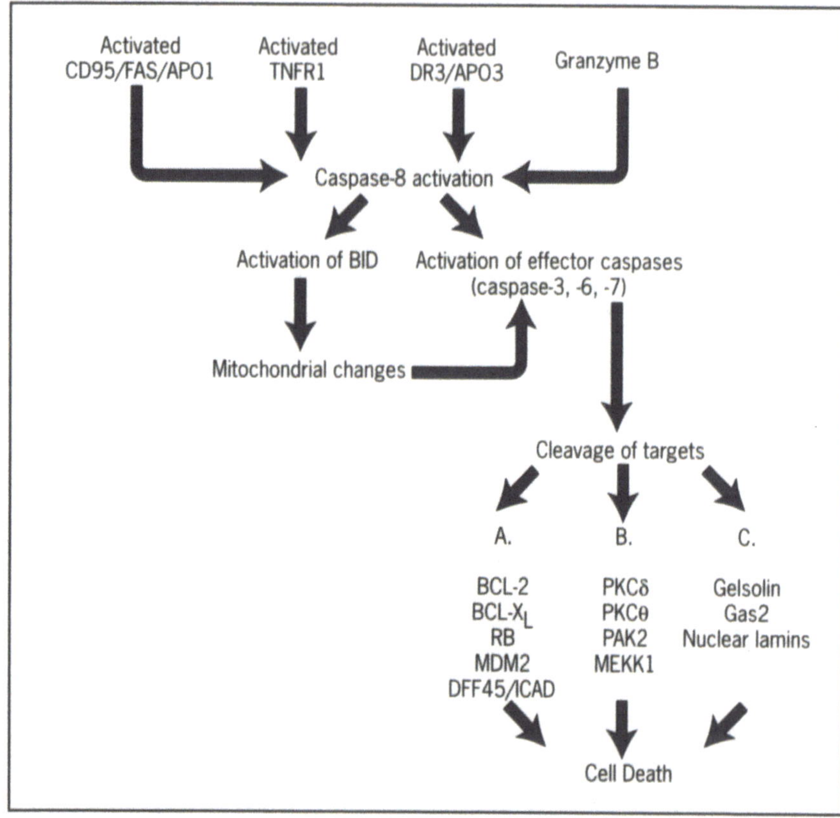

Figure 11-3. Caspase-8 relay of upstream apoptotic signals to downstream mediators. Caspase-8 is activated by a variety of killing signals as indicated. Activated caspase-8 cleaves and activates effector caspase-3, -6, and -7 as well as BID. Listed in groups are some of the targets of the effector caspases. A more detailed list can be found in [8]. Different aspects of cell killing are represented by each category: inhibitors of killing that are inactivated by cleavage (*A*); enzymes that are cleaved and activated (*B*); and proteins controlling structural integrity (*C*). With the exception of MDM2, RB, nuclear lamins, and DFF45/ICAD all the cleaved products of the listed proteins strongly induce killing. The cleavage of BCL-2 and $BCL\text{-}X_L$ convert the proteins from antiapoptotic to proapoptotic. Some changes in the cytoskeleton are mediated by cleavage of gelsolin and GAS2, whereas changes in the nuclear envelope result from cleavage of nuclear lamins. The cleavage of BID strongly enhances its proapoptotic functions. The mitochondrial changes induced by BID and the cleavage of structural proteins and enzymes by caspases eventually lead to the dismantling of the cell.

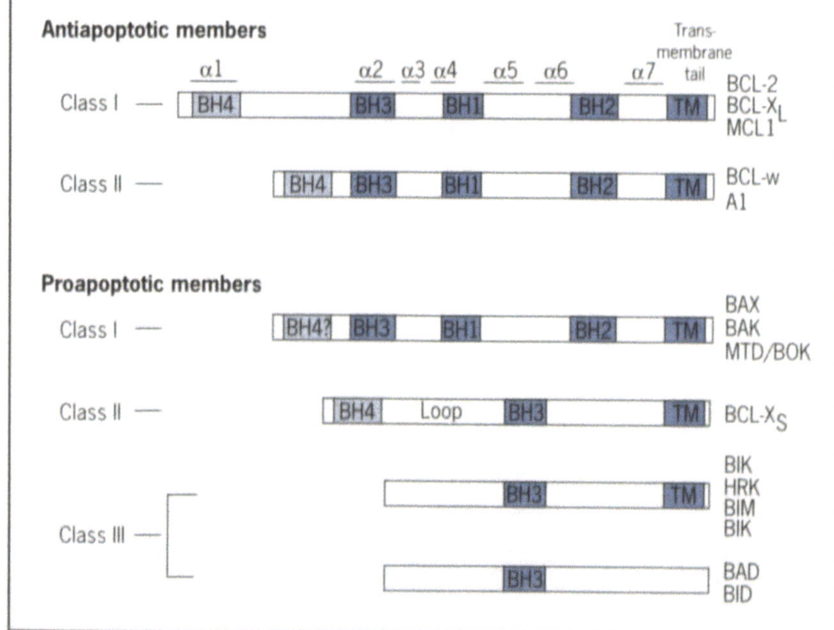

Figure 11-4. Structural characteristics of the BCL-2 family of proteins. The BCL-2 family proteins are classified on the basis of their function, *ie*, proapoptotic or antiapoptotic. Each of the groups is further classified based on domain organization. Indicated (not to scale) are BCL-2 homology domains, BH1-BH4. All antiapoptotic members contain BH1-BH4, whereas the minimal proapoptotic members contain only a BH3. The predicted α-helical segments $\alpha 1$-$\alpha 7$, and the membrane anchoring region (TM) is indicated. (*Adapted from* Kelekar and Thompson [25]; with permission.)

[22,23], and the null cells derived from the embryos show a significantly reduced sensitivity to many, but not all apoptotic inducers. This phenotype is similar, but more severe than that of caspase-3 or caspase-9 knockout mice [17–19].

CED-9 Like Family

BCL-2 was the first identified mammalian homolog of CED-9. Upon introduction into *C. elegans*, BCL-2 can substitute for CED-9 in blocking developmental cell death, again emphasizing the functional similarities between the worm and mammalian killing mechanisms [24]. The BCL-2 family is rapidly growing and includes 15 members with either antiapoptotic or proapoptotic functions. The multiple activities of the various members and their complicated levels of regulation are being investigated, but thus far, the mechanisms by which these proteins carry out either function are not completely defined.

The mammalian BCL-2 family members can be classified according to their function or structural features as shown in Figure 11-4 [25]. Shown are the BCL-2 homology (BH) domains 1 through 4 that represent the highest level of homology between the various members and the seven α-helical domains. Several members contain membrane–anchoring domains that tether the protein to the mitochondria, endoplasmic reticulum, or nuclear membrane. The antiapoptotic proteins contain all four BH domains, BH1-BH4, and a transmembrane domain. All of the proapoptotic proteins contain the BH3 domain.

The activities of the BCL-2 members are related to the structural domains as follows. The BH4 domain is involved in protein–protein interactions with cellular signaling molecules, such as the protein kinase RAF1 and the protein phosphatase calcineurin. Interaction of BCL-2 with RAF1 results in relocalization of the protein kinase to the mitochondrial membrane [26] where it presumably phosphorylates proteins involved in cell killing, leading to protection of cells from apoptosis. BH4 binding to the protein phosphatase calcineurin may protect T cells from killing by regulating the activation of T cells. BH4 binding sequesters calcineurin to the mitochondria where it can no longer regulate nuclear factor of activated T cells (NFAT) activity [27] required for T cell activation. Fully activated T cells are very sensitive to killing compared to nonactivated T cells. Thus, in this context BH4 may regulate killing through the regulation of transcription. The crucial role of the BH4 domain is highlighted by the finding that its removal from antiapoptotic proteins abrogates their antiapoptotic function [28].

Crystallography and nuclear magnetic resonance studies of BCL-X_L indicate that BH1, BH2, and BH3 domains fold to generate an extended hydrophobic cleft to which BH3 binds [29,30]. Alterations in the BH1 and BH2 domains of BCL-2 and BCL-X_L that interfere with antiapoptotic function also interfere with BAX binding. The members that contain only BH3 are proapoptotic, presumably by virtue of their binding and interference with the antiapoptotic BH1, BH2, and BH3 containing members such as BCL-2 [25]. Understanding the functions that are altered by BH3 binding is crucial for the understanding of cell killing because the antagonistic actions of proapoptotic and antiapoptotic proteins are mediated by binding of BH3 to the hydrophobic cleft.

A channel forming activity of the helices exerts an additional level of regulation of cell killing. The α5 and α6 helices, located between the BH1 and BH2 domains in BCL-2, BCL-X_L, and BAX, form ion conducting channels in vitro [29]. The properties of the ion channels derived from BCL-2, BCL-X_L, and BAX are different and depend on the in vitro conditions in which they are tested, suggesting that the properties of the channels govern their function, *ie*, protection from killing (BCL-2, BCL-X_L) or promotion of killing (BAX) [31–33]. The potential role of the channel formation in regulating apoptosis is being investigated. In the case of BAX-induced apoptosis, BAX induces mitochondrial swelling and rupture, leading to the release of cytochrome *c* and apoptosis inducing factor (AIF). Because this killing is inhibited by BCL-X_L, it is hypothesized that a pore formed by BCL-X_L acts to regulate osmotic swelling, preventing mitochondrial rupture [34]. In summary, the various BCL-2 family members regulate apoptosis by the activation of caspases or by a caspase independent mechanism [9,35].

MITOCHONDRIAL CHANGES ASSOCIATED WITH CELL DEATH

In addition to the processing of caspases and the network of protein–protein interaction involving the BCL-2 family members, mitochondrial dysfunction plays an important role in cell killing. During the induction of apoptosis, three changes in the mitochondria are frequently observed [35]. First there is the release of two proapoptotic factors, namely, cytochrome *c* and AIF. The second alteration is the collapse of the mitochondrial transmembrane potential (ΔY_m), which results in loss of mitochondrial function, including ATP production. The third alteration is the production of reactive oxygen species (ROS), causing protein and lipid damage.

Cytochrome *c* and AIF normally reside in the mitochondria, and apoptotic triggers such as activated caspase-8, BID, and BAX induce their release by an unknown mechanism [36]. Once released, they serve as mediators of caspase signaling by activating downstream caspases. The ΔY_m collapse is likely a result of the opening of the permeability transition pore (PTP), also known as the megachannel or multiple conductance channel. The PTP is a transmembrane complex composed of the adenine nucleotide translocator (ANT) on the inner mitochondrial membrane and possibly the voltage-dependent anion channel on the outer membrane [35,37]. The opening of the PTP is regulated by a variety of apoptosis inducing signals, including calcium fluxes and ROS. Although the pore can adopt a variety of conductance states, the high conductance state induces a collapse of the ΔY_m, leading to inhibition of ATP production in the mitochondria. It has been suggested that the release of cytochrome *c* and AIF is regulated by opening of the PTP, although there are situations in which the loss of cytochrome *c* precedes collapse of the ΔY_m [35,37]. The involvement of PTP in apoptosis is further supported by the recent findings that BAX directly interacts with ANT and that ANT is essential for BAX-induced killing in yeast [38]. The mode of killing induced by BAX in yeast is controversial, but it does not involve the activation of caspases. Similarly, overexpression of BAX induces caspase independent apoptosis in mammalian cells [8]. Because BAX can form a transmembrane channel and interacts with ANT, it is possible that BAX affects the PTP by forming an extended channel or by modulating the properties of the ANT channel. The PTP has been reconstructed in vitro using synthetic membranes and in such a system, the induction of the high conductance state is blocked by the addition of BCL-2 [39]. Similarly, in cultured cells, the collapse of the ΔY_m is blocked by overexpression of BCL-X_L or BCL-2 [37,40].

Low levels of ROS are normally generated by the mitochondria as byproducts in the electron transport chain, which is tightly coupled to the generation of ΔY_m. The ΔY_m is used to generate ATP through the action of the FOF1 ATPase. Processes that affect this coupling, such as PT-induced dissipation of ΔY_m, can lead to increased ROS production. It should be noted that this increase is often a late event in killing and likely contributes to the completion of killing [35].

Taken together, the mitochondria have two distinct functions in killing. First, early in the killing process, they serve as integration points where proapoptotic and antiapoptotic signals are received and processed. When a strong proapoptotic signal (such as BAX) is received in the absence of a strong antiapoptotic signal (such as BCL-X_L), the proapoptotic signal is amplified by the release of cytochrome *c* and AIF, which in turn initiates the caspase cascade. In addition, mitochondria respond to proapoptotic signals such as activated caspase-8. The second role of mitochondria in killing is the production of ROS and the shut off of ATP production, both of which also contribute to cell death.

SIGNALLING VIA DEATH RECEPTORS

Apoptotic signals can originate either from internal cellular sensing systems or from external stimuli that are transmitted through members of the superfamily of TNF death receptors. The best characterized death receptors, FAS and TNFR1 [14,16,41], will be described as models for apoptosis signaling. Recent work has indicated that the FAS pathway is triggered by internal events as well, such as the induction of *p53* [42].

A schematic representation of apoptosis signaling by FAS is shown in Figure 11-5. Binding of FAS ligand to FAS results in trimerization of the receptor and binding of the adaptor FADD to its cytoplasmic tail

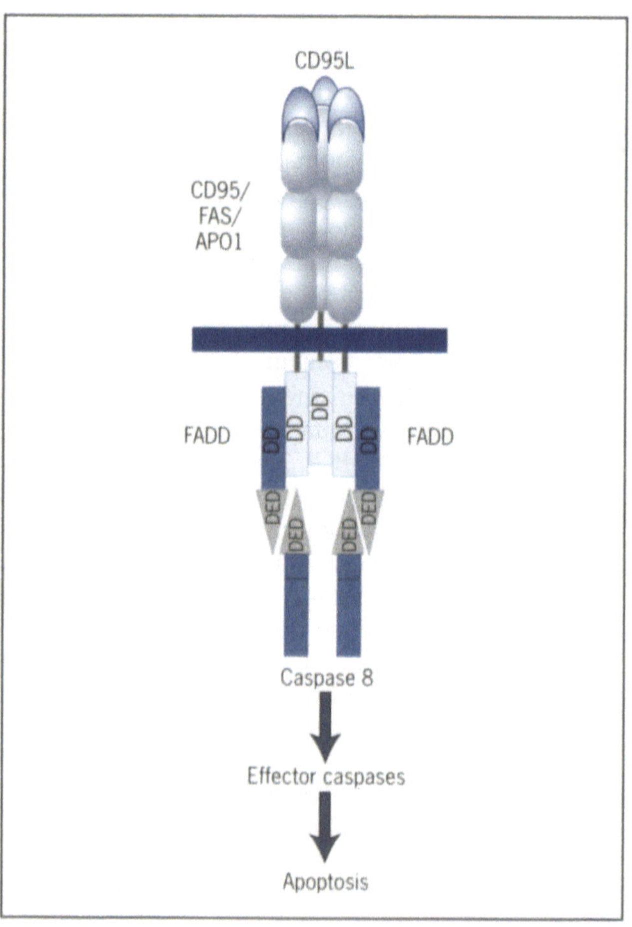

Figure 11-5. Apoptosis signaling by FAS. The binding of the FAS ligand indicated in green induces trimerization and clustering of the receptor. The death domain (DD) present on the cytoplasmic tail of the receptor binds to the DD present on the adaptor molecule FAS-associated protein with death domain (FADD). The death effector domain (DED) present on FADD binds to the DED present on caspase-8, leading to the proteolytic activation of caspase-8, downstream effector caspases, and cell killing. (*Adapted from* Ashkenazi and Dixit [14]; with permission.)

through DDs that are present on both molecules [43]. Subsequent interaction between the DED of FADD and the DED of caspase-8 induces proteolytic activation of caspase-8, initiating the caspase cascade, and the cleavage of BID into a fragment that induces the release of cytochrome *c* and AIF [13,44–46] leading to activation of downstream caspases and death. In addition to FADD, DAXX (Fas-death domain associated protein) interacts independently with the cytoplasmic tail of FAS, leading to activation of the c-JUN NH2-terminal kinase (JNK) followed by cell killing [47]. The contribution of DAXX signaling to the FAS induced killing is still being investigated.

Recent work has demonstrated two modes of FAS induced killing, depending on the cell type [40]. In type I cells, FAS activation results in rapid and strong activation of caspase-8, followed by the release of cytochrome *c* and subsequent activation of the caspase cascade. Overexpression of BCL-2 inhibits cytochrome *c* release but does not prevent killing. In type II cells, FAS induced killing is characterized by a weak activation of caspase-8 and a delayed activation of downstream caspases which follow the release of cytochrome *c* from the mitochondria, consistent with the model of caspase activation by the APAF1/caspase-9/cytochrome *c* complex. Whereas in both modes of killing, overexpression of BCL-2 inhibits cytochrome *c* release, only in the second mode does BCL-2 protect the cells from killing. Thus, a rapid activation of caspases through a strong activation of caspase-8 leads to killing that is independent of cytochrome *c* release and BCL-2. Alternatively, in some cells, killing requires mitochondrial perturbations and is inhibited by BCL-2.

Proapoptotic and antiapoptotic signaling by TNFR1 and death receptor 3 (DR3, also called APO3 or WSL1) is demonstrated in Figure 11-6. Binding of TNF to TNFR1 induces trimerization of the receptor and recruitment of a set of adaptor molecules that mediates the induction of NF-κB and killing. The adaptor molecule TNFR-associated death domain (TRADD) binds to the TNFR1 cytoplasmic tail through DD, which is present on both proteins [15]. Interaction between TRADD and FADD is followed by the activation of the caspase-8 pathway as described earlier for FAS [15,48]. TRADD recruits the receptor interacting protein (RIP), inducing a phosphorylation cascade that results in the activa-

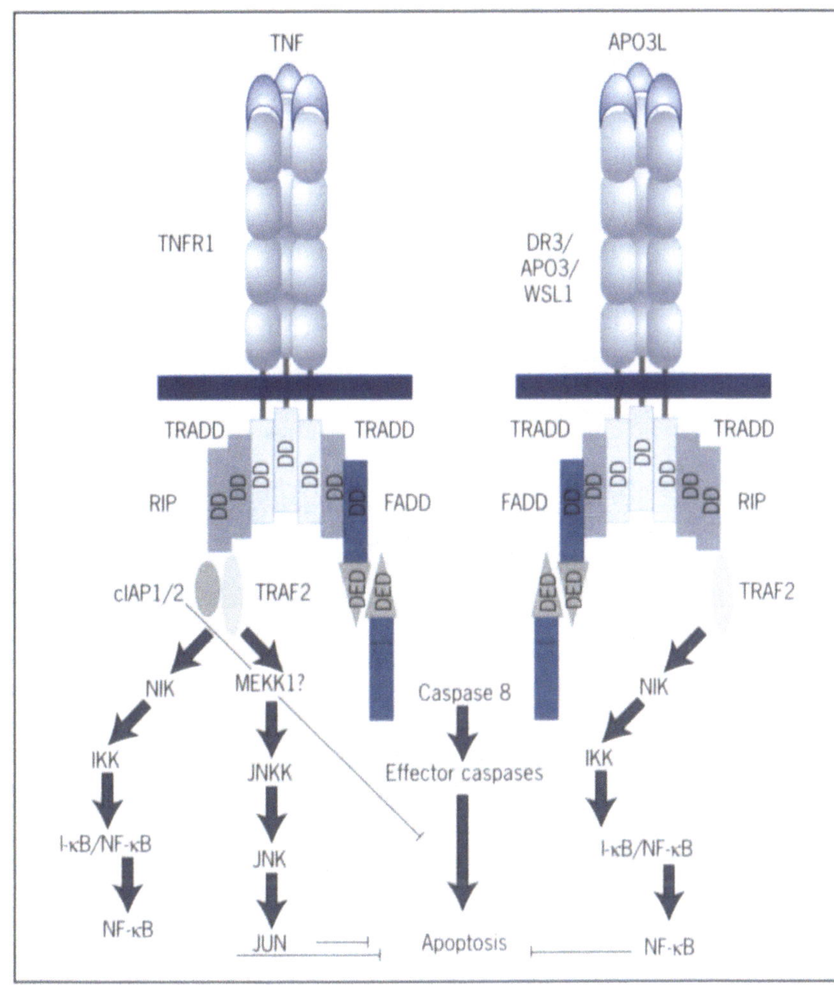

Figure 11-6. Proapoptotic and antiapoptotic signaling by TNFR1 and DR3. The trimerized receptors interact with the TNFR1 adaptor molecule (TRADD), which binds to FAS-associated protein with death domain (FADD), leading to caspase-8 activation and apoptosis. RIP, TRAF2, c-IAP1, and c-IAP2 also are recruited to the receptors. RIP recruitment is linked to the activation of NF-κB and protection from apoptosis through a phosphorylation cascade involving NIK, IKK, and the phosphorylation of I-κB. TRAF2 is required for the activation of JUN mediated by JNK, JNKK, and perhaps MEKK1. The activation of JUN also modulates apoptosis. Thus, the cell response to TNF and APO3L is determined by the balance between activation of proapoptotic and antiapoptotic pathways. DD—death domain; DED—death effector domain. (*Adapted from* Ashkenazi and Dixit [14]; with permission.)

tion of NF-κB, which protects cells from killing [49]. This protection is in part due to upregulation of the cellular inhibitors of apoptosis (c-IAPs) 1 and 2 that are recruited into a TNFR1 signaling complex as well [50]. In addition, TRADD binding recruits TNFR-associated factor 2 (TRAF2), which leads to activation of JNK [14]. DR3 induced killing resembles TNFR1 signaling as follows: binding of APO3 ligand to DR3 induces both NF-κB activation and killing; the cytoplasmic tail of DR3 binds to the adaptor TRADD, which then binds to FADD, leading to caspase-8 activation and killing, and; TRADD binds to RIP as well, leading to NF-κB activation [14].

A novel level of regulation of cell death has been described for the ligand APO2L/TRAIL, which binds to the DR4 or DR5 receptor and induces caspase-dependent, FADD-independent killing [51,52] as illustrated in Figure 11-7. APO2L/TRAIL also binds to a set of "decoy receptors," DCR1 or DCR2, which do not elicit a killing response [53]. DCR1 is a glycosyl phosphatidylinositol-linked receptor, whereas DCR2 is a transmembrane receptor that resembles DR4 and DR5 but with a truncated cytoplasmic domain. Overexpression of DCR1 in an APO2L/TRAIL sensitive cell line results in reduced levels of killing induced by APO2L/TRAIL due to competitive binding [54].

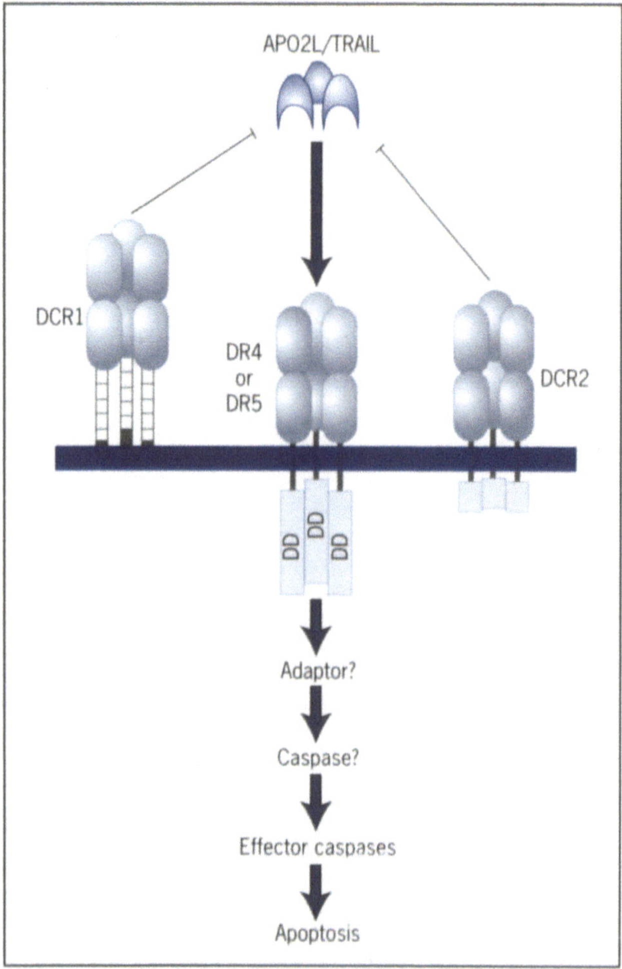

Figure 11-7. Apoptosis signaling by DR4 and DR5 and its inhibition by decoy receptors. Binding of APO2L/TRAIL to DR4 or DR5 leads to the activation of caspases by an unknown mechanism that is blocked by caspase inhibitors. The competitive binding to the decoy receptors DCR1 or DCR2 does not induce an apoptotic response. Thus, binding of APO2L/TRAIL to DCR1 or DCR2 prevents the binding to DR4 or DR5 and cell killing. DR—death receptor. (*Adapted from* Ashkenazi and Dixit [14]; with permission.)

The killing response is regulated by a variety of control mechanisms, many of which involve the CED-3 and CED-9 family members as illustrated in Figure 11-8. A simple response to a death signal such as FAS ligand binding is regulated in a layered manner. A primary control point is the abundance of the receptor, which is regulated both transcriptionally and post-transcriptionally. Another level of regulation involves protein–protein interactions. For example, FLIP (FADD-like ICE inhibitory protein), which contains two DEDs but does not induce downstream signaling [55], competes with FADD for binding to caspase-8. The release of cytochrome *c* induced by activated BID or by the effector caspases is negatively regulated by overexpression of BCL-2 or BCL-X_L [8,25,40]. As discussed, the cellular environment provides another level of regulation of the killing process. The activity of all caspases is blocked by nitric oxide, and the activity of caspase-3 and caspase-7 is inhibited by the binding of XIAP, a member of the growing family of IAPs that include c-IAP1, c-IAP2, NIAP, survivin, and viral IAPs [8,56,57]. Thus, the core killing events that consist of alteration of mitochondrial functions and activation of caspases are integrated and regulated by many different mechanisms.

STRATEGIES FOR CLONING AND IDENTIFYING MEDIATORS OF APOPTOSIS

Several strategies have been used to identify mediators of apoptosis, including the Technical KnockOut (TKO) method, genetic suppressor element (GSE) method, death trap method, and transient expression of plasmids [58]. TKO, which successfully employs functional genetic screening, is diagrammed in Figure 11-9 [59]. It is based on the random inactivation of human genes mediated by expression of an antisense complimentary DNA (cDNA) library, followed by selection for a specific phenotypic alteration. The antisense constructs responsible for the phenotypic change are easily extracted and shuttled into bacteria by virtue of the episomal vector in which the library is constructed. The recovered plasmids are tested individually for their ability to confer the phenotypic alteration. The sequence of the positive antisense cDNA is determined and used to identify its corresponding inactivated gene.

The TKO selection has been successfully used to identify seven mediators of interferon-γ (IFN-γ)–induced cell killing [58–60]. Analysis of the cloned genes is ongoing, and to date, two of the cloned genes have been shown to be involved in cell killing and tumor suppression. One of the identified proteins, death associated protein (DAP) kinase, mediates apoptosis induced by IFN-γ, TNF, FAS, and matrix detachment. It was reported to be absent in 21 of 39 diverse human tumor derived cell lines examined [58]. More importantly, DAP kinase was shown to mediate suppression of metastasis in a mouse metastasis model [61]. DAP kinase expression inversely correlated with the metastatic potential of a set of Lewis lung carcinomas and its reintroduction into a highly metastatic variant led to suppression of metastasis. Thus, DAP kinase mediates cell killing that is associated with suppression of metastasis. Further work is required to determine whether DAP kinase controls metastasis of human tumors. Another gene identified in this screen, cathepsin D, mediates IFN-γ, FAS, TNF, and p53 induced killing [58,62].

APOPTOSIS, ONCOGENES, AND TUMOR SUPPRESSOR GENES

Because apoptosis is a tightly regulated process that suppresses tumorigenicity, the accumulation of genetic alterations that abrogate cell death leads to the development of tumors. Figure 11-10 is a schematic representation of tumor formation, illustrating side-by-side the inducers of apoptosis and the corresponding cellular changes that abolish cell killing. The inducers include developmental signals, c-*MYC* overexpression, inadequate blood supply, immune response, loss of contact with matrix, chemotherapy, and radiation treatment. Several mechanisms, such as overexpression of *BCL-2* and other oncogenes, or the loss of some tumor suppressor genes have been adopted by tumor cells to override the killing signals. The key role for oncogenes and tumor suppressors in the regulation of apoptosis will be demonstrated by describing the oncogenes *BCL-2*, c-*MYC*, and *AKT/PKB* and the tumor suppressor genes *p53*, *RB*, *PTEN*, *BCL-2* and DAP kinase.

The *BCL-2* oncogene was originally identified as a gene overexpressed in follicular lymphoma and some diffuse large cell lymphomas due to chromosomal translocation. In vivo and in vitro studies demonstrated that BCL-2 does not transform cells, but renders them more resistant to killing induced by a wide range of triggers, as summarized in Table 11-1 [63]. Survival of cells that have escaped cell killing permits the accumulation of additional alterations that ultimately result in malignant transformation. One such alteration is overexpression of the oncogene c-*MYC*. Transgenic mice overexpressing both c-*MYC* and *BCL-2* exhibit higher levels of tumor formation than mice overexpressing either gene alone (Fig. 11-11). Overexpression of c-*MYC* and *BCL-2* act in synergy to promote survival and proliferation as follows: overexpression of *BCL-2* protects cells from killing, but can result in growth arrest, depending on the cellular envi-

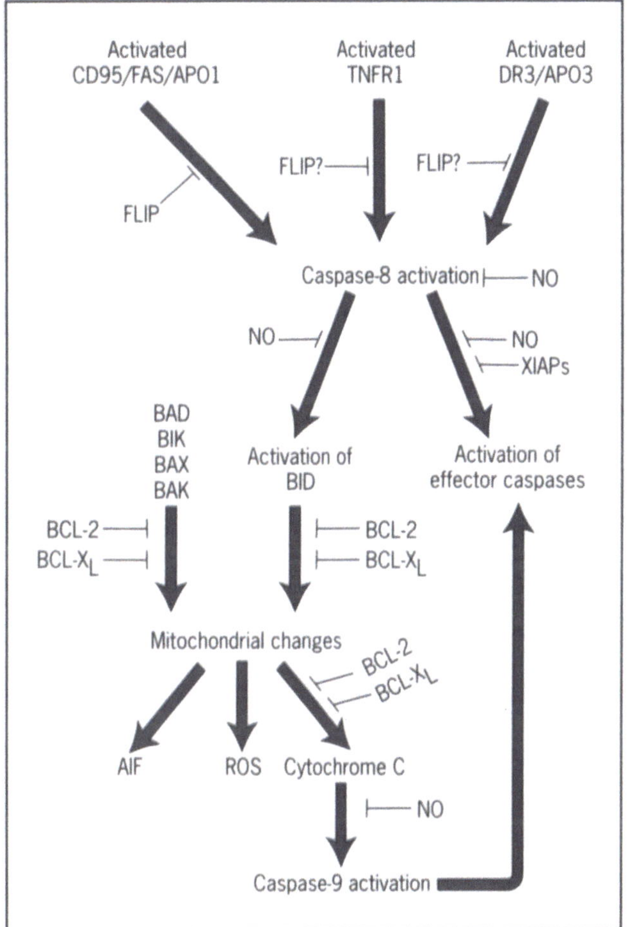

Figure 11-8. Modulation of apoptotic signaling. Many of the steps in apoptosis are tightly regulated and are blocked by overexpression of various inhibitors as indicated (*bars*). Illustrated are the regulators of caspases. FLIP competes with caspase-8 for binding to FADD. While the activation of every caspase is blocked by NO, the activity of effector caspases-3 and -7 is inhibited by XIAPs. Both the release of cytochrome *c* and the activity of the proapoptotic BCL-2 family members are blocked by overexpression of BCL-2 and BCL-X$_L$. NO—nitric oxide.

ronment; overexpression of c-*MYC* exerts a strong proliferation signal and a strong killing signal [64]. Whereas the proliferation signal of c-*MYC* abrogates the growth arrest signal of *BCL-2*, the cell killing signal induced by c-*MYC* is inhibited by *BCL-2* [65–67].

Another example that highlights the requirement for survival signals to counteract killing signals in tumorigenesis is the formation of solid tumor metastases, in which cells detach from the primary tumor and travel to a distal site. The detachment process sensitizes the cells to killing because attachment to matrix is a survival signal [68,69]; therefore, successfully metastasized tumor cells require a survival signal. In a mouse model for metastasis, one such survival signal is the loss of DAP kinase, a mediator of cell killing of metastatic cells [60,61].

Not only oncogenes such as c-*MYC* exert antagonistic effects on tumor formation. The loss of the tumor suppressor RB results in proliferation because RB negatively regulates the transcription of cell cycle progression genes. RB inhibits killing induced by p53, INF-γ, TGF-β, and irradiation, and its loss sensitizes cells to killing [70–73].

The apoptosis signal generated by c-MYC overexpression is blocked by insulin-like growth factor 1 (IGF1), activated AKT/PKB, or loss of p53 [74–79]. As shown in Figure 11-12, IGF1 and interleukin 3 (IL3) transmit survival signals by binding to their receptors and initiating a cascade of phosphorylation events that leads to the phosphorylation and activation of phosphatidylinositol 3- (PI3) kinase. PI3 kinase phosphorylates phosphoinositides (PtdIns) on position three of the inositol ring to generate PtdIns(3,4)P2 and PtdIns(3,4,5)P3, which have pleiotropic effects that include activation of the protein kinase AKT/PKB. Activation is achieved directly by binding to AKT/PKB and translocating it to the plasma membrane and indirectly by binding and activating phospholipid dependent kinases 1 and 2 (PDK1, PDK2) which phosphorylate and activate AKT/PKB. Activated AKT/PKB phosphorylates the proapoptotic BAD which is then sequestered and inactivated by a member of the 14-3-3 family [80,81]. The inactive BAD no longer antagonizes the antiapoptotic BCL-X_L, leading to protection of the mitochondria from proapoptotic BAX and to survival. The tumor suppressor lipid phosphatase PTEN antagonizes the AKT/PKB pathway by dephosphorylating PtdIns(3,4)P2 and PtdIns(3,4,5)P3 [82]. Thus, loss of the tumor suppressor PTEN results in higher levels of PtdIns(3,4)P2 and PtdIns(3,4,5)P3, higher levels of activated AKT/PKB and protection from apoptosis.

The tumor suppressor p53 mediates numerous proapoptotic signals, including chemotherapeutics, gamma radiation, ultraviolet radiation, hypoxia, matrix detachment and overexpression of MYC, as described in Figure 11-13. These signals are transduced by a p53 dependent transcription mode or by a transcription independent pathway. Four genes that are transcriptionally activated by p53 and mediate death have been described, namely, IGF binding pro-

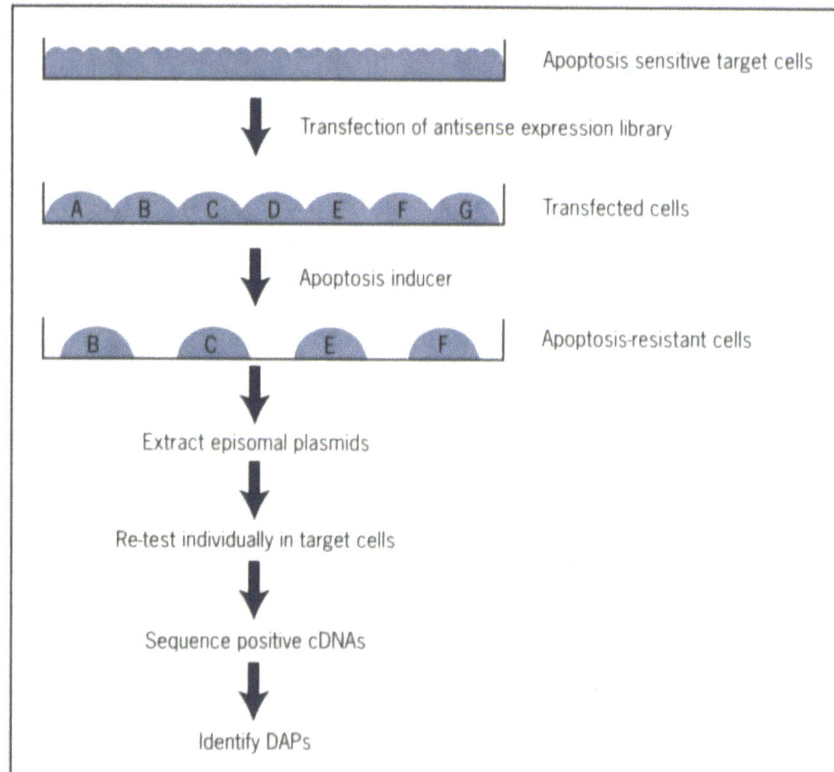

Figure 11-9. Identification of death associated protein (*DAP*) genes using the Technical KnockOut (TKO) method. A sensitive target cell population is transfected with an antisense complimentary DNA (cDNA) expression library followed by exposure to an apoptosis inducer. The surviving transfected cells are expanded, and the antisense carrying plasmids are recovered from the resistant cells. Individual plasmids are tested for their ability to confer resistance to apoptosis. cDNAs of positive clones are sequenced and the gene that is inactivated in the resistant population is identified. By using TKO, a group of DAPs have been identified that includes two putative tumor suppressors.

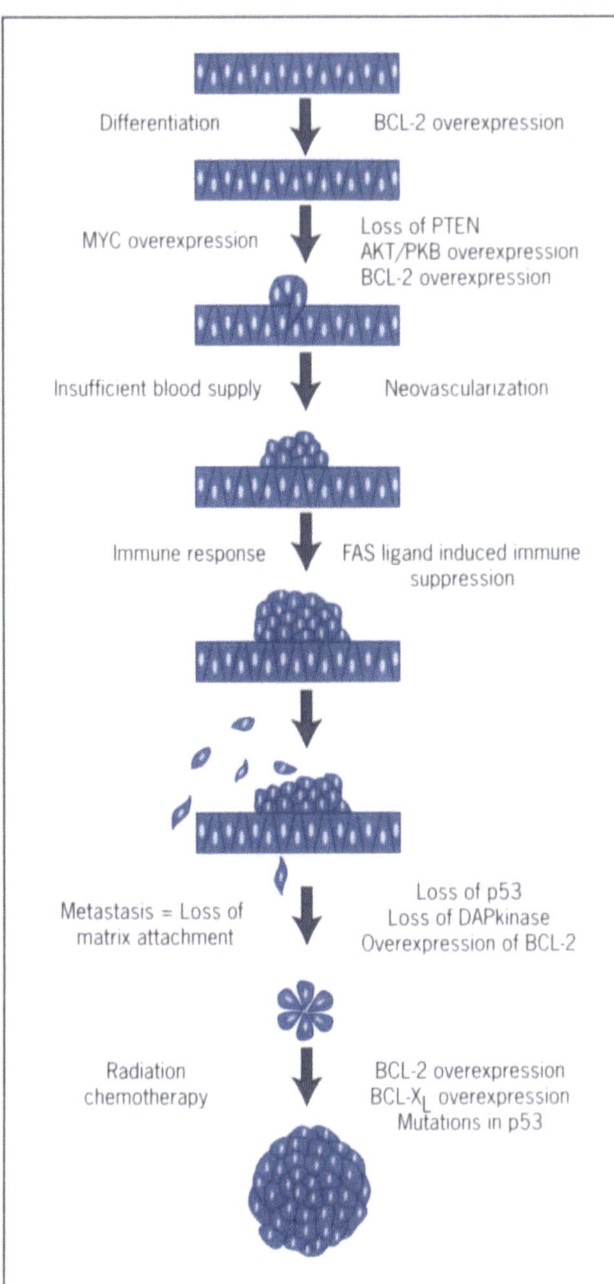

Figure 11-10. Killing signals and survival signals in tumorigenesis. Listed on the left are apoptosis inducers that restrict tumor progression, while on the right are the cellular alterations that abrogate killing. Differentiation and MYC overexpression induce cell killing. Absence of an adequate blood supply that provides oxygen as well as growth and survival factors to the growing tumor is lethal. In addition, tumors are targeted for killing by the immune system. In some cases, tumor cells detach and travel to a distal site, *ie*, metastasize. Because interaction with the extracellular matrix is a strong survival signal, detachment from the main tumor induces killing. Finally, clinically applied chemotherapeutics and radiation therapy induce a strong killing response in sensitive tumors. The genetic alterations that abrogate these killing signals include overexpression of oncogene products, loss of tumor suppressors, neovascularization, and immune suppression.

tein 3 (*IGF-Bp3*), *BAX*, *DR5*, and cathepsin D [62,83–85]. While IGF-Bp3 reduces the protective effect of IGF by binding and inactivating IGF, BAX mediates cell killing by altering mitochondrial function. It was shown that DR5 induces killing by activating caspases [14], but the mechanism of killing by overexpression of cathepsin D is unknown [58]. In addition, p53 induced the transcription of the onco-

Table 11-1. Cell deaths repressed by BCL-2

Lymphoid
Factor withdrawal—IL-2, IL-3, IL-4, IL-6, GM-CSF
Glucocorticoid
γ Irradiation
Phorbol esters
Calcium
Cross-linking by anti-CD3
Neuronal
Factor withdrawal—NGF, BDNF, Neurotrophin-3
Serum withdrawal
Calcium
Infarction
Axotomy
Naturally occurring cell death
Fibroblasts
Serum deprivation and MYC induction
Oncogene-related
MYC-induced
E1A-induced
p53-mediated
Viral infections
Adenovirus
Sindbis virus
HTLV-1
Chemotherapeutic drugs
DNA synthesis inhibitors
Alkylating agents
Topoisomerase inhibitors
Microtubule inhibitors
Antimetabolites
Oxidant stress
H_2O_2
Menadione
Membrane peroxidation
Others
TGF-β
Staurosporine
Loss of extracellular matrix

Adapted from Yang et al. [63].

gene *MDM2*, which negatively regulates p53. The FAS pathway is induced by activated p53 in a transcription independent fashion by rapid re-localization of FAS from internal pools to the cell surface [42].

In summary, the core killing machinery consisting of caspases, BCL-2 family members, and mitochondria regulates the activities of oncogenes and tumor suppressor genes, and in turn is controlled by their actions.

APOPTOSIS AND CANCER

The current understanding of apoptosis already is being used to design and test new approaches for improving the prevention, diagnosis, and treatment of cancer. The field of prevention can immediately benefit from the fact that mediators of apoptosis, such as DAP kinase and *p53*, are potential tumor suppressor genes. Similar to screening for mutations in *p53* that predispose carriers to cancer, individuals from families with hereditary cancer should be screened for the status of mediators of cell killing. Identified carriers should be placed on more aggressive preventative regimens and should be more carefully monitored for the appearance of early clinical signs of cancer. Improved molecular diagnosis of cancer can emerge from the field of apoptosis as well. Ideally, the expression of proapoptotic and antiapoptotic genes should be used to predict tumor progression and the response of various tumors to chemotherapy induced killing.

At present, the levels of expression of two antiapoptotic proteins, namely survivin and BCL-2, have been evaluated in human tumors in an

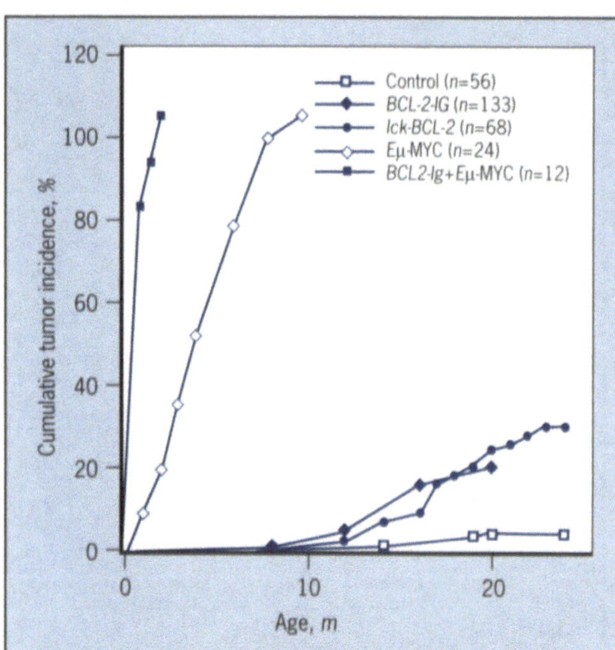

Figure 11-11. *BCL-2* and *MYC* synergize to induce tumors. Shown is the cumulative tumor incidence in transgenic mice overexpressing *BCL-2*, *MYC*, or both. The expression of *BCL-2* is driven by either the immunoglobulin promoter or the lck promoter. *MYC* expression is driven by the Eμ promoter. Mice expressing both *BCL-2* and *MYC* show an increased rate of tumor formation compared with mice expressing only one transgene. (*Adapted from* Yang and Korsmeyer [63]; with permission.)

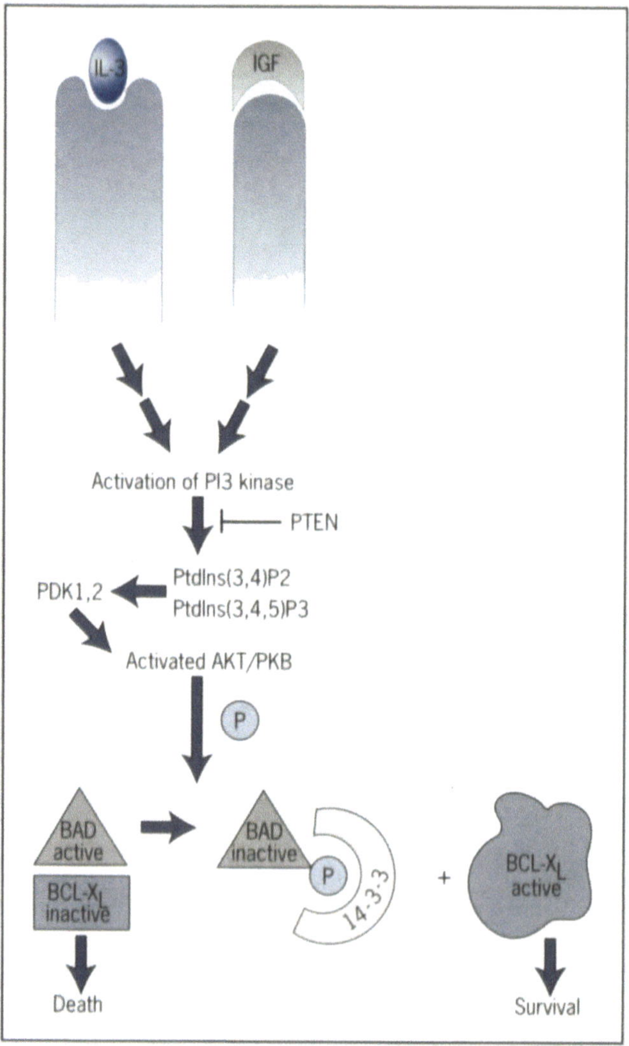

Figure 11-12. Survival pathway involving Phosphatidylinositol 3- (PI3) kinase, AKT/PKB, and the tumor suppressor PTEN. Binding of the survival factors IGF and IL3 to their receptors transduces a phosphorylation cascade leading to the activation of PI3 kinase. PI3 kinase phosphorylates lipids to generate PtdIns(3,4)P2 and PtdIns(3,4,5)P3, which are dephosphorylated by PTEN. PtdIns(3,4)P2 and PtdIns(3,4,5)P3 activate AKT/PKB directly by translocating it to the plasma membrane and indirectly by activating PDK1 and PDK2, which then phosphorylate and activate AKT/PKB. Activated AKT/PKB phosphorylates and inactivates the proapoptotic protein BAD, resulting in activation of the antiapoptotic BCL-X_L.

attempt to correlate them with tumor prognosis [86]. The levels of expression of survivin, which is a member of the IAP family, is associated with high tumor grade and poor prognosis in neuroblastoma and colon tumors. Elevated levels of BCL-2 correlate with high grade or poor prognosis of neuroblastoma, non-Hodgkin's lymphoma, and prostate tumors. Conversely, in breast, colon, kidney, ovary, and pancreas tumors, high levels of BCL-2 may correlate with lower grade or better prognosis. BCL-2 may possess antiapoptic activity or growth-suppressing activity in different cell types. Whereas the antiapoptotic activity may be required for tumor initiation, BCL-2 may be detrimental for cell proliferation and tumor progression. Another explanation for the lack of universal correlation between levels of BCL-2 and poor prognosis is additional alterations in the levels of expression of other members of the BCL-2 family. Because apoptosis is regulated by the balance of pro- and antiapoptotic proteins, the ratio of BCL-2 to Bax expression could be used in predicting the sensitivity of tumor cells to apoptosis and their response to therapy. Indeed, a high ratio of BCL-2 to Bax is an accurate indicator of poor response to therapy in acute myelogenous leukemia (AML) and a marker of poor prognosis in chronic lymphocytic leukemia (CLL). Thus, the long-term approaches for improving the prevention, diagnosis, and treatment of cancer will become more practical as additional mediators of cell killing are identified and fully characterized.

The most challenging goal is to harness apoptosis in an effort to develop effective cancer treatments. A thorough understanding of cell death is required in order to tailor a specific response in the tumor with limited collateral damage to the surrounding organs. Based on our current knowledge, several strategies are being considered.

Induction of Death in Tumor Cells

In 50% of human tumors p53 is mutated or lost. In these tumors, triggering FAS or TNF induced apoptosis that is independent of p53 will provide a direct mechanism for tumor killing that bypasses the need for a functional p53. While induction of the FAS pathway or administration of TNF can cause substantial side effects, the death ligand APO2L/TRAIL is an apoptosis inducer candidate that appears to preferentially kill tumor cells without substantial side effects [14]. Triggering of additional death receptors is being clinically evaluated. An additional approach should involve designing and delivering to tumor cells, potent inducers of death such as the proapoptotic BH3 domain. Because tumor cells become dependent on the inhibition of apoptosis [64,66], downregulation of antiapoptotic genes such as *BCL-2* by interventional drugs should be tested. One major advantage of killing tumor cells by inducing apoptosis is that often only a transient treatment with an inducer is sufficient to commit cells to die.

Antiangiogenic Strategies

The pioneering work of Folkman and coworkers [87] demonstrated that the growth of solid tumors is dependent on a robust blood supply that is furnished by the generation of new blood vessels via the secretion of factors that induce neovascularization, as well as by the downregulation of genes that prevent neovascularization. In the human body, the rate of neovascularization is very low, and actively proliferating vascular endothelial cells are predominantly found at tumor sites. Because tumor growth requires this neovascularization, two strategies have been designed to inhibit the formation of new vasculature or to disrupt tumor recruited vasculature; the development of agents that specifically kill or arrest growing but not

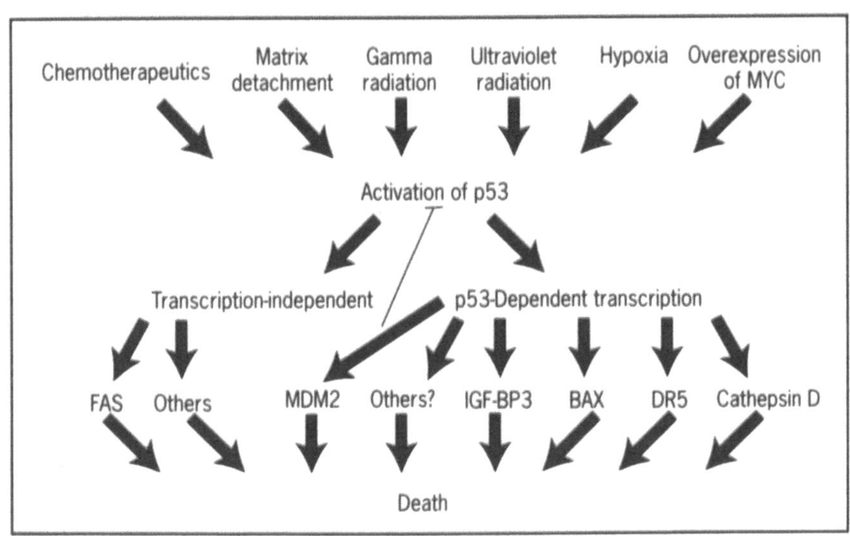

Figure 11-13. The p53 protein as a mediator of apoptotic signaling. Shown are inducers of apoptosis that require p53 to elicit killing and the transduction of the signals by p53.

arrested vascular endothelial cells [88–92], and the targeting of a thrombolytic agent(s) to tumor derived vasculature [93]. In both approaches the end result is the disruption of a tumor induced blood supply followed by rapid killing of tumor cells. Thus far these approaches, which represent an alternative use of apoptosis to limit tumor growth, have been very promising in animal models.

Anti-Immune Suppression Strategies

Tumor formation is regulated by a variety of suppressing mechanisms, including immune mediated tumor suppression. Immune suppression naturally occurs at immune privileged sites such as the retina and testis, and it is enforced by the expression of FAS ligand on the cell surface of cells at these sites [94]. Cytotoxic T lymphocytes (CTLs) and natural killer (NK) cells directed against cells at these sites are killed following the binding to FAS ligand. A number of tumors have adapted this mechanism of killing tumor-directed CTLs and NK cells by expressing FAS ligand [95]. The elimination of antitumor CTLs and NK cells reduces the antitumor immune response [96]. Thus, transient inhibition of FAS induced killing by inhibitors of caspases or by anti-FAS antagonistic antibodies could enhance the antitumor immune response.

Summary

Tremendous progress has been made in revealing the role of apoptosis in cancer. Because apoptosis is crucial in regulating tumor initiation and progression, major efforts are invested in the identification of genes and mechanisms that control cell response to apoptosis. Eventually it will be possible to predict the response of a tumor to apoptotic induction by measuring the expression of positive or negative regulators of apoptosis. Mechanistic studies have identified a number of genes that are good pharmacologic targets for selective killing of tumor cells. We are entering an exciting era in which initial strategies designed to harness apoptosis are in clinical trial and our knowledge of the process is expanding daily. We expect many more improvements in cancer prevention, diagnosis, and treatment, based on this young and exciting field.

Acknowledgments

I acknowledge my colleagues for stimulating discussions, and I apologize to those whose works were not cited due to length limitations.

References:

1. Kerr JF, Wyllie AH, Currie AR: Apoptosis: a basic biological phenomenon with wide-ranging implication in tissue kinetics. *Br J Cancer* 1972, 26:239–257.
2. Thompson CB: Apoptosis in the pathogenesis and treatment of disease. *Science* 1995, 267:1456–1462.
3. Hengartner MO, Horvitz HR: Programmed cell death in *Caenorhabditis elegans*. *Curr Opin Genet Dev* 1994, 4:581–586.
4. Yuan J, Horvitz HR: The *Caenorhabditis elegans* cell death gene ced-4 encodes a novel protein and is expressed during the period of extensive programmed cell death. *Development* 1992, 116:309–320.
5. Yuan J, Shaham S, Ledoux S, *et al.*: The *C. elegans* cell death gene ced-3 encodes a protein similar to mammalian interleukin-1 beta-converting enzyme. *Cell* 1993, 75:641–652.
6. Hengartner MO, Ellis RE, Horvitz HR: *Caenorhabditis elegans* gene ced-9 protects cells from programmed cell death. *Nature* 1992, 356:494–499.
7. Shaham S, Horvitz HR: Developing *Caenorhabditis elegans* neurons may contain both cell-death protective and killer activities. *Genes Dev* 1996, 10:578–591.
8. Cryns V, Yuan J: Proteases to die for. *Genes Dev* 1998, 12:1551–1570.
9. Adams JM, Cory S: The Bcl-2 protein family: arbiters of cell survival. *Science* 1998, 281:1322–1326.
10. Hengartner M: Death by crowd control. *Science* 1998, 281:1298–1299.
11. Yang X, Chang HY, Baltimore D: Essential role of CED-4 oligomerization in CED-3 activation and apoptosis [see comments]. *Science* 1998, 281:1355–1357.
12. Conradt B, Horvitz HR: The *C. elegans* protein EGL-1 is required for programmed cell death and interacts with the Bcl-2-like protein CED-9. *Cell* 1998, 93:519–529.
13. Cohen GM: Caspases: the executioners of apoptosis. *Biochem J* 1997, 326:1–16.
14. Ashkenazi A, Dixit VM: Death receptors: signaling and modulation. *Science* 1998, 281:1305–1308.
15. Hsu H, Xiong J, Goeddel DV: The TNF receptor 1-associated protein TRADD signals cell death and NF-κ B activation. *Cell* 1995, 81:495–504.
16. Nagata S: Apoptosis by death factor. *Cell* 1997, 88:355–365.
17. Kuida K, Zheng TS, Na S, *et al.*: Decreased apoptosis in the brain and premature lethality in CPP32-deficient mice. *Nature* 1996, 384:368–372.
18. Kuida K, Haydar TF, Kuan CY, *et al.*: Reduced apoptosis and cytochrome c-mediated caspase activation in mice lacking caspase 9. *Cell* 1998, 94:325–337.
19. Hakem R, Hakem A, Duncan GS, *et al.*: Differential requirement for caspase 9 in apoptotic pathways in vivo. *Cell* 1998, 94:339–352.
20. Zou H, Henzel WJ , Liu X, *et al.*: Apaf-1, a human protein homologous to *C. elegans* CED-4, participates in cytochrome c-dependent activation of caspase-3 [see comments]. *Cell* 1997, 90:405–443.

21. Pan G, O'Rourke K, Dixit VM: Capsase-9, Bcl-XL, and Apaf-1 form a ternary complex. *J Biol Chem* 1998, 273:5841–5845.

22. Cecconi F, Alvarez-Bolado G, Meyer BI, *et al.*: Apaf1 (CED-4 homolog) regulates programmed cell death in mammalian development. *Cell* 1998, 94:727–737.

23. Yoshida H, Kong YY, Yoshida R, *et al.*: Apaf1 is required for mitochondrial pathways of apoptosis and brain development. *Cell* 1998, 94:739–750.

24. Hengartner MO, Horvitz HR: *C. elegans* cell survival gene ced-9 encodes a functional homolog of the mammalian proto-oncogene bcl-2. *Cell* 1994, 76:665–676.

25. Kelekar A, Thompson CB: Bcl-2-family proteins: the role of the BH3 domain in apoptosis. *Trends Cell Biol* 1998, 8:324–330.

26. Wang H-G, Rapp UR, Reed JC: Bcl-2 targets the protein kinase Raf-1 to mitochondria. *Cell* 1996, 87:629–638.

27. Shibasaki F, Kondo E, Akagi T, McKeon F: Suppression of signalling through transcription factor NF-AT by interactions between calcineurin and Bcl-2. *Nature* 1997, 386:728–731.

28. Hunter JJ, Bond BL, Parslow TG: Functional dissection of the human Bc12 protein: sequence requirements for inhibition of apoptosis. *Mol Cell Biol* 1996, 16:877–883.

29. Muchmore SW, Sattler M, Liang H, *et al.*: X-ray and NMR structure of human Bcl-xL, an inhibitor of programmed cell death. *Nature* 1996, 381:335–341.

30. Sattler M, Liang H, Nettesheim D, *et al.*: Structure of Bcl-xL-Bak peptide complex: recognition between regulators of apoptosis. *Science* 1997, 275:983–986.

31. Minn AJ, Velez P, Schendel SL, *et al.*: Bcl-x(L) forms an ion channel in synthetic lipid membranes. *Nature* 1997, 385:353–357.

32. Schendel SL, Xie Z, Montal MO, *et al.*: Channel formation by antiapoptotic protein Bcl-2. *Proc Natl Acad Sci U S A* 1997, 94:5113–5118.

33. Schlesinger PH, Gross A, Yin XM, *et al.*: Comparison of the ion channel characteristics of proapoptotic BAX and antiapoptotic BCL-2. *Proc Natl Acad Sci U S A* 1997, 94:11357–11362.

34. Vander Heiden MG, Chandel NS, Williamson EK, *et al.*: Bcl-xL regulates the membrane potential and volume homeostasis of mitochondria [see comments]. *Cell* 1997, 91:627–637.

35. Green DR, Reed JC: Mitochondria and apoptosis. *Science* 1998, 281:1309–1312.

36. Green DR: Apoptotic pathways: the roads to ruin. *Cell* 1998, 94:695–698.

37. Kroemer G, Zamzami N, Susin SA: Mitochondrial control of apoptosis. *Immunol Today* 1997, 18:44–51.

38. Marzo I, Brenner C, Zamzami N, *et al.*: Bax and adenine nucleotide translocator cooperate in the mitochondrial control of apoptosis. *Science* 1998, 281:2027–2031.

39. Antonsson B, Conti F, Ciavatta A, *et al.*: Inhibition of Bax channel-forming activity by Bcl-2. *Science* 1997, 277:370–372.

40. Scaffidi C, Fulda S, Srinivasan A, *et al.*: Two CD95 (APO-1/Fas) signaling pathways. *EMBO J* 1998, 17:1675–1687.

41. Nagata S: Fas-induced apoptosis, and diseases caused by its abnormality. *Genes Cells* 1996, 1:873–879.

42. Bennett M, Macdonald K, Chan SW, *et al.*: Cell surface trafficking of fas: a rapid mechanism of p53-mediated apoptosis. *Science* 1998, 282:290–293.

43. Chinnaiyan AM, O'Rourke K, Tewari M, Dixit VM: FADD, a novel death domain containing protein, interacts with the death domain of Fas and initiates apoptosis. *Cell* 1995, 81:505–512.

44. Luo X, Budihardjo I, Zou H, *et al.*: Bid, a BCL-2 interacting protein, mediates cytochrome c release from mitochondria in response to activation of cell surface death receptors. *Cell* 1998, 94:481–490.

45. Boldin MP, Goncharov TM, Goltsev YV, Wallach D: Involvement of MACH, a novel MORT1/FADD-interacting protease, in Fas/APO-1- and TNF receptor-induced cell death. *Cell* 1996, 85:803–815.

46. Muzio M, Chinnaiyan AM, Kischkel FC, *et al.*: FLICE, a novel FADD-homologous ICE/CED-3-like protease, is recruited to the CD95 (Fas/APO-1) death-inducing signaling complex. *Cell* 1996, 85:817–827.

47. Yang X, Khosravi-Far R, Chang HY, Baltimore D: Daxx, a novel Fas-binding protein that activates JNK and apoptosis. *Cell* 1997, 89:1067–1076.

48. Hsu H, Shu HB, Pan MG, Goeddel DV: TRADD-TRAF2 and TRADD-FADD interactions define two distinct TNF receptor 1 signal transduction pathways. *Cell* 1996, 84:299–308.

49. Ting AT, Pimentel-Muinos FX, Seed B: RIP mediates tumor necrosis factor receptor 1 activation of NF-κB but not Fas/APO-1-initiated apoptosis. *Embo J* 1996, 15:6189–6196.

50. Wang CY, Mayo MW, Korneluk RG, Goeddel DV, Baldwin A, Jr.: NF-kappaB antiapoptosis: induction of TRAF1 and TRAF2 and c-IAP1 and c- IAP2 to suppress caspase-8 activation. *Science* 1998, 281:1680–1683.

51. Yeh WC, Pompa JL, McCurrach ME, *et al.*: FADD: essential for embryo development and signaling from some, but not all, inducers of apoptosis. *Science* 1998, 279:1954–1958.

52. Zhang J, Cado D, Chen A, *et al.*: Fas-mediated apoptosis and activation-induced T-cell proliferation are defective in mice lacking FADD/Mort1. *Nature* 1998, 392:296–300.

53. Marsters SA, Sheridan JP, Pitti RM, *et al.*: A novel receptor for Apo2L/TRAIL contains a truncated death domain. *Curr Biol* 1997, 7:1003–1006.

54. Sheridan JP, Marsters SA, Pitti RM, *et al.*: Control of TRAIL-induced apoptosis by a family of signaling and decoy receptors [see comments]. *Science* 1997, 277:818–821.

55. Irmler M, Thome M, Hahne M, *et al.*: Inhibition of death receptor signals by cellular FLIP [see comments]. *Nature* 1997, 388:190–195.

56. Ambrosini G, Adida C, Altieri DC: A novel anti-apoptosis gene, survivin, expressed in cancer and lymphoma. *Nat Med* 1997, 3:917–921.

57. Deveraux QL, Takahashi R, Salvesen GS, Reed JC: X-linked IAP is a direct inhibitor of cell-death proteases. *Nature* 1997, 388:300–304.

58. Kimchi A: DAP genes: novel apoptotic genes isolated by a functional approach to gene cloning. *Biochim Biophys Acta* 1998, 1377:F13–33.

59. Deiss LP, Kimchi A: A genetic tool used to identify thioredoxin as a mediator of a growth inhibitory signal. *Science* 1991, 252:117–120.
60. Deiss LP, Feinstein E, Berissi H, *et al.*: Identification of a novel serine/threonine kinase and a novel 15-kD protein as potential mediators of the gamma interferon-induced cell death. *Genes Dev* 1995, 9:15–30.
61. Inbal B, Cohen O, Polak-Charcon S, *et al.*: DAP kinase links the control of apoptosis to metastasis. *Nature* 1997, 390:180–184.
62. Wu GS, Saftig P, Peters C, El-Deiry WS: Potential role for cathepsin D in p53 dependent tumor suppression and chemosensitivity. *Oncogene* 1998, 16:2177–2183.
63. Yang E, Korsmeyer SJ: Molecular thanatopsis: a discourse on the BCL-2 family and cell death. *Blood* 1996, 88:386–401.
64. Evan GI, Wyllie AH, Gilbert CS, *et al.*: Induction of apoptosis in fibroblasts by c-myc protein. *Cell* 1992, 69:119–128.
65. Bissonnette RP, Echeverri F, Mahboubi A, Green DR: Apoptotic cell death induced by c-myc is inhibited by bcl-2. *Nature* 1992, 359:552–554.
66. Fanidi A, Harrington EA, Evan GI: Cooperative interaction between c-myc and bcl-2 proto-oncogenes. *Nature* 1992, 359:554–556.
67. Wagner AJ, Small MB, Hay N: Myc-mediated apoptosis is blocked by ectopic expression of Bcl-2. *Mol Cell Biol* 1993, 13:2432–2440.
68. Frisch SM, Francis H: Disruption of epithelial cell-matrix interactions induces apoptosis. *J Cell Biol* 1994, 124:619–626.
69. Frisch SM, Ruoslahti E: Integrins and anoikis. *Curr Opin Cell Biol* 1997, 9:701–706.
70. Berry DE, Lu Y, Schmidt B, *et al.*: Retinoblastoma protein inhibits IFN-gamma induced apoptosis. *Oncogene* 1996, 12:1809–1819.
71. Fan G, Ma X, Kren BT, Steer CJ: The retinoblastoma gene product inhibits TGF beta1 induced apoptosis in primary rat hepatocytes and human HuH-7 hepatoma cells. *Oncogene* 1996, 12:1909–1919.
72. Haupt Y, Rowan S, Oren M: p53-mediated apoptosis in HeLa cells can be overcome by excess pRB. *Oncogene* 1995, 10:1563–1571.
73. Haas-Kogan DA, Kogan SC, Levi D, *et al.*: Inhibition of apoptosis by the retinoblastoma gene product. *EMBO J* 1995, 14:461–472.
74. Hermeking H, Eick D: Mediation of c-Myc-induced apoptosis by p53. *Science* 1994, 265:2091—2093.
75. Wagner AJ, Kokontis JM, Hay N: Myc-mediated apoptosis requires wild-type p53 in a manner independent of cell cycle arrest and the ability of p53 to induce p21waf/cip1. *Genes Dev* 1994, 8:2817–2830.
76. Kauffmann-Zeh A, Rodriguez-Viciana P, Ulrich E, *et al.*: Suppression of c-Myc-induced apoptosis by Ras signalling through PI(3)K and PKB. *Nature* 1997, 385:544–548.
77. Kennedy SG, Wagner AJ, Conzen SD, *et al.*: The PI 3-kinase/Akt signaling pathway delivers an anti-apoptotic signal. *Genes Dev* 1997, 11:701–713.
78. Cantley LC, Neel BG: New insights into tumor suppression: PTEN suppresses tumor formation by restraining the phosphoinositide 3-kinase/AKT pathway. *Proc Natl Acad Sci U S A* 1999, 96:4240–4205.
79. Coffer PJ, Jin J, Woodgett JR: Protein kinase B (c-Akt): a multifunctional mediator of phosphatidylinositol 3-kinase activation. *Biochem J* 1998, 335 (Pt 1):1–13.
80. Zha J, Harada H, Yang E, *et al.*: Serine phosphorylation of death agonist BAD in response to survival factor results in binding to 14-3-3 not BCL-X(L) [see comments]. *Cell* 1996, 87:619–628.
81. Datta SR, Dudek H, Tao X, *et al.*: Akt phosphorylation of BAD couples survival signals to the cell- intrinsic death machinery. *Cell* 1997, 91:231–241.
82. Maehama T, Dixon JE: The tumor suppressor, PTEN/MMAC1, dephosphorylates the lipid second messenger, phosphatidylinositol 3,4,5-trisphosphate. *J Biol Chem* 1998, 273:13375-13378.
83. Deiss LP, Galinka H, Berissi H, *et al.*: Cathepsin D protease mediates programmed cell death induced by interferon-gamma, Fas/APO-1 and TNF-α. *Embo J* 1996, 15:3861–3870.
84. Buckbinder L, Talbott R, Velasco-Miguel S, *et al.*: Induction of the growth inhibitor IGF-binding protein 3 by p53. *Nature* 1995, 377:646–649.
85. Miyashita T, Reed JC: Tumor suppressor p53 is a direct transcriptional activator of the human bax gene. *Cell* 1995, 80:293–299.
86. Jaattela M: Escaping cell death: survival proteins in cancer. *Exp Cell Res* 1999, 248:30–43.
87. Folkman J: Angiogenesis in cancer, vascular, rheumatoid and other disease. *Nat Med* 1995, 1:27–31.
88. O'Reilly MS, Holmgren L, Chen C, Folkman J: Angiostatin induces and sustains dormancy of human primary tumors in mice. *Nat Med* 1996, 2:689–692.
89. Parangi S, O'Reilly M, Christofori G, *et al.*: Antiangiogenic therapy of transgenic mice impairs de novo tumor growth. *Proc Natl Acad Sci U S A* 1996, 93:2002–2007.
90. Brooks PC, Montgomery AM, Rosenfeld M, *et al.*: Integrin alpha v beta 3 antagonists promote tumor regression by inducing apoptosis of angiogenic blood vessels. *Cell* 1994, 79:1157–1164.
91. Brooks PC, Stromblad S, Klemke R, *et al.*: Antiintegrin alpha v beta 3 blocks human breast cancer growth and angiogenesis in human skin [see comments]. *J Clin Invest* 1995, 96:1815–1822.
92. Brooks PC, Silletti S, von Schalscha TL, *et al.*: Disruption of angiogenesis by PEX, a noncatalytic metalloproteinase fragment with integrin binding activity. *Cell* 1998, 92:391–400.
93. Huang X, Molema G, King S, *et al.*: Tumor infarction in mice by antibody-directed targeting of tissue factor to tumor vasculature [see comments]. *Science* 1997, 275:547–550.
94. Strand S, Hofmann WJ, Hug H, *et al.*: Lymphocyte apoptosis induced by CD95 (APO-1/Fas) ligand expressing tumor cells–a mechanism of immune evasion? [see comments]. *Nat Med* 1996, 2:1361–1366.
95. Hahne M, Rimoldi D, Schroter M, *et al.*: Melanoma cell expression of Fas(Apo-1/CD95) ligand: implications for tumor immune escape [see comments]. *Science* 1996, 274:1363–1366.
96. Nagata S: Fas ligand and immune evasion [news; comment]. *Nat Med* 1996, 2:1306–1307.

CHAPTER

12

Approaches to New Drug Discovery

Lawrence M. Kauvar

For this survey, current approaches to the discovery of new anticancer drugs are discussed in three categories: tumor-directed delivery vehicles, screens for specific protein modulators, and mechanism-blind assays. These approaches are intertwined in several respects (Fig. 12-1). New methods for identifying tumor markers provide novel delivery "addresses" as well as novel targets for drug inhibition or activation. Conversely, proteins identified by genetic epidemiology or cell biology studies as potential intervention points may also provide new addresses. In addition, random screening of novel compounds in cell-based assays, especially natural products, continues to uncover new drug targets. Moreover, cell-based cytotoxicity screening has reached a level of sophistication that allows compounds to be evaluated for novelty in their spectrum of activity before committing to the full expense of clinical development. Closing the loop, gene-transfer technology has provided cell-based screening with new power as a target validation tool, conveniently extendable to animal models via tumor-directed delivery approaches. An important conclusion from this survey is that the logic of current research is increasing the desirability of tailoring treatment protocols to patients stratified by multiple criteria.

TUMOR-DIRECTED DELIVERY

TUMOR ANTIGENS

Tumor-specific antigens have long been recognized in mice. Figure 12-2 illustrates that the transfer of killed cells from chemically induced tumor 1 to syngeneic (genetically identical) mice provides immunologic protection against tumor 1 but not against tumors 2, 3, or 4. From numerous repetitions of this experiment, it is clear that most tumors differ significantly in their antigenic composition. Identifying such antigens in outbred human populations is much more difficult, however. Ex vivo expansion of tumor-infiltrating lymphocytes, although still a cumbersome and controversial technique for the immunologic treatment of cancer, is in principle a way to circumvent the difficulties in direct identification of antigens. Pending progress on identifying truly tumor-specific antigens, primary emphasis is currently on a few antigens that are known to be at least strongly tumor associated [1].

Hybridoma technology has played a prominent role in the study of tumor antigens. About a decade ago, such monoclonal antibodies appeared to be one of the most promising new cancer treatment approaches (Fig. 12-3). Although results to date have not provided the desired universal cure, the technology continues to have great potential as many of the obstacles to the simplistic hopes for these "magic bullets" are becoming understood and overcome. One of the subtle obstacles is the ease with which monoclonal antibodies can be prepared using the original hybridoma technology and subsequent variations. A rational approach is still not in place for prioritizing drug development on the estimated 100,000 monoclonal antibodies already raised against human tumor specimens worldwide. The most tumor-specific antigens generally are found in only a small number of patients, creating further obstacles to commercial development.

Hybridoma technology was initially developed using murine myelomas fused to antigen-primed murine B cells. The resulting murine antibodies are recognized as foreign proteins by the human immune system. Techniques for "humanizing" antibodies by replacing murine constant region motifs with corresponding human motifs are providing antibodies that are far less subject to the human antimouse antibody response [2]. Alternatively, transplanting human hematopoietic progenitor cells into immune-deficient mice promises to provide fully human monoclonal antibodies [3]. Finally, recombinant human antibodies are now being developed (Fig. 12-4). Because this last

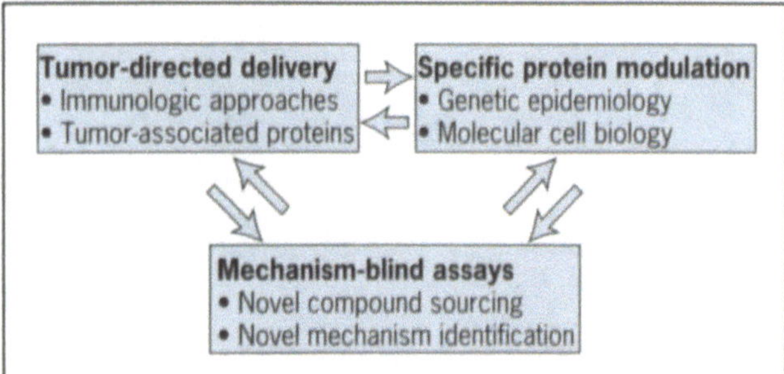

Figure 12-1. Interconnections among cancer therapy approaches.

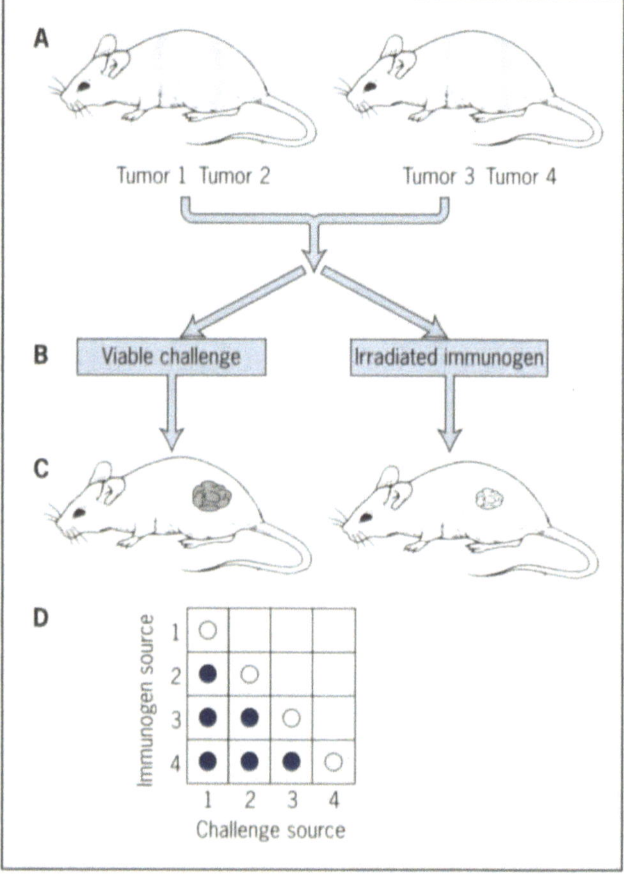

Figure 12-2. Tumor-specific antigens. **A**, Sarcomas are induced by painting a carcinogen (methyl cholanthrene) on the skin. **B**, The resulting tumors are sampled to provide live "challenge" cells as well as "immunogen" cells (irradiated sufficiently to prevent replication). **C**, Genetically identical hosts that have mounted an immune response to tumor-specific antigens in the immunogen are protected against tumor formation by the challenge. **D**, Almost all tumors, even those induced at two different sites on the same mouse, only provide protection against themselves, not against other challenge cells.

technique does not provide preferential growth of immunogen-responsive clones as in hybridoma methods, more efficient selection methods are required, *eg*, using phage display technology [4].

Figure 12-5 illustrates the degree of antibody localization that can be achieved clinically, in this case using a humanized murine monoclonal to carcinoembryonic antigen, a fetal protein often expressed on epithelial cell tumors. Antigens such as carcinoembryonic antigen, as opposed to truly unique antigens, are more readily evaluated using the standard regulatory paradigm than are highly specific targeting reagents that apply to only small numbers of patients. As another example, nearly all B-cell lymphomas retain surface expression of the CD20 antigen found on mature B cells, thus providing a convenient targeting address for antibody-dependent cell-mediated lysis or delivery of a radioisotope. Although not tumor specific, this antigen is absent on the immature precursor cells, allowing normal immune cells to

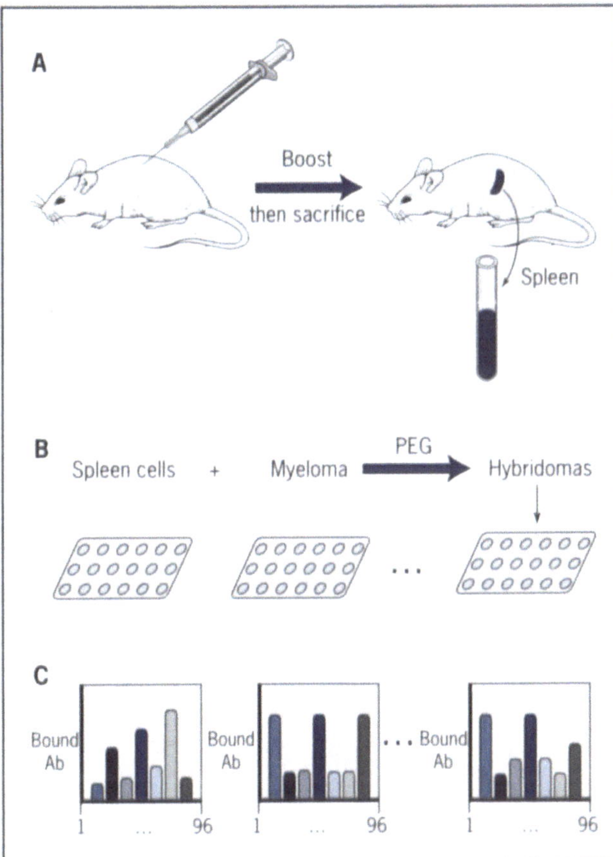

Figure 12-3. Hybridoma technology. **A**, Hybridoma creation begins with immunization of a mouse and collection of the splenocytes. **B**, These splenocytes are immortalized by fusion with an established myeloma line and plated out. Each clone secretes a distinctive (monoclonal) antibody. **C**, Because B cells proliferating in response to immunization are highly preferential fusion partners, a substantial proportion of the clones secrete an antibody that can bind to the immunogen.

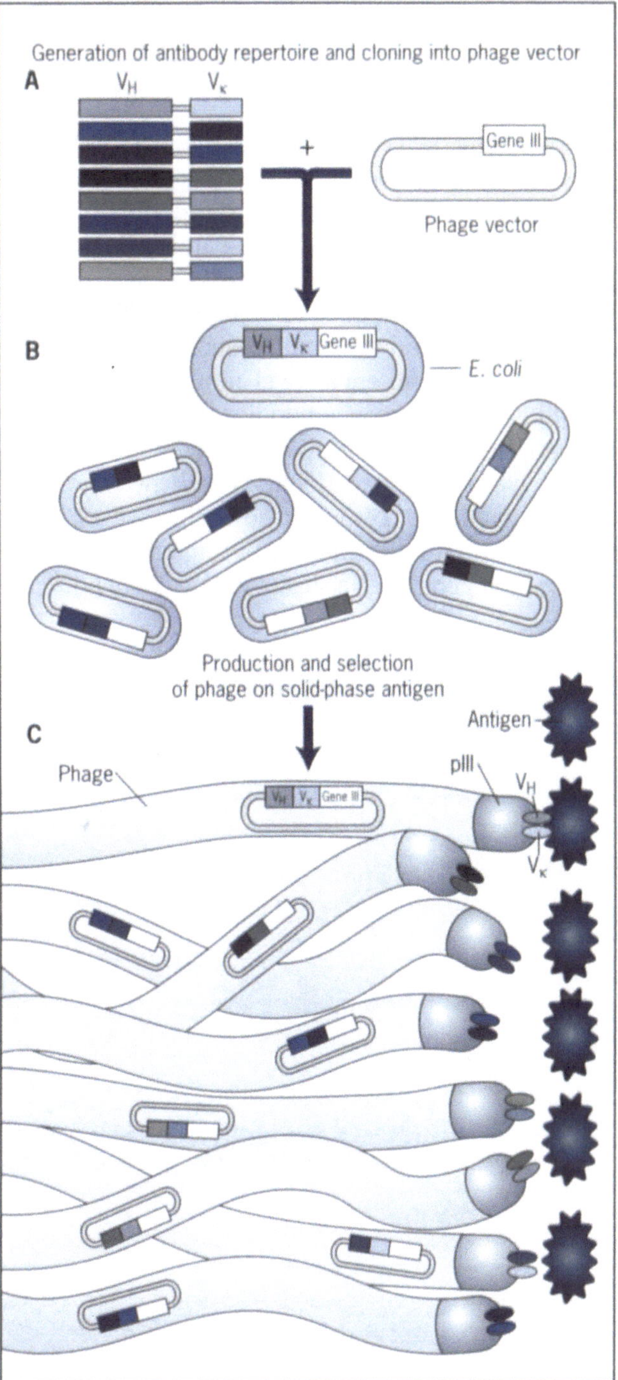

Figure 12-4. Antibody production with phage libraries. **A**, Using appropriate linkers, a repertoire of single-chain Fv genes (*scFv*) from human B cells is generated by reverse transcriptase polymerase chain reaction cloning into a phage vector that fuses the antibody combining site to a protein expressed on the surface of the phage. **B**, Billions of phage grow up, each expressing one of a wide variety of antibodies on the phage surface. **C**, Phage that express antibodies that can stick to the target antigen are extracted and expanded by standard viral growth methods. Typically, the enrichment for true positive clones is 20- to 1000-fold at each round, depending on the affinity and wash stringency. Thus, even very rare clones can be isolated after repeated rounds of selection. (*Adapted from* Marks and Marks [4]; with permission.)

repopulate the blood after depletion of all B cells, both normal and malignant [5]. Even for a common antigen, certain epitopes may be enriched in a broad population of tumors, such as abnormally glycosylated breast epithelial mucin [6].

Optimizing delivery of antibodies into a solid tumor mass has been a difficult art, in part because only the newly forming blood vessels at the periphery of the mass are sufficiently leaky for the antibody to escape and thus binding is preferentially seen on the periphery. Fusion proteins combining an antibody with a protein that promotes blood vessel permeation (interleukin-2 in the initial test) represent a novel approach to this problem [8]. Another reason antibodies appear localized on the periphery is that the addressing antigenic determinants have been degraded in the highly necrotic interior of the mass. The necrotic tissue itself, however, can be turned into a useful address by targeting abundant exposed antigens, such as histones (Fig. 12-6) [9].

Biodistribution

Simply making smaller antibody fragments to improve tumor penetration is often problematic because the systemic clearance time drops to a few minutes, whereas optimal localization at the tumor site typically takes a minimum of 24 to 48 hours. Higher affinity and specificity for the "address" helps in this regard (Fig. 12-7) [10]. To achieve targeted delivery across the whole tumor mass, it is also important that the methods for radioisotope chelation and conjugation to the antibody be secure enough to survive extended periods in the circulation [11].

Nonradioactive toxins can also be delivered in a way that bathes the vicinity of an addressing tumor marker. For example, antibodies have been conjugated to a cytotoxin such as doxorubicin via a linkage that is broken following uptake of the bound complex

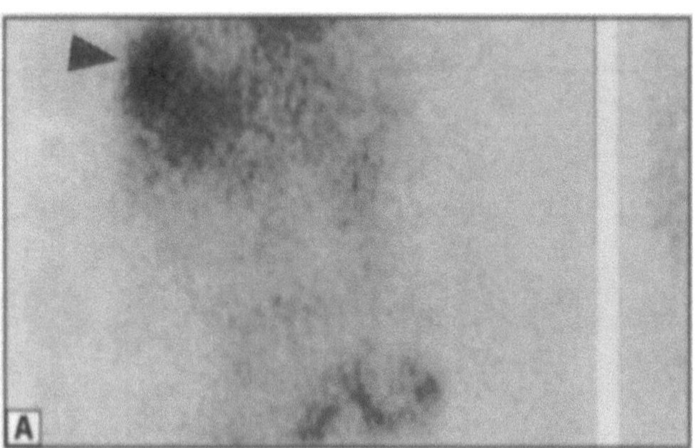

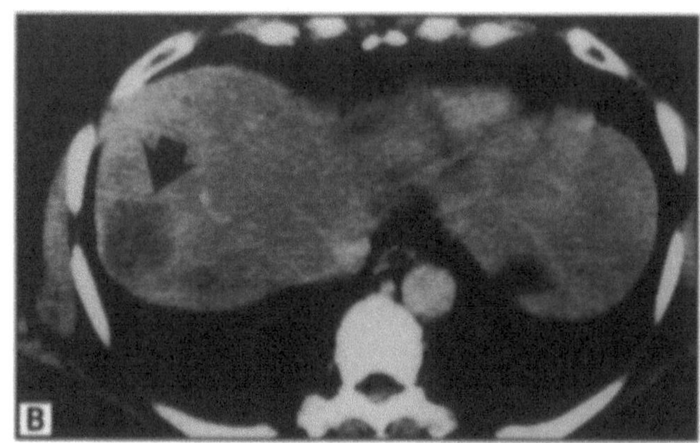

Figure 12-5. In vivo antibody localization. **A**, Anterior abdomen imaged 192 hours after ^{131}I-labeled anti–carcinoembryonic antigen antibody injection, collating gamma ray detector data from 64 projections, shows a metastasis to the liver (*arrowhead*). **B**, Computed tomographic scan of the liver confirms the metastasis (*arrow*). (*From* Sharkey *et al.* [7]; with permission.)

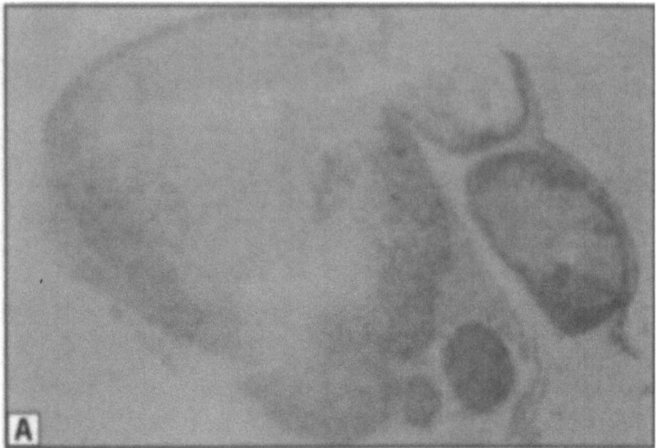

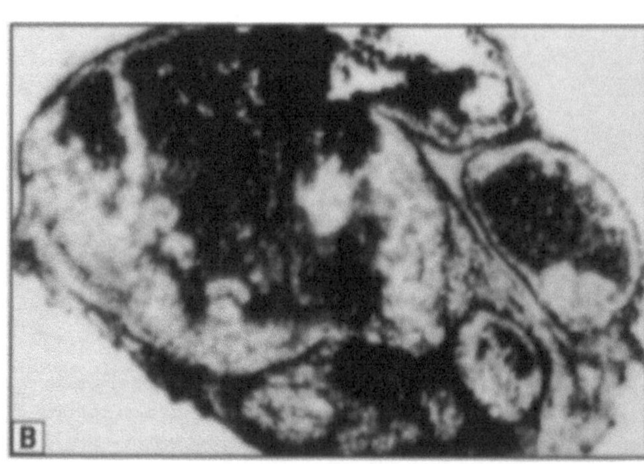

Figure 12-6. Addressing necrotic tissue. ^{125}I-TNT antihistone antibody accumulates throughout the necrotic interior of a cervical carcinoma xenograft tumor mass, seen here 48 hours after injection. **A**, Hematoxylin-eosin stain. **B**, Macroautoradiograph of tissue section directly exposed to radiographic film. (*From* Chen *et al.* [9]; with permission.)

into intracellular lysosomes, after which the active drug can leak into the surrounding tissue [12].

Another approach to targeting "bystander" cells is to conjugate antibodies to an enzyme that activates a subsequently delivered prodrug (Fig. 12-8) [13]. Still another means of attacking the whole tumor mass, applicable to internal or external surface-exposed tumors, is to coat the site with an

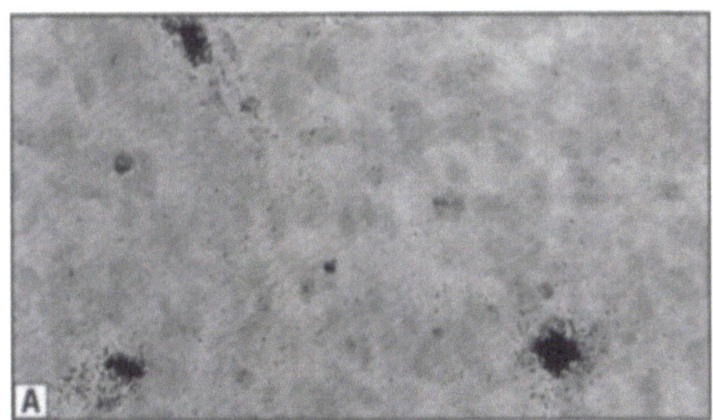

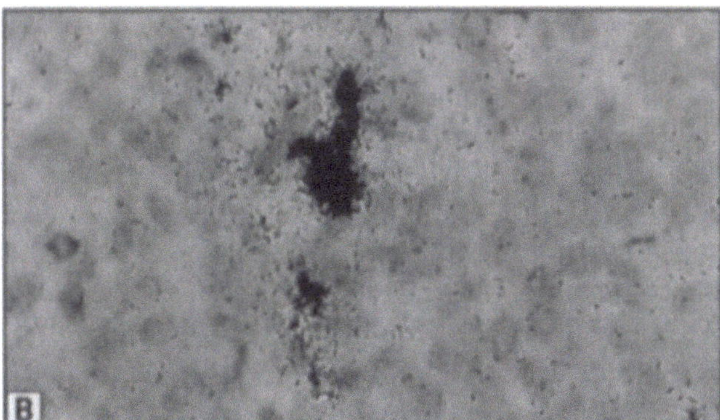

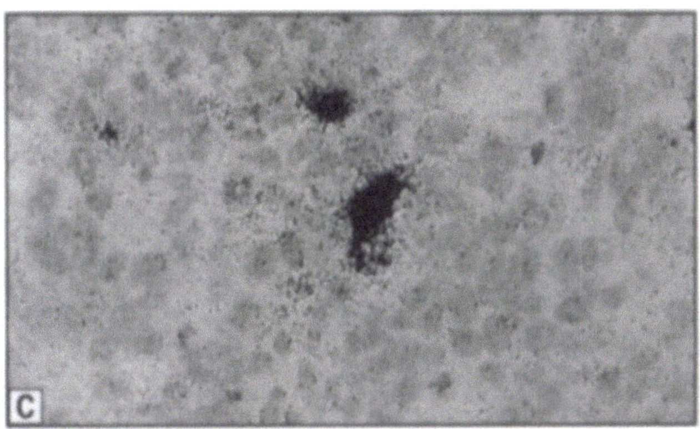

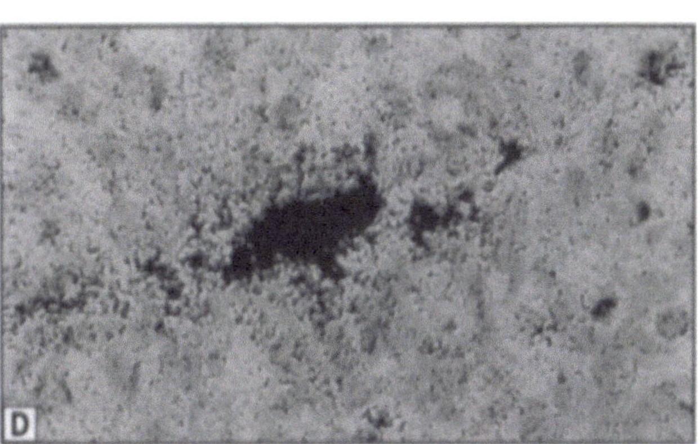

Figure 12-7. Antibody pharmacodynamics. **A–D**, Visualizing bound radiolabeled IgG antibody (*panel 7A*) and smaller fragments (*panels 7B–7D*) on a cross-section of a colon carcinoma xenograft at 6 hours after intravenous injection shows that the smaller fragments accumulate to a higher absolute level, even though a lower percentage of the injected dose ends up at the tumor site due to more rapid clearance from the circulation. The antibody combining site for this series of homologs has high affinity (approximately 10^9 to 10^{10}) for the pancarcinoma antigen TAG-72. (*From* Yokota *et al.* [10]; with permission.)

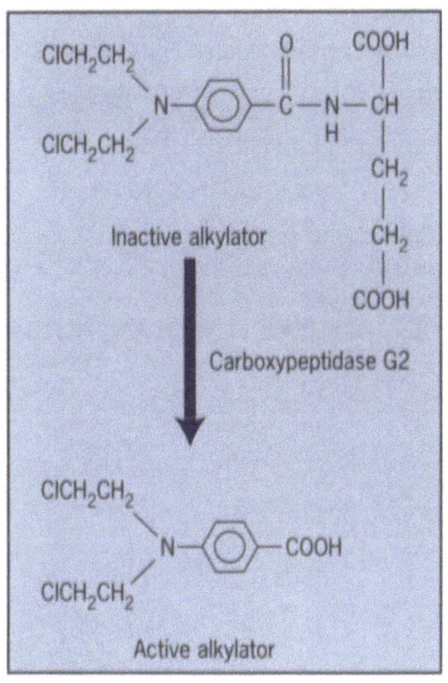

Figure 12-8. Drug activation at a tumor address. A prodrug conjugate of chlorambucil and glutamate is inactive until cleaved by carboxypeptidase G2. If the protease is linked to an antibody that has been allowed to accumulate at a tumor mass, the active alkylator drug will be generated preferentially in the vicinity of tumor cells, which might not otherwise be accessible to the antibody.

"antenna" for collecting light energy (photodynamic therapy) [14].

Prodrugs traditionally have been used to improve oral availability by removal of a masking moiety, in the liver or in tissues generally. Activation by enzymes at the tumor site, enriched artificially via antibody conjugation, takes the prodrug concept to a qualitatively more sophisticated level. In the extreme case, there is no need for an antibody as a targeting vehicle at all. For example, a "latent drug" form of the widely used cytotoxic nitrogen mustard motif has been developed [15], which is activated by glutathione S-transferase, an intracellular enzyme elevated in many tumors and associated with poor prognosis (Fig. 12-9).

During the 24 to 48 hours it typically takes for optimal localization of an antibody to a tumor site, normal tissues are exposed to any linked toxin, which generally has a finite rate of release from the antibody as a result of serum proteases. One approach to avoiding the resulting systemic exposure is to use a prelocalized antibody to capture a rapidly cleared small-molecule toxin (Fig. 12-10) [17]. Care must be taken in implementing this approach because it will be less effective to the extent that the bound antibody becomes internalized, a consideration that does not apply to antibodies directly conjugated to a toxin.

Tumor Physiology

Molecular cell biology and genetic epidemiology studies are documenting an increasing variety of proteins as tumor associated. As the function of these

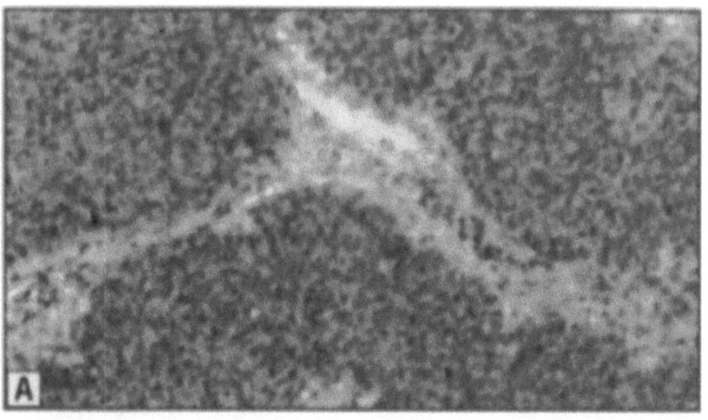

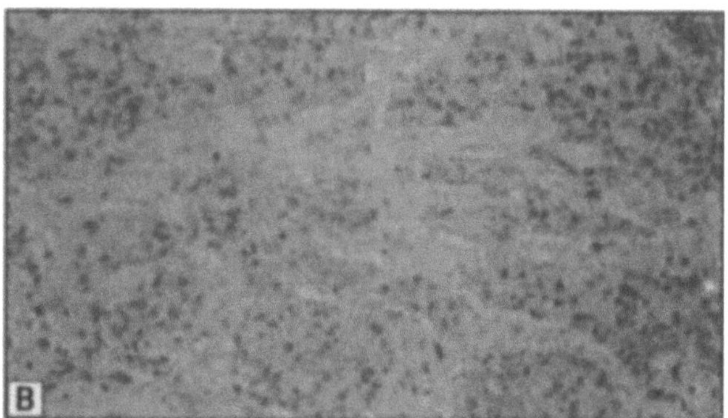

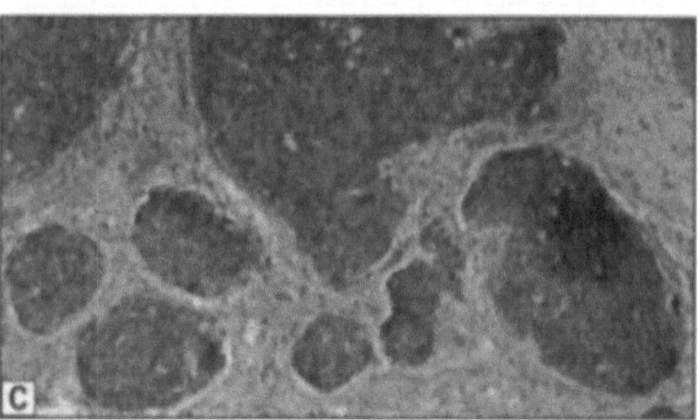

Figure 12-9. A tumor address useable for drug activation. **A**, Glutathione S-transferase (GST) P1-1 in a tissue specimen taken at primary presentation from a laryngeal cancer. *Brown color* indicates immunohistochemical staining. The tumor was responsive to chemotherapy. **B**, A specimen taken following a relapse 2 years later shows elevated levels of GST P1-1. Salvage surgery was performed. **C**, The levels of GST P1-1 were highly elevated the following year, at which point the tumor was resistant to conventional chemotherapy [16]. Elevated GST, however, can activate a novel class of prodrugs [15]. (*From* Nishimura *et al.* [16]; with permission.)

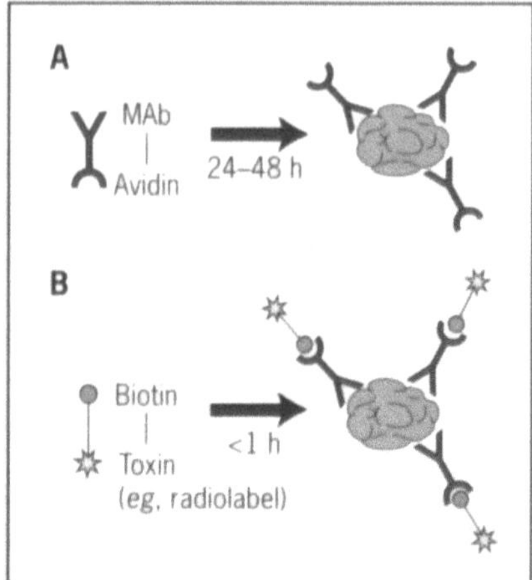

Figure 12-10. Pharmacokinetics. **A**, A conjugate of a monoclonal antibody (MAb) to avidin has slow systemic clearance and minimal systemic toxicity, allowing optimal localization to the tumor site. **B**, Conjugating a toxin, *eg*, a chelated radioisotope, to biotin provides a very high affinity capture mechanism for the toxin at the site of antibody localization. Rapid clearance of the small molecule minimizes systemic exposure. MAb–monoclonal antibody.

proteins becomes better understood, it may be possible to redirect the dysfunctional growth program in tumor cells into a more benign differentiation program [18]. Independent of their causal role in cancer, however, such tumor-associated proteins can provide an addressing mechanism for antibodies, for latent drugs, or for their natural ligand conjugated to a toxin (Fig. 12-11). Small-molecule mimics of the natural ligand should prove even more effective. Particularly attractive targets are autocrine growth factor receptors because mutations that abolish the address will concomitantly select for poorly growing cells [19]. A caveat on this approach is the toxicity associated with targeting a widely expressed protein such as the epidermal growth factor receptor.

Another approach to targeting a physiologic function associated with tumors relies on the need for solid tumors to induce the creation of new blood vessels (angiogenesis) in order to grow. Inhibition of this process is a promising approach to arresting tumor growth. Specific targeting of angiogenesis inhibitors to tumors promises to provide desirable chronic cytostatic activity without blocking normal angiogenesis. A demonstration experiment has used thrombus formation to abort angiogenesis, thereby inducing necrosis in a mouse neuroblastoma (Fig. 12-12) [20].

An even more abstract aspect of tumor physiology, which can nonetheless be targeted, arises from the fact that solid tumors are hostile environments for cells, being enriched in toxic products resulting from cell necrosis. Tumors commonly overuse the relatively inefficient pentose shunt, as compared with mitochondrial glucose catabolism, most likely because it directly increases cytoplasmic reducing power to offset the oxidative stress of the necrotic environment. The controversial role of oxidative damage in cancer, associated with claims for vitamin C as a cure, should not discourage the search for rational intervention in this key area of physiology. In particular, local changes in oxidation-reduction potential and lower pH from increased lactic acid production provide opportunities to target drugs to tumors without any specific protein as the addressing mechanism (Fig. 12-13). Amifostine (Ethyol; US Bioscience, West Conshohocken, PA), for example, provides reducing power to detoxify chemotherapeutic agents and is thus a chemoprotectant. It acts preferentially to protect normal cells, apparently because it is poorly absorbed at the lower pH that is characteristic of solid tumors.

Gene Transfer

Generalized biologic response modifiers have a long history in cancer treatment. Modern versions of this approach include the use of specific recombinant factors, notably interferon and interleukin-2. A targeted gene delivery concept offers the possibility of achieving local production of immunomodulators at far higher levels than could be tolerated systemically (Fig. 12-14) [1].

Genes that more directly address unique aspects of tumor physiology can also be delivered. Viral transformation of cells with a gene regulated by tumor-associated proteins offers the potential to deliver a lethal protein to cells expressing commonly mutated genes. For example, requiring abnormal p53 function to achieve viral replication should kill only cells expressing this phenotype, namely a majority of tumors (Fig. 12-15). Further specificity in initial trials of this idea is being sought by preferentially infecting tumor cells through tomography-guided injection of the virus into the tumor mass [22].

Engineered genes can also be used to inhibit particular genes. Such antisense drugs still face significant obstacles to commercial use, including the cost of synthesis, bioavailability, and the extent to which the targeted gene's expression is reduced; similar issues apply to ribozymes. Even before these challenges are fully

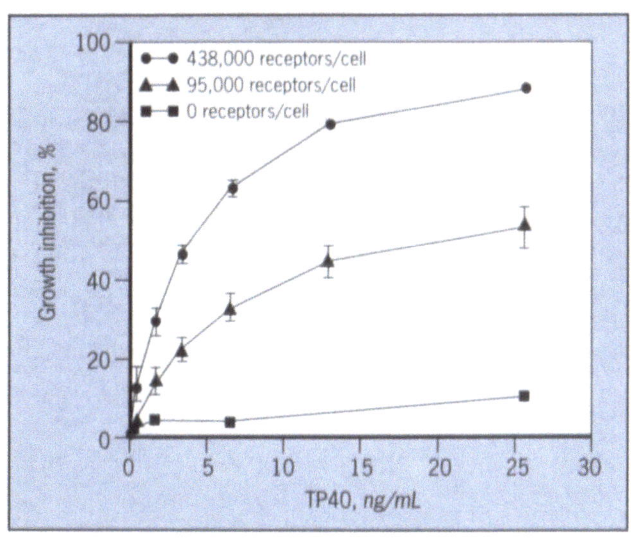

Figure 12-11. Targeting autocrine receptors. TP40 is a chimeric protein comprising a fusion of transforming growth factor-α and a modified *Pseudomonas* bacterial toxin (PE40), which inhibits protein synthesis following internalization and release from endosomes. It is minimally toxic to a parental Chinese hamster ovary (CHO) line lacking epidermal growth factor receptors (*squares*) but is toxic in proportion to receptor level on epidermal growth factor–receptor transfected CHO cells: 95,000 receptors per cell (*triangles*), 438,000 receptors per cell (*circles*). PE40 alone is far less toxic. (*Adapted from* Baldwin *et al.* [19]; with permission.)

overcome, however, these nucleic acid constructs can be used in model systems and for proof of principle in the clinic. A promising example now being tested clinically is the use of a protein kinase C antisense construct at low micromolar concentrations, which largely blocks expression of the alpha isozyme (Fig. 12-16) [23].

Encapsulation of a drug or gene in liposomes or other microdroplets protects it from degradation in the bloodstream while shielding normal tissues from inappropriate exposure. Dissolution of liposomes to release the drug preferentially at the tumor site has been achieved in model systems by focusing physical energy on the tumor site, *eg*, using hyperthermia [24] or ultrasound [25]. Under the proper conditions, antibody targeting can itself also accomplish localized release (Fig. 12-17) [26].

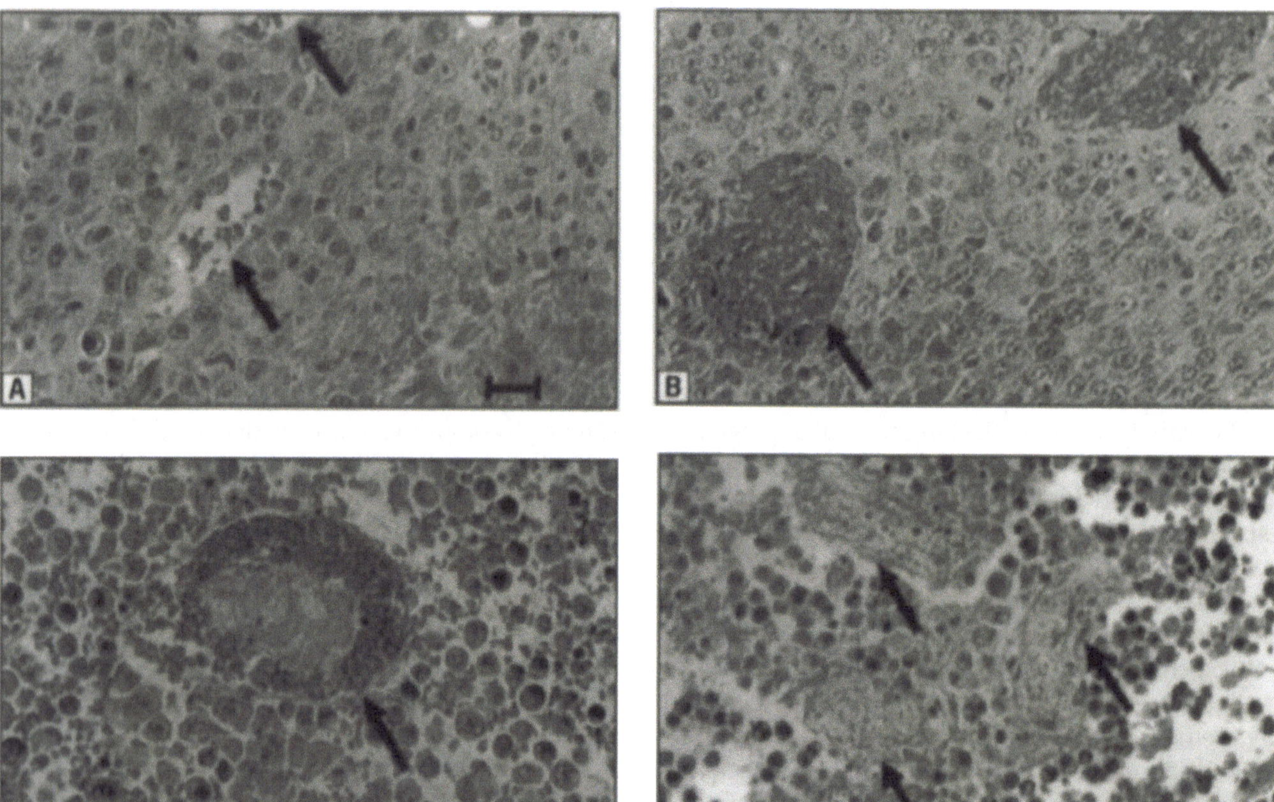

Figure 12-12. Targeting angiogenesis. An antibody conjugated to tissue factor (an activating agent for clotting) is targeted to a genetically engineered tumor vascular antigen. **A**, Prior to treatment, blood vessels within the tumor mass are intact and the tumor cells appear viable by histologic analysis. *Arrows* indicate vessels; *bar*=50 μM. **B**, Within 30 minutes, the blood vessels are thrombosed. **C**, By 4 hours, dense thrombi are present in all tumor vessels, and erythrocytes can be seen in the degenerating tumor interstitium. **D**, At 24 hours, there is advanced necrosis throughout the tumor. (*From* Huang *et al.* [20]; with permission.)

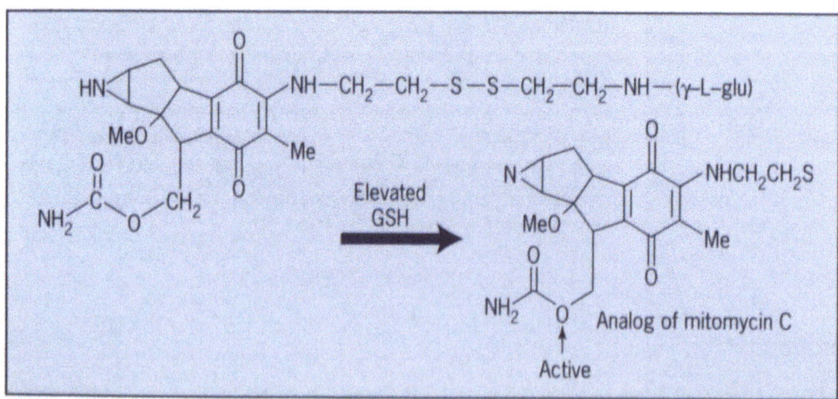

Figure 12-13. Redox activation. An analog of mitomycin C is activated by high levels of glutathione (GSH) in cells [21], a tumor phenotype particularly noticeable in some drug-resistant tumors.

SPECIFIC PROTEIN MODULATION

SCREENING CHEMICAL LIBRARIES

Genetic epidemiology is now identifying numerous oncogenes for which mutations are associated with particular cancers, thus extending the molecular biology paradigm, which was previously focused on normal cellular homologues of genes from transforming viruses. With the widened definition of oncogenes, the proteins identified are not necessarily involved in cell growth regulation, but may affect other clinically relevant processes such as invasiveness and metastasis. Clonal chromosomal breakpoints associated with cancer have been mapped for the whole genome, with chromosome 1 illustrated (Fig. 12-18) [27]. The tumor types are listed in which a breakpoint at the indicated band position has been found. For approximately 5% of these breakpoints, there are several recurrences in the Swedish database drawn from approximately 27,000 patients (biased in favor of hematologic cancers), often as the only karyotype abnormality. Although it is exciting to identify each potential intervention target, their sheer number poses a challenge for drug discovery. Enough of these breakpoints have been mapped to a specific gene of known function to make it likely that most of them are functionally relevant to causing cancer, rather than secondary epiphenomena. As an added complication, many of the mutants represent loss of function for genes whose normal role is thus considered to include tumor suppression. Specific modifications of normal function, including changes in amount or subcellular localization, are also found, sometimes by creation of novel fusion proteins. Both loss of function and subtle gain of function defects are intrinsically more difficult to target pharmacologically than is a purely tumor-specific function.

The large number of newly identified oncogenes is creating pressure to accelerate the discovery of drug candidates for evaluation. For investigators with access to a large, structurally diverse chemical library, direct screening of a target to find lead compounds is a proven technology that is being intensively automated. With today's robotic equipment, focused on 96-well microplates, more than 100,000 compounds a

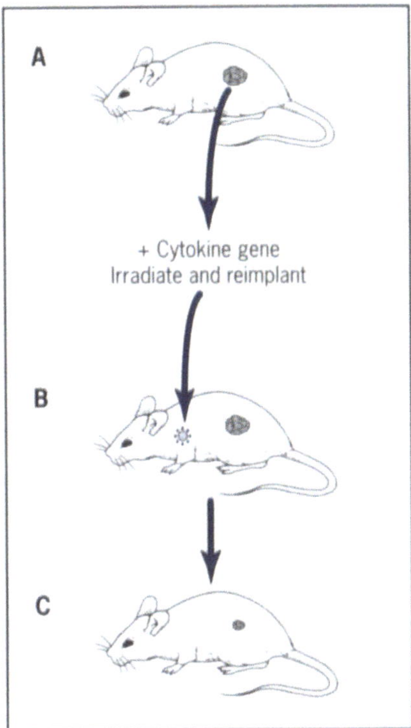

Figure 12-14. Targeted immunostimulation. **A**, A tumor cell line is created by ex vivo transfection of cytokine genes. **B**, Following irradiation to destroy proliferative capacity, the cells are then reintroduced into the body, where they present tumor-specific antigens within a halo of high-concentration cytokines. **C**, The enhanced immunologic response against the tumor-specific antigens causes regression of the parental tumor cells throughout the body.

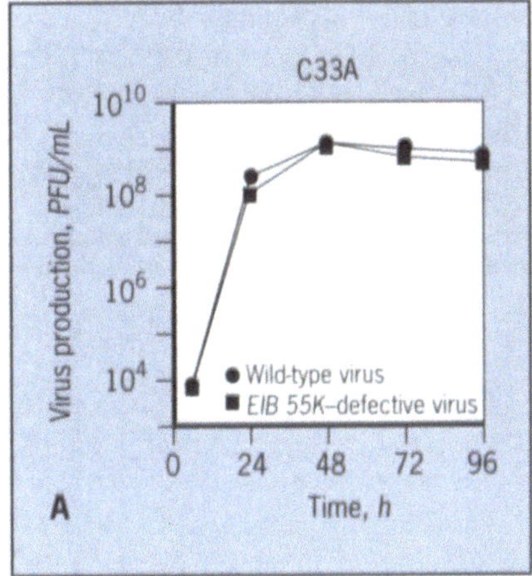

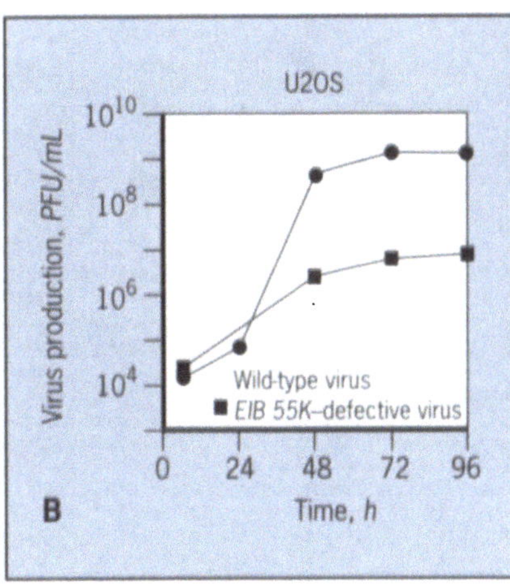

Figure 12-15. Gene therapy. An engineered adenovirus, defective in the *E1B 55K* gene, cannot prevent *p53*-mediated apoptosis induced by the *E1A* gene. **A**, In C33A cervical carcinoma with defective *p53*, the engineered virus (*squares*) is as lethal as the wild-type virus (*circles*). **B**, In U2OS cells with normal *p53*, the engineered virus is much less cytotoxic than the wild-type virus, presumably due to elimination of the viral replicative burst in cells undergoing *p53*-mediated apoptosis. PFU—plaque-forming unit. (*Adapted from* Bischoff *et al.* [22]; with permission.)

year can be screened against at least 25 targets. Technology under development for miniaturizing the screening format promises to increase this screening capacity greatly, *eg*, using ink jet technology to generate microdroplets that can be screened in a fluorescence-activated cell sorter (Fig. 12-19).

A continuing obstacle to success with high-throughput screening is the need to simplify a complex biologic process to create an assay that is compatible with high-volume screening. The simplifications required to create an in vitro biochemical assay are more extensive than those needed for screening within the context of a whole cell, using genetically engineered constructs. The extensive family of seven-transmembrane domain G-protein–coupled receptors, for example, is being studied as a source of cancer drug targets, using cells in which the receptor is coupled to a signal transduction pathway that leads to a readily detectable signal (Fig. 12-20) [28]. Compound screening is thus directed at the target in a more physiologic context than might be the case in vitro using detergent-solubilized receptors and a competitive binding assay.

The most extensive chemical libraries being used for high-throughput screening exist as the legacy from the past century of chemical research, primarily

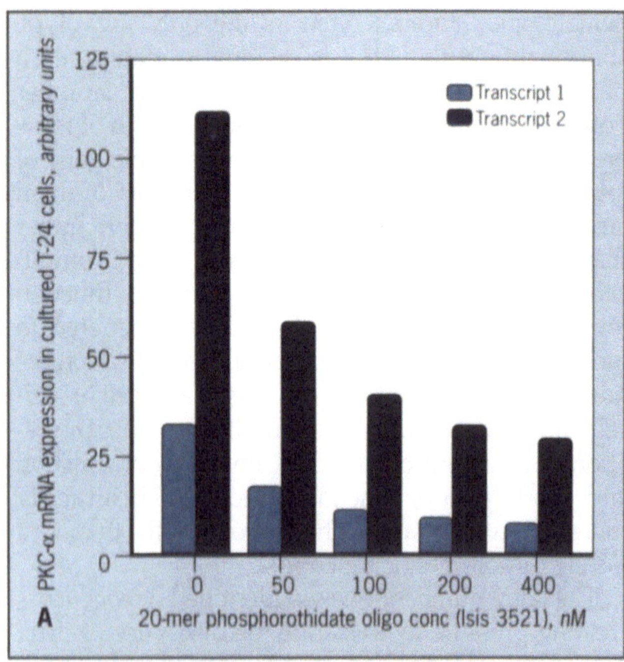

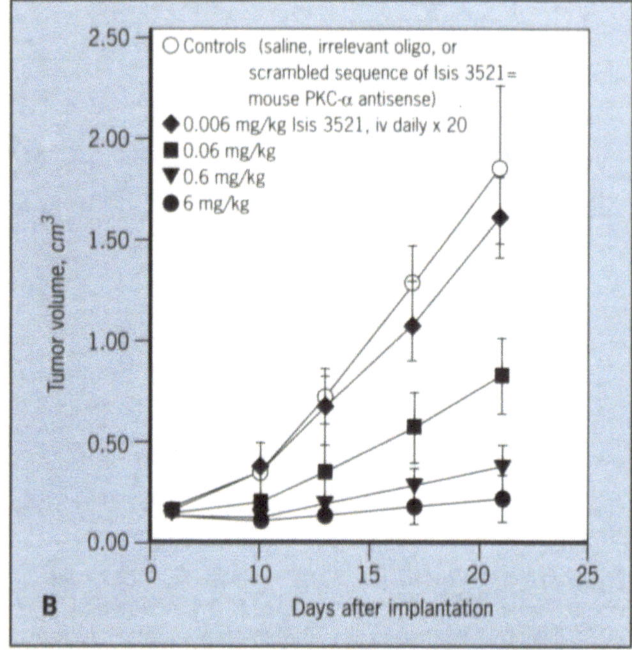

Figure 12-16. Antisense drugs. **A**, The expression of both splicing variants of protein kinase C (PKC)-α mRNA in cultured T-24 human bladder carcinoma cells is reduced in proportion to the dose of ISIS 3521, a 20mer phosphorothioate oligonucleotide. **B**, T-24 xenografts in nude mice show dose-dependent tumor growth arrest when the antisense compound is delivered daily for 20 days. (*Adapted from* Dean *et al.* [23]; with permission.)

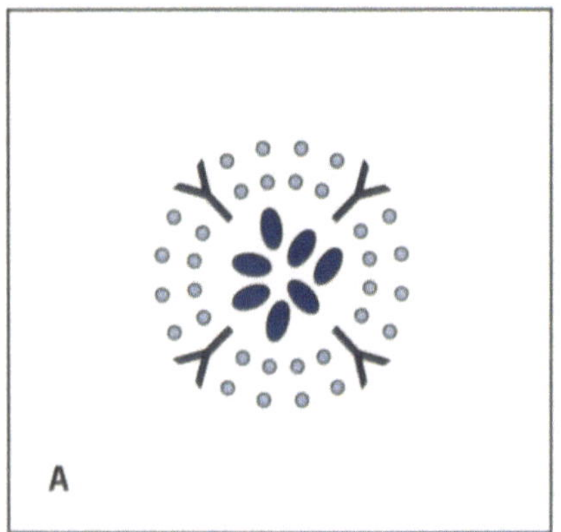

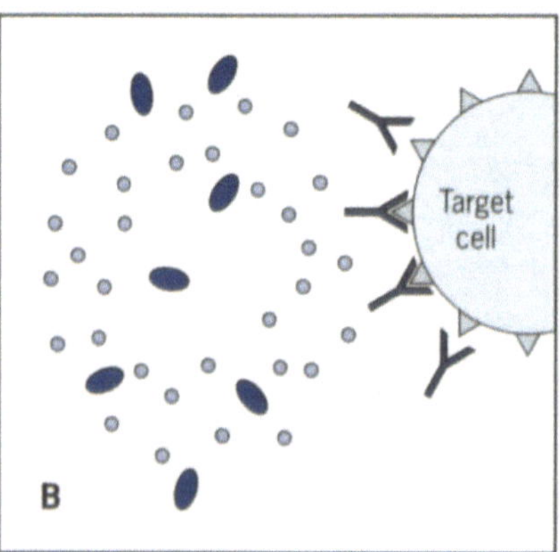

Figure 12-17. Liposomes. **A**, A drug is encapsulated in a liposome incorporating targeting antibodies within the fluid liposome surface. **B**, When antibodies aggregate at the target site, the structural integrity of the liposome is compromised, allowing the drug to diffuse out.

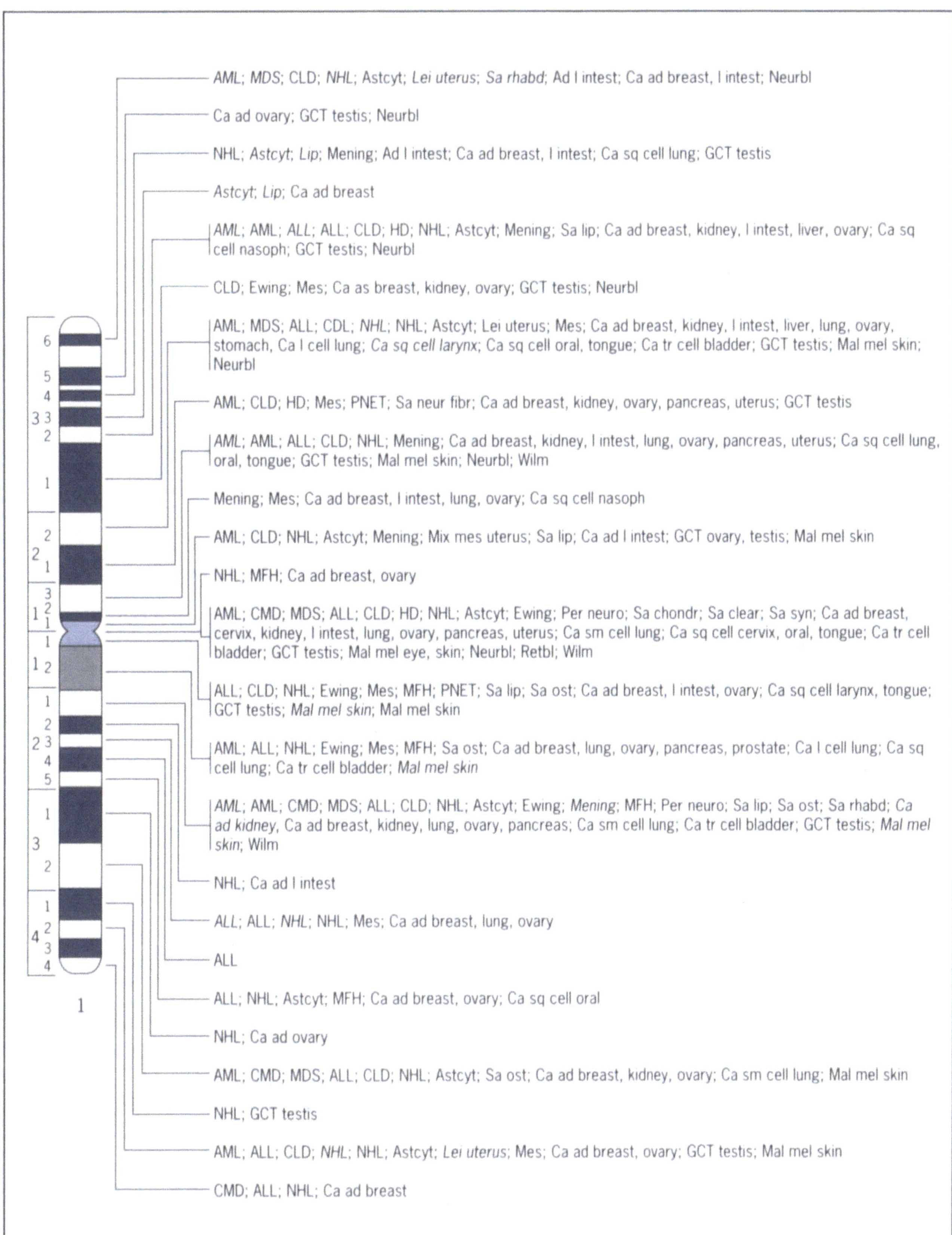

Figure 12-18. Karyotype abnormality map correlated with tumor types. (*From* Mitelman *et al.* [27]; with permission.)

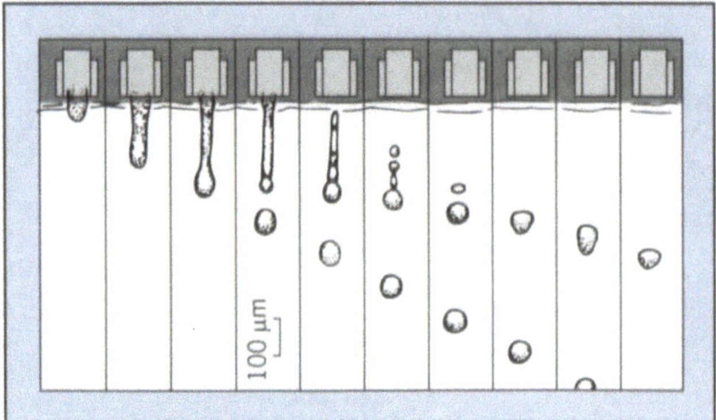

Figure 12-19. Assay miniaturization. Microdroplet dispensing using a piezoelectric valve on a small orifice can deliver a drop size of 0.5 nL, with a deviation of <3%. Dispensing rate can be as high as 3000 droplets per second. Running screening assays in this format thus represents a miniaturization factor of approximately 10^5 compared with standard 96-well microplates.

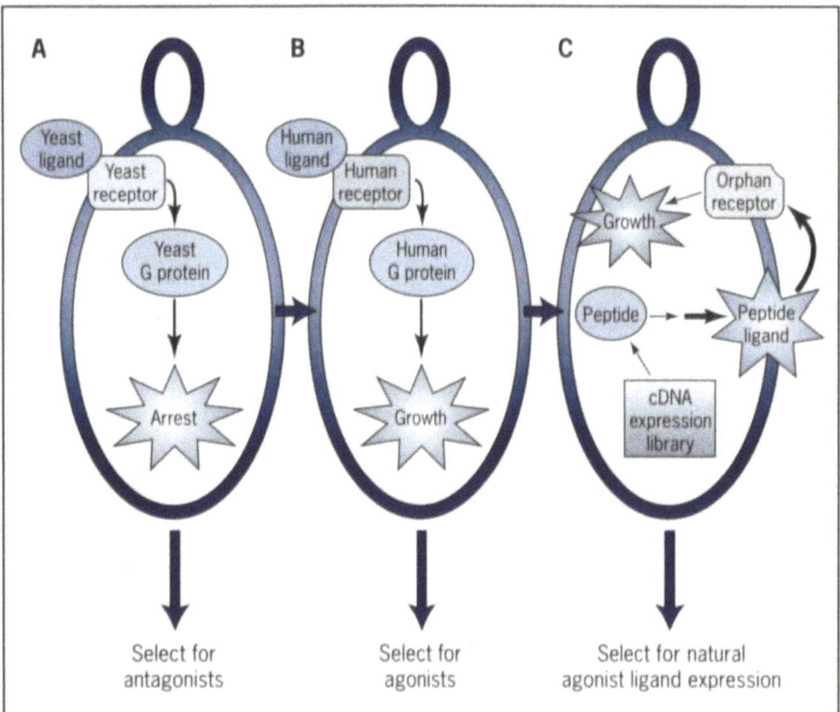

Figure 12-20. Assays using engineered cells. **A** and **B**, Stimulation of an endogenous or transfected G-coupled receptor in yeast stimulates production of a readily measured response, such as growth arrest (*panel 20A*) or growth stimulation (*panel 20B*), allowing screening for antagonists or agonists, respectively. **C**, By coupling the agonist readout to expression of cDNA-derived peptides, natural ligands for orphan receptors can be identified. (*Adapted from* Broach and Thorner [28]; with permission.)

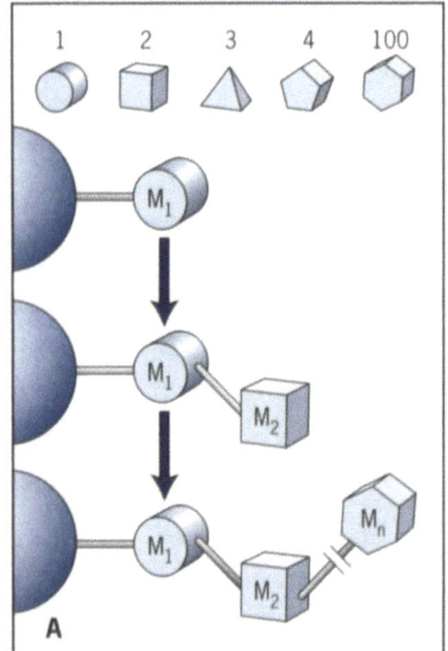

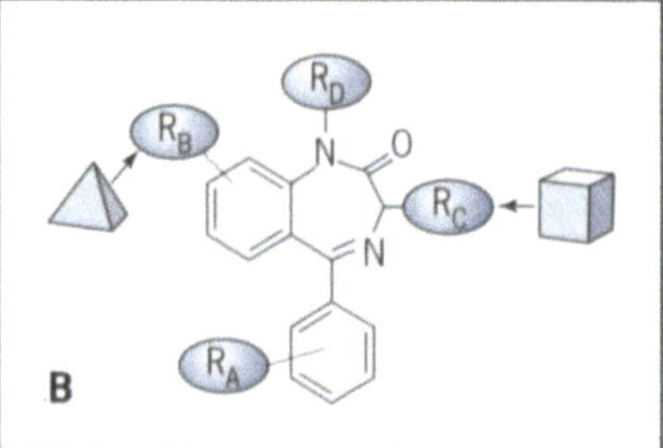

Figure 12-21. Combinatorial chemistry. **A**, A pool of 100 monomers can be oligomerized by n stepwise additions to create 100^n combinations. **B**, Alternatively, if the 100 monomers are coupled to three discrete positions on a scaffold, 10^6 combinations can be created. (*Adapted from* Mitchison [29]; with permission.)

in the major pharmaceutical companies. An increasingly popular alternative is the use of combinatorial chemistry libraries [29], the underlying principles of which are based on solid-phase peptide synthesis. A variety of building blocks are chosen that can be assembled in a mix-and-match process (Fig. 12-21). Several different techniques are in use to decode the identity of any compound that scores positive in the assay. Increasing emphasis is being placed on assessing diversity of such libraries, in part to determine if they can truly match that of historical archives and in part to reduce the frequency of false positives and redundant positives, which can impose a heavy burden on secondary screens [30].

Computer-Aided Drug Design

Another alternative for identifying hits against a target in the absence of an extensive chemical library is to determine the structure of the protein, typically by x-ray crystallography, although nuclear magnetic resonance imaging is becoming increasingly useful as are purely computational-based homology modeling methods. Docking compounds from a virtual library into the protein's active site can be used to select promising candidates for synthesis and direct testing (Fig. 12-22).

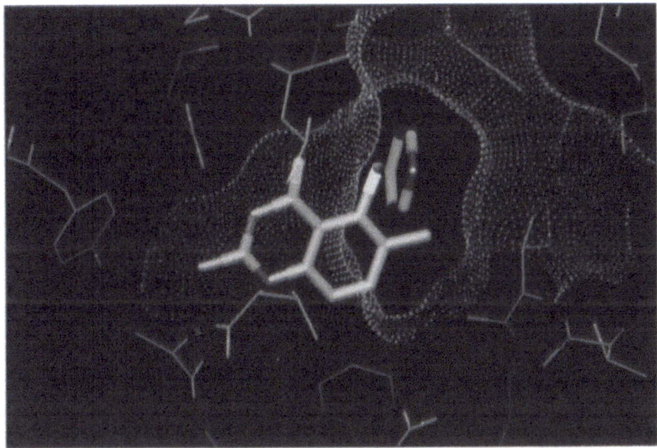

Figure 12-22. Rational drug design. The structure of AG337 (Thymitaq; Agouron Pharmaceuticals, San Diego, CA) is shown docked into the folate binding site of thymidylate synthase [31]. The dots demarcate the surface of the protein; the drug's structure is drawn using thick lines.

Because a high-resolution protein structure is too costly to obtain for the numerous emerging targets, computational chemistry is also being applied to the design of compounds that mimic known ligands, particularly peptides. Peptidomimetics are compounds in which portions of a peptide structure are replaced with similar structures that offer more rigidity or are more resistant to proteolysis. Computational analysis of the structure–activity relationships from such compounds can direct the synthesis of even less peptide-like compounds (Fig. 12-23). Mimics of the RGD peptide motif are of special interest because one such ligand binds to the IIb/IIIa receptor (also called her-2), for which an antibody is being explored as a treatment for breast cancer.

Computational chemistry, applied to both ligands and proteins, calculates the properties of molecules by using a combination of fundamental physical chemical theory and empirically derived parameters. A new set of empiric parameters has been developed to aid in this task (Fig. 12-24). It has been shown that a reference panel of fewer than 20 proteins can be selected, which accounts for the statistical binding properties of small molecules to a much larger set of proteins. By referring to a stored database, comprising the binding properties of a chemical library against such a reference panel, a computational surrogate of the target can be created from very limited data that enables prediction of the target's binding to the much larger number of compounds in the database [33]. This technique is particularly useful when the target is in limited supply or the assay is complex. Both conditions apply to most early-stage research projects.

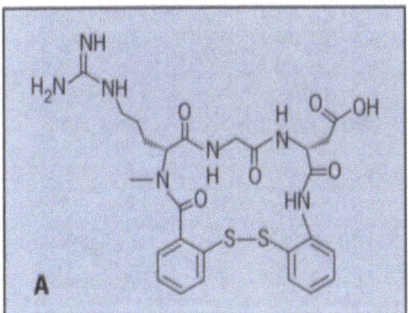

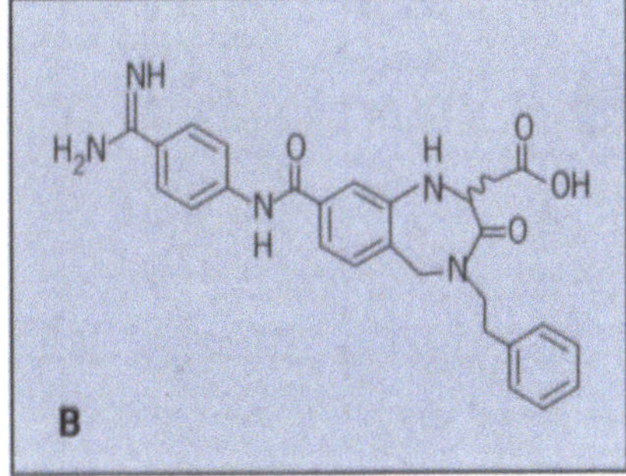

Figure 12-23. Peptidomimetics. An RGD-containing peptide was placed within an antibody variable loop CDR and used to derive structural information for searching a database of compounds previously screened directly against the αIII/β3 receptor. **A,** This compound (4 nM affinity) is from a peptidomimetic library with arginine side chains, for which the structural data yielded active compounds at an 11% success rate. This rate is significantly enriched over the known 0.4% success rate from direct screening. **B,** This compound (2.3 nM affinity) is from a focused library incorporating a benzamidine mimic of an arginine side chain, and in this case the success rate was 93% [32].

Macromolecular Interactions

The vast majority of current drugs for all diseases are directed to enzymes, ion channels, and small-molecule hormone receptors. Because many oncogenes are involved in signal transduction based on protein associations, designing drugs that specifically affect protein–protein interactions is of special interest to oncologists. Only one face of a drug candidate is likely to be involved in high-affinity binding to one of the proteins (Fig. 12-25). If the opposite face has sufficiently repellent steric or electronic properties, it should block the entire protein–protein interaction. Because the functions required for this kind of drug differ from most current drugs, the effective chemical classes may be sufficiently novel to enable strong patent positions on composition, with broad applications.

Because many oncogenes are tumor suppressors, reversing the effects of their loss may be achievable by creating agonists of parallel signaling pathways via small molecules that can promote the interaction of two proteins. Such effects are certainly possible. Taxol, for example, works by stabilizing the interaction of tubulin monomers, thus creating a different set of problems for the cell than colchicine, which destabilizes the

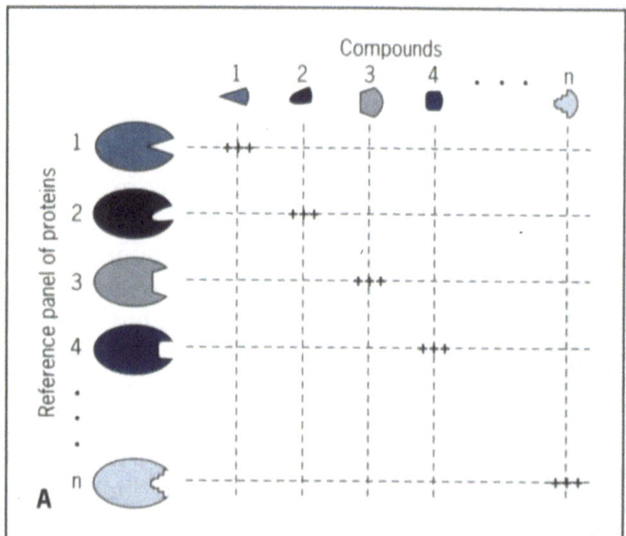

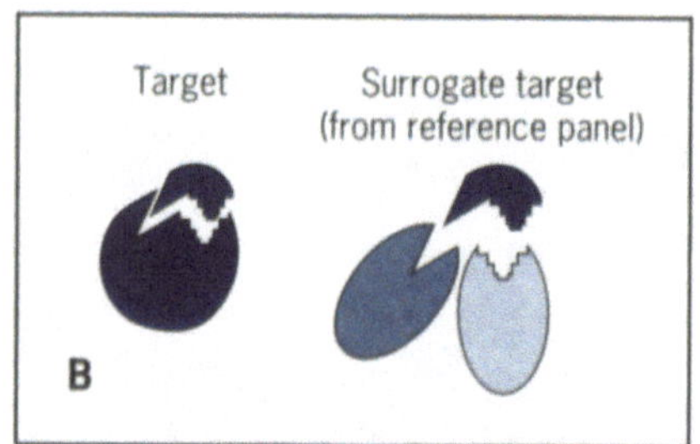

Figure 12-24. Affinity fingerprinting. **A**, The relative affinities of a small reference panel of generic proteins for a wide range of compounds is measured using high-throughput assays. Type specimen "training" compounds are selected for maximal diversity against the panel. **B**, Assaying the training compounds against a new target allows a subset of reference proteins to be selected, which together mimic the binding characteristics of the target. This subset can then be used to extract from the database those compounds most likely to bind the target.

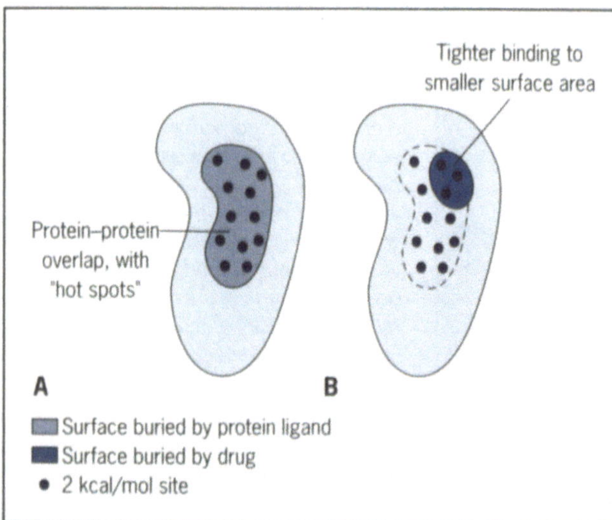

Figure 12-25. Inhibiting dimerization. **A**, Protein–protein binding involves a large surface area of interaction and thus can achieve high-binding energies due to the summation of numerous relatively weak contacts. **B**, Each of the individual contact sites provides an opportunity for designing an antagonist that binds better at that site than the natural protein ligand. Smaller ligands are preferred due to improved chances of oral availability. (*Adapted from* R. Spencer, Pfizer Central Research, Groton, CT.)

same protein–protein interaction. Using random peptide phage display technology (Fig. 12-4), a peptide has been discovered that promotes dimerization of the erythropoietin receptor. It has shown activity comparable to erythropoietin in mice, even prior to any optimization of formulation or dosing regimen (Fig. 12-26) [34]. Even if this particular peptide proves to be difficult to translate to an orally active small organic molecule, its discovery demonstrates that binding sites exist on the receptor that can be used to accomplish dimerization by a relatively small molecule.

An approach that incorporates elements of gene therapy as well as protein–protein interaction involves the creation of artificial signal transduction pathways. For example, the protein product of the oncogene ras normally initiates a mitogen-activated protein kinase signaling cascade by binding to the ser/thr kinase raf, which then phosphorylates the protein MEK. Artificially induced dimerization of raf is sufficient to initiate the cascade, however (Fig. 12-27) [35]. This technology can be used to elucidate signaling pathways in normal and cancerous tissues. Improved understanding at this level offers hope for rational selection of targets for differentiation therapy. The experience with retinoids, which have expanded the definition of hormonal therapy, is particularly informative in this regard. Based on the complex clinical results in both chemoprevention and therapeutic applications, the spectrum of utility and side effects for modulators of differentiation is expected to be distinct from cytotoxins [36].

Designing differentiation inducers and other signaling modulators is likely to require substantial effort, however. Although cancer has been a recognizable disease for thousands of years in highly disparate cultures, with numerous herbal remedies attempted that presumably address all aspects of cancer physiology, killing tumor cells remains the most effective adjunct to surgical debulking. The high failure rate of current cytotoxins, although frustrating, should not discourage efforts to find more effective cytotoxins, because this approach clearly can work well in many instances. The natural product calicheamicin provides an example of a compound whose very high potency as a cytotoxin is attributable to its distinctive ability to damage DNA [37]. Calicheamicin (Fig. 12-28) consists of two moieties, one of which binds DNA with modest sequence specificity. As a result, the other moiety, activated by thiols, is then well positioned to attack the sugar phosphate backbones of both strands of DNA, resulting in strand scission, which is very difficult for the cell to repair.

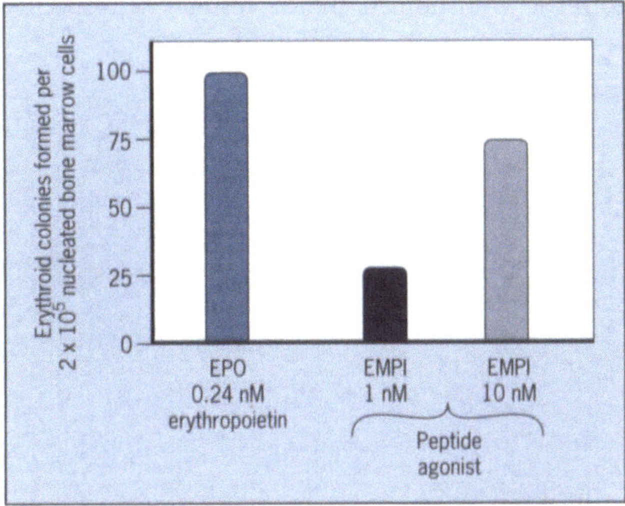

Figure 12-26. Peptide mimics. EMP1 is a 14-mer disulfide-bonded cyclic peptide, which acts in a dose-dependent manner as a full agonist of the erythropoietin receptor in bone marrow cell culture. The peptide was discovered through phage display technology. (*Adapted from* Wrighton *et al.* [34]; with permission.)

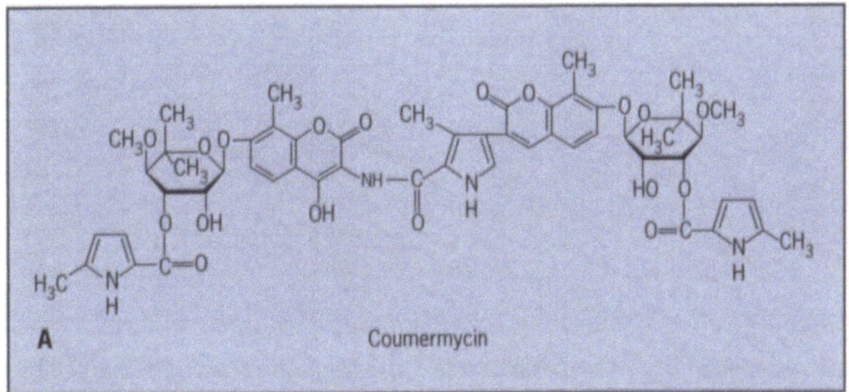

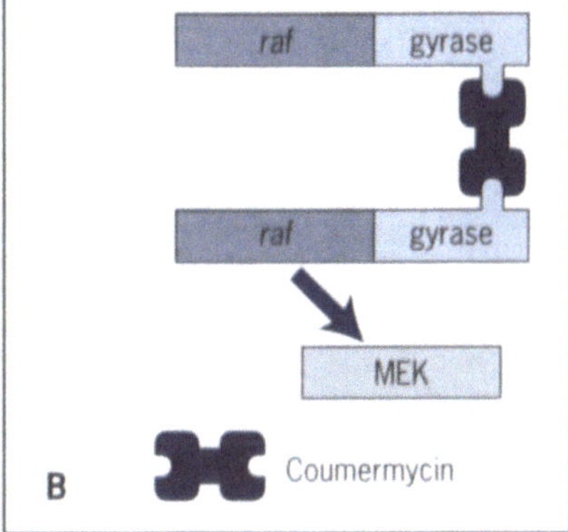

Figure 12-27. Induced dimerization. **A**, The natural product coumermycin, which binds to the protein gyrase in a 1:2 stoichiometry. **B**, Genetically fusing gyrase to *raf* induces dimerization in the presence of coumermycin, which thus acts as an artificial hormone to initiate a signal cascade.

Telomerase has drawn a great deal of attention as a strongly tumor-associated protein whose role in chromosome maintenance suggests it would be a useful target for developing novel cytotoxins. Telomeres are characterized by a very distinctive short DNA sequence that is repeated hundreds to thousands of times. Normal DNA replication results in a loss of a small amount of this telomeric repeat located at the end of the chromosome. To restore this lost telomeric DNA, telomerase uses an intrinsic complementary template RNA sequence. Because telomerase is thus mechanistically a reverse transcriptase, nucleotide analogs developed for antiviral work have been tested as inhibitors of the telomerase enzymatic activity. Low micromolar hits have indeed been found, but they have not shown significant growth arrest properties (Fig. 12-29) [38]. Because other mechanisms apparently also participate in the recognition and repair of shortened telomeres, better understanding of the full spectrum of telomere interactions may be needed for effective drug discovery efforts.

MECHANISM-BLIND ASSAYS

Lead Optimization

Traditional medicinal chemistry has a successful record in optimizing leads with regard to potency, bioavailability, and cost of manufacture. A less often discussed obstacle to effective optimization is the limited degree to which cell and animal cancer models correlate with human clinical results. Retrospective

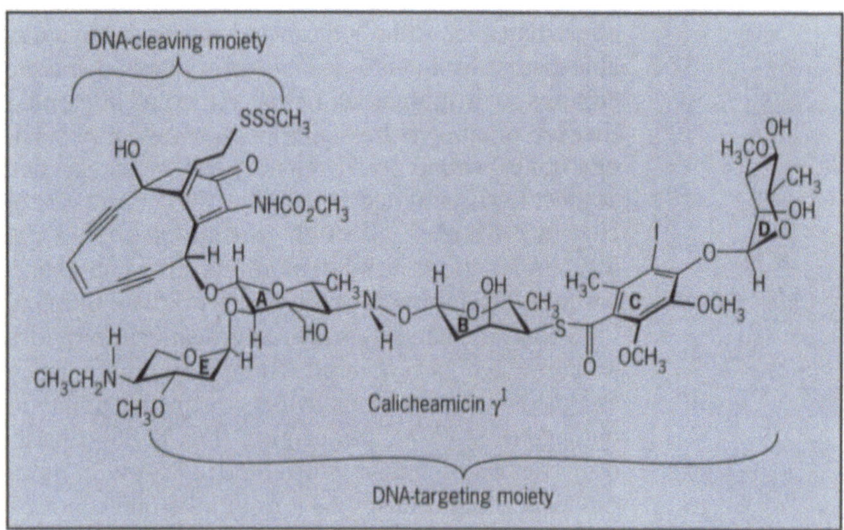

Figure 12-28. A novel cytotoxin. Structure of calicheamicin, showing the carbohydrate portion that binds to the minor groove of DNA and the aglycone diyne-ene portion that cleaves DNA following an internal rearrangement initiated by thiols, which yields a 1, 4-benzenoid diradical.

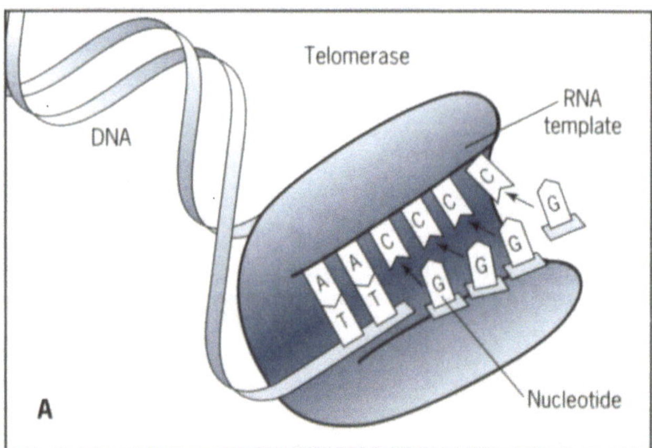

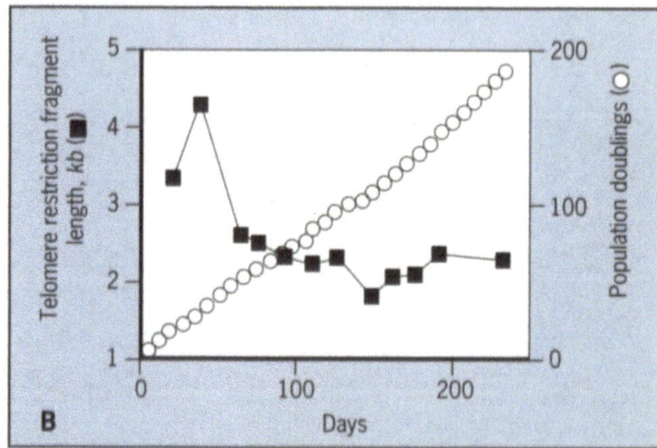

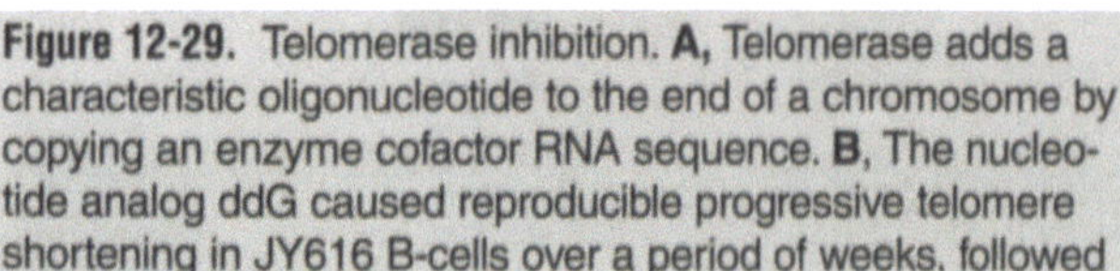

Figure 12-29. Telomerase inhibition. **A**, Telomerase adds a characteristic oligonucleotide to the end of a chromosome by copying an enzyme cofactor RNA sequence. **B**, The nucleotide analog ddG caused reproducible progressive telomere shortening in JY616 B-cells over a period of weeks, followed by stabilization of telomere length. No effect on growth of the cells or indication of senescence was observed even after 9 months and more than 200 passages in 10 μM ddG. (*Adapted from* Strahl and Blackburn [38]; with permission.)

analysis of primary tumor clonogenic assays (Fig. 12-30) indicates that this method is quite reliable for predicting which of the known drugs will fail in particular patients (approximately 90% correlation), although the technique is not yet as reliable for predicting efficacy (approximately 70% correlation) [39]. Extending this work to prospective drug models may be critical to effective exploitation of the flood of new targets arising from molecular biology research. Preservation of the cytoarchitecture of the tumor in vitro would probably improve the predictions, although this introduces difficulties with regard to visualizing effects of the drug on the tumor cells compared with stromal cells [40]. As tumor-associated markers become available as addresses for visualization reagents, however, it should become technically feasible to use model systems that more accurately mimic the in vivo physiology.

Because many cancer drugs are intended to be toxic, issues of safety versus efficacy are quite different in oncology compared with other areas of medicine. Some of the most successful new oncology drugs of the past decade, such as antinausea drugs and myelostimulants, have in fact not been developed as antineoplastic agents per se, but rather are used to ameliorate the toxicity of existing drugs. Several approaches to directly enhancing tumor-specific toxicity are also in development, including inhibitors of DNA repair enzymes (such as topoisomerase) and of drug-resistance modulators (such as the multidrug-resistant efflux pump). A wide variety of other detoxication enzymes are also known [41] and may provide useful targets. They may also provide insights into individual variation in drug metabolism. The major enzymes of detoxication are listed in Table 12-1. Many of these enzymes comprise multiple isoforms, which can sometimes provide tumor specificity. Glutathione transferase, for example, includes at least 10 major isoforms, with one form (P1-1) being the most strongly tumor associated (Fig. 12-9) [42].

Along with the steady increase in potential targets with well-characterized functions, the rapid progress of molecular genetics, including random sequencing, is providing an abundance of new proteins with no known function. One approach to dealing with this problem is to build rough models of biochemical pathways that can be refined as proteins are identified that fit the predicted properties of missing elements.

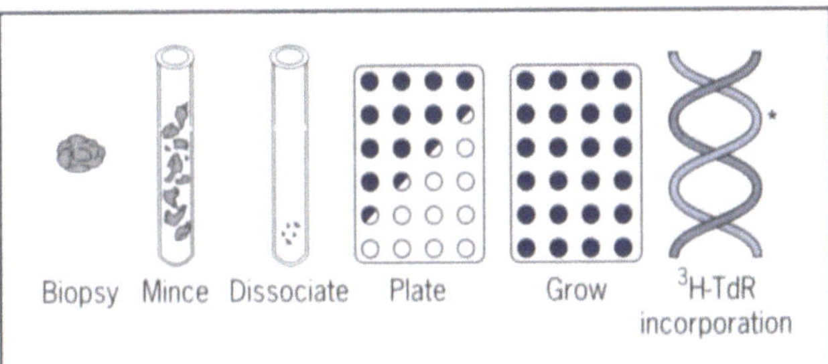

Figure 12-30. In vitro determination of drug response. A solid tumor specimen (1–5 g) is shipped in sterile media to a central laboratory, where mincing and enzyme action dissociates single cells for plating in soft agar. Treatment with drugs is followed by incubation for 3 days. Cells still able to replicate are quantitated by incorporation of tritiated thymidine over the next 24 hours. (*Adapted from* Fruehauf and Bosanquet [40]; with permission.)

Table 12-1. The enzymes of detoxication

Flavin-containing monooxygenases	Glutathione transferase
P-450–dependent monooxygenases	UDP-glucuronyl transferase
Alcohol dehydrogenases	Phenol sulfotransferase
Aldehyde dehydrogenase	Tyrosine-ester sulfotransferase
Carbonyl reductase	Alcohol sulfotransferase
Dihydrodiol dehydrogenase	Amine *N*-sulfotransferase
Glutathione peroxidase	Cysteine conjugate *N*-acetyltransferase
Monoamine oxidase	Catechol *O*-methyltransferase
Aldehyde oxidase	Amine *N*-methyltransferase
Xanthine oxidase	Thiol *S*-methyltransferase
D-Amino acid oxidase	Thiol transferase
Quinone reductase	Acetyltransacetylase
Epoxide hydrolase	Rhodanese
Esterases/amidases	

A promising embodiment of this idea, adapted from Petri net models used in macroscopic manufacturing process control, has been explored for the well-studied pathway of protein coagulation (Fig. 12-31) [43].

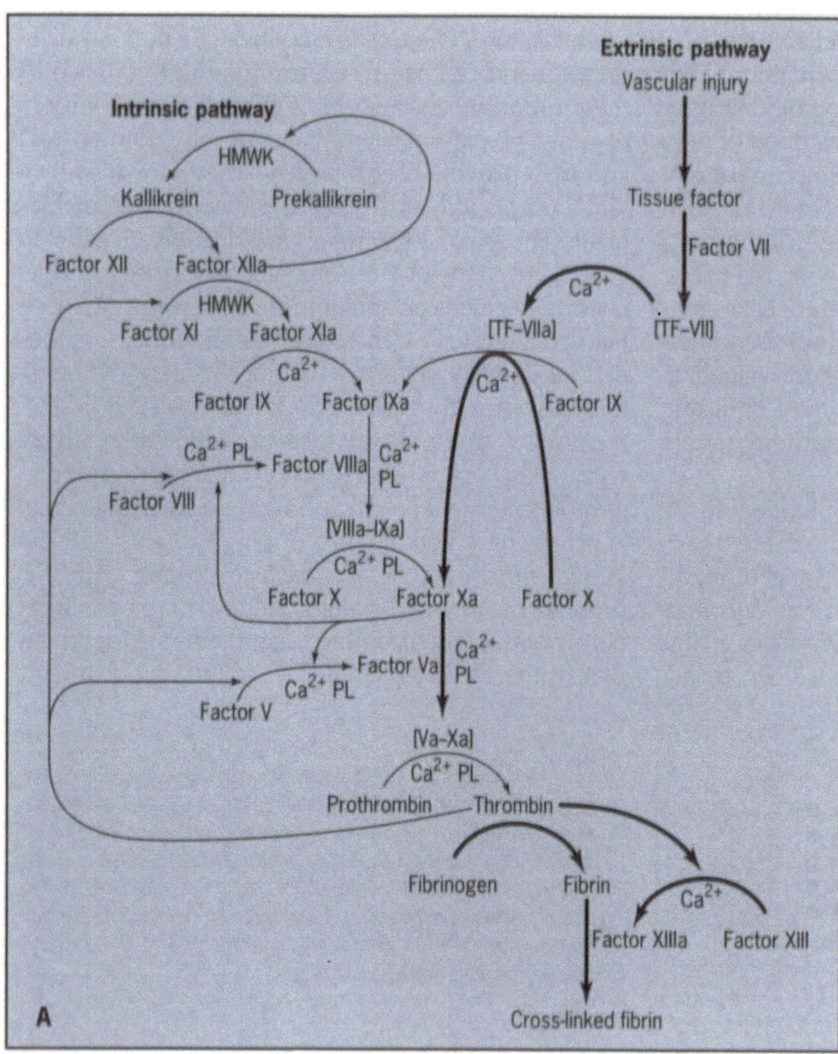

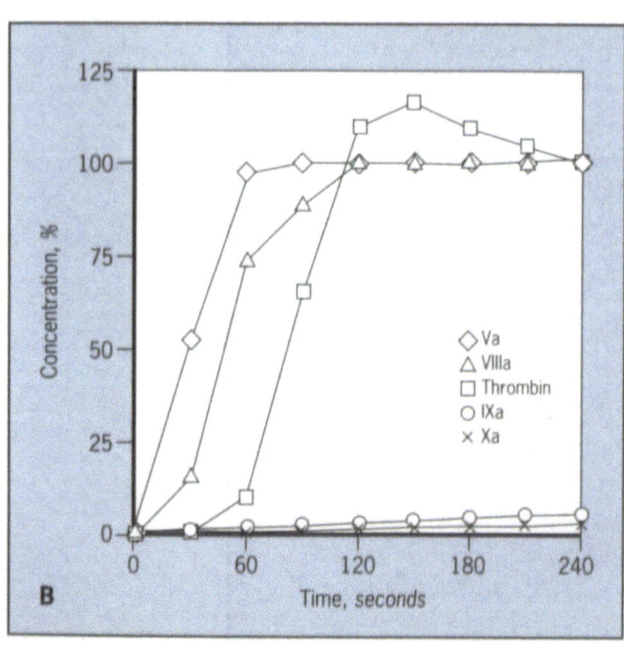

Figure 12-31. Pathway modeling. **A**, Standard view of the clotting pathway. **B**, Experimental kinetics of key clotting components. (*continued*)

The model has not only matched the empirical data quite well but has also provided insights into clotting disorders. It is now being extended to signal transduction pathways. Understanding a pathway may allow identification of compensating intervention points that can ameliorate loss of function mutations. Differential display of mRNA has identified a large class of tumor suppressors to which this approach might be usefully applied [44]. Specifically, hundreds of proteins have been found whose expression is extinguished in breast cancer without structural alteration of the encoding DNA, and in some cases it has been shown that resupplying the protein arrests tumor growth.

Cell-Based Screening

Since the discovery of cellular oncogenes, considerable effort has been devoted to cloning genes based on assays of cell transformation in culture. More

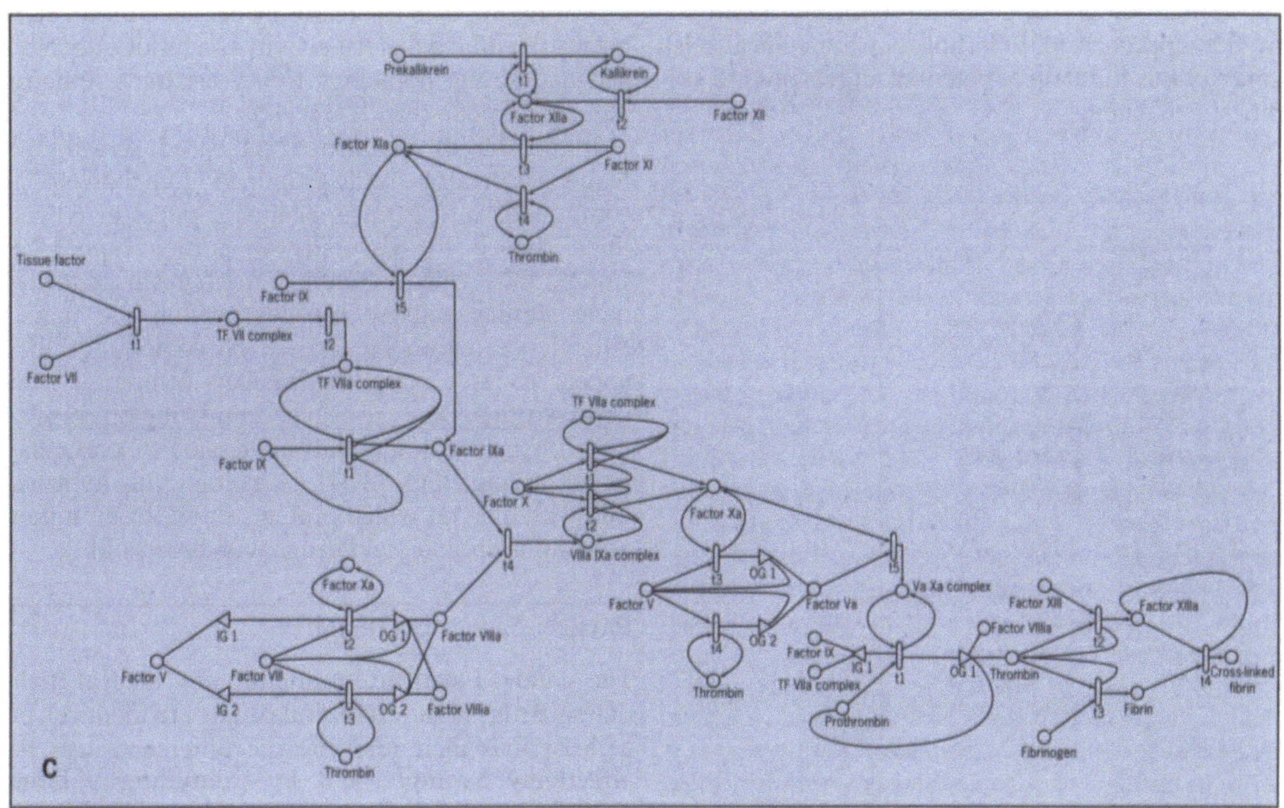

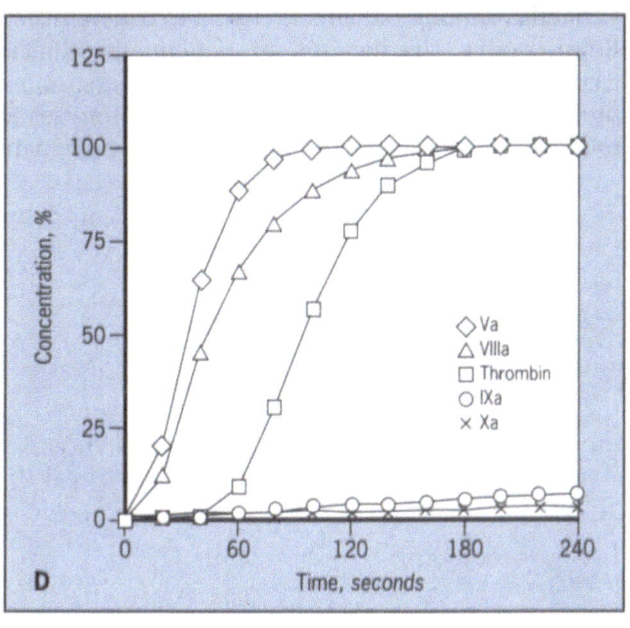

Figure 12-31. *(continued)* **C**, The pathway as modeled using Petri net formalism. **D**, The kinetics predicted from the model. (*Adapted from* Mounts and Liebman [43]; with permission.)

broadly, random genomic DNA can be shotgun-cloned in expression vectors and used to select for interesting phenotypes, such as drug resistance (Fig. 12-32). The method was verified using the topoisomerase gene as the DNA source to overcome etoposide selection and then applied to total HeLa cDNA. Three genes were thereby discovered that can also contribute to etoposide resistance, two of which were completely novel sequences. The expressed DNA can act by coding for a protein that provides a positive function or one that inhibits some other function, or it can act by an antisense mechanism. A substantial variety of genes are typically identified by this approach [45]. Sorting out the clinical relevance of this fountain of potential targets poses a significant challenge.

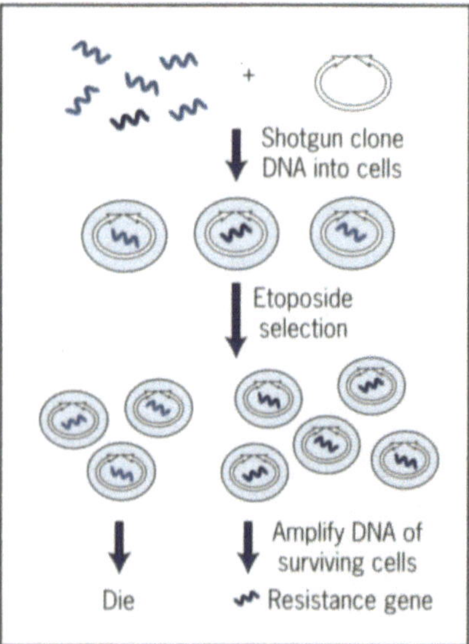

Figure 12-32. Shotgun cloning for target identification. An expression library is made from random DNA fragments inserted into a viral vector. Infected cells are selected for etoposide resistance or any other selectable phenotype. DNA from surviving cells is extracted and recloned for testing individually.

Natural products, which have been the starting point for many of today's drugs in all fields of medicine, are synthesized by the producing organisms in a highly intentional fashion, generally targeting particular proteins [46]. Because most human proteins have homologues extending across vast phylogenetic distances, a natural product has a good chance of showing activity against some human protein. Direct screening of such compounds for anticancer activity in cell-based assays can lead to the identification of novel mechanisms of action. For example, trapoxin, a novel microbial toxin, causes cell cycle arrest between G1 and G2. Using trapoxin as an affinity ligand, a protein target was identified that has activity as a histone deacetylase and strong homology to a yeast transcriptional regulator, Rpd3p (Fig. 12-33) [47].

In the largest published cell-based screen, the National Cancer Institute examined more than 60,000 compounds and extracts against a panel of 60 cell lines chosen for diversity in tumor type [48]. Compounds with a common mechanism of action have similar activity profiles against the panel. Attention can thus be focused on compounds that appear to have novel mechanisms compared with known drugs. Data are also accumulating on correlations of drug efficacy with expression of particular target proteins (Fig. 12-34). Combining this information with data on which proteins show strong tumor association should yield drugs with broad utility.

Patient-Specific Therapy

The standard statistical foundation for clinical trials of new drugs assumes that all people are identical, or at least that their idiosyncratic differences can be effectively averaged out by examining a large enough population. For anticancer drugs, however, variability among patients is crucial to drug efficacy. Retrospective stratification of patients in clinical trials, based on a wide range of tumor-associated proteins, is now becoming possible and promises to rationalize the choice of discovery targets. Movement

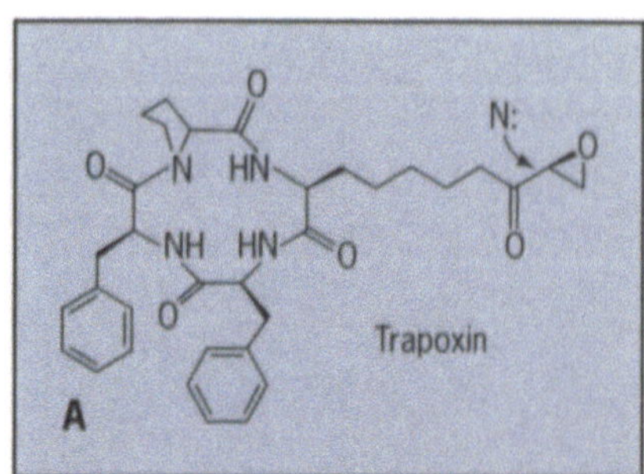

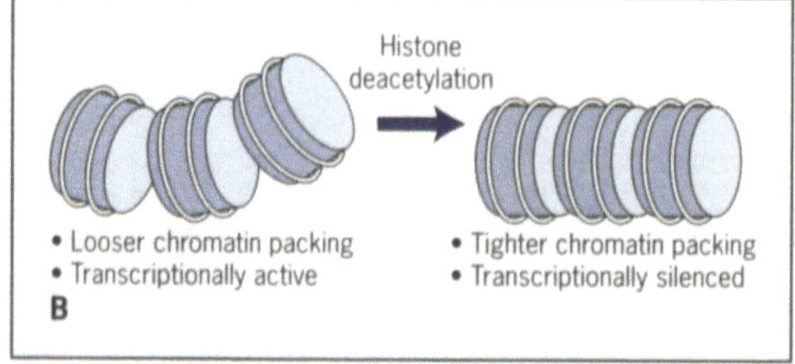

Figure 12-33. Natural products for target identification. **A**, Structure of the cyclotetrapeptide trapoxin. **B**, Trapoxin's inhibition of histone deacetylase is believed to maintain the chromatin in a transcriptionally active loose-packing form, preventing the normal mitotic S phase.

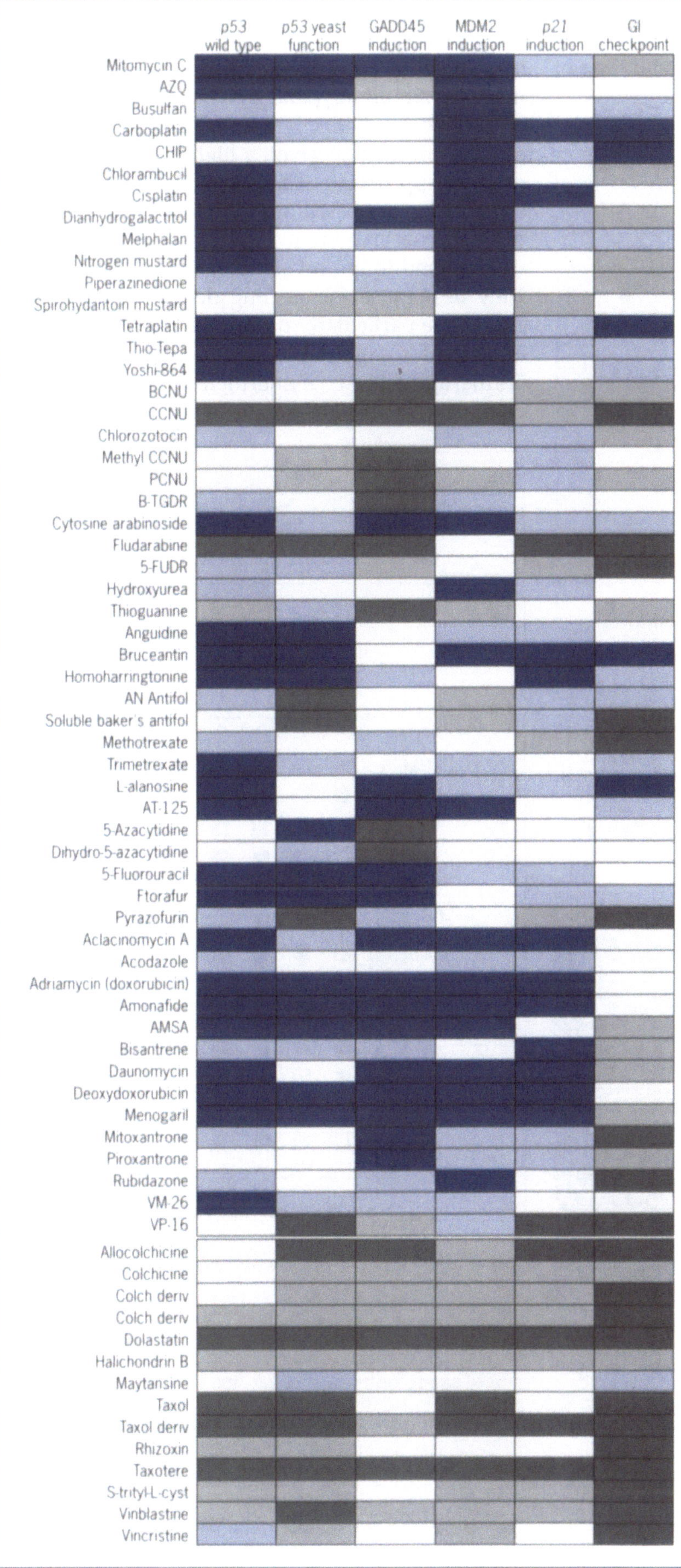

Figure 12-34. Multivariate statistics. Normality of *p53*, assayed directly or by examination of proteins known to be regulated by *p53*, shows a strong positive correlation for efficacy of most current drugs from several classes, with the exception of agents targeting tubulin. Correlation coefficients are color-coded from strongly positive (*dark blue, r*= -0.5 to 0.9) to moderately positive (*light blue, r*= 0.2 to 0.4) to neutral (*white, r*= 0 to 0.2; *light gray, r*= -0.2 to 0) to negative (*dark gray, r*= -0.5 to -0.3). Correlations are between the protein or cell cycle phenotype and the efficacy of the drug averaged over the National Cancer Institute 60 cell line panel. (*Adapted from* Weinstein *et al.* [48]; with permission.)

toward individually tailored treatment should accelerate as diagnostic capability improves, with initial emphasis likely to be on improved understanding of the metabolism of existing drugs [49].

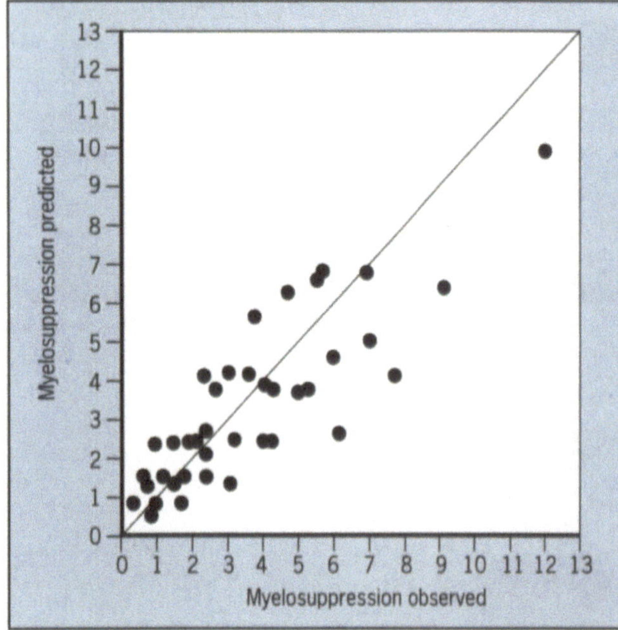

Figure 12-35. Patient stratification. Assay for the metabolism of caffeine is highly predictive of the activation of amonafide, which in turn correlates well with the clinically observed toxic side effect of myelosuppression. (*Adapted from* Ratain *et al.* [50]; with permission.)

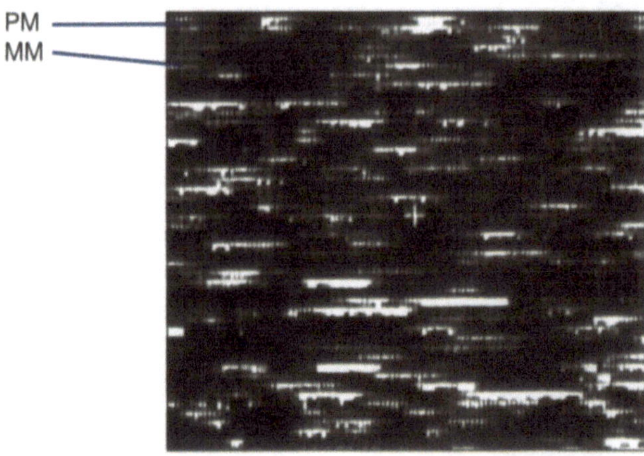

Figure 12-36. Expression profiling. Arrays of 20-mer oligonucleotide probes are synthesized on a glass wafer and used to capture fluorescently labeled probes prepared from cellular mRNA. Overlapping sequences provide sufficient redundancy to identify rare mRNA in the presence of more abundant partially cross-hybridizing sequences. Each *box*=100 μM on a side and has a different sequence. MM—the same 20-mer as in the position above it but with one mismatched base; PM—perfect match sequences. (*From* Lockhart *et al.* [51]; with permission.)

For example, an easily performed assay for the metabolism of caffeine is being used in clinical trials of amonafide, a novel alkylating agent prodrug, as a means of stratifying patients with regard to efficiency of the enzyme that activates the drug [50]. Treatment groups can then be given a high or low dose of the drug, as appropriate. The predicted damage to white blood cell count based on this stratification correlates well with observed retrospective data (Fig. 12-35).

The trend to improved diagnostics is accelerating. New techniques for creating dense arrays of DNA probes are particularly promising as a means of generating information on large numbers of genes from normal and diseased tissue, thereby permitting analysis of the flood of new targets by multivariate statisti-

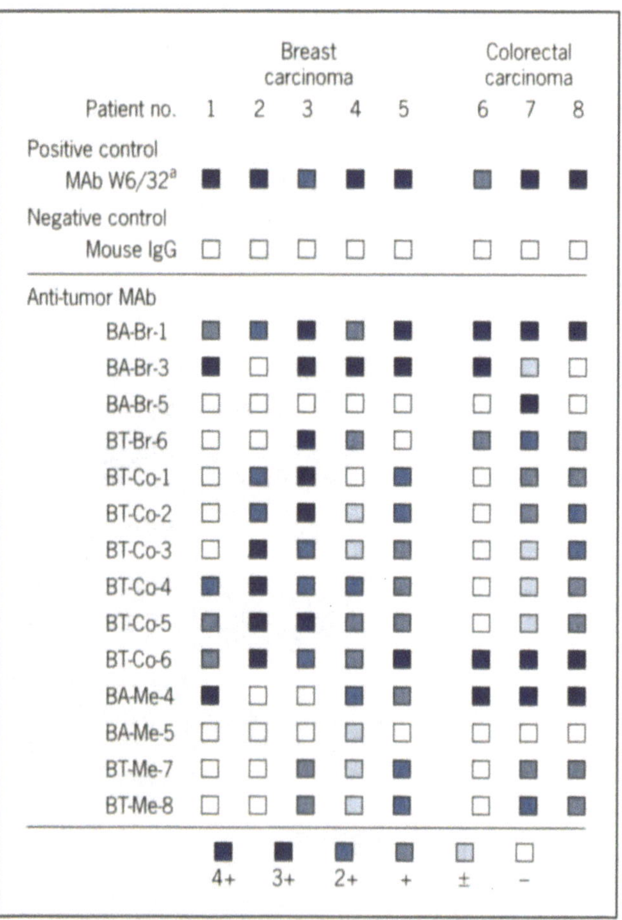

Figure 12-37. Patient-specific therapy. A panel of 14 monoclonal antibodies raised against various tumor types (breast, colon, melanoma) was used to phenotype tumor biopsy specimens from 110 patients by immunohistochemistry. For the eight representative specimens illustrated, some specific subset of these antibodies provides staining of essentially all the tumor cells at levels comparable to the positive control anti-HLA antibody (W6/32) that stains both tumor and normal cells. Intensity of staining is color-coded from strong to weak or null. (*Adapted from* Liao *et al.* [52]; with permission.)

cal methods (Fig. 12-36). Sequence abundance can be accurately quantitated from a few copies per cell to more than 10,000 copies per cell, and the next generation of wafers under development should allow measuring the entire genome at the same time [51].

Perhaps the most far-reaching prospect for patient-specific therapy is selection of a unique combination of antibodies for each tumor (Fig. 12-37). Such mixtures should provide substantially improved tumor specificity compared with normal tissue as well as help in overcoming tumor heterogeneity. The approximately 100,000 monoclonal antibodies already raised against human tumor specimens can in principle be classified by the kind of multivariate methods already in use for defining histocompatibility-typing reagents. As tools for antibody staining of tumor biopsy specimens improve, more categories can be prospectively evaluated in order to choose the most appropriate cocktail of antibodies for the individual patient [52]. The active agent delivered by such antibodies can of course encompass a wide range of categories.

ACKNOWLEDGMENTS

I would like to thank my colleagues at Terrapin Technologies, the members of Terrapin's Science Advisory Board, and a broad range of consultants and colleagues who have been instrumental over the past 5 years in helping to organize my thoughts on cancer treatment. Special thanks go to Ken Tew, PhD, and Jordan Gutterman, MD, for their critical review of the manuscript.

REFERENCES

1. Chang AE, Shu S: Current status of adoptive immunotherapy of cancer. *Crit Rev Oncol Hematol* 1996, 22:213–228.
2. Rosok MJ, Yelton DE, Harris LJ, *et al.*: A combinatorial library strategy for the rapid humanization of anticarcinoma BR96 Fab. *J Biol Chem* 1996, 271:22611–22618.
3. Jakobovits A: Production of fully human antibodies by transgenic mice. *Curr Opin Biotechnol* 1995, 6:561–566.
4. Marks C, Marks JD: Phage libraries: a new route to clinically useful antibodies. *N Engl J Med* 1996, 335:730–733.
5. Maloney DG, Liles TM, Czerwinski DK, *et al.*: Phase I trial using escalating single dose infusion of chimeric anti-CD20 monoclonal antibody (IDEC-C2B8) in patients with recurrent B-cell lymphoma. *Blood* 1994, 84:2457–2466.
6. Peterson JA, Couto JR, Taylor MR, Ceriani RL: Selection of tumor-specific epitopes on target antigens for radioimmunotherapy of breast cancer. *Cancer Res* 1995, 55:5847s–5851s.
7. Sharkey RM, Juweid M, Shevitz J, *et al.*: Evaluation of a complementarity-determining region grafted (humanized) anti-carcinoembryonic antigen monoclonal antibody in preclinical and clinical studies. *Cancer Res* 1995, 55:5935s–5945s.
8. Hu P, Hornick JL, Glasky MS, *et al.*: A chimeric Lym-1/interleukin 2 fusion protein for increasing tumor vascular permeability and enhancing antibody uptake. *Cancer Res* 1996, 56:4998–5004.
9. Chen FM, Epstein AL, Li Z, Taylor CR: A comparative autoradiographic study demonstrating differential intratumor localization of monoclonal antibodies to cell surface (Lym-1) and intracellular (TNT-1) antigens. *J Nucl Med* 1990, 31:1059–1066.
10. Yokota T, Milenic DE, Whitlow M, Schlom J: Rapid tumor penetration of a single chain Fv and comparison with other immunoglobulin forms. *Cancer Res* 1992, 52:3402–3408.
11. Larson SM, Divgi CR, Scott AM: Overview of clinical radioimmunodetection of human tumors. *Cancer* 1994, 73(3 suppl):832–835.
12. Trail PA, Willner D, Knipe J, *et al.*: Effect of linker variation on the stability, potency, and efficacy of carcinoma-reactive BR64-doxorubicin immunoconjugates. *Cancer Res* 1997, 57:100–105.
13. Melton RG, Sherwood RF: Antibody-enzyme conjugates for cancer therapy. *J Natl Cancer Inst* 1996, 88:153–165.
14. Schuitmaker JJ, Baas P, van Leengoed HL, *et al.*: Photodynamic therapy: a promising new modality for the treatment of cancer. *J Photochem Photobiol B* 1996, 34:3–12.
15. Satyam A, Hocker MD, Kane-Maguire KA, *et al.*: Design, synthesis, and evaluation of latent alkylating agents activated by glutathione *S*-transferase. *J Med Chem* 1996, 39:1736–1747.
16. Nishimura T, Newkirk K, Sessions RB, *et al.*: Immunohistochemical staining for glutathione *S*-transferase predicts response to platinum-based chemotherapy in head and neck cancer. *Clin Cancer Res* 1996, 2:1859–1865.
17. Sung C, van Osdol WW: Pharmacokinetic comparison of direct antibody targeting with pretargeting protocols based on streptavidin-biotin binding. *J Nucl Med* 1995, 36:867–876.
18. Sachs L: The control of growth and differentiation in normal and leukemic blood cells. *Cancer* 1991, 65:2196–2206.
19. Baldwin RL, Kobrin MS, Tran T, *et al.*: Cytotoxic effects of TGF-α-*Pseudomonas* exotoxin A fusion protein in human pancreatic carcinoma cells. *Pancreas* 1996, 13:16–21.
20. Huang X, Molema G, King S, *et al.*: Tumor infarction in mice by antibody-directed targeting of tissue factor to tumor vasculature. *Science* 1997, 275:547–550.
21. Lee JH, Naito M, Tsuruo T: Non-enzymatic reductive activation of a mitomycin analog by thiols. *Cancer Res* 1994, 54:2398–2403.

22. Bischoff JB, Kirn DH, Williams A, *et al.*: An adenovirus mutant that replicates selectively in *p53*-deficient human tumor cells. *Science* 1996, 274:373–376.
23. Dean N, McKay R, Miraglia L, *et al.*: Inhibition of human tumor cell lines in nude mice by an antisense oligonucleotide inhibitor of protein kinase C-α expression. *Cancer Res* 1996, 56:3499–3507.
24. Ning S, Macleod K, Abra RM, *et al.*: Hyperthermia induces doxorubicin release from long-circulating liposomes and enhances their anti-tumor efficacy. *Int J Radiat Oncol Biol Phys* 1994, 29:827–834.
25. Vyas SP, Singh R, Asati RK: Liposomally encapsulated diclofenac for sonophoresis induced systemic delivery. *J Microencapsul* 1995, 12:149–154.
26. Ho RJY, Rouse BT, Huang L: Target sensitive immunoliposomes. *Biochemistry* 1986, 25:5500–5506.
27. Mitelman F, Mertens F, Johansson B: A breakpoint map of recurrent chromosomal rearrangements in human neoplasia. *Nat Genet* 1997, 15:417–474.
28. Broach JR, Thorner J: High-throughput screening for drug discovery. *Nature* 1996, 7(suppl):14–16.
29. Mitchison TJ: Towards a pharmacological genetics. *Chem Biol* 1994, 1:3–6.
30. Lyttle MH: Combinatorial chemistry: a conservative perspective. *Drug Dev Res* 1995, 35:230–236.
31. Raymond E, Djelloul S, Buquet-Fagot C, *et al.*: Synergy between the non-classical thymidylate synthase inhibitor AG337 (Thymitaq) and cisplatin in human colon and ovarian cancer cells. *Anticancer Drugs* 1996, 7:752–757.
32. Zhao B, Helms LR, des Jarlais RL, *et al.*: A paradigm for drug discovery using a conformation from the crystal structure of a presentation scaffold. *Nature Struct Biol* 1995, 12:1131–1137.
33. Kauvar LM, Higgins DL, Villar HO, *et al.*: Predicting ligand binding to proteins by affinity fingerprinting. *Chem Biol* 1995, 2:107–118.
34. Wrighton NC, Farrell FX, Chang R, *et al.*: Small peptides as potent mimetics of the protein hormone erythropoietin. *Science* 1996, 273:458–463.
35. Farrar MA, Alberola-Ila J, Perlmutter RM: Activation of the *Raf*-1 kinase cascade by coumermycin induced dimerization. *Nature* 1996, 383:178–181.
36. Arnold A: Moving promising research findings to the clinic: methodological issues in the design and conduct of clinical trials of retinoids. *Int J Cancer* 1997, 70:467–469.
37. Walker S, Landovitz R, Ding WD, *et al.*: Cleavage behavior of calicheamicin γ^1 and calicheamicin T. *Proc Natl Acad Sci U S A* 1992, 89:4608–4612.
38. Strahl C, Blackburn EH: Effects of reverse transcriptase inhibitors on telomere length and telomerase activity in two immortalized human cell lines. *Mol Cell Biol* 1996, 16:53–65.
39. Von Hoff DD: He's not going to talk about in vitro predictive assays again, is he? *J Natl Cancer Inst* 1990, 82:96–101.
40. Fruehauf JP, Bosanquet AG: In vitro determination of drug response: a discussion of clinical applications. In *Cancer, Principles and Practice of Oncology*, 4th ed. Edited by DeVita VT Jr, Hellman S, Rosenberg SA. Philadelphia: JB Lippincott; 1993:1–16.
41. Jakoby WB, Ziegler DM: The enzymes of detoxication. *J Biol Chem* 1990, 265:20715–20718.
42. Montali JA, Wheatley JB, Schmidt DE Jr: Comparison of GST levels in predicting the efficacy of a novel alkylating agent. *Cell Pharmacol* 1996, 2:241–247.
43. Mounts WM, Liebman MN: Qualitative modeling of normal blood coagulation and its pathological states using stochastic activity networks. *Int J Biol Macromol* 1997, 20:265–281.
44. Sager R: Expression genetics in cancer. *Proc Natl Acad Sci U S A* 1997, 94:952–955.
45. Roninson IB, Gudkov AV, Holzmayer TA, *et al.*: Genetic suppressor elements: new tools for molecular oncology. *Cancer Res* 1995, 55:4023–4028.
46. Meinwald J, Eisner T: The chemistry of phyletic dominance. *Proc Natl Acad Sci U S A* 1995, 92:14–18.
47. Taunton J, Hassig CA, Schreiber SL: A mammalian histone deacetylase related to the yeast transcriptional regulator Rpd3p. *Science* 1996, 272:408–411.
48. Weinstein JN, Myers TG, O'Connor PM, *et al.*: An information intensive approach to the molecular pharmacology of cancer. *Science* 1997, 275:343–349.
49. Tew KD: Genetic polymorphisms of detoxification enzymes. *Cell Pharmacol* 1996, 3:143–152.
50. Ratain MJ, Mick R, Janisch L, *et al.*: Individualized dosing of amonafide based on a pharmacodynamic model incorporating acetylator phenotype and gender. *Pharmacogenetics* 1996, 6:93–101.
51. Lockhart DJ, Dong H, Byrne MC, *et al.*: Expression monitoring by hybridization to high-density oligonucleotide arrays. *Nature Biotech* 1996, 14:1675–1680.
52. Liao SK, Meranda C, Avner BP, *et al.*: Immunohistochemical phenotyping of human solid tumors with monoclonal antibodies in devising biotherapeutic strategies. *Cancer Immunol Immunother* 1989, 28:77–86.

CHAPTER

13

Pharmacogenetics and Cancer

Warren D. Kruger
Kenneth D. Tew

It has been known for more than 30 years that individuals vary in their ability to metabolize therapeutically useful molecules. This variation is due in large part to genetic differences among individuals. Humans are exposed to thousands of natural and synthetic compounds, in addition to drugs, that must be metabolized to become carcinogenic. Genetic variation in the encoded enzymes involved in this metabolism is thought to be the basis for some of the differences in cancer susceptibility among individuals. The study of how genetic variation affects the metabolism of drugs and other compounds is called pharmacogenetics.

In this chapter we discuss how pharmacogenetics may be an important factor in determining who gets cancer and how genes and the environment interact to determine cancer risk. The emerging role of pharmacogenetics in cancer treatment is also examined.

METABOLIC ACTIVATION OF XENOBIOTICS

Metabolism of drugs or carcinogens can usually be classified into two distinct phases (Fig. 13-1; Table 13-1). In phase I, carcinogens can be activated by the cytochrome P450 family of monooxygenases. The resulting molecules are frequently highly reactive and are often powerful mutagens. These mutagens can cause alterations in DNA that can result in cancer. In phase II, these activated metabolites are primarily converted into more soluble products by conjugation reactions at functional sites (Table 13-1). The conjugated metabolite is then excreted from the body [1]. As a result of this scheme, it is easy to see how variation in expression of either phase I or phase II enzymes could influence cancer susceptibility or response to drugs (Fig. 13-2). For example, individuals overexpressing phase I enzymes produce higher levels of reactive products and thus are at increased risk for DNA damage and, ultimately, of developing cancer. Conversely, individuals with increased expression of phase II enzymes may be at decreased risk for developing cancer because the concentration of activated intermediates is decreased.

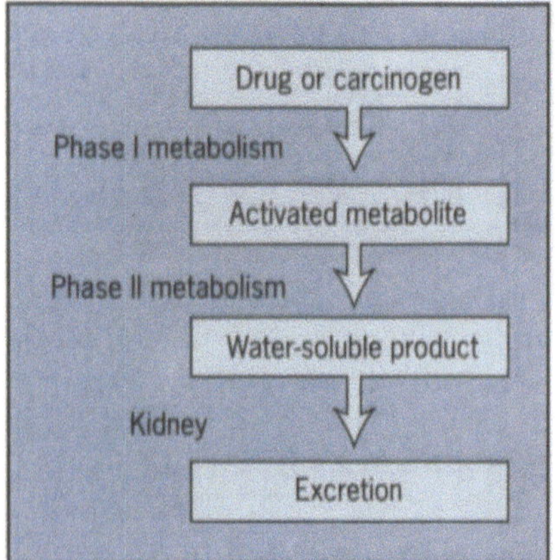

Figure 13-1. Phase I and II drug and carcinogen metabolic pathway.

Phase I metabolism involves the action of the P450 family of monooxygenases. All P450 monooxygen-

Table 13-1. Classification of metabolism reactions

Phase I		
	Oxidation involving cytochrome P450	
	Oxidation (others)	
	Reduction	
	Hydrolysis	
	Hydration	
	Dethioacetylation	
	Isomerization	
Phase II		
Reaction	**Enzyme**	**Functional group**
Glucuronidation	UDP-glucuronosyltransferase	–OH, –COOH, $-NH_2$, –SH
Glycosidation	UDP-glycosyltransferase	–OH, –COOH, –SH
Sulfation	Sulfotransferase	$-NH_2$, $-SO_2NH_2$, –OH
Methylation	Methyltransferase	–OH, NH_2
Acetylation	Acetyltransferase	NH_2, $-SO_2NH_2$, –OH
Amino acid conjugation		–COOH
Glutathione conjugation	Glutathione-*S*-transferase	Epoxide
		Organic halide
		Peroxides
		Aryl/alkyl groups
		Electrophilic centers
Fatty acid conjugation		–OH
Condensation		Various

Phase I: Functionalization reactions—small changes in structure producing reactive functional groups.
Phase II: Conjugation reactions—larger "addition" reactions changes characteristics and solubility of the drug.

ases have the ability to insert an atom of molecular oxygen into their substrates, which leads to an increase in hydrophilicity and facilitates excretion from the cells. However, when carcinogens are acted on by P450 monooxygenases, highly mutagenic electrophiles may be the catalytic product. The P450 proteins are encoded by the *CYP* genes. At present, 11 distinct *CYP* gene families, each of which has a distinctive pattern of substrate specificity, have been described in humans (Table 13-2) [2]. Each gene family has several members that tend to have overlapping, but not identical, substrate specificities. The expression of many of the *CYP* genes is induced by substrates and related molecules. For example, the aryl hydrocarbon (Ah) receptor induces expression of some of the *CYP1* family members but not others (Fig. 13-3) [3].

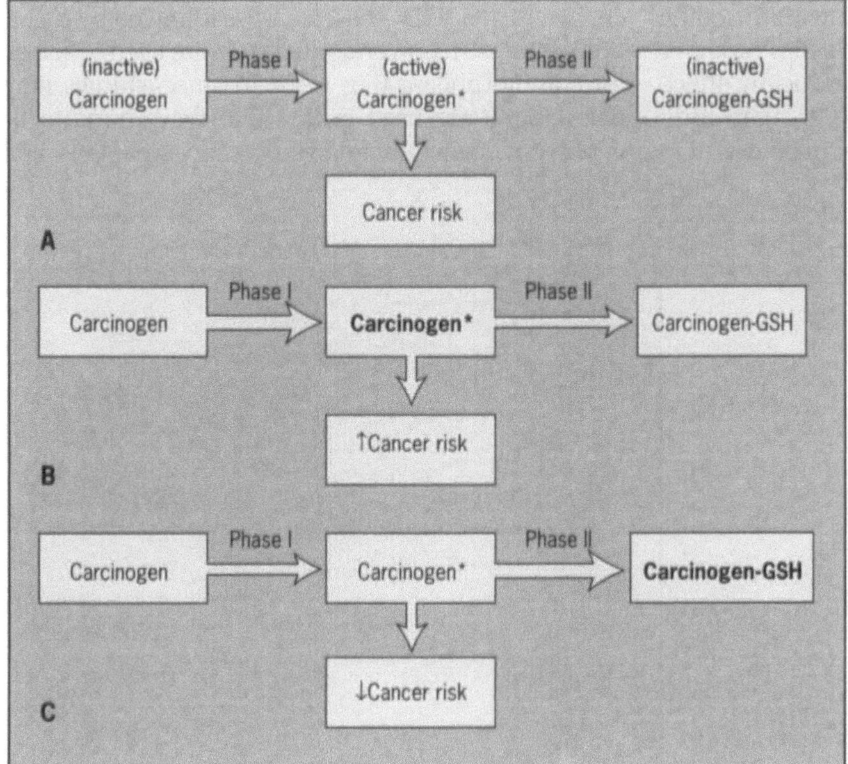

Figure 13-2. Variation in phase I and phase II expression levels and cancer risk. **A,** Carcinogens frequently are activated by phase I enzymes to become mutagenic (*) and increase cancer risk. The mutagenic form is also the substrate for phase II enzymes, such as glutathione-*S*-transferase, which, when conjugated, make the mutagenic form inactive. **B,** Increased expression or activity of phase I enzymes results in more activated carcinogen and therefore increased cancer risk. **C,** Increased level of activity of phase II enzymes results in decreased active carcinogen concentrations and therefore decreased cancer risk.

Table 13-2. Human *CYP* gene family members

Gene family	Number of functional genes	Chromosomal location	Example substrates
CYP1A	2	15q22-qter	Polycyclic aromatic hydrocarbons
CYP1B	>2	?	Steroid hormones
CYP2A	>3	19q13.1-13.3	Aflatoxin B_1
CYP2B	2–3	19q13.1-13.3	Nicotine
CYP2C	4	10q24.1-24.3	Benzpyrene
CYP2D	1	22q11.2-qter	Debrisoquine
CYP2E	1	10	Acetaldehyde
CYP2F	1–2	19	Unknown
CYP3A	3–5	7q21.3-q22	Doxorubicin
CYP4A	2–4	1	Phenobarbitone
CYP4B	1	1p12-q34	Phenobarbitone

(Adapted from Smith et al. [1]; with permission.)

GENETIC POLYMORPHISMS IN *CYP* GENES

Among any distantly related individuals, it is estimated that there is about one nucleotide difference every 1000 base pairs. These differences are called DNA polymorphisms. Because most of the human DNA sequence is noncoding, most of the polymorphisms are thought to have no phenotypic effect. However, DNA alterations that lie within coding sequences or regulatory sequences of genes can have an effect on the underlying protein product by affecting protein function or expression (Fig. 13-4). In addition, even "neutral" polymorphisms can be useful as markers for functional polymorphisms because of linkage disequilibrium (Fig. 13-5).

Polymorphisms within the *CYP* genes and their role in pharmacogenetics is an intensely studied area. Most of these studies are conducted as association studies with cases and controls. For example, in pharmacogenetic studies of drug metabolism, individuals are divided into "high-metabolizer" and "low-metabolizer" groups and are screened for the DNA polymorphism of interest. Usually, polymerase chain reaction (PCR)-based assays followed by digestion with restriction endonucleases are used to screen for polymorphisms (Fig. 13-6). In cancer studies, similar designs are used except that the groups to be genotyped generally represent cancer patients and

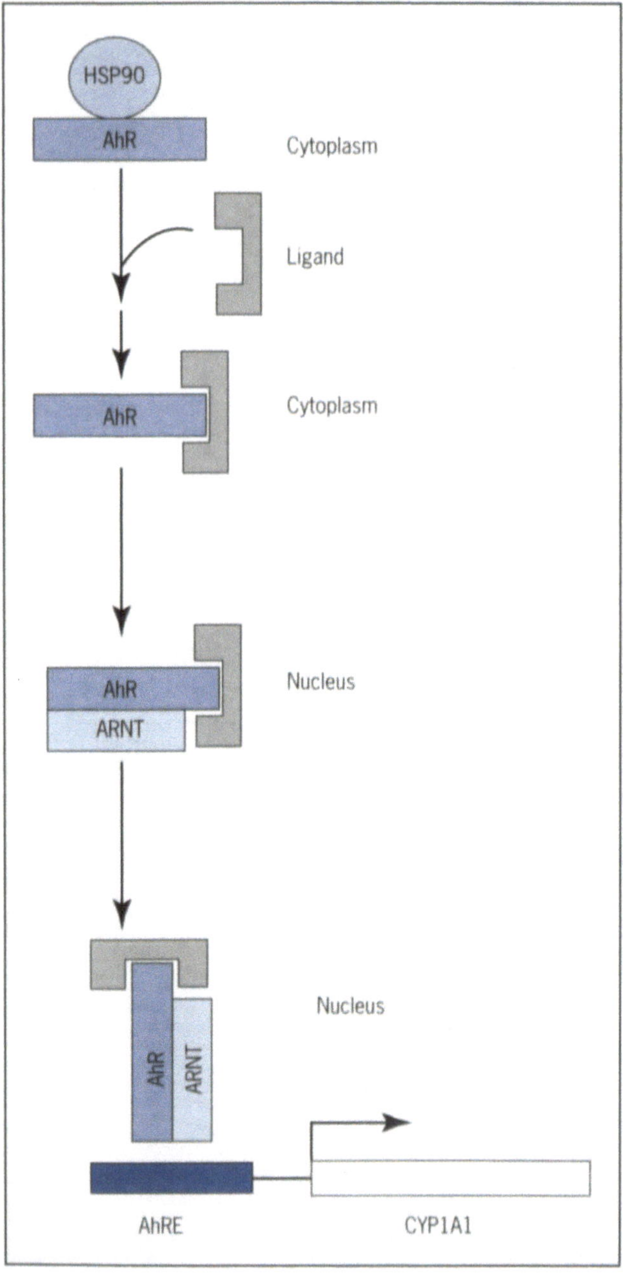

Figure 13-3. Proposed mechanism of aryl-hydrocarbon receptor (AhR) mediated transcriptional activation. The receptor is kept inactive in the cytoplasm by being bound to HSP90. On induction by aryl-hydrocarbons, HSP90 is released, and the AhR migrates to the nucleus where it forms a heterodimer with the AhR nuclear translocator (ARNT). The dimeric complex then binds to DNA sequences called aryl-hydrocarbon response elements (AhRE) that are found in front of inducible genes. The bound complex then acts to stimulate transcription (*Adapted from* Gonzalez [3]; with permission.)

age-matched controls. The rationale is that if a specific polymorphism in a gene is associated with an increased risk of a particular kind of cancer, the polymorphisms should be over-represented in cancer patients relative to the respective controls. Table 13-3 presents a summary of data showing the association of specific *CYP* gene polymorphisms with specific cancers.

Differential activity of *CYP* genes due to polymorphisms may also be important in determining the aggressiveness of different types of tumors. In Japan, a large study looked at clinical measures of non–small cell lung cancer outcome versus presence or absence of the *Msp*I polymorphism in the *CYP1A1* gene [4]. This polymorphism is in linkage disequilibrium with another alteration, I462V, which is located in the protein itself. The variant appears to be hyperinducible in response to carcinogens [5]. As shown in Figure 13-7, individuals with at least one allele containing the *Msp*I restriction site have significantly decreased survival.

One hypothesis to explain these findings involves the role of mutation in the *P53* gene in lung cancer. The P53 gene product is a transcription factor important in both cell cycle control and apoptosis. It has been observed that the presence of *P53* mutations in non–small cell lung cancers is associated with shorter survival [6,7]. Thus, the presence of a *P53* mutation is a hallmark of a more aggressive cancer. In addition, a larger percentage of non–small cell tumors from patients containing at least one *Msp*I restriction site have inactivating *P53* mutations [8]. Thus, the shorter survival time may reflect the fact that individuals with increased *CYP1A1* activity are exposed to higher internal mutagen levels that may be associated with an increased likelihood of a *P53* mutation (Fig. 13-8). Furthermore, the *P53* gene is

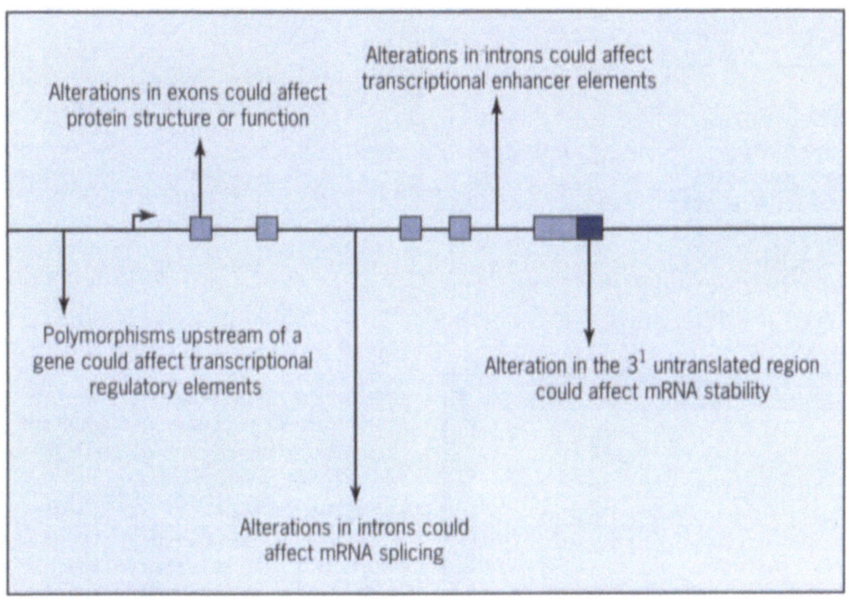

Figure 13-4. How polymorphisms or mutations can effect gene function. The *thin line* represents intronic sequences, and the *solid boxes* represent exons. The *open box* represents the 3 prime untranslated region of a gene. The *horizontal arrow* indicates the start site, and the *vertical arrows* show the results of different kinds of mutations.

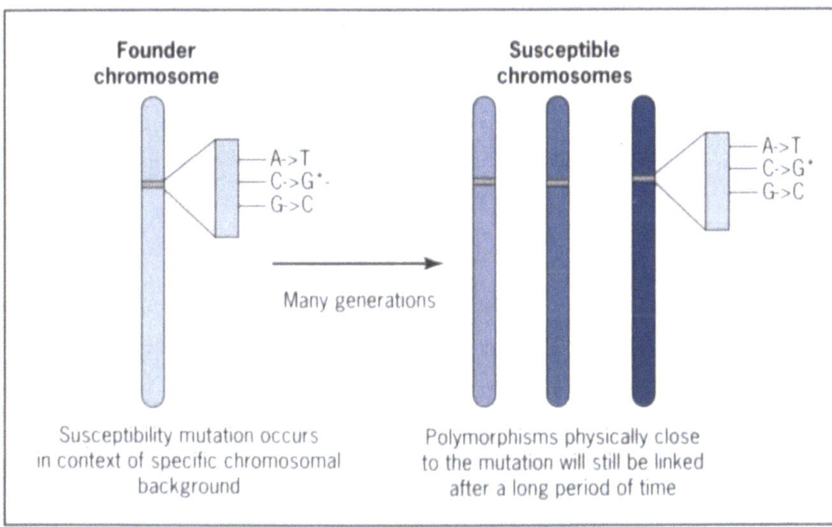

Figure 13-5. Linkage disequilibrium. The original cancer susceptibility mutation (asterisk) occurs on the founder chromosome (*left*). This chromosome also contains two other polymorphisms flanking the susceptibility mutation. Because the distance between the flanking polymorphisms and the cancer susceptibility mutation is small, they are still linked after many generations. Thus, the flanking polymorphisms show association with the cancer susceptibility phenotype, even though they are not functionally important in the promotion of cancer.

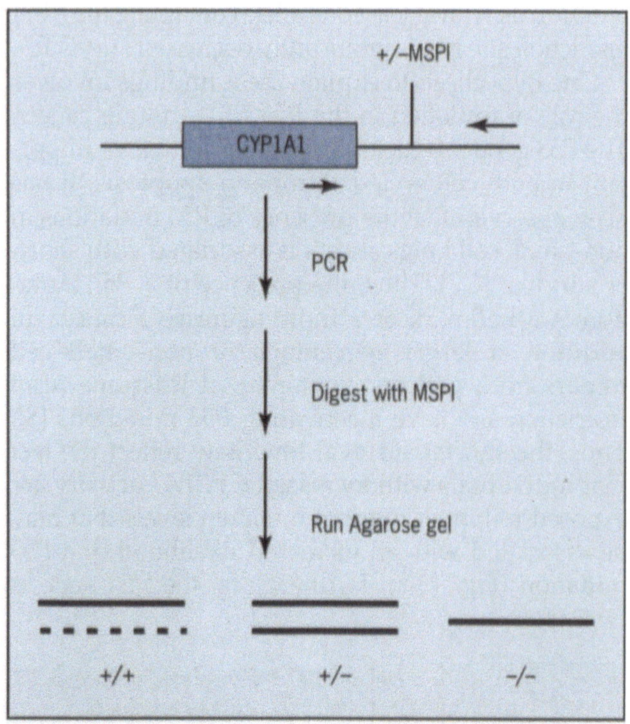

Figure 13-6. Detection of a *CYP1A1 MSPI* polymorphism. *Horizontal arrows* show the location of primers used for polymerase chain reaction amplification of genomic DNA. The polymorphic *MSPI* restriction site is shown. The *bottom* of the figure shows the expected agarose gel electrophoresis pattern observed for each of the three genotypes.

Table 13-3. Significant associations between CYP polymorphisms and cancer

	Polymorphism	Risk
CYP1A1	3'-MspI/I462V	Increased lung and oral cancer
CYP2D6	Poor metabolizer alleles	Decreased bladder cancer
		Decreased lung cancer
CYP2E1	*DraI*	Increased non-small cell lung cancer
CYP1A2	High activity alleles	Increased bladder cancer

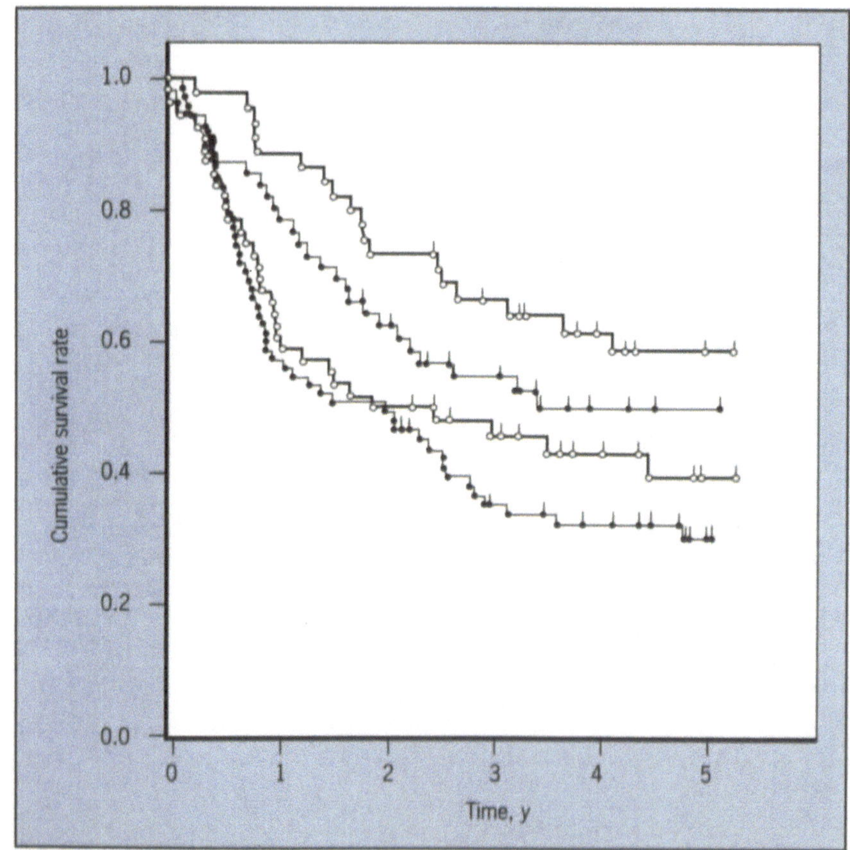

Figure 13-7. Differential survival curves for patients with non–small cell lung cancer based on their *CYP1A1* and *GSTM1* genotypes. For *CYP1A1*, "+" refers to the presence of the *MspI* site, while "-" indicates its absence. For GSTM1, "+" indicates wt, while "-" indicates the null allele. The *open square* is -/- for both *CYP1A1* and +/+ or +/- for *GSTM1*. The *darkened square* is -/- for *CYP1A1* and -/- for *GSTM1*. The *open circle* is +/- or +/+ for *CYP1A1* and +/+ or +/- for *GSTM1*. The *darkened circle* is +/- or +/+ for *CYP1A1* and -/- for *GSTM1*. (*From* Goto *et al.* [4]; with permission.)

polymorphic in the human population, encoding either a proline or an arginine at codon 72. Recent data [9] indicate that individuals with human papillomavirus-associated cervical cancer are much more likely to have the arginine form of P53 than the rest of the population ($\chi^2 = 10.5$; $P < 0.0005$; Fig. 13-9). Based on this study, individuals homozygous for the arginine polymorphism are predicted to have a sevenfold risk of developing cervical carcinoma that is associated with human papilloma virus. Although the direct relevance of this polymorphism to treatment outcome has yet to be studied, the amino acid change lies within a domain of *P53* that is important in determining apoptotic response.

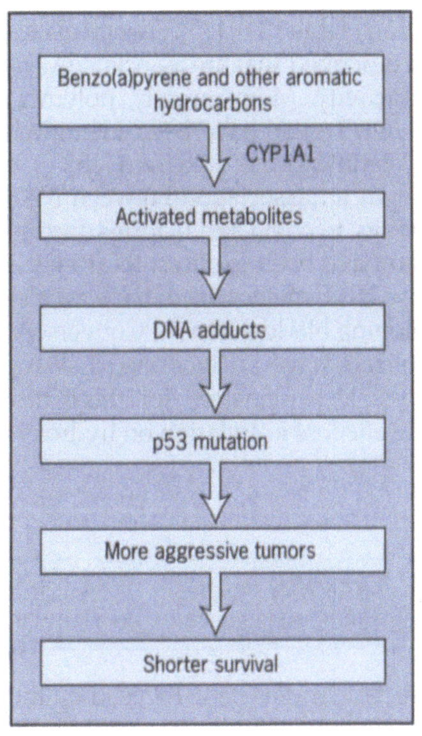

Figure 13-8. Hypothesis for the association of *CYP1A1* polymorphism with decreased survival rates in lung cancer patients.

GENETIC POLYMORPHISMS IN PHASE II GENES

GLUTATHIONE-*S*-TRANSFERASES

Polymorphisms in phase II detoxification enzymes also are thought to play an important role in cancer susceptibility. Among the most studied phase II enzymes are the glutathione-*S*-transferases (GSTs). These enzymes catalyze the conjugation of glutathione to electrophilic substrates, some of which have been formed during phase I metabolism. Four major families of GST enzymes have been described in humans (GSTα, GSTμ, GSTπ, and GSTθ), each of which are encoded for by multiple genes (Table 13-4). Although polymorphic loci have been identified in genes encoding each of the GST class members, the therapeu-

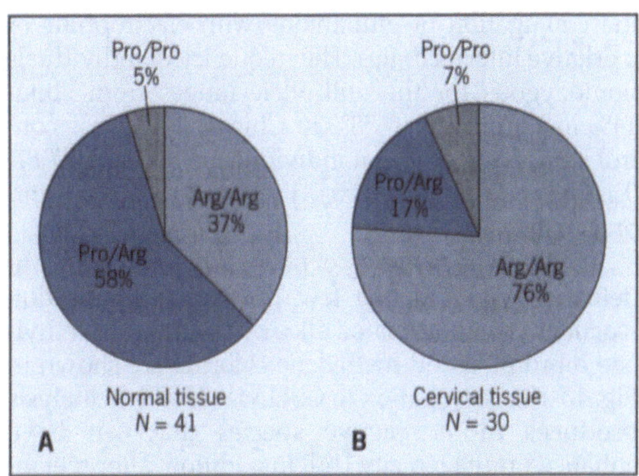

Figure 13-9. Frequency of *P53* alleles in the normal population (*A*) and in individuals with human papillomavirus–associated cervical cancer (*B*).

Table 13-4. Glutathione-*S*-transferases in humans

Glutathione-*S*-transferase family	Number of genes	Chromosomal location	Substrates
α	>2	6	Aromatic amines, anticancer drugs
μ	5	1p13	Lipid peroxidation products
π	1	11	Polycyclic aromatic hydrocarbons
θ	>2	?	Solvents
Microsomal	1	12	?

(From Smith et al. [1]; with permission.)

tic and pathologic consequences of most of this variation remains unclear.

The most studied polymorphism in this family of genes is in the *GSTM1* gene. There are three common M1 alleles, M1*a, M1*b, and M1*-0 (Table 13-5). The M1-0 allele is a large deletion of the M1 locus, therefore GSTM1 is not produced in individuals homozygous for this allele [10]. Homozygosity for the deletion allele is surprisingly frequent in human populations, ranging from 22% in Nigerians to 67% in Australians. A meta-analysis of studies examining the association of the M-0 genotype and lung cancer suggests that homozygotes have about a 40% increased risk for developing lung cancer [11]. Interestingly, this risk appears to be greater among Asians than among whites. Convincing associations between *GSTM1*-0* and bladder and colon cancer also have been reported [10].

A null mutation also has been observed in another member of the GST family, *GSTT1*. Like *GSTM1*, *GSTT1* encodes a cytosolic enzyme that can catalyze the conjugation of glutathione with electrophilic or oxidative intermediates. The frequency of individuals homozygous for the null allele ranges from about 14% in Europeans to 58% in Chinese [10]. Case-control studies suggest that individuals with the *GSTT1-0* allele may be at increased risk for colorectal and brain cancer [12,13].

Although the majority of phase II reactions serve to detoxify xenobiotics, a few produce a toxification reaction. For halogenated alkanes and alkenes (ethylene dibromide and methylene chloride are shown in Fig. 13-10), conjugation to GSH via *GSTT1-1* catalysis produces more reactive species that can have enhanced mutagenicity [14]. In addition, after metabolism by cysteine conjugate beta-lyase, a nephrotoxic product can be formed. These observations predict that the theta polymorphism may significantly impact the metabolism of chemicals and therapeutics with a similar halogenated structure in ways that are difficult to predict.

N-Acetyltransferases

Another phase II enzyme family that has been implicated in carcinogenesis is the family of *N*-acetyltransferases (*NAT* genes). *NAT* genes catalyze the acetylation of amino groups of xenobiotics, facilitating their detoxification and excretion from the cell. Early in the study of these genes, it was appreciated that there was wide variation in *NAT* activity between individuals, and family studies soon revealed that this variation was genetic in origin. These so-called slow acetylators were hypothesized to be homozygous for a recessive gene [1].

Modern molecular studies have identified two *NAT* genes, *NAT1* and *NAT2*. Genetic variation in *NAT2* appears to be responsible for most of the individual variation in acetylation (Table 13-6) [15]. Several alleles of *NAT2* have been described that are associated with decreased enzyme activity. More recently, polymorphisms within the *NAT1* gene have been identified, but their functional significance is unknown [15].

Studies have shown an association between *NAT* status and susceptibility to colon and bladder cancers [3]. Individuals who have been exposed to aromatic amines and are slow NAT metabolizers have an elevated risk for developing bladder cancer. Conversely, rapid NAT metabolizers have an increased risk for colon cancer. A possible explanation for these discrepant results is the effect of acetylation on hydroxylated amines (Fig. 13-11).

GENE-ENVIRONMENT INTERACTIONS

Many of the most recent studies have focused on the interaction between environmental exposure to specific carcinogens and polymorphic variation in phase I and phase II enzyme–encoding genes. The

Table 13-5. Common GSTM1 alleles and association with cancer risk

GSTM			
Allele	Molecular change	Allele frequency	Cancer risk
*M1*a*	172K	≈0.20	Decreased risk of bladder cancer
*M1*b*	172N	≈0.10	
M1-0*	Large deletion	≈0.70	Increased risk of lung, colon, and bladder cancer

rationale behind these studies is that specific polymorphisms may only play a role in the development of a particular cancer when there is exposure to a specific carcinogen. A strong example of this logic is found in studies examining the relation between the *CYP2D6* "debrisoquine" polymorphism, smoking, and lung cancer.

The *CYP2D6* gene encodes a P450 protein that has specificity for a number of substances, including debrisoquine (an antihypertensive drug) and 4-(methylnitrosamino)-1-(3-pyridyl)-1-butanone (NNK), a substance found in cigarette smoke. More than 20 years ago, it was discovered that 5% to 7% of whites lack the ability to metabolize debrisoquine

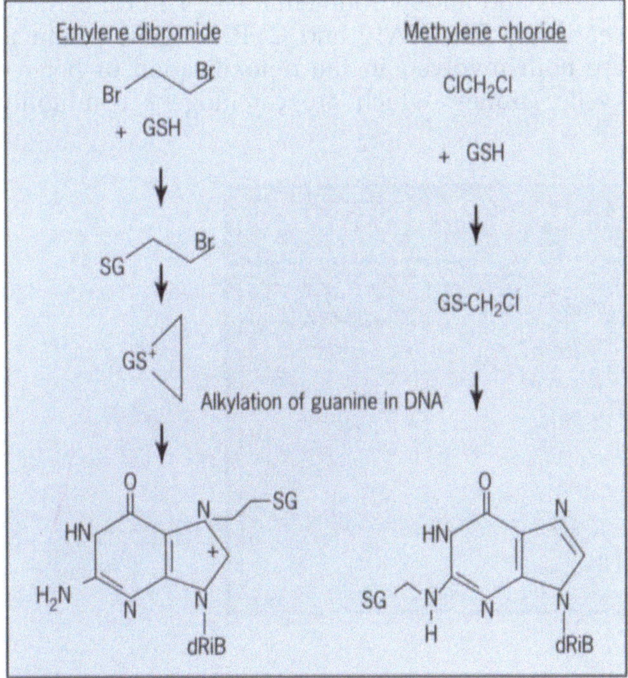

Figure 13-10. Activation of alkylhalides to more toxic products. (From Tew [29]; with permission.)

Table 13-6. Common NAT2 alleles

Mutation	Allele designation	Phenotype	Frequency (whites), %
None	NAT2*4	Rapid	≈22
T341C, C481T, A803G	NAT2*5B	Slow	≈40
C282T, G590A	NAT2*6A	Slow	≈25
T341C, T481T	NAT2*5A	Slow	≈3.0
T341C, A803G	NAT2*5C	Slow	≈2.5
C282T, G857A	NAT2*7B	Slow	≈1.5
C282T	NAT2*13	Slow	≈1.5

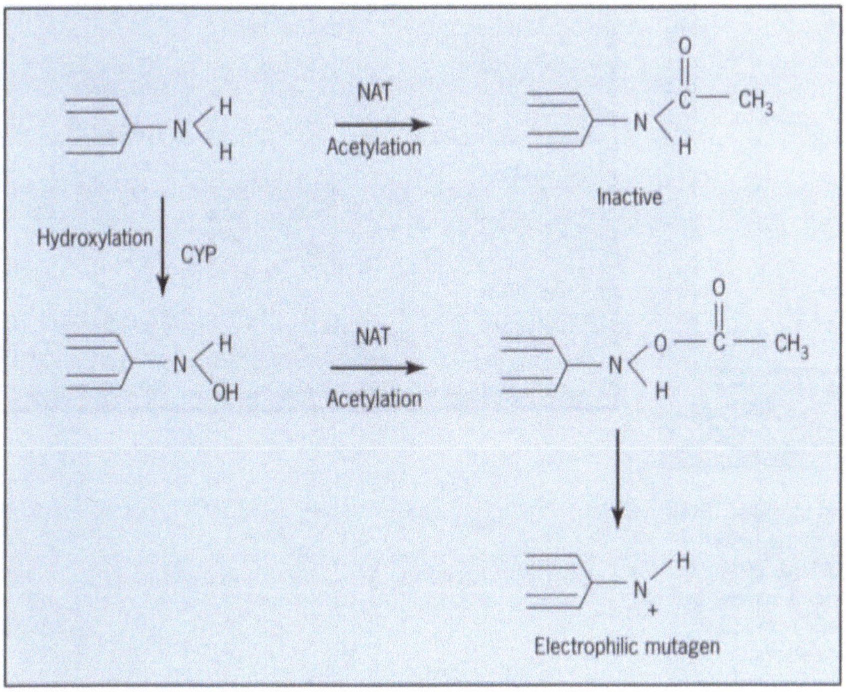

Figure 13-11. Competition between CYP1A1 and NAT2. An arylamine can be acetylated by NAT2 directly, or it can be first hydroxylated by CYP1A2 and then acetylated by NAT2. In the former case, NAT2 inactivates the arylamine, whereas in the latter case, acetylation causes the production of a mutagenic metabolite. Thus, increased NAT2 activity can be protective or damaging, depending on the *CYP1A2* status of an individual. (*Adapted from* Kadlubar *et al.* [28]; with permission.)

[16]; later studies showed that this ability was owing to lack of a functional CYP2D6 gene product [17]. Molecular studies have revealed the existence of at least 12 different alleles at this locus (Table 13-7) [1]. Some of these alleles produce inactive proteins and are associated with the "poor metabolizer" (PM) phenotype observed in specific individuals.

A large number of studies conducted in various patient groups have examined whether individuals with PM alleles of *CYP2D6* are at decreased risk for lung cancer. The hypothesis is that these individuals activate the carcinogens found in cigarette smoke to a lesser degree than other individuals. Some of these studies found that individuals with the PM phenotype did appear to be at decreased risk, whereas other studies did not. However, when the smoking history of each of the cohorts was taken into account, a clearer picture emerged [18]. The highest odds ratios were found in those individuals with the greatest smoking history (Fig. 13-12) and the highest *CYP2D6* activity.

Even more complexity can be observed when considering the effect of two different polymorphisms and an environmental factor in cancer susceptibility. The NAT2 and CYP1A2 gene products are both involved in the detoxification of heterocyclic amines, which are carcinogens commonly

Table 13-7. CYP2D6 alleles in humans

Allele	Mutation	Enzyme activity	Allele frequency, %
CYP2D6*1	None	Normal	≈36
CYP2D6*2	CT2938	Normal	≈32.4
CYP2D6*3	2397delA	Inactive	≈2
CYP2D6*4	CT188, GA1934, GC4268	Inactive	≈20.7
CYP2D6*6	1795delT	Inactive	≈0.9
CYP2D6*10	188C>T, 4268G>C	Reduced	≈1.5

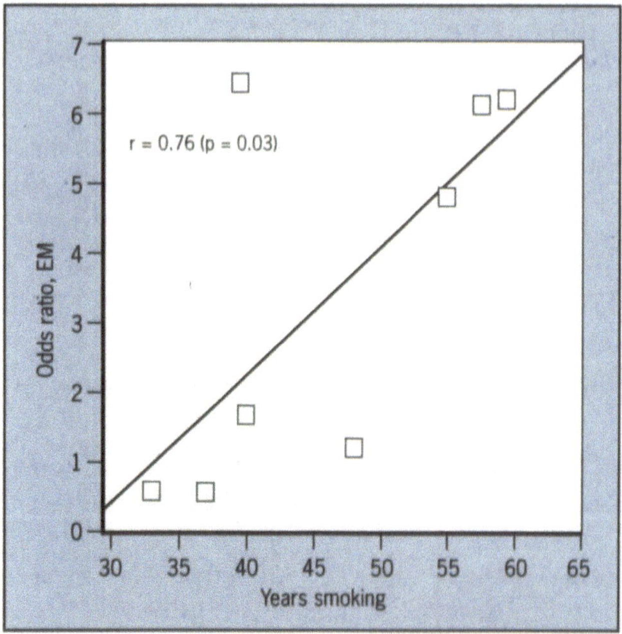

Figure 13-12. Odds ratios for the extensive metabolizer (EM) and lung cancer. Each *open square* represents the odds ratio found in a specific study. Although the studies seem to have very different odds ratios, these differences are largely explained when factoring pack per year history in the study. (*Adapted from* Caporaso *et al.* [18]; with permission.)

Table 13-8. Interactions between phenotype and dietary exposure.

Phenotypes (NAT2 and CYP1A2)	Meat cooking preference	Odds ratio
Slow-slow	Rare/medium	1.00
Rapid-slow		0.91
Slow-rapid		1.39
Rapid-rapid		3.13
Slow-slow	Well done	2.06
Rapid-slow		1.87
Slow-rapid		2.86
Rapid-rapid		6.45

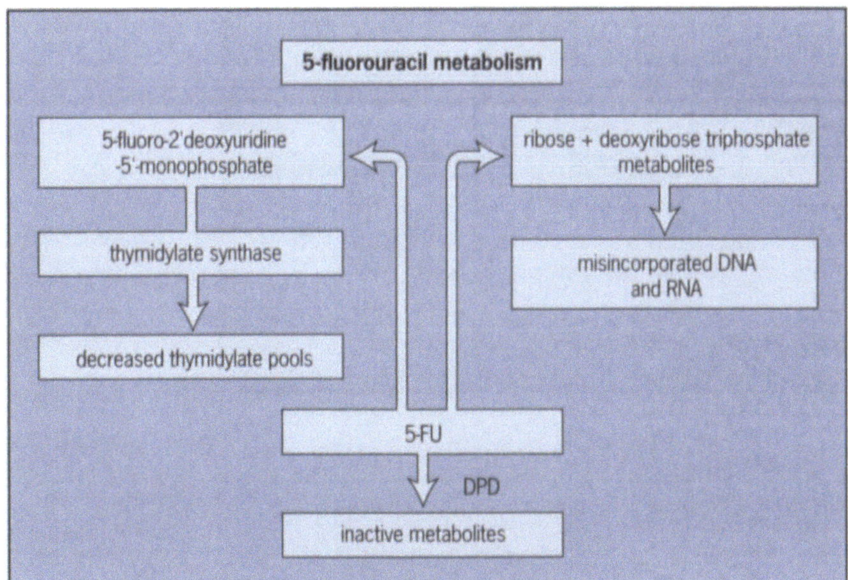

Figure 13-13. 5-Fluorouracil (5-FU) metabolism. The three potential pathwys for 5-FU metabolism are shown. The upper two pathways produce cytotoxic effects, whereas the lower pathway produces inactive metabolites. DPD— dihydropyrimidine dehydrogenase.

Table 13-9. 5-Fluorouracil toxicity and dihydropyrimidine dehydrogenase (DPD) levels

Patient	Cancer	Toxicity grade	DPD %
1	Breast	V	7.0
2	Colon	V	6.0
3	Colon	V	6
4	Rectal	II	18
5	Rectal	II	28
6	Colon	III	17
7	Breast	II	10
8	Colon	II	26
9	Colon	III	19

found in cooked food. In looking at the risk of colon cancer, it was found that the highest odds ratios were obtained in individuals who liked to eat meat well done and had rapid *NAT2* and *CYP1A2* phenotypes (Table 13-8) [19].

PHARMACOGENETICS AND CANCER TREATMENT

An individual's pharmacogenetic characteristics also play an important role in determining response to cancer treatment. Most chemotherapeutic drugs are metabolized and cleared from the body in relatively short periods of time. However, individuals can differ in their inherent ability to clear these drugs. These differences are controlled at least in part by genetic factors and can have important clinical ramifications.

5-Fluorouracil (5-FU) is a uracil analog that is commonly used in the treatment of colon, breast, head and neck, and ovarian cancer. 5-FU inhibits nucleotide biosynthesis and thus kills dividing cells. Most 5-FU is cleared metabolically (Fig. 13-13). The rate-limiting enzyme in this clearance process appears to be dihydropyrimidine dehydrogenase (DPD) [20]. There is a wide range of variation in DPD levels in normal populations [21]. It was first recognized in the mid-1980s that some cancer patients undergoing treatment with 5-FU reported extreme toxicities, with patients occasionally dying as a result. Examination of these individuals indicated that they had undetectable or extremely low levels of DPD activity (Table 13-9) [21]. This low level of DPD appears to be due in part to mutations in the DPD-encoding gene. Individuals who are homozygous and some who are heterozygous exhibit severe 5-FU–induced toxicity. A number of mutations in the DPD gene have been identified (Table 13-10) [22–25]. It is estimated that up to 3% of the human population may be at increased risk for 5-FU toxicity.

The prodrug cyclophosphamide is one of the most frequently used anticancer alkylating agents. Figure 13-14 shows the metabolic scheme for activation and detoxification of cyclophosphamide. Each reaction step provides an opportunity for differences in metabolism premised on polymorphic expression of either phase I or phase II enzymes.

Using the rationale that *GSTP1-1* is overexpressed in tumors compared with normal tissues, a new anticancer alkylating agent has been tested preclinically [26]. Figure 13-15 shows that pharmacologically active chloroethylating species are released following

Table 13-10. Dihydropyrimidine dehydrogenase mutations

Mutation	Resultant protein	5-Fluorouracil toxicity	Allele frequency, %
Splice donor GT>AT	55–Amino acid deletion	Yes, heterozygous	≈1.2
Missense	N974V	Yes, heterozygous	<1.0
Missense	I543V	No	26
Missense	S534R	No	≈2.0

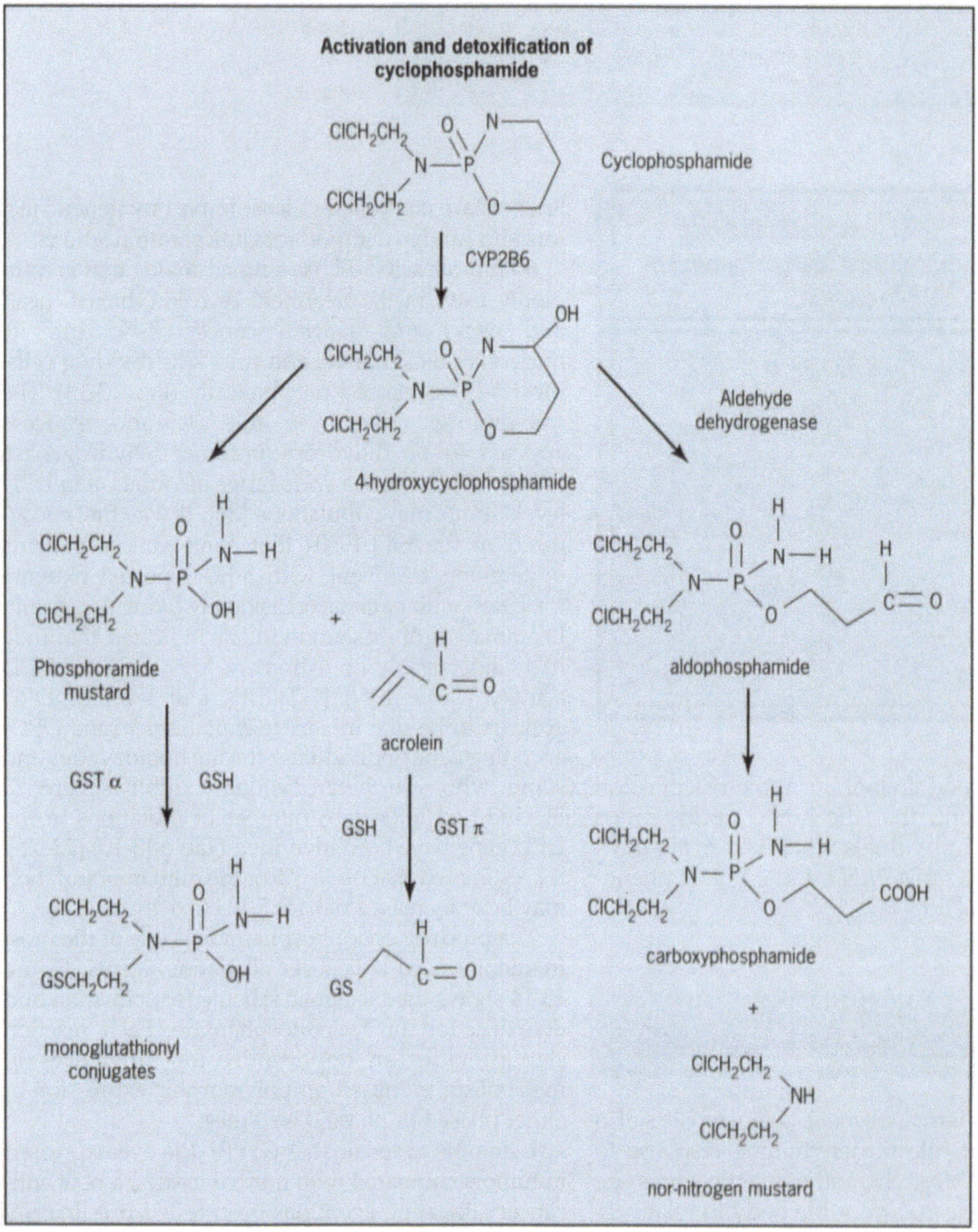

Figure 13-14. Activation and detoxification of cyclophosphamide.

proton abstraction by the tyrosine in the catalytic site of *GSTP1-1*. Because polymorphic forms of *GSTP* are known to exist, there is the possibility of individual differences in drug activation.

FUTURE PROSPECTS

The potential clinical application of pharmacogenetic information to the management of cancer seems enormous (Fig. 13-16). In cancer prevention, pharmacogenetics can be used to identify individuals who are at increased risk for developing specific cancers. Individuals with susceptible phenotypes could be counseled to avoid particular carcinogens that are hazardous for their individual genotype. For example, people with rapid metabolizer alleles of *CYP1A1* and *NAT2* could be advised to avoid eating overcooked meats, because they would be at increased risk for colon cancer. With the advent of so called DNA-chips and other DNA sequencing technologies, hundreds of pharmacogenetically related polymorphisms potentially could be tested in each individual at a reasonable cost. As the population of genotyped individuals is followed over time and their cancer outcomes are recorded, more precise associations between cancer risks and genotypes could be determined. It seems plausible that in the future each individual will have their own risk assessment based on their own specific pharmacogenetic makeup.

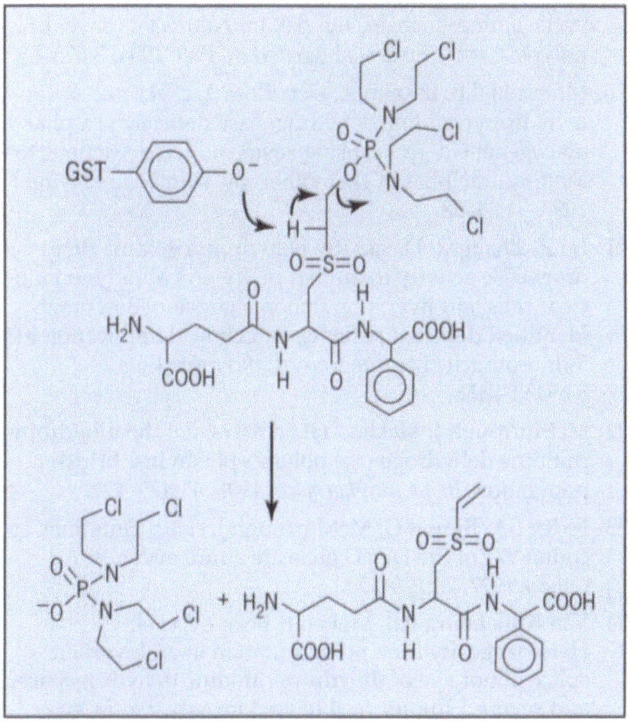

Pharmacogenetic knowledge may also provide new targets for the development of novel drugs that may be useful in cancer treatment or chemoprevention. After susceptibility genes are identified, drugs that alter the expression or function of these gene products could be sought. For example, oltipraz, a compound that causes induction of GST enzymes in certain normal tissues, is presently being tested for its efficacy in reducing the risk for colon cancer. Such treatments might augment the activity in individuals with exceptionally "weak" or "strong" alleles. In addition, the identification of new targets may emerge from a fuller understanding of those genes that are critical to drug metabolism. As more polymorphisms (such as, DPD) are identified, it should be possible to select a priori the best agent and dosage, for an individual. Potentially, pharmacogenetic knowledge could reduce much of the uncertainty involved in chemotherapy and thereby minimize the toxicity or morbidity associated with cancer treatment. Although this research is still in its infancy, it seems rife with clinical potential.

Figure 13-15. Activation of Ter 286, an alkylating prodrug. (*From* Morgan *et al.* [26]; with permission.)

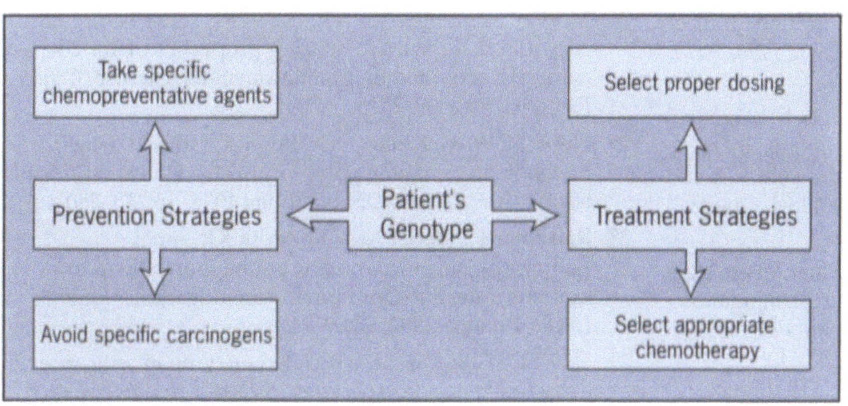

Figure 13-16. Clinical uses of pharmacogenetic information.

REFERENCES

1. Smith G, Stanley LA, Sim E, *et al.*: Metabolic polymorphisms and cancer susceptibility. *Cancer Surv* 1995, 25:27–65.
2. Nelson DR, Koymans L, Kamataki T, *et al.*: P450 superfamily: update on new sequences, gene mapping, accession numbers and nomenclature. *Pharmacogenetics* 1996, 6:1–42.
3. Gonzalez FJ: The role of carcinogen-metabolizing enzyme polymorphisms in cancer susceptibility. *Reprod Toxicol* 1997, 11:397–412.
4. Goto I, Yoneda S, Yamamoto M, Kawajiri K: Prognostic significance of germ line polymorphisms of the CYP1A1 and glutathione S-transferase genes in patients with non-small cell lung cancer. *Cancer Res* 1996, 56:3725–3730.
5. Crofts F, Taioli E, Trachman J, *et al.* Functional significance of different human CYP1A1 genotypes. *Carcinogenesis* 1994, 15:2961–2963.
6. Horio Y, Takahashi T, Kuroishi T, *et al.* Prognostic significance of p53 mutations and 3p deletions in primary resected non-small cell lung cancer. *Cancer Res* 1993, 53:1–4.
7. Mitsudomi T, Oyama T, Kusano T, *et al.*: Mutations of the p53 gene as a predictor of poor prognosis in patients with non-small-cell lung cancer. *J Natl Cancer Inst* 1993, 85:2018–2023.
8. Kawajiri K, Eguchi H, Nakachi K, *et al.*: Association of CYP1A1 germ line polymorphisms with mutations of the p53 gene in lung cancer. *Cancer Res* 1996, 56:72–76.
9. Storey A, Thomas M, Kalita A, *et al.*: Role of a p53 polymorphism in the development of human papillomavirus-associated cancer. *Nature* 1998, 393:229–234.
10. Rebbeck TR: Molecular epidemiology of the human glutathione S-transferase genotypes GSTM1 and GSTT1 in cancer susceptibility. *Cancer Epidemiol Biomarkers Prev* 1997, 6:733–743.
11. McWilliams JE, Sanderson BJ, Harris EL, *et al.*: Glutathione S-transferase M1 (GSTM1) deficiency and lung cancer risk. *Cancer Epidemiol Biomarkers Prev* 1995, 4:589–594.
12. Deakin M, Elder J, Hendrickse C, *et al.*: Glutathione S-transferase GSTT1 genotypes and susceptibility to cancer: studies of interactions with GSTM1 in lung, oral, gastric and colorectal cancers. *Carcinogenesis* 1996, 17:881–884.
13. Elexpuru-Camiruaga J, Buxton N, Kandula V, *et al.*: Susceptibility to astrocytoma and meningioma: influence of allelism at glutathione S-transferase (GSTT1 and GSTM1) and cytochrome P-450 (CYP2D6) loci. *Cancer Res* 1995, 55:4237–4239.
14. Dekant W, Vamvaka S, Anders MW: Formation and fate of nephrotoxic and cytotoxic glutathione S-conjugates: cysteine conjugate beta-lyase pathway. *Adv Pharmacol* 1994, 27:114–162.
15. Meyer UA, Zanger UM: Molecular mechanisms of genetic polymorphisms of drug metabolism. *Annu Rev Pharmacol Toxicol* 1997, 37:269–296.,
16. Mahgoub A, Idle JR, Dring LG, *et al.*: Polymorphic hydroxylation of Debrisoquine in man. *Lancet* 1977, 2:584–586.
17. Gonzalez FJ, Skoda RC, Kimura S, *et al.*: Characterization of the common genetic defect in humans deficient in debrisoquine metabolism. *Nature* 1988, 331:442–446.
18. Caporaso N, DeBaun MR, Rothman N: Lung cancer and CYP2D6 (the debrisoquine polymorphism): sources of heterogeneity in the proposed association. *Pharmacogenetics* 1995, 5:S129–134.
19. Lang NP, Butler MA, Massengill J, *et al.*: Rapid metabolic phenotypes for acetyltransferase and cytochrome P4501A2 and putative exposure to food-borne heterocyclic amines increase the risk for colorectal cancer or polyps. *Cancer Epidemiol Biomarkers Prev* 1994, 3:675–682.
20. Morrison GB, Bastian A, Dela Rosa T, *et al.*: Dihydropyrimidine dehydrogenase deficiency: a pharmacogenetic defect causing severe adverse reactions to 5-fluorouracil-based chemotherapy. *Oncol Nurs Forum* 1997, 24:83–88.
21. Lu Z, Zhang R, Diasio RB: Dihydropyrimidine dehydrogenase activity in human peripheral blood mononuclear cells and liver: population characteristics, newly identified deficient patients, and clinical implication in 5-fluorouracil chemotherapy. *Cancer Res* 1993, 53:5433–5438.
22. McMurrough J, McLeod HL: Analysis of the dihydropyrimidine dehydrogenase polymorphism in a British population. *Br J Clin Pharmacol* 1996, 41:425–427.
23. Ridge SA, Brown O, McMurrough J, *et al.*: Mutations at codon 974 of the DPYD gene are a rare event. *Br J Cancer* 1997, 75:178–179.
24. Van Kuilenburg AB, Vreken P, Beex LV, *et al.*: Heterozygosity for a point mutation in an invariant splice donor site of dihydropyrimidine dehydrogenase and severe 5-fluorouracil related toxicity. *Eur J Cancer* 1997, 33:2258–2264.
25. Wei X, McLeod HL, McMurrough, J, *et al.*: Molecular basis of the human dihydropyrimidine dehydrogenase deficiency and 5-fluorouracil toxicity. *J Clin Invest* 1996, 98, 610–615.
26. Morgan AS, Sanderson PE, Borch RF, *et al.*: Tumor efficacy and bone marrow sparing properties of Ter 286, a cytotoxin activated by glutathione S-transferase. *Cancer Res* 1998, 58:2568–2575.
27. Nebert DW, McKinnon RA, Puga A: Human drug-metabolizing enzyme polymorphisms: effects on risk of toxicity and cancer. *DNA Cell Biol* 1996, 15:273–280.
28. Kadlubar FF, Butler MA, Kaderlik KR, *et al.*: Polymorphisms for aromatic amine metabolism in humans: relevance for human carcinogenesis. *Environ Health Perspect* 1992, 98:69–74.
29. Tew KD: Glutathione associated enzyme in anticancer drug resistance. Perspectives in cancer research. *Cancer Res* 1994, 54:4313–4320.